W9-BMI-398

Medication Errors

2nd Edition

Medication Errors

2nd Edition

Edited by

Michael R. Cohen, RPh, MS, ScD, DPS

President
Institute for Safe Medication Practices
Huntingdon Valley, Pennsylvania

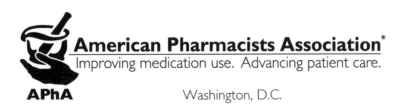

American Pharmacists Association®
Improving medication use. Advancing patient care.
APhA

Washington, D.C.

Editor: Nancy Tarleton Landis
Acquiring Editor: Julian I. Graubart
Layout and Graphics: Roy Barnhill
Proofreading: Kathleen K. Wolter
Indexing: Jen Burton, Columbia Indexing Group
Cover Design: Daniel Kohan, Sensical Design and Communication
Credits for Cover Photography: Stockbyte Royalty-Free Photos (top photograph), G. Schuster/zefa/Corbis
   (bottom photograph)

© 2007 by the American Pharmacists Association
APhA was founded in 1852 as the American Pharmaceutical Association.

Published by the American Pharmacists Association
1100 15th Street, NW, Suite 400
Washington, DC 20005-1707

To comment on this book via e-mail, send your message to the publisher at aphabooks@aphanet.org.

Library of Congress Cataloging-in-Publication Data

Medication errors / edited by Michael R. Cohen. -- 2nd ed.
      p. ; cm.
    Includes bibliographical references and index.
    ISBN-13: 978-1-58212-092-8
    ISBN-10: 1-58212-092-7
    1. Medication errors.   I. Cohen, Michael R. (Michael Richard),
  1944-   . II. American Pharmacists Association.
    [DNLM: 1. Medication Errors.   QZ 42 M489 2006]
  RM146.M415 2006
  615.5'8--dc22

                                                              2006022484

How to Order This book
Online: www.pharmacist.com
By phone: 800-878-0729 (from the United States and Canada)
VISA®, MasterCard®, and American Express® cards accepted

To my wife, Hedy;
our children, Rachel and Neil Brown and Jennifer and Mitchell Gold;
and our grandchildren, Brett and Sydney Brown and Ethan and Alec Gold.
I love you all with all my heart.

In memory of my parents, Elinore and Victor Cohen,
and my uncle, Jerome Orman.

Contents

Part I: Preparing for Action

Part II: Understanding the Causes of Medication Errors

Part III: Preventing Medication Errors: A Shared Responsibility

Part IV: Preventing Medication Errors: Specific Medications, Patients, and Conditions

Part V: Reducing Risks and Creating a Just Culture of Safety

Foreword

During medical school and residency, I don't remember hearing anything about safety in general or medication safety in particular. We were taught about the pathophysiology of disease, with a special focus on rare diseases. Although I noticed that things didn't always go the way they were supposed to, and that patients were sometimes injured as a result, we took this as a matter of course, as just a part of delivering care.

I first got interested in medication safety when the results of the Harvard Medical Practice Study (HMPS) were released. At the time, I was finishing my fellowship in clinical epidemiology, and our hospital was thinking about implementing computerized physician order entry (CPOE). I knew from my training that there were many opportunities to improve clinical decision-making, and it seemed to me that computerizing orders could make a big difference. The HMPS had shown that drugs were the leading cause of injuries in the hospital. I approached Lucian Leape, one of the HMPS investigators, and we decided to undertake a study of adverse drug events and serious errors caused by drugs in hospitalized patients, to be followed closely by interventions to improve medication safety.

The studies that followed were my introduction to medication safety, but many people had been working in this area for a long time. One of the first people I met was Michael Cohen, president of the Institute for Safe Medication Practices (ISMP). Michael has devoted his entire career to improving medication safety and has made enormous contributions. For many years, his was a voice crying out in the wilderness—one of the few voices speaking out about the problem. Despite repeated warnings by ISMP, medication-related problems—including many deaths and serious injuries—occurred again and again. But over time, important changes have been made because of ISMP's efforts, such as removing concentrated potassium solutions from most clinical settings and relabeling cisplatin and carboplatin to prevent confusion between the two. Still, more and more data indicate that medication safety is a major problem in all areas of health care in the United States and around the world.

The good news is that, especially in the years since the Institute of Medicine's *To Err Is Human* report, we've learned a lot about how to improve patient safety. It should soon be possible to improve medication safety to a level previously unattainable, through technologies such as CPOE and bar coding. Yet major challenges remain. The many new drugs coming to market can both help and harm patients. More important, most organizations haven't yet assimilated proven safety strategies, which can be expensive and difficult to implement. Furthermore, achieving a high level of medication safety requires doing many things well; it's a lot more complicated than just purchasing some new technology. For technologies—especially those as complex as bar coding or CPOE—to have the desired effect, they must be implemented well and incorporate the right rules, and a strong safety culture and clinician buy-in are essential.

No group has deeper and more practical knowledge of how to improve medication safety than ISMP. Cohen and his colleagues have gained this knowledge through more than 30 years of experience and hundreds of visits to health care organizations, often after a serious accident has occurred. This book attempts to summarize what has been learned from those experiences and to give providers a detailed blueprint for improving medication safety. The book includes much new information gained since the 1999 edition. It should be required reading for anyone interested in or working on improving medication safety.

It is now within our grasp to make a huge improvement in medication safety. Doing so will require understanding the magnitude of the problem, studying our medication systems, engaging all the disciplines involved, choosing the right solutions, and building a culture of safety—in sum, a daunting task for any organization. This book provides the tools for that task.

David W. Bates
September 2006

Preface

Medications are a blessing if health care providers prescribe, prepare, dispense, and administer them to patients safely and appropriately. Yet, health care providers are human and, as such, fallible. Despite their expertise and commitment to quality, errors and other adverse events with medications occur and sometimes cause human suffering. Administering the wrong drug, strength, or dose; mistaking one look-alike or sound-alike drug name for another; giving medications by the incorrect route of administration; miscalculating doses; misusing medical equipment; prescribing or transcribing the wrong medication; or choosing the wrong patient from a list on the computer screen—despite our best efforts, these things happen every day, to every kind of person, in every health care setting. The large number of new drugs and technologies introduced each year further complicates medication use, as does a growing elderly population with chronic and acute conditions that require complex treatment strategies. Each error can be tragic and costly in both human and economic terms.

Since 1975, I have had the privilege of working in the field of medication safety and participating in the development of a voluntary practitioner error reporting program that capitalizes on people's willingness to share their experiences after involvement in an error or report hazardous conditions that could lead to patient harm. This work led to the formation of a nonprofit organization, the Institute for Safe Medication Practices (ISMP), and to collaboration between ISMP and the United States Pharmacopeia (USP) on the nation's oldest and most beneficial voluntary practitioner medication error reporting program—the only one devoted entirely to medication safety. Called the USP-ISMP Medication Errors Reporting Program (MERP), this program also functions cooperatively with the Food and Drug Administration (FDA) MedWatch program, maximizing the value of both of these voluntary practitioner reporting programs.

After a number of highly publicized medical errors in the 1990s, serious concern about patient safety has grown in the past 1½ decades. Public pressure led to a federally mandated investigation into the quality of health care in America by the Institute of Medicine (IOM); the findings were published at the end of 1999. That report, *To Err Is Human: Building a Safer Health System,*[1] noted that as many as 98,000 people die each year as a result of medical errors, 7,000 from medication errors alone. The report captured widespread media attention and stimulated renewed professional and public dialogue about patient safety.

Has all this attention to safety actually resulted in improvements? Five years after *To Err Is Human,* two of the nation's leading safety experts (and contributors to that report), Lucian Leape, MD, of the Harvard School of Public Health, and Donald Berwick, MD, of the Institute for Healthcare Improvement, found it difficult to substantiate an overall national impact.[2] "The groundwork for improving safety has been laid in these past five years, but progress is frustratingly slow," they said. Still, they clearly believe that health care providers have changed the way they think about medical errors. They note that providers have come to appreciate the seriousness of the problem, demonstrated an understanding of the system-based causes of medication errors, and made a commitment to improvement. A new IOM report released in July 2006, *Preventing Medication Errors,*[3] agrees that we still have much work to do. The report calls the frequency of medication errors and related injuries "a serious concern" and suggests numerous error-prevention strategies that will require our undivided attention, including electronic prescribing, improved pharmacy leaflets and medication-related information on the Internet for consumers, better communication of patient information to those who need it, and collaboration among industry,

FDA, and patient safety organizations to address problems with drug naming, labeling, and packaging.

Although we still have a great deal to accomplish, I see unquestionable signs that we're making headway. Thanks to the participation of frontline practitioners who have reported errors to MERP, we have been able to identify many important medication system deficiencies and publicize these, along with error prevention recommendations and other ideas for improving safety. We have been heartened to learn just how many facilities use this information. These organizations establish a process for regular, interdisciplinary review of the *ISMP Medication Safety Alert!* newsletter and ISMP Action Agenda (a quarterly "to do" list for addressing ongoing safety issues) to identify and implement proactive error-reduction strategies.

A 2004 survey completed by 748 subscribers provided evidence that the newsletter has spurred numerous changes to reduce the risk of medication errors. Most pharmacy directors (95%), quality/risk management staff (90%), and nurse executives (87%) responding reported that information in the newsletter had prompted organizationwide changes. More than 70% of frontline practitioners, such as staff nurses and pharmacists, reported frequent changes in their individual practices in response to newsletter articles. Many readers reported use of the newsletter to increase patient and staff education.[4] In addition, two-thirds of the respondents to a recent survey of readers of the *ISMP Nurse Advise-ERR* newsletter said it had influenced them to make changes in the workplace.[5]

Collaborative efforts involving practitioners, the pharmaceutical industry, FDA, the National Quality Forum, USP, accrediting agencies, the public, and many other organizations are also making a difference. The work of the Joint Commission on Accreditation of Healthcare Organizations (JCAHO) is a prime example of how the IOM report helped to engage, in new ways, the nation's patient safety organizations and other stakeholders to drive necessary changes. Rarely have oversight organizations dedicated time and effort to bringing national experts together to recommend safety goals, inform practitioners and health care organizations about specific error types, and hold organizations accountable for proactively implementing evidence-based system changes that are known to enhance patient safety. But that is exactly what JCAHO has accomplished, most recently through the adoption of National Patient Safety Goals (NPSGs) and medication management standards for accreditation.

Working with safety experts around the United States, JCAHO has set forth new requirements for accredited organizations that address recognized causes of sentinel events (unexpected occurrences involving death or serious injury). Many of the same issues ISMP has written about, such as discouraging the use of dangerous abbreviations, preventing free-flow of IV infusions, labeling drug containers in the sterile field and other clinical areas, and removing potassium chloride injection concentrate from patient care areas, have been addressed in NPSGs.

Regarding the inadvertent IV administration of concentrated potassium chloride, it seems clear that efforts by JCAHO, ISMP, and Dr. Leape, an early advocate of constraining this drug's availability, have had a preventive effect. JCAHO received reports of eight deaths related to this product in 1997 through its voluntary sentinel event reporting program. Subsequently, JCAHO began to require accredited institutions to remove potassium chloride from patient care areas. From 2000 to the present, despite an increasing volume of sentinel event reports (from just over 100 in 1997 to nearly 600 per year in 2005), there have been no reports of events involving concentrated potassium chloride (see Figure 19-4). In fact, in what may be another hopeful sign, the number of serious medication errors reported to JCAHO has leveled off in recent years. These improvements have come about, I believe, because of efforts aimed specifically at preventing well-known, repetitive errors in medication prescribing, dispensing, and administration, such as serious events involving high-alert drugs and errors associated with abbreviations and look-alike/sound-alike names.

In my many visits to health care organizations in the United States and other countries, I continue to be amazed at providers' commitment and innovative efforts to improve patient safety. I have yet to walk out of a single organization without at least one success story that I wanted to share immediately with other health care providers. And it is not just facilities such as the *U.S. News & World Report* top 100 hospitals that are making great progress in creating safer health care environments. From the smallest critical-access hospital to the largest university hospital, providers of every size and setting are taking steps to make patients safer.

As I wrote in the preface to the first edition of this book, if we are going to prevent errors, we must start by acknowledging that human beings make mistakes and that medication errors are not typically made or prevented by one person in isolation. Fail-safe systems are at the heart of prevention. In **Chapter 1**, Systems Analysis and Redesign: The Foundation of Medical Error Prevention, we've again called upon Harvard's Lucian Leape to give readers a basic understanding of the role of human error and systems failures in health care and how they can be addressed.

A common question asked of ISMP staff is "How often do medication errors happen?" In order to assess the current level of safety and understand the impact of system changes, it is important to be familiar with research on the frequency of medication errors. As in our first edition, we've called upon Elizabeth Allan Flynn and Kenneth N. Barker of Auburn University for a review of the major studies published to date, including their own observational studies in hospitals, long-term care facilities, and community pharmacies (**Chapter 2**).

ISMP Trustee Zane Robinson Wolf, Dean and Professor of Nursing at La Salle University School of Nursing, Philadelphia, is world renowned for her work in identifying the effects of medication errors on the practitioners who make them. In **Chapter 3**, she discusses this often overlooked but important subject. Emphasizing that people who make errors are usually devastated and in need of psychological support, Dr. Wolf believes we can help by creating an environment that fosters open and honest discussion about errors.

Medication errors happen because of breakdowns in the systems that have been developed for handling and processing drugs, from prescribing and ordering to distribution and administration. The systems involved cross every discipline and spread beyond arbitrary boundaries of responsibility. Teamwork is vital. In **Chapter 4**, I cover some of the most common reasons that errors reach patients. **Chapters 9** covers prescribing errors, and in **Chapters 10 and 11**, ISMP colleague Judy Smetzer joins me in writing about errors in dispensing and drug administration—and the interdisciplinary cooperation needed to address them. We illustrate these chapters with examples of actual errors that have come to our attention through the error reporting programs.

If we've learned one thing over the years from investigating medication errors, it's that causation is always multifactorial. Never can an incident be blamed on a single factor. There is always a story behind the story, and multiple opportunities to make improvements. **Chapter 5**, by pharmacist Mary Burkhardt, formerly of the Department of Veterans Affairs (VA) National Center for Patient Safety (now Chief Medication Safety Officer at Medco Health Solutions, Inc.) and her colleagues Caryl Lee, Lesley Taylor, Rodney Williams, and James Bagian, present the complex topic of root cause analysis in a very understandable fashion.

Chapter 6 takes a look at safety issues related to drug nomenclature. ISMP trustee George Di Domizio, a well-known expert in trademark and drug nomenclature issues, and Robert E. Lee, Jr., Assistant General Patent Counsel at Eli Lilly and Company and Chairman of the Trademark and Copyright Focus Group within the Pharmaceutical

Research and Manufacturers of America, join me in reviewing nomenclature issues and approaches under way within the global industry and regulatory communities to improve medication safety. In **Chapter 7**, I review the role that unsafe drug packaging, labeling, and advertising have played in errors. My hope is that the examples of past errors and the suggestions for improvement will help both industry and practitioners to recognize features of labeling, packaging, and marketing that can cause or prevent errors.

Chapter 8 reviews and identifies the many problems that have been reported when unsafe medical abbreviations, symbols, and dose designations confuse practitioners. An effective way to control and standardize vocabulary and nomenclature is to maintain a list of prohibited abbreviations, which, when misinterpreted, can cause significant harm to patients. The JCAHO NPSG prohibits the use of certain dangerous abbreviations, mainly in medication orders, but these are only a small number of the confusing designations that students and practitioners should refrain from using. In Chapter 8, ISMP's Michael Gaunt and I present background information about the problem, detail many of the unsafe designations reported over the years, and compile them in a useful table.

Health care professionals, particularly nurses, use a wide variety of devices to help administer medications, from IV administration sets and oral syringes to sophisticated infusion pumps. Appropriate safety assessment of these drug delivery devices prior to purchase and during use is key to error prevention. Competency in using the devices is also paramount. In **Chapter 12**, Judy Smetzer and I review many pitfalls we've learned about over the years and offer recommendations to managers and practitioners.

Patients have a role in ensuring their own safety. In **Chapter 13**, Stacy Aimette, a former ISMP Safe Medication Management Fellow (now at excelleRx, Inc. in Philadelphia) joins ISMP nurse Nancy Tuohy and me in describing how practitioners can partner with patients, family, and the community to reduce the risk of medication errors.

The chapter on high-alert medications was popular in the first edition of this book. To improve safety, it is especially important to be aware of the medications most frequently involved in harmful events and the precautions that should be taken to avoid such errors. ISMP and others have developed a strong foundation of research in this area, and ISMP coined the term "high-alert medications" close to a decade ago. These are drugs and drug categories that bear a heightened risk of causing significant patient harm when they are used in error. Although mistakes may or may not be more common with these drugs, the consequences of an error with these medications are clearly more devastating to patients. On the basis of error reports submitted to MERP, literature reports of harmful errors, and a survey of over 350 U.S. practitioners, ISMP created a list of high-alert medications. In **Chapter 14**, Judy Smetzer, Nancy Tuohy, and I, along with physician Charles Kilo, review these drugs and drug categories and offer strategies for preventing harmful errors.

Incorporating technology across the whole medication management spectrum should be a strategic goal for every organization. Evidence is building to demonstrate the value of technologies such as order scanning systems, computerized prescribing, "smart" pumps, and bedside scanning. But implementing technology in health care organizations can be a daunting task. Too many organizations have purchased various forms of automation without sufficient planning and a solid foundation on which to apply the technology; in such cases, staff will work around the safety features offered by the technology. In **Chapter 15**, ISMP pharmacists Allen Vaida and Matthew Grissinger and nurse Hedy Cohen discuss applications of technology for error prevention, new types of errors that may be associated with technology, and actions needed to ensure safe use of these systems.

Some specialty areas of drug therapy are especially fraught with risk when dosing is inaccurate; several chapters are devoted to these areas. In **Chapter 16**, I discuss error prevention in cancer chemotherapy. ISMP pediatric safety expert Stuart Levine takes the lead in **Chapter 17**, on preventing errors in pediatric and neonatal patients, and in

Chapter 18 pharmacist John Grabenstein, of the Army's Military Vaccine Agency, and I address the prevention of errors with immunologic drugs.

In the wake of *To Err Is Human*, a number of medical error reporting programs have been implemented or refined around the world. Our medication error reporting program has been in existence since 1975, and we have learned a great deal about success and failure in the operation of these programs. In **Chapter 19**, lead author Judy Smetzer and I share our experiences and discuss how what we have learned can be applied in organizations' internal reporting programs. Judy has provided direct input to congressional staff and contributed to the Patient Safety and Quality Improvement Act of 2005.

Within the health care community, ISMP was the first organization to promote the use of failure mode and effects analysis (FMEA),[6] a tool used for proactive risk assessment. Organizations can use FMEA to look at medication therapy or device use as a process, pinpoint all the ways in which it might fail, and analyze why failures might occur and how to avoid them. Three sets of authors cover this subject in detail in **Chapter 21**. In Part I, John Senders, an internationally known expert in human factors and consulting scientist at ISMP, along with Stefan Senders, provides an introduction to the subject. In Part II, Judy Smetzer and I show how FMEA can be applied as a risk management tool. In Part III, a team from the VA National Center for Patient Safety, headed by Mary Burkhardt, reviews an FMEA method specifically designed for use in health care—Healthcare Failure Mode and Effects Analysis. Examples of FMEA and HFMEA are included.

In **Chapter 22**, an important chapter for health care practitioners and students alike, ISMP Trustee J. Russell Teagarden makes the case for rooting safe medication practices in what he refers to as "clinical bioethics." He establishes links among bioethics concepts, safe medication practices, and current views of health care. He shows how clinical bioethics concepts can be used to support safe medication practices, and how they can help to explain and justify the strong stance on safety required in health care.

Two chapters, 20 and 23, address the culture of safety in health care. Organizations that have exemplary records in patient safety exhibit a particular set of characteristics, including a strategic emphasis on safety, workforce mindfulness, teamwork, outward focus, and a just culture. In **Chapter 23**, Judy Smetzer of ISMP describes each characteristic and provides examples related to medication safety and more broad-based patient safety. A culture of safety supports disclosure of medical errors to patients and families, as discussed in **Chapter 20** by ISMP nurses Nancy Tuohy and Judy Smetzer.

The development and implementation of safety improvements must be given the highest priority in health care. Such efforts must be aimed specifically at preventing well-known and repetitive categories of prescribing, dispensing, and administration errors, which erode patient confidence in our health care system. My hope is that this book will provide practical guidance to the health care community—in any setting, be it acute care, long-term care, community practice, industry, regulatory affairs, or academia—to make patients who take or receive medications safer as we work collectively toward a six-sigma level of performance (3.4 errors per million medications).

1. Kohn LT, Corrigan JM, Donaldson MS, eds. *To Err Is Human: Building a Safer Health System.* Washington, DC: National Academies Press; 2000.
2. Leape LL, Berwick DM. Five years after *To Err Is Human*: what have we learned? *JAMA.* 2005;293:2384–90.
3. Committee on Identifying and Preventing Medication Errors; Aspden P, Wolcott J, Bootman JL, et al., eds. *Preventing Medication Errors.* Washington, DC: National Academies Press; 2006. Prepublication copy available at http://darwin.nap.edu/books/0309101476/html/R2.html. Accessed July 21, 2006.
4. Institute for Safe Medication Practices. *Safety Alert* readers tell us how we are doing. *ISMP Medication Safety Alert!* June 17, 2004. Available at: www.ismp.org/Survey/Survey200405.asp.
5. Institute for Safe Medication Practices. Readership survey for *Nurse Advise-ERR. ISMP Medication Safety Alert!* August 2005. Available at: www.ismp.org/Survey/NurseSurvey200508R.asp.
6. Cohen MR, Senders J, Davis NM. Failure mode and effects analysis: a novel approach to avoiding dangerous medication errors and accidents. *Hosp Pharm.* 1994;29:319–24, 326–8, 330.

THE INSTITUTE FOR SAFE MEDICATION PRACTICES (ISMP)

Who We Are

We are a nonprofit health care agency comprising pharmacists, nurses, and physicians. Founded in 1994, our organization is dedicated to learning about medication errors, understanding their system-based causes, and disseminating practical recommendations that can help health care providers, consumers, and the pharmaceutical industry prevent errors.

Who We Are NOT

We are not a governmental, regulatory, licensing, inspecting, or membership organization, or an accrediting agency. While we work collaboratively with these types of agencies to influence medication safety, we do not set health care standards or require individual organizations to implement the recommendations we make.

How We Are Funded

As a nonprofit agency, we rely on charitable donations, unrestricted grants, subscriptions to our newsletters, and fees from our consulting and educational services. We are not funded by the pharmaceutical industry and do not accept advertising in any of our publications.

How We Learn about Medication Errors

More than 30 years ago, we started a voluntary error reporting program to learn about medication errors that were occurring across the nation. In January 1994, ISMP was chartered as a nonprofit agency to further this work. Today, the program, now called the USP-ISMP Medication Errors Reporting Program (MERP), continues to thrive. Each year, hundreds of health care professionals trust us enough to report errors to this program to help us learn about errors, understand their causes, and share the "lessons learned" with others. You, too, can report errors through our Web site (www.ismp.org) or e-mail (ismpinfo@ismp.org) or by calling 1-800-FAIL-SAF(E).

How We Keep Error Reports Confidential

While we share stories about medication errors in our publications and through other educational efforts, we have never disclosed the specific location of an event, the people involved, or the person who reported the error. When necessary, less important details about an error may be changed to ensure that inadvertent recognition of the error is not possible. In addition, if health care facilities seek our advice about a medication error or other medication safety issue, facility-specific recommendations are not disclosed publicly, even in a blinded manner.

How We Learn about Error-Reduction Strategies

Many years of analyzing medication error reports have enabled us to suggest credible error-reduction strategies. We are in constant contact with an advisory panel of practicing health care professionals, researchers, and experts in human factors and medication safety, who collectively help us offer evidence-based and practical error-reduction strategies that work. In addition, our staff spends considerable time in health care facilities learning firsthand about innovative medication safety practices so we can share these ideas with others.

What's Available on Our Web Site

We offer a wide variety of free educational materials and services on our Web site (www.ismp.org):

- ❑ Special medication hazard alerts
- ❑ Searchable information on a wide variety of medication safety topics
- ❑ Answers to frequently asked questions about medication safety
- ❑ FDA patient safety videos
- ❑ Three Pathways for Medication Safety tools:
  - − A model strategic plan for medication safety
  - − Risk assessment tools and questions for clinicians
  - − Readiness assessment for bedside bar coding
- ❑ White papers on bar coding technology and electronic prescribing
- ❑ A monitored message board to share questions, answers, and ideas
- ❑ Other medication safety tools, products, and resources

Other Ways We Can Help

Over the years, we've developed numerous publications, programs, and tools designed to help health care professionals prevent medication errors. For example, we

- ❑ Publish three professional newsletters and one consumer newsletter (collectively reaching millions of readers)
- ❑ Conduct frequent educational programs, including teleconferences, on medication safety issues
- ❑ Offer posters, videos, patient brochures, books, and other drug safety tools
- ❑ Conduct on-site risk assessments of medication safety in health care facilities and respond to sentinel events
- ❑ Provide support for implementing medication safety technologies such as bar coding, electronic prescribing, pharmacy systems, and automated dispensing cabinets

Acknowledgments

In the first edition of *Medication Errors,* I started by noting that although I've devoted my professional life as a pharmacist to medication error prevention, I've always recognized that I must never pretend I could do this work alone. My work at the Institute for Safe Medication Practices (ISMP), and any successes we've had, are shared with many, and I realize this even more today.

First and foremost, I must give very special recognition to those who have placed enough trust in us to share their stories, and sometimes their grief, in the hope that some good would come from it—that patients would be kept out of harm's way. Their only motivation is a hope that the information they share will make a difference. Thank you. Humankind owes you the deepest gratitude. You have, in fact, made a difference.

I would also like to acknowledge my wife of 40 years, Hedy Cohen, a registered nurse and passionate advocate for patient safety. Hedy has been an active participant in the work of ISMP since the early days, having typed my first columns, which were handwritten on a yellow pad, while offering advice and suggestions that have been instrumental in shaping our approach to safety. Much credit is also deserved by other members of my family for the support they've given me over the years and their forgiveness during my frequent absences for ISMP activities. Thanks to Rachel, Neil, Brett, Sydney (she's Little Sydney Snodgrass to me), Jennifer, Mitch, Ethan, Alec, Rosanne, Paul, Lauren, Chad, Olivia, and Tyler.

I cannot adequately express the gratitude I feel toward the ISMP professional and clerical staff and the fellows and students who have worked at ISMP since our founding. It would simply not be possible to assemble a more dedicated group of individuals in the field of patient safety. Each of them eats, lives, and breathes safety, as anyone who interacts with them can readily recognize. Thanks to Renee Brehio, MA; Hedy G. Cohen, BSN, MS; Rachel L. Cohen, MS, RD; William Cunningham; Matthew Fricker, RPh, MS; Michael J. Gaunt, PharmD; Nancy J. Globus, PharmD; Nicole Graser; Matthew Grissinger, RPh; Reuben Grubb; Karyn Hetzel, RPh, MBA; Donna Horn, RPh, DPh; Russell Jenkins, MD; Kate Kelly, PharmD; Lena Khavinson; Marci Lee, PharmD; Stuart Levine, PharmD; Michelle Mandrack, RN, BSN, MSN; Renee Mandrack; Kristine Needleman, RPh; Susan Paparella, RN, MSN; Susan M. Proulx, PharmD; Andrea Rothbart, PharmD; Judy Smetzer, RN, BSN; Mimi Spiegel; Kelly Stanforth, PharmD; Kelly Stever; Kellie A. Taylor, PharmD, MPH; Nancy Tuohy, RN, MSN; Allen J. Vaida, PharmD, FASHP; and Michelle Walker.

Thanks to the ISMP Board of Trustees for the oversight they provide for our activities, and especially to Louis Martinelli, PharmD, PhD, who serves as chairperson. Thanks also to the management team: Susan Proulx, PharmD, president of our Med-ERRS Division; Russell Jenkins, MD, our medical director; Hedy Cohen, RN, vice president; Judy Smetzer, RN, vice president; and Allen Vaida, PharmD, our executive vice president. Each of you has gone well beyond any expectation I could ever have, in terms of your work excellence and the friendship you've extended to me. Without the contributions all of these people have made and their incredible dedication, we clearly would not be successful in our work.

I would also especially like to mention my friends Jerry Phillips, formerly of the Food and Drug Administration (FDA), Carol Holquist of FDA, and Diane Cousins of the United States Pharmacopeia (USP). Jerry, who is now at the Drug Safety Institute but who formerly headed FDA's Division of Medication Errors and Technical Support, and his replacement, Carol Holquist, have worked hard within the agency to address specific medical product errors. Diane and her staff at USP's Center for Patient Safety have been instrumental in furthering the development of the USP-ISMP Medication Errors Reporting Program (MERP) and the USP MEDMARX Program. She has provided steadfast leadership on patient safety issues and reporting programs at USP for many years, and she also established the National Coordinating Council on Medication Error Reporting and Prevention, which has had many accomplishments. We should be indebted to all of them for the progress made to date and the advances that are now under way.

Let me also give thanks to those who volunteer their services on our various editorial review boards. Every issue of our *ISMP Medication Safety Alert!* Acute Care and Community/Ambulatory editions and our consumer *(Safe Medicine)* and nursing *(Nurse Advise-ERR)* newsletters is reviewed by at least 10 outside reviewers as well as our own staff. The reviewers' input and willingness to share their expertise is what has made these publications so successful. Our circulation is among the widest in health care; each month our publications, including the four newsletters and the columns and features we publish in professional journals, reach more than 3.5 million people. Our own Web site and Epocrates alerts and Medscape columns reach many more.

I would also like to acknowledge the important work of our international sister organizations. Pharmacist David U and the staff at the Institute for Safe Medication Practices–Canada, in Toronto, and pharmacist María José Otero, PhD, and her staff at ISMP–Spain have made great progress in improving medication safety in their respective countries. Each organization works collaboratively with the health care community, regulatory agencies, policy makers, and international patient safety organizations to promote safe medication practices. Thanks to David and Maria, and to pharmacist colleague Mário Borges Rosa, who is working with nurses, pharmacists, and physicians throughout Brazil to establish ISMP–Brasil. We look forward to the ongoing success of these organizations and others internationally.

I am indebted to my colleague Neil M. Davis, PharmD. It was Neil's idea to start a medication error column in the journal *Hospital Pharmacy*, the focus of which was to be what went wrong, never who did it. Neil taught me that errors are not really about being careless or lazy, but instead are caused by poor systems and processes that set people up to make errors. The first column was printed in March 1975, and the column is still published today by Facts and Comparisons in *Hospital Pharmacy*. It was this column that eventually developed into MERP. Along the way I have been blessed to meet many terrific people in medicine, nursing, pharmacy, and the consumer movement—some of the world's top experts in the field of patient safety. Therefore, I especially thank Neil for the opportunity afforded me and the ability to do this work.

Finally, I am extremely grateful for all the hard work, research, and timely management and writing skills that Judy Smetzer, RN, BSN, and Nancy Tuohy, RN, MSN, put into this book. They somehow were always able to get me back on track, despite frequent derailments. It's not likely that this book would have been completed without their support.

Contributors

Stacy A. Aimette, PharmD, MS
excelleRx, Inc.
Philadelphia, Pennsylvania

James Bagian, MD, PE
Department of Veterans Affairs
Veterans Health Administration
National Center for Patient Safety
Ann Arbor, Michigan

Kenneth N. Barker, PhD
Center of Pharmacy Operations and Designs
Auburn University
Auburn, Alabama

David W. Bates, MD, MSc
Chief, Division of General Internal Medicine,
    Brigham and Women's Hospital
Professor, Harvard Medical School
Professor of Health Policy and Management,
    Harvard School of Public Health
Boston, Massachusetts

Mary Burkhardt, MS, RPh, FASHP
Medco Health Solutions, Inc.
Franklin Lakes, New Jersey

Hedy Cohen, RN, BSN, MS
Institute for Safe Medication Practices
Huntingdon Valley, Pennsylvania

Joseph DeRosier, PE, CSP
Department of Veterans Affairs
Veterans Health Administration
National Center for Patient Safety
Ann Arbor, Michigan

George Di Domizio
Gemini Trademark Services
Green Lane, Pennsylvania

Elizabeth Allan Flynn, PhD, RPh
Center of Pharmacy Operations and Designs
Auburn University
Auburn, Alabama

Michael J. Gaunt, PharmD
Institute for Safe Medication Practices
Huntingdon Valley, Pennsylvania

John D. Grabenstein, PhD, FASHP
Military Vaccine Agency
U.S. Army Medical Department
Falls Church, Virginia

Matthew Grissinger, RPh, FASCP
Institute for Safe Medication Practices
Huntingdon Valley, Pennsylvania

Charles M. Kilo, MD, MPH
Chief Executive Officer
GreenField Health
Portland, Oregon

Lucian L. Leape, MD
Adjunct Professor of Health Policy
Department of Health Policy and Management
Harvard School of Public Health
Boston, Massachusetts

Caryl Lee, RN, MSN
Department of Veterans Affairs
Veterans Health Administration
National Center for Patient Safety
Ann Arbor, Michigan

Robert E. Lee, Jr.
Assistant General Patent Counsel
Trademarks, Copyrights, and Information
    Technology
Eli Lilly and Company
Chairman, Trademark and Copyright Focus Group
Pharmaceutical Research and Manufacturers
    of America

Stuart Levine, PharmD
Institute for Safe Medication Practices
Huntingdon Valley, Pennsylvania

J. W. Senders, PhD
Professor Emeritus, University of Toronto
Toronto, Ontario, Canada
Consulting Scientist, ISMP
Huntingdon Valley, Pennsylvania
Trustee, ISMP Canada, Toronto, Ontario

S. J. Senders, PhD
Assistant Professor of Writing and Rhetoric
Hobart and William Smith Colleges
Geneva, New York

Judy L. Smetzer, RN, BSN
Institute for Safe Medication Practices
Huntingdon Valley, Pennsylvania

Erik Stalhandske, MPP, MHSA
Department of Veterans Affairs
Veterans Health Administration
National Center for Patient Safety
Ann Arbor, Michigan

Lesley Taylor, BS
Department of Veterans Affairs
Veterans Health Administration
National Center for Patient Safety
Ann Arbor, Michigan

J. Russell Teagarden, MA, RPh
Vice President, Clinical Practices and
  Therapeutics
Medco Health Solutions, Inc.
Franklin Lakes, New Jersey

Nancy R. Tuohy, RN, MSN
Institute for Safe Medication Practices
Huntingdon Valley, Pennsylvania

Allen J. Vaida, PharmD, FASHP
Institute for Safe Medication Practices
Huntingdon Valley, Pennsylvania

Rodney Williams, MPA, JD, LLM
Department of Veterans Affairs
Veterans Health Administration
National Center for Patient Safety
Ann Arbor, Michigan

Zane Robinson Wolf, PhD, RN, FAAN
Dean and Professor
La Salle University School of Nursing
Philadelphia, Pennsylvania

PART I

PREPARING FOR ACTION

CHAPTER 1

SYSTEMS ANALYSIS AND REDESIGN: THE FOUNDATION OF MEDICAL ERROR PREVENTION

Lucian L. Leape

An error can be defined as an unintended act (either of omission or commission) or as an act that does not achieve its intended outcome. Until recently, medical errors were seldom discussed. The public preferred to believe that errors in medical practice were rare. Health professionals, fearing loss of trust and impaired reputation, sought to perpetuate that misconception. The adversarial climate produced by the threat of malpractice litigation exacerbated this "see nothing, do nothing" approach.

All this has changed in the past 10 years. A new "movement" for patient safety began in 1995, when a series of apparently egregious errors resulting in death or inappropriate surgery were widely publicized. Hospitals began to recognize that they could do more to prevent patient injuries by using a nonpunitive approach to errors. The result has been substantial increases in both research on the causes of medical error and implementation of preventive mechanisms.

EXTENT OF MEDICAL INJURY

The toll of medical error is substantial. A significant number of patients suffer treatment-caused injuries while in the hospital.[1-5] The Harvard Medical Practice Study (HMPS),[1,2] a population-based study of iatrogenic injuries in patients hospitalized in 1984 in New York State, is the most comprehensive examination to date. Nearly 4% of patients suffered an injury that prolonged their hospital stay or resulted in measurable disability. Approximately 14% of these injuries were fatal.

If these findings are typical of the United States as a whole, each year an estimated 1.3 million people are injured by treatment intended to help them, and 180,000 people die as a result of medical accidents. More than two-thirds of the injuries found in the HMPS were due to errors and thus, by definition, were preventable.[6] Other researchers have reported similar findings.

The HMPS has been replicated in Australia,[7] New Zealand,[8] Denmark,[9] the United Kingdom,[10] and Canada,[11] and significantly higher rates of adverse events (9% to 13%) have been found. In all of these studies, approximately half of the adverse events were deemed preventable.

In 1991, Bedell et al.[5] reported that 64% of cardiac arrests at a teaching hospital were caused by errors. Misuse of medications was the leading cause. Many studies have found medication errors to be common. The rate of dosing errors by nurses is reportedly as high as 20%.[12] Most of these errors are minor, such as giving a medication late or failing to watch the patient take the dose. However, a study of adverse drug events (ADEs) in two Harvard teaching hospitals showed that serious, injury-producing errors in the use of medications occurred in nearly 2% of patients, while an additional 5.5% of patients were exposed to "near misses," errors with potential for injury that were intercepted or, by luck, failed to cause harm.[13]

Other studies[14–18] have shown that medication errors account for 10% to 25% of all errors. Most do not result in serious injury.[19] Given the complex nature of medical practice and the multitude of interventions with each patient, a high error rate is perhaps not surprising. Delivery of a single dose of a medication is the end result of a complicated process involving 30 to 40 steps, each of which offers an opportunity for error. Using process steps instead of patient admissions as a denominator suggests that the medication error rate in hospitals may be as low as 1 in 1,000 to 1 in 10,000 (0.01%).[20] Even a failure rate of 0.01%, however, is substantially higher (10 to 100 times) than that tolerated in other industries, particularly in hazardous fields such as aviation and nuclear power. Health care can, and must, do better.

TRADITIONAL APPROACH TO ERROR

Health professionals—physicians, nurses, and pharmacists, in particular—have difficulty dealing with human error, in part because of the emphasis during their training on error-free practice.[21] In everyday practice, they continue to hear the message that mistakes are unacceptable. Physicians, nurses, and pharmacists are expected to function without errors, which means that they feel ashamed and inadequate when errors inevitably do occur. Their laudable striving for perfection is consistent with another goal of professional training: developing a sense of responsibility for the patient. If one is responsible for the patient, one also feels personally responsible for any errors that occur.

The high standards of practice that are taught to nurses, pharmacists, and physicians have often been reinforced in hospital practice by an unforgiving system of censure and discipline. Attempts are made to eliminate errors by requiring perfection and responding to failure (error) by blaming individuals. Errors are regarded as someone's fault, caused by a lack of sufficient attention or, worse, a lack of caring. In severe cases, the person at fault may be fired or subjected to retraining.

Not surprisingly, this "blame and train" approach to medical error has created strong pressure on individuals to cover up mistakes rather than admit them.[22] Even if punishment is not overt, the realization that colleagues will regard them as incompetent or careless makes many health professionals reluctant to admit or discuss their errors. The threat of malpractice litigation provides an additional incentive to keep silent.

Students of error and human performance reject the blame and train approach to error prevention. Although the nearest error leading to an accident is usually a human one, the causes of that error often are beyond the individual's control. Systems that rely on perfect performance by individuals to prevent errors are doomed to fail, for the simple reason that all humans err, and frequently. If physicians, nurses, pharmacists, and administrators are to succeed in reducing errors in health care, they must change the way they think about why errors occur. Fortunately, much has been learned about error prevention in other disciplines, and this information is relevant to the hospital practice of medicine.

PSYCHOLOGICAL AND HUMAN-FACTORS RESEARCH

Cognitive psychologists and human-factors specialists have been concerned with the biology, psychology, and sociology of errors for several decades. By developing models of human cognition and studying complex environments such as airplane cockpits and nuclear power plant control rooms, they have learned a great deal about why people make errors and how to prevent them.[23] The principles developed by experts in these fields are pertinent to the redesign of health care systems to reduce errors. In simple terms, there are two modes of mental functioning: automatic and problem-solving.

Most mental functioning is automatic—effortless and rapid. We don't have to think about the process of eating or driving to work, for example. These "unconscious" functions are performed in a parallel-processing mode. We have to pay attention only when there is a change or interruption in the process.

Problem solving, on the other hand, requires intense mental activity. To solve problems we have to recall stored knowledge and apply rules. In contrast to the automatic mode, problem-solving thought processes are conscious, slow, and sequential, and therefore difficult.

Errors in the Automatic Mode

Errors that occur when an individual is functioning in the automatic mode are called "slips." They usually result from distractions or failure to pay attention at critical moments. An example is setting out in an automobile to go shopping and finding that one has driven to work instead. Psychologists' term for this phenomenon is "capture." Another common error mechanism is loss of activation, in which attention is distracted and a thought process is lost. An example is entering a room and failing to remember why.

Both physiological and psychological factors can divert attentional control and make slips more likely. Physiological factors include fatigue, sleep loss, alcohol, drugs, and illness. Psychological factors include other activity ("busyness") as well as emotional states such as boredom, frustration, fear, anxiety, and anger. All lead to preoccupations that divert attention. Psychological factors, though considered internal or endogenous, may be triggered by external factors such as overwork, interpersonal relations, and other forms of stress. Environmental factors such as noise, heat, visual stimuli, and motion can also divert attention and lead to slips.

Errors in the Problem-Solving Mode

Errors of problem-solving thought ("mistakes," in human-factors jargon) are more complex. They include rule-based mistakes, which occur when a wrong rule is chosen—either because one misperceives the situation and applies the wrong rule or because one simply misapplies a rule. Knowledge-based mistakes occur when the problem solver confronts a situation for which he or she possesses no programmed solutions. Errors arise because of lack of knowledge or because of misinterpretation of the problem.

Familiar patterns are assumed to have universal applicability because they usually work. We see what we know. It is simpler to apply a pattern than to rethink each situation. Errors can arise from discrepancies in pattern matching; sometimes we unconsciously match the wrong patterns. One form of pattern mismatching is caused by biased memory. Decisions are based on what is in our memory, but memory is biased toward overgeneralization and overregularization of the commonplace.[24]

Another aberration of thought that leads to error is the availability heuristic. This is the human tendency to grab the first answer that comes to mind and to stick with it despite evidence to the contrary. This tendency may be compounded by another mechanism, confirmation bias, which is the natural inclination to accept evidence that confirms one's hypothesis and to reject evidence that negates it. Many other mechanisms have been described. The important point is that these things happen every day to all of us. Rule-based and knowledge-based functioning are affected by the same physiological, psychological, and environmental influences that produce slips.

Stress is often cited as a cause of errors. Although it is often difficult to establish a causal link between stress and specific accidents, there is little question that both slips and mistakes are increased when people are under stress.

Three clear lessons emerge from this research. First, errors are normal. Everyone errs every day. To err is indeed to be human. Second, errors result from well-known cognitive mechanisms—mechanisms that are complex but understandable. Third, distractions are a common cause of errors. Errors truly result from a "normal" pathology.

SYSTEMS CAUSES OF ERRORS

Although insights from cognitive psychology and human-factors research help us understand how and why people make mistakes, they offer limited help in devising methods for preventing errors. It may be possible to avoid distractions, for example, or at least to recognize when one is at risk of being distracted, but individuals have a limited ability to "think straight" all the time. Successful methods of preventing errors require additional insight and understanding.

The major breakthrough in thinking about errors was the recognition that systems factors play a major role in increasing the likelihood that an individual will make an error. A watershed event in this understanding was the nuclear power plant accident at Three Mile Island in 1979. Although initial investigations revealed the expected operator errors (i.e., "human error"), it became clear that preventing many of these errors was beyond the capabilities of the specific individuals operating the system at the moment the accident occurred. Many of the errors were caused by faulty interface design or breakdowns that were not discernible by the operators or their instruments. The errors were the result of major failures of design and organization that occurred long before the accident.

Investigations following the accident at Three Mile Island revealed that faulty design provided gauges that gave a low pressure reading both when pressure was low and when the gauge was not working. Therefore, the operator thought the pressure was low when actually the gauge was broken. Also, the system had a control panel on which 100 lights started flashing simultaneously; faulty maintenance had disabled a safety backup system. Operators had been trained in how to respond to each light individually but not in how to prioritize should multiple lights go on at once. Thus, although an operator error may have been the proximal cause of the accident, the root causes had been present in the system for a long time.

Faulty systems design has two effects: It causes operator errors, and it makes them impossible to detect in time to prevent an accident. The operators at Three Mile Island were "set up" for failure by poor design, faulty maintenance, inadequate training, and poor management decisions. Together, these factors created a situation in which a minor operator error could result in a serious injury.

Reason[23] terms errors resulting from these situations "latent" errors—errors whose effects are delayed. Latent errors can be described as accidents waiting to happen. The effects of active errors, in contrast, are felt immediately.

Psychological precursors, one type of latent error, are working conditions that predispose to errors.[23] Inappropriate work schedules, for example, can result in high workloads and undue time pressures, two conditions that induce errors. Poor training can lead to inadequate recognition of hazards or inappropriate procedures that may lead to accidents. A precursor can be the product of more than one management or training failure. For example, excessive time pressure can result from poor scheduling, but it can also result from inadequate training or faulty division of responsibilities. Because they can affect all cognitive processes, precursors can cause an immense variety of errors that result in unsafe acts.

The primary objective of systems design for safety is to make it difficult for individuals to err. Even with the best system, however, errors will inevitably occur. A mechanism is needed for recognizing and correcting errors before they cause accidents. Ideally, systems should be designed to automatically correct errors when they occur. If this cannot be done, mechanisms should be in place to detect errors as soon as possible so that corrective action can be taken to minimize patient injury. In addition to designing the work environment to minimize psychological precursors, designers should provide feedback mechanisms in the form of monitoring instruments. They must also build in buffers and make provisions for redundancy. Buffers are design features that automatically correct for human or mechanical error. Redundancy is duplication (or triplication or quadruplication) of critical mechanisms and instruments. If a system is redundant, a single failure does not result in loss of the function.

Accident prevention efforts must focus on systems failures—on errors in design and implementation of systems. Most errors result from failure to use basic human-factors principles in the design of tasks and systems. Excessive reliance on memory, lack of standardization, inadequate availability of information, and poor work schedules all create situations in which individuals are more likely to make mistakes.

INDUSTRIAL MODELS

Aviation, nuclear power generation, and space travel employ technology that is at least as complicated and risky as that used in health care. Nonetheless, these industries have developed highly reliable systems for minimizing human error. For example, airline travel in the United States is indeed safe: The statistical chance of dying when you board a scheduled airliner is less than 1 in 3 million.

The difference between the approach used in the aviation industry and that used in medicine is that the aviation industry designs its systems for safety. Preventing accidents is a principal objective of aircraft design and flight procedures. First, aircraft designers assume that errors and failures are inevitable. They therefore design systems to absorb them by building in multiple buffers, automation, and redundancy. Second, procedures are standardized to the maximum extent possible. Specific protocols must be followed for trip planning, operations, and maintenance. Pilots go through a checklist before each takeoff.

Third, the training, examination, and certification process is highly developed and strictly enforced. Airline pilots take proficiency examinations every 6 months. Much of the content of these examinations is directly concerned with safety procedures. Finally, safety in aviation has been institutionalized. The Federal Aviation Administration regulates all aspects of flying and prescribes safety procedures, and the National Transportation Safety Board investigates every accident. The adherence of airlines and pilots to safety standards is closely monitored.

A unique feature of the aviation industry is the Aviation Safety Reporting System, which provides immunity against disciplinary action for pilots, controllers, or others who report a dangerous situation, such as a near-miss midair collision. This program has been highly successful in ensuring the prompt reporting of unsafe conditions, communication problems, and traffic control inadequacies. The Aviation Safety Reporting System receives more than 5,000 notifications each year.[25]

THE MEDICAL MODEL

In contrast, accident prevention has not been a primary focus of hospital medicine. Health care personnel typically react to a specific accident and focus on the error rather than attempting to understand the systemic cause. For example, a typical response to a dosing error is the institution of an additional checking stage. Human-factors experts recognize the futility of concentrating on solutions to the unsafe acts themselves. Other errors, unpredictable and infinitely varied, will soon occur if the underlying systems failure goes uncorrected. Correcting systems failures will not eliminate all errors, because individuals still bring various abilities and work habits to the workplace. Nonetheless, correcting systems failures will substantially reduce the probability of error.

Most important, rather than designing systems to prevent or absorb errors, designers of medical systems rely largely on faultless performance by individuals to prevent errors. They expect individuals not to make errors, rather than assuming that they will.

There are, of course, exceptions. For example, unit dose drug distribution was a major systems change in medication dispensing that has markedly reduced medication dosing errors. In intensive care units, monitoring is sophisticated and extensive (though perhaps not sufficiently redundant). Equipment and procedures for anesthesia have been developed that make it difficult for personnel to commit errors. Mortality from anesthesia has been estimated at less than 1 in 200,000, compared with 1 in 10,000 to 20,000 a decade earlier.[26] Anesthesiologists have led the medical profession in recognizing systems factors as causes of errors, in the design of fail-safe systems, and in training to avoid errors.[27–29]

MEASURING ERRORS

Health care organizations that want to reduce errors need to develop reliable methods for measuring them. The errors that occur provide clues as to which systems need to be targeted for redesign. Changes in the error rate are the measure of the effectiveness of system changes. Accurate and reproducible measurement of errors is difficult, but the purpose of measuring is to discover errors, quantify the extent and types of errors, and document trends.

Discovering Errors

Most health care organizations rely on spontaneous reporting to identify errors. This method is not only inadequate but also misleading, because the punitive nature of most hospitals' responses to error reporting stifles such reporting. Typical incident reports identify only 2% to 5% of reportable ADEs.[30] This is beginning to change as more and more hospitals implement a nonpunitive approach to errors. When immunity is provided, the yield is sometimes astonishing.[13]

Identification of errors, as well as investigation of all errors that cause injuries, should be a routine part of hospital practice. Only when errors are accepted as an inevitable, though manageable, part of everyday practice will it be possible for hospital personnel to shift from a punitive to a creative frame of mind that seeks out and identifies the underlying systems failures.

Quantifying Types of Errors

It is neither feasible nor necessary to measure all types of errors on a continuous basis. Periodic, focused data collection is sufficient. Once systems changes have been selected, specific indicator errors can be identified and measured intensively over a short period to determine the base error rate.

Documenting Trends

Once indicator errors have been identified and systems changes have been introduced, errors or adverse events should be measured periodically to assess the effectiveness of the systems changes. It is helpful to present such data over time in the form of control charts that show the baseline rate, upper and lower control limits (usually three standard deviations), the error rate after the intervention, and maintenance of the improvement over time. Chapter 23 provides more information on measuring medication safety.

Measuring errors may be expensive, but the consequences of errors are more so. In industry, the savings from reduction of errors and accidents more than make up for the costs of data collection and investigation. In hospitals, the additional savings from reduced patient care and liability costs for hospitals and physicians are substantial. In one hospital, the average cost of each preventable ADE has been estimated to be $4,685.[31]

FRAMEWORK FOR SYSTEMS ANALYSIS

Once the extent of errors is known in a health care system (e.g., the medication system, the radiology department, or the emergency room), the next question is to determine where remedial efforts can be most profitably targeted. Systems failures can be grouped into two broad categories: design failures and organizational and environmental failures.

Design Failures

Many hospital systems were never "designed" in the true sense; they just grew. Errors occur because the processes used in these systems have not been well thought out. Basic human-factors principles have been disregarded in the design of these systems. Design failures can be classified into three categories: process design, task design, and equipment design.

Process design failures result from failure to analyze the purposes of the system and how best to achieve them. What are the objectives of the system? How can it best meet users' needs? What are its potential hazards? One must think through the system and determine the consequences of actions that can go wrong at each point.

In a study of medication errors causing ADEs, my colleagues and I[20] found that failures in just three systems accounted for more than half of the errors that either caused an ADE or were near misses (intercepted errors). These three systems were drug knowledge dissemination, checking dose and identity of drugs, and making patient information available.

Drug knowledge dissemination is a major problem. Because of the number, variety, and complexity of drugs, it is impossible for any individual to recall all that he or she needs to know in order to use a drug appropriately and safely. Health professionals need to have drug information available at the time decisions are made and in a form they can easily use.

Methods for tracking and identifying drug, dose, and patient are often primitive compared with those used in industry. Supermarkets keep better track of groceries than many hospitals do of medications. Creative ways need to be developed for making patient information more readily available: displaying it where it is needed, when it is needed, and in an accessible form. Computerizing the medical record, for example, would facilitate bedside display of patient information, including test results and medications.

Task design failures result from the failure to incorporate human-factors principles into planning tasks. Norman[24] has pointed out the importance of designing tasks to minimize errors and has recommended a set of principles that have general applicability. Tasks should be simplified to minimize the load on the weakest aspects of cognition (i.e., short-term memory, planning, and problem solving). The power of constraints should be exploited. One way to do this is with forcing functions. These are design features that make it impossible to perform a specific erroneous act (e.g., the lock that prohibits release of the parking gear of a car unless the brake pedal is depressed). Standardization of procedures, displays, and layouts reduces errors by reinforcing the pattern recognition that humans perform well. Finally, where possible, operations should be easily reversible or, when not reversible, difficult to carry out.

Checklists, protocols, and computerized decision aids could be used more widely. For example, physicians should not have to rely on their memories to retrieve a laboratory test result, nor should nurses have to remember the time a medication dose is due. Computers can do these tasks more reliably than humans.

Standardization is one of the most effective ways to prevent errors; examples in the airline industry include maintenance protocols and pilot checklists. The advantages of standardizing drug doses and administration times, for example, are obvious. Is it acceptable to ask nurses to follow six different "K scales" (directions for how much potassium to give according to the patient's serum potassium level) solely to satisfy idiosyncratic physician prescribing patterns? Other areas in which standardization would be beneficial include information displays, methods for common practices (e.g., surgical dressings), and the location of equipment and supplies in a patient care unit.

Forcing functions can be used to structure critical tasks so that errors cannot be made. For example, a computerized system for medication orders can be designed so that a physician cannot enter an order for a lethal overdose of a drug or prescribe a medication to which a patient is known to be allergic.

Equipment design failures result from failure to apply basic human-factors principles to the design of equipment displays and controls. It is astonishing that most people using most of the equipment in hospitals do not understand how that equipment works. This is primarily a design problem; manufacturers have not seen to it that equipment offers the user information and controls that are readily understandable. In other words, the manufacturers, too, have failed to apply basic human-factors principles. It is also remarkable that it is possible to connect an epidural catheter to a syringe with medication prepared only for intravenous use. A simple forcing function design, such as has long been used with oxygen and nitrous oxide connections in anesthesia, could prevent this error.

Organizational and Environmental Failures

Organizational and environmental failures, unlike design failures, can often be remedied through changes at the departmental or unit level (i.e., the pharmacy or nursing unit). Institutionwide changes may not be needed. Three types of organizational failures may induce errors: psychological precursors, inadequate team building, and training failures.

Psychological precursors are conditions in the workplace, such as schedules, work assignments, and interpersonal relationships, that cause stress and lead to errors. These include environmental factors, such as excessive heat, inadequate light, crowded space, and high noise levels, as well as excessive workloads, long working hours, and poor managerial styles. Although the influence of the stresses of everyday life on human behavior cannot be eliminated, stresses caused by a faulty work environment can be. Eliminating fear and creating a supportive working environment are powerful methods for preventing errors.

Team building requires a supportive environment and skilled leaders who can encourage individuals to work together effectively, help each other avoid mistakes, intercept errors, and reduce psychological precursors. Hospitals have historically been poor team builders because physicians and nurses have functioned semiautonomously and autocratically.

Training is essential. If personnel neither understand their responsibilities nor possess adequate skills, they will be more likely to make errors. Health professionals need more training in error prevention and identification. They need to learn to think of errors primarily as symptoms of systems failures. Many interns need more rigorous instruction and supervision than is currently provided. Young physicians need to be taught that safe practice is as important as effective practice.

RETROSPECTIVE SYSTEMS ANALYSIS

Most hospitals consider systems analysis, if they consider it at all, only in response to a serious adverse event. A root cause analysis (see Chapter 5) may be carried out, focusing on the specific error. Vincent et al.[32] caution against such a simplistic approach: "While it is sometimes straightforward to identify a particular action or omission as the immediate cause of an incident, closer analysis usually reveals a series of events leading up to adverse outcome. The identification of an obvious departure from good practice is usually only the first step of the investigation." Instead, they counsel, one should look broadly for all potential contributing factors. These include task factors, such as availability of protocols; environmental factors, such as staffing levels and workloads; team factors, such as communication and supervision; and organizational and management factors.

Systems analysis of an adverse event is difficult and time-consuming. However, it can be extremely rewarding. Investigation almost always reveals a host of contributing factors (e.g., poor work schedules, inappropriate protocols, poor labels on drugs, and inadequate training or supervision) that are the underlying causes of the event. For example, investigation of a fatal medication error in an infant (see Chapter 5 appendix) revealed more than 50 systems failures.[33]

PROSPECTIVE SYSTEMS ANALYSIS

An organization that is seriously committed to patient safety will not wait for tragedy to strike before identifying systems failures. It will adopt a practice widely observed in engineering, the prospective search for potential systems failures, or "accidents waiting to happen"—also known as failure mode and effects analysis (FMEA). A small group of frontline caregivers identifies a potential hazard and then brainstorms about all of the possible things that could go wrong, diagramming relationships in a "fishbone" or similar diagram (see Chapter 21).

OBSTACLES TO SYSTEMS REDESIGN

Like any established institution, the modern hospital presents significant barriers to those who seek to change its practices. These barriers appear to be both extensive and daunting, but recognizing them is the first step in designing methods to overcome them. The following obstacles are found in most hospitals:

1. A culture of shame and blame. Often, there still are strong sanctions (overt or covert) against those who make mistakes. Because errors are thought to be due to carelessness, workers are punished when they make mistakes. For physicians, punishment is likely to be covert (i.e., disapproval or shunning). As a result of this culture, most failures are not reported.[30] They are also not discussed, which makes improvement (i.e., systems redesign) impossible.

2. Infrequent occurrence of events. Despite the alarming statistics, serious errors are uncommon in the experience of most hospital professionals. For example, the widely quoted estimate from the Institute of Medicine of 98,000 preventable deaths annually works out, on average, to only 1 death every 7 years for a physician. Evidence abounds that most errors are not recognized, so it is likely that an average physician is aware of a preventable death only two or three times in a lifetime. Similarly, nonfatal errors are often unrecognized. This perceived low error rate leads to complacency. It also means that a change targeted at a low-frequency problem can potentially result in an increase in overall work for a relatively low yield.

3. Complexity and lack of ownership. Hospital systems are complex, involving a wide variety of personnel and interlocking flows of materials and information. Many individuals have interests in multiple operations, and each system and subsystem has multiple stakeholders, but none of the stakeholders has complete control of any of the systems; there are no owners. The system for ordering, dispensing, and administering medications is a good example of the challenges posed by complex systems. This system is characterized by multiple actors (physicians, nurses, pharmacists, clerks, and technicians), multiple choices (drugs, names, routes, doses), multiple handoffs that are frequent and fragile, no ownership, no natural team, and no one with hospitalwide authority to make changes and ensure quality.

4. Unavailability of information. Because of the complexity of processes, information transfer can pose a major challenge to knowledge-based problem solving. A systems analysis of ADEs showed that lack of information about the patient and lack of knowledge of drugs were the most common systems failures, accounting for 40% of the serious, injury-producing errors.[20] Modern medicine is complicated; it is difficult to remember everything one needs to know to diagnose, treat, and monitor care in all kinds of patients. It is also difficult to ensure that all the pertinent information about each patient is readily available to all who are involved in decisions about care. Physicians, nurses, pharmacists, and others need to have information available when it is needed, where it is needed, and in a form that can be readily used.

5. Physician resistance. Physicians have been reluctant participants in the modern safety movement. Why? An obvious and often-cited reason is the fear of inciting malpractice litigation. Many physicians do not believe that state peer-review statutes provide adequate protection. But there are no studies demonstrating that internal review of mishaps increases malpractice risk. Those hospitals that are making major strides in safety do not have a greater frequency of lawsuits. Still, many physicians choose not to take the chance.

A second reason is that many physicians do not accept the systems concept. It seems like a vague and complicated solution to a simple problem: you made a mistake, so take your punishment. It goes against all we've been taught: that if we're careful and do our homework, we won't make mistakes. And, it smacks of irresponsibility: "Don't blame me; it's the system." Finally, as suggested above, many do not believe the numbers; the high rates of injury and death are not consistent with their personal experience.

6. Lack of leadership. It is not just physicians who have not signed on to the safety movement; neither have the chief executive officers (CEOs) of most hospitals and health care systems. CEOs do not believe the numbers and are caught in the blaming approach to safety. Like physicians, they are not sure they believe in the systems approach. They are leery of getting ahead of their physicians, since they have limited control over the physicians' practices. Finally, they do not feel much pressure from the public or from their boards to change.

7. Tolerance of individualistic practices. One manifestation of the lack of leadership is hospitals' tendency to cater to the idiosyncrasies and special demands of individual physicians. In drug prescribing, for example, tolerance of illegible and nonstandard orders and catering to prescribing differences contribute to the likelihood of error. Noncompliance with safety practices, such as hand-disinfecting and "sign your site" policies, is also tolerated. No other business or industry would tolerate such flagrant disregard of its policies. Following rules is basic. Safe practice cannot be achieved in such an environment. Changing such long-standing practices can be a challenge.

CONCLUSION

Few American institutions are as ripe for systems redesign as hospitals. The current drive for efficiency will necessitate reexamination of the most serious form of inefficiency: injury-producing errors. Significant improvements will require major commitments to error reduction by each organization's leadership, as well as acceptance by all professionals and administrators that error is an inevitable aspect of the human condition. Until errors are recognized as symptoms of systems flaws, not of character flaws, substantial progress in reducing medical errors is unlikely.

REFERENCES

1. Brennan TA, Leape LL, Laird N, et al. Incidence of adverse events and negligence in hospitalized patients: results from the Harvard medical practice study I. *N Engl J Med.* 1991;324:370–6.
2. Leape LL, Brennan TA, Laird NM, et al. The nature of adverse events in hospitalized patients: results from the Harvard Medical Practice Study II. *N Engl J Med.* 1991;324:377–84.
3. Schimmel E. The hazards of hospitalization. *Ann Intern Med.* 1964;60:100–10.
4. Steel K, Gertman P, Crescenzi C, Anderson J. Iatrogenic illness on a general medical service at a university hospital. *N Engl J Med.* 1981;304:638–42.
5. Bedell S, Deitz D, Leeman D, et al. Incidence and characteristics of preventable iatrogenic cardiac arrests. *JAMA.* 1991;265:2815–20.
6. Leape LL, Lawthers AG, Brennan TA, et al. Preventing medical injury. *QRB Qual Rev Bull.* 1993;19:144–9.
7. Wilson R, Runciman W, Gibberd R, et al. The quality in Australian Health Care Study. *Med J Aust.* 1995;163:458–71.
8. Davis P, Lay-Yee R, Briant R, et al. *Adverse Events in New Zealand Public Hospitals: Principal Findings from a National Survey.* Wellington, New Zealand: Ministry of Health; 2001.
9. Schioler T, Lipczak H, Pedersen BL, et al. Incidence of adverse events in hospitals. A retrospective study of medical records [Danish]. *Ugeskrift Laeger.* 2001; 163:5370–8.
10. Vincent C, Neale G, Woloshynowych M. Adverse events in British hospitals: preliminary retrospective record review. *BMJ.* 2001; 322:517–9.
11. Baker GR, Norton PG, Flintoft V, et al. The Canadian Adverse Events Study: the incidence of adverse events among hospital patients in Canada. *Can Med Assoc J.* 2004;170:1678–86.
12. Barker KN, Flynn EA, Pepper GA, et al. Medication errors observed in 36 health care facilities. *Arch Intern Med.* 2002;162:1897–903.
13. Bates DW, Cullen DJ, Laird N, et al. Incidence of adverse drug events and potential adverse drug events. *JAMA.* 1995;274:29–34.
14. Barker K, Allan E. Research on drug-use system errors. *Am J Health Syst Pharm.* 1995;52:400–3.
15. Lesar T, Briceland L, Delcoure K, et al. Medication prescribing errors in a teaching hospital. *JAMA.* 1990;263:2329–34.
16. Raju T, Thornton J, Kecskes S, et al. Medication errors in neonatal and paediatric intensive-care units. *Lancet.* 1989:374-79.
17. Classen D, Pestonik S, Evans R, et al. Computerized surveillance of adverse drug events in hospital patients. *JAMA.* 1991;266:2847–51.
18. Folli H, Poole R, Benitz W, et al. Medication error prevention by clinical pharmacists in two children's hospitals. *Pediatrics.* 1987;79:718–22.
19. Bates DW, Boyle DL, Vander Vliet MB, et al. Relationship between medication errors and adverse drug events. *J Gen Intern Med.* 1995;10:199–205.
20. Leape LL, Bates DW, Cullen DJ, et al. Systems analysis of adverse drug events. *JAMA.* 1995;274:35–43.
21. Hilfiker D. Facing our mistakes. *N Engl J Med.* 1984;310:118–22.
22. McIntyre N, Popper K. The critical attitude in medicine: the need for a new ethics. *BMJ.* 1989;287:1919–23.
23. Reason J. *Human Error.* Cambridge, Mass: Cambridge University Press; 1990.
24. Norman D. *To Err Is Human: The Psychology of Everyday Things.* New York: Basic Books; 1988.

25. Billings CE. The NASA aviation safety reporting system: lessons learned from voluntary incident reporting. Enhancing Patient Safety and Reducing Errors in Health Care. Annenberg Conference, Rancho Mirage, Calif, November 8–10, 1998.

26. Orkin F. Patient monitoring during anesthesia as an exercise in technology assessment. In: Saidman L, Smith N, eds. *Monitoring in Anesthesia*. Boston: Butterworth-Heinemann; 1993:439–55.

27. Gaba D. Human error in anesthetic mishaps. *Int Anesth Clin*. 1989;27:137–47.

28. Cooper J, Newbower R, Kitz R. An analysis of major errors and equipment failures in anesthesia management: considerations for prevention and detection. *Anesthesiology*. 1984;60:34–42.

29. Cullen D, Nemeskal R, Cooper J, et al. Effect of pulse oximetry, age, and ASA physical status on the frequency of patients admitted unexpectedly to a postoperative intensive care unit and the severity of their anesthesia-related complications. *Anesth Analg*. 1992;74:181–8.

30. Cullen DJ, Bates DW, Small SD, et al. The incident reporting system does not detect adverse drug events. *Jt Comm J Qual Improv*. 1995;21:541–8.

31. Bates DW, Spell N, Cullen DJ, et al. The costs of adverse drug events in hospitalized patients. *JAMA*. 1997;277:307–11.

32. Vincent C, Taylor-Adams S, Chapman EJ, et al. How to investigate and analyse clinical incidents: clinical risk unit and association of litigation and risk management protocol. *BMJ*. 2000;320:777–81.

33. Smetzer J, Cohen M. Lesson from the Denver medication error/criminal negligence case: look beyond blaming individuals. *Hosp Pharm*. 1998;33:640–57.

CHAPTER 2

RESEARCH ON ERRORS IN DISPENSING AND MEDICATION ADMINISTRATION

Elizabeth Allan Flynn and Kenneth N. Barker

Progress toward an error-free medication distribution system has been charted in studies over nearly half a century. The goals of this research have been to measure medication error rates, compare the accuracy of different drug distribution systems, identify the causes of errors, and evaluate the effectiveness of error detection techniques. Studies have revealed how often errors occur, what changes in the medication distribution system can decrease errors, what factors affect error rates, and the effects of automated drug dispensing devices.

Medication administration errors in inpatient settings and dispensing errors in inpatient, outpatient, and community pharmacy are the focus of this chapter. Its objectives are to (1) describe the frequency and significance of administration and dispensing errors, (2) summarize the terminology used in the medication error literature and the methods used to study errors, (3) critique published medication error studies, (4) review factors associated with medication errors that have been identified through research, (5) summarize findings on the effects of automated dispensing technologies and other interventions, and (6) describe how error detection techniques have been applied in practice. The chapter concludes with some research-based recommendations for error prevention.

CLINICAL SIGNIFICANCE OF MEDICATION ERRORS

Most studies of the clinical significance of medication administration errors have focused on error (incident) reports and on evidence of harm found in patients' charts. Some studies have used the National Coordinating Council for Medication Error Reporting and Prevention (NCCMERP) index to classify the severity of reported errors.[1] This index categorizes errors according to the risk of harm to the patient. Several investigators have rated the clinical significance of errors according to the potential for harm from drugs in particular pharmacologic categories. Barker and colleagues[2] classified 66.1% of 653 detected errors (excluding wrong-time errors) as serious, meaning that the drugs involved were deemed harmful (when misused) by a two-pharmacist panel. Other investigators have used this method for rating the severity of errors, with similar results.[3–5]

Schnell[6] rated the severity of individual errors on a scale of 0 to 100 according to the error category to which each error was assigned. For example, all wrong-dose errors were given a clinical significance rating of 80, whereas wrong-time errors were assigned a value of 20. The clinical significance indices ranged from 28.0 to 47.1, and from 63.0 to 73.5 when wrong-time errors were excluded. Schnell used combined data from four hospitals; the results for traditional and unit dose drug distribution systems were similar. In an observational study, Barker et al.[7] adjusted the potential for harm by considering not only the drug involved in each error, but also the patient's condition as judged by a panel of three physicians. Excluding wrong-time errors, they found that 10% of the errors were potentially serious.

ECONOMIC IMPACT

Economic consequences of medication administration errors include extended hospital stays, additional treatment, and malpractice litigation. Schneider and colleagues[8] reported that the mean costs of medication-related problems (medication errors and adverse drug reactions[ADRs]) at a university hospital ranged from $95 for extra laboratory tests to $2,640 for intensive care. The total cost of medication-related problems at that hospital in 1994 was $1.5 million. In a study at a teaching hospital, the cost per medication error during a 3-month period averaged $55 to $146, depending on the severity; this included labor, room, and laboratory costs.[9] Error-related hospital costs for an outpatient who received glyburide 5 mg instead of diazepam 5 mg were $13,941.72.[10]

Hynniman and co-workers[11] calculated the cost benefits of various drug distribution systems. They proposed that the ultimate criterion for evaluating the expense of a medication system is the cost per dose delivered correctly. The unit dose system had a cost per dose of $0.33 and an error rate of 3.5%. A floor-stock system had a similar cost per dose of $0.32 and an error rate of 11.5%. At three hospitals using a prescription order system, the cost per dose ranged from $0.38 to $0.54 and error rates were 8.3% to 20.6%. Data from other cost comparisons of drug distribution systems indicate that when nursing and pharmacy costs are considered, the unit dose system is the least expensive to operate.[12,13]

The average indemnity payment for claims related to medication errors between 1985 and 1992 was $99,721.[14] Most medication error-related claims are settled out of court for much larger amounts, because they are so hard for the provider to defend.[15]

FREQUENCY OF MEDICATION ERRORS

Administration Errors

Medication errors in 36 hospitals and skilled-nursing facilities occurred at the rate of two per patient day in an observational study published in 2002.[7] Administration errors occurred at a rate of 19% (605 errors detected in 3,216 doses). Excluding wrong-time errors, the rate was 10%. The most frequent errors by category were wrong time (43%), omission (30%), wrong dose (17%), and unauthorized drug (4%). Seven percent of the errors, or more than 40 per day in a typical 300-patient facility, were judged potential ADEs. The researchers concluded that facilities' medication administration systems are often defective.

Error rates found in other observational studies of the medication administration process are summarized in Table 2-1.[16–37] Because of differences in error category definitions and methods, caution should be used in comparing error rates between studies. Although errors, excluding wrong-time errors, have been estimated to occur at a rate of about one per patient per day, rates of two or three per patient per week have been achieved by installing unit dose systems.[27]

Administration errors in particular patient care areas have been studied. Croskerry and colleagues[38] described errors in adults and children in an emergency department and discussed prevention.

TABLE 2-1 Inpatient Medication Administration Error Rates in Observation-Based Research

Date	Hospital, Facility, or Type of Unit	TOE[b]	Error Rate (%)[a] With Wrong Time Errors	Error Rate (%)[a] Without Wrong Time Errors	Drug Distribution System Unit Dose	Drug Distribution System Unit Dose with Automation	Drug Distribution System Other
1962[16]	University of Florida	572	16.2	14.7			X
1964[17]	UAMC pilot before unit dose	1,313	16.1	14.4			X
	UAMC pilot after unit dose	1,124	7.2[c]	1.8[c]	X		
1966[2]	General hospital	9,789	15.0	6.7			X
1967[18]	University of Iowa before DUDD	6,806	17.7[d,e]	0.4			X
	University of Iowa after DUDD	11,001	8.8[d,e]	0.9	X		
1969[19]	UAMC before unit dose	11,015	25.9	13.0			X
	UAMC after unit dose	3,043	12.0[c]	1.9[c]	X		
1970[3]	University of Kentucky	6,061	f	3.5	X		
	Kentucky Hospital A	1,921	f	8.3			X
	Kentucky Hospital B	788	f	9.9			X
	Kentucky Hospital C	1,432	f	11.5			X
	Kentucky Hospital D	1,279	f	20.6			X
1971[20]	N.C. nursing home	235	59.1	24.7	X		X
	N.C. nursing home	289	49.5	21.1	X		X
	N.C. nursing home after unit dose	351	1.7	1.4	X		
1973[21]	Ohio State: Nurse administration	3,678	f	5.3	X		
	Ohio State: Pharmacy technician administration	3,447	f	0.6[c]	X[g]		
1975[22]	Johns Hopkins Hospital before unit dose	1,428	f	7.3[h]			X
	Johns Hopkins Hospital after unit dose	1,243	f	1.6[c,h]	X		
1976[6]	Canadian Hospital A before unit dose	3,123	37.2	8.9[c]			X
	Canadian Hospital A after unit dose	3,235	38.5	14.6	X		
	Canadian Hospital B before unit dose	3,443	42.9	14.5			X
	Canadian Hospital B after unit dose	3,069	23.3[c]	12.9[i]	X		
	Canadian Hospital C before unit dose	3,103	20.1	7.7			X
	Canadian Hospital C after unit dose	2,883	7.8[c]	2.0[c]	X		
	Canadian Hospital D before unit dose	3,134	38.5	9.6			X
	Canadian Hospital D after unit dose	4,445	23.1[c]	3.7[c]	X		

TABLE 2-1 Inpatient Medication Administration Error Rates in Observation-Based Research (continued)

Date	Hospital, Facility, or Type of Unit	TOE[b]	Error Rate (%)[a]		Drug Distribution System		
			With Wrong Time Errors	Without Wrong Time Errors	Unit Dose	Unit Dose with Automation	Other
1976[23]	16 Hospitals <100 beds	1,197	24.6	17.5	j		
1982[24]	58 Long-term care facilities	3,051	f	12.2	j		
	10 Hospitals with < 150 beds	425	f	11.0	j		
1982[25]	Skilled-nursing facility	415	34.2	4.8			X
	Skilled-nursing facility	417	18	4.8			X
1984[15]	Sinai Hospital	2,018	36.8	9.0	X		
1984[26]	Sinai Hospital re-evaluation	781	41.8	10.2	X		
	Sinai Hospital re-evaluation, after improvements	1,003	40.3	12.3[j]	X		
1984[27]	Hospital with decentralized pharmacy system	873	15.9	6.7	X		
	Automated bedside device	902	10.6[c]	5.2[i]		X	
1986[5]	Intensive care nursery	389[k]	17.0	6.9			X
	Pediatric intensive care	231[k]	35.1	10.8			X
1988[28]	Ohio State: Administration by a technician	2,028	4.4	1.6	X		
1991[29]	Pediatric hospital before unit dose (included left at bedside doses)	282	37.2[h]	10.3[h]			X
	Pediatric hospital after unit dose (included left at bedside doses)	241	21.2[h]	2.9[h]	X		
1994[30]	Long-term care facility, blister card	286[l]	2.1	1.4		ATC Plus[m]	X
	Long-term care facility, single unit dose packaging	287	0	0		ATC Plus	
	Long-term care facility, multidose packaging	265	0	0			
1995[31]	Teaching hospital	873	16.9	6.5		Medstation[n]	
	Teaching hospital	929	10.4	2.0		Medstation Rx	
1995[32]	Long-term care facilities before nurse education	NR	10.6	NR	NR	NR	NR
	Long-term care facilities after nurse education	NR	2.9	NR	NR	NR	NR
1995[33]	British hospital, ward-based floor stock	2,756	NS	3.0			X
	American hospital	919	NS	6.9		X	
1998[34]	Pediatric intensive care unit, university hospital, Switzerland	275	26.9	18.2			FS
1999[35]	Intensive care unit, France	2,009	6.6	6.1			FS
1999[36]	Medical units (2), hospital in UK	842	NS	8.0			FS
	Surgery and rehabilitation units, hospital in Germany	973	NS	5.1			FS
	Respiratory and urology units, hospital in Germany	1,318	NS	2.4		ATC-212	FS
2003[37]	Geriatric and cardiovascular-thoracic surgery units, university hospital, France	523	14.9	11.1			FS

DUDD = decentralized unit dose dispensing; NR = not reported; NS = not studied; FS = floor stock.

a Percentage of total opportunities for error.

b Total opportunities for error.

c Indicates that this value is significantly lower than the measurement for other drug distribution systems in the study at the p ≤ 0.05 level of significance.

d In order to increase comparability with other studies, these figures combine errors and discrepancies, but they exclude "Left at bedside" discrepancies.

e Statistical analyses were not performed in this study.

f Wrong time errors were not measured.

g 50% of the packages used by nurses were in unit dose form.

h Excludes omission errors.

i No significant difference between this value and its comparison value.

j Multiple drug distribution systems included. The error rate is an average value.

k Total opportunities for error modified: number of omission errors added to doses administered and error rates recalculated from data in the study.

l Number of routine orders reported. Number of total opportunities for error calculated by dividing the number of errors by the error rate reported (6 errors divided by 0.021 = 286 opportunities for error).

m Baxter Healthcare Corporation, Chicago, Illinois.

n Pyxis Corporation, San Diego, California.

TABLE 2-2 Dispensing Error Rates in Prescription-Filling Operations

Type of Pharmacy	No. Errors	No. Prescriptions	Dispensing Error Rate (%)
Community pharmacy, patient follow-up[52]	29	223	13
Ambulatory pharmacy, pharmacists[53]	48	929	5
Ambulatory pharmacy, technicians[53]	44	1,055	4
Ambulatory pharmacy, teaching hospital[54]	1,085	9,394	12
High-volume military ambulatory pharmacy[55]	369	10,889	3
Ambulatory pharmacy[56]	37	3,227	1
Ambulatory pharmacy[57]	195	5,072	3
Ambulatory pharmacy[58]	552	9,846	6
Community pharmacies[59]	24	100	24

Inpatient Dispensing Errors

Rates of inpatient pharmacy dispensing errors during the cart-filling process (termed *picking errors*) range from 0.04% to 2.9%.[39–46] Some states allow technicians to check other technicians' filling of patient medication drawers, instead of requiring that a pharmacist do so.[47] A comparison of pharmacists' versus technicians' checking of filled unit dose medication drawers showed that error detection did not differ significantly.[48] Both pharmacists and technicians found a 1.2% cart-fill error rate. However, pharmacists overlooked more errors: 107 errors in 49,718 doses (0.21% error rate) versus 50 errors overlooked by technicians in 55,470 doses (0.09% error rate). Although the percentage of missed errors that could have resulted in patient harm was not significantly different (25.2% for pharmacists versus 32.0% for technicians), pharmacists overlooked 27 potentially serious errors and technicians, 16. Campbell and Facchinetti[49] used process control charts to monitor errors in dispensing and checking in an inpatient pharmacy; to help evaluate accuracy, they introduced artificial errors.

The source of information on medication profiles used in cart checking has also been studied. The rate of missing doses decreased from 0.93% to 0.33% when nursing and pharmacy personnel checked the cart against the patient's medication administration record (MAR).[50]

Outpatient and Community Pharmacy Dispensing Errors

In a national, observation-based study of prescription dispensing accuracy in 50 pharmacies, dispensing error rates ranged from 0% to 13%, with an overall error rate of 1.7% (77 errors in 4,481 prescriptions).[51] For example, a pharmacy dispensing 250 prescriptions per day would dispense 4 of them in error. Most deviations from the prescription were label errors (51 of 77 errors), followed by wrong quantity (9), wrong strength (8), wrong drug (6), omission (2), and wrong dosage form (1). In previous studies of prescription-filling operations, summarized in Table 2-2,[52–59] error rates ranged from 1% to 24%. The rate of errors that could potentially have harmed patients was reported for some of these studies and ranged from 1.5% to 4%.[54,57,58]

A study of dispensing errors reported over a 4-year period found 82 errors, most of which were wrong drugs and wrong doses.[60] This study, in contrast to observation-based studies of dispensing errors, led to the conclusion that error prevention efforts should focus on selecting the correct drug and patient.

A study in a mail order pharmacy serving a correctional health care system evaluated dispensing errors reported before and after implementation of an automated system for sorting prescription batches by delivery location.[61] Dispensing errors went from 6.3 to 4.1 per 100,000 orders filled.

TERMINOLOGY

Various terms and definitions have been used in medication error research over the past 45 years. In comparing studies, it is important to note the definitions used. In the past, the term *medication error* referred to administration errors; today, it refers to errors at any stage of the medication use process. A *medication administration error* is defined as a deviation from the prescriber's order as written on the patient's chart or as entered into the hospital's computer system by the prescriber.[2] *Drug misadventure* is a broad term applied to adverse drug reactions and medication errors.[62,63] The Food and Drug Administration (FDA) Adverse Event Reporting System (AERS) uses the Medical Dictionary for Regulatory Activities term *drug maladministration* for medication errors.[64] An *adverse drug event* (ADE) is defined as an injury from a drug-related intervention; ADEs can include adverse drug reactions and can result from errors in prescribing, dispensing, and administration.[1] ADEs have been categorized as preventable, nonpreventable, and potential.

The term *medication error* typically is associated with drug administration in the hospital, whereas *dispensing error* is associated with mistakes in distributing medications to nursing units or distributing prescriptions directly to patients in an ambulatory care pharmacy setting.

The definition of medication error includes errors in the process of ordering or delivering a medication.[65] Errors in ordering alone are commonly called prescribing errors.

Barker et al.[2] coined the term *opportunity for error* (OE) for use as the basic unit of data in medication administration error studies. An OE includes any dose given as well as any dose ordered but omitted. Because the dose in any given OE must be either correct or incorrect (i.e., either it is or is not an error), the error rate cannot exceed 100%. An OE includes only those doses of medication whose preparation and administration both are witnessed by an observer; the observer must actually see the patient receive the medication. The following situations typically are not counted as OEs: a drug left at the patient's bedside for self-administration (its consumption is not observed) and a dose associated with an uninterpretable written order.

Total opportunity for error (TOE) is the sum of all doses ordered plus all unordered doses that are given.[2] Some studies have defined TOE as all doses given plus all doses omitted (ordered, but not given); this definition yields the same result.[66]

The *medication error rate* is calculated as the number of OEs that are incorrect (in one or more ways) divided by the TOE. This figure is multiplied by 100 to arrive at a percentage. To calculate the rate of medication accuracy, the number of doses administered correctly would be divided by the TOE.

TYPES OF ERRORS

Definitions Used in Observational Studies

The categories of errors used in observational studies of medication administration are defined in this section. The error types are not mutually exclusive, so the rates for different types of error usually cannot be summed to obtain an overall error rate.

An *unordered* or *unauthorized drug error* (also called a *wrong-drug error*) is the administration of a dose of medication that was never ordered for that patient.

An *extra-dose error* is a dose given in excess of the total number of times ordered by the physician, such as a dose given on the basis of an expired order, after a drug has been discontinued, or after a drug has been put on hold. For example, if a physician ordered a drug to be given every morning and the patient receives a dose in the evening as well, an extra-dose error has occurred.

An *omission error* is noted if a patient fails to receive a dose of medication that was ordered by the time the next dose is due. If the patient refuses the medication, neither an error nor an OE is counted. Doses withheld according to policy (e.g., "nothing by mouth before surgery") are not counted as errors or OEs. The observer detects omissions by comparing the medications administered at a given time with doses that should have been given at that time according to the prescriber's written orders. If a dose was not given, an omission error is counted, barring another explanation.

Some studies may use a *wrong-patient* category, as listed in the NCCMERP taxonomy of errors (www.nccmerp.org/pdf/taxo2001-07-31.pdf.). This can be both an unordered drug error for the patient who received the dose and a possible omission error for the patient for whom the dose was intended.

A *wrong-dose error* occurs when any dose is given that contains the wrong number of preformed dosage units (e.g., tablets) or is, in the judgment of the observer, more than 17% greater or less than the correct dosage (e.g., of an oral liquid). Judgments about dosage are based on the measuring devices routinely used by the institution, such as graduations on syringes and on medicine cups. Some researchers have used a narrower definition for injectable doses; any dose that differs by more than 10% from the correct dosage would be in error. Wrong-dose errors are counted for ointments, topical solutions, and similar medications only when the dose was quantitatively specified by the prescriber (e.g., in inches of ointment).

Wrong-route errors occur when a medication is administered via a different location or site on the patient's body than was ordered. Examples are oral administration of a drug ordered for intramuscular use and a dose given in the right ear instead of the left ear.

Wrong-time errors are typically defined as administration of a dose more than 60 minutes before or after the scheduled administration time in the absence of an acceptable reason. Acceptable reasons include situations where a physician has ordered that the patient not consume anything by mouth or when the patient is undergoing a procedure elsewhere in the hospital. As-needed (prn) doses should be administered no closer together than ordered. The time of the previous prn dose is determined from the observer's notes, the MAR, or information in an automated drug dispensing device. The time frame should be based on how long it takes nurses to prepare and administer medications during a medication pass.

The hospital's standard dose administration schedule should be followed. If the physician did not record the time an order was written, wrong-time errors should not be recorded for doses given that day until a second dose is given. The first dose given according to the standard schedule establishes the schedule in effect, and subsequent doses on the same day can then be examined for wrong-time errors. Hospitals can define the acceptable time range within which doses can be administered; 60 minutes before or after is often used, because of the observation that nurses usually can administer all of their medications within 1 hour. Some hospitals using bar codes to verify administration use an interval of 90 minutes before or after, to accommodate the assessment and documentation requirements of such systems. Because opinions differ on the seriousness of wrong-time errors, error rates often are stated with and without wrong-time errors (but based on the same number of TOEs).

A *wrong dosage-form error* is the administration of a dose in a form different from the form that was ordered. Examples are giving a tablet when a suspension was ordered and administering plain aspirin instead of enteric-coated aspirin. Instances in which tablets are crushed are not considered wrong dosage-form errors because of the lack of information about the effect of crushing on the effectiveness of some tablets.

A *wrong technique error* is an incorrect or omitted action during dose preparation or administration that does not result in another type of error. For example, if the wrong infusion rate is used but the patient receives the correct dose, a wrong technique error has occurred. If the prescriber ordered that the patient's heart rate or blood pressure be determined to fall within certain limits prior to drug administration and this verification was omitted, this is a wrong technique error. If the heart rate is measured and found to be too low but the dose is administered, an extra-dose error has occurred.

A study in the United Kingdom defined an *intravenous drug error* as "any deviation in the preparation or administration of a drug from a doctor's prescription, the hospital's intravenous policy, or the manufacturer's instructions."[67] The authors added, however, that "all errors had to have the potential to adversely affect the patient, so deviations from hospital procedure were not errors if the correct drug was given to the patient."

To enable comparison of new results with past findings, it is recommended that future studies use the error categories that have been used and tested in previous studies.[68]

Definitions for Pharmacy Dispensing Error Studies

This section defines categories that have been used in studies of pharmacy dispensing errors. A *wrong-drug error* occurs when a medication different from that named in writing on a prescription is used to fill the prescription. A *wrong-strength* error occurs when a dosage unit containing an amount of medication different from what the prescriber specified is used to fill a prescription; an exception is when a pharmacist adjusts the dosing instructions so that the patient receives the prescribed amount. A *wrong dosage-form (correct drug)* error is counted when the form of the medication used to fill the prescription differs from what the prescriber wrote, such as the use of an enteric-coated or an extended-release version of a product when that form was not specified. *Wrong-quantity* errors occur when the amount of medication dispensed to a patient differs from the amount ordered and there is no acceptable reason, such as what quantity a third-party payer will reimburse.

Label errors can be divided into two types: instructions, and all other label information. *Wrong label-instruction* errors occur when directions to the patient on the prescription label deviate in one or more ways from what was prescribed; the exception is changes based on good pharmacy practice, such as adding the indication (e.g., "for pain") at the end of the instructions. Auxiliary label information added to the prescription label or vial may or may not be evaluated in studies. For example, it would be an error if a physician wrote "for 14 days" on the prescription and this was omitted from the label instructions, but it would not be an error if "for 14 days" was added at the end of the directions for an antibiotic that should be taken for a complete course of therapy.

Errors involving *wrong prescription label information* (excluding instructions) are determined by comparing the prescription with federal or state requirements for the following label contents:

- Name and address of dispenser (pharmacy),
- Serial number of prescription,
- Date of prescription or date of filling,
- Name of prescriber,
- Name of patient, if stated in the prescription,
- Drug name,
- Drug strength (if more than one strength was available),
- Quantity dispensed,

- Expiration date, and
- Manufacturer or distributor (principal labeler).

Deteriorated-drug errors occur when a medication is beyond its expiration date or is stored in a location that is not in accordance with the manufacturer's recommendations (for example, outside a refrigerator).

Omission errors occur when a patient fails to receive a prescribed medication. For example, if calcium carbonate is dispensed when calcium carbonate with vitamin D was prescribed, the omission of vitamin D is an error even though calcium carbonate was dispensed correctly.

Wrong-time errors can occur in ambulatory care settings that fill blister cards for long-term care or mental health facilities. The medication might be placed in a location on the card that is different from what is conveyed on the prescription. For example, a medication might be placed in the time "bubble" for use at bedtime instead of that for administration with dinner.[51]

METHODS FOR DETECTING ERRORS

Six techniques for detecting medication administration errors and ADEs are discussed in this section:

1. Anonymous self-reports (questionnaires),
2. Incident reports, including voluntary reports,
3. The critical incident technique,
4. Chart review,
5. Computer-assisted monitoring, and
6. Direct observation.

Other error detection methods include stimulated self-report using interview;[14,15] attending medical rounds to listen for clues that an error has occurred;[69] detecting omission errors on the basis of doses returned on the medication cart;[45,70,71] urine testing as evidence of omitted drugs and unauthorized drug administration;[72] examining death certificates;[73] attending nurse change-of-shift report;[74] comparing MARs with physician orders;[75,76] comparing drugs removed from an automated dispensing device for a patient with physician orders, including overrides;[77,78] and data mining.[79] A review of methods for detecting adverse events is available.[80]

Anonymous Self-Reports

Anonymous self-reporting methods such as questionnaires provide a means by which the person committing or witnessing an error can report the mistake but not be associated with it.[16] Advantages of the self-report method are low cost and the ability of staff to avoid the fear of disciplinary action. A limitation is that the person witnessing an error can report it only if he or she is aware that a mistake was made.

According to one study, a nurse who knows that an error has been made may be reluctant to report it if a physician advises against reporting, if the nurse believes the drug involved will not lead to patient harm, or if the error involved is an omission or a wrong-time error.[16] An ethnomethodological study by Baker[74] revealed that nurses may "redefine" errors to justify not reporting them, as follows:

1. If it's not my fault, it's not an error.
2. If everyone knows, it's not an error.

3. If you can make it right, it's not an error.
4. If a patient has needs that are more urgent than the accurate administration of medication, it's not an error.
5. A clerical error is not a medication error.
6. If an irregularity is carried out to prevent something worse, it is not an error.

A recent survey of 1,105 staff nurses at 25 hospitals found three factors related to reporting: administrative response to reports, personal fears, and unit quality management.[81] Barker and McConnell[16] found in an early study that only six anonymous reports of medication errors were filed over a 7-month period in a teaching hospital; 40% of the nurses said they opposed this type of reporting.

Incident Reports

An incident report is a legally recognized report of a medication error that is written by a hospital staff member who detects a medication error or other untoward incident. Incident reports are required by the hospital and cannot be submitted anonymously. Guidelines, recommendations, and forms for reporting incidents are available.[82,83]

Many groups, including the Joint Commission on Accreditation of Healthcare Organizations, FDA, the U.S. Pharmacopeia (USP), and the Institute for Safe Medication Practices, advocate a "culture of safety" that promotes voluntary reporting of medication errors without threat of disciplinary action. In this approach, aspects of the medication use system that may have led to the error are examined for the purpose of preventing similar errors in the future.[84] The advantages and disadvantages of such reporting systems are discussed in Chapter 19.

Incident reports have been used as a source of data in studies of the clinical significance and possible causes of medication errors. Studies have focused on anesthesia,[85,86] pediatrics,[34,87,88] hospitals,[89] and community pharmacy.[90,91] An analysis of FDA AERS data for 1993–1998 showed that improper doses represented 41% of the fatal errors.[65] USP publishes analyses of data from its national voluntary medication error reporting program and MEDMARX database.[92,93] A recent examination suggests that medication error reports to MEDMARX apply definitions inconsistently; agreement in the use of definition codes between MEDMARX users and experts was poor, ranging from 37% to 93%.[94]

One advantage of incident reports is that they provide an ongoing reporting mechanism for an entire hospital.[95] In contrast, observational studies of medication errors sample only selected time periods in certain patient care areas. Low cost has been cited as another advantage of incident report use.[96] However, Shannon and DeMuth[97] found that the time per patient in observational studies was significantly less than the time per patient for reviewing incident reports. From staff estimates of the time spent, Brown[98] in 1979 calculated a cost of $6.71 for completing and analyzing one incident report.

The primary disadvantage of using internal incident reports is gross underreporting of errors (in part because staff is not aware of errors), which produces a false sense of security. Barker and McConnell[16] demonstrated the inadequacy of incident reports as an error detection method. They found that incident reports documented 36 errors over a 1-year period. In comparison, 2 weeks' worth of data collected by direct observation and extrapolated to the same time period indicated that 51,200 errors may have occurred (including 600 wrong-time errors). In brief, the observation technique is capable of detecting far more errors than are detected through incident reports.

Shannon and DeMuth compared a combination of reviews of charts and incident reports with the observation method.[97] Each method was performed simultaneously in long-term care facilities. Their results confirmed the earlier work of Barker and McConnell.[16] Their observation method detected a mean error rate of 9.6%, whereas the paper review method yielded a mean error rate of 0.2%. Flynn and colleagues[99] more recently compared chart and incident report reviews with observation for error detection in 2,557 medication doses at 36 hospitals and skilled-nursing facilities. Observation detected 456 errors and incident reports, 1.

Other investigators have compared the number of incident reports filed with the number of errors detected by observation and have produced similar results.[2,15,31,66] The investigators in one study concluded that it would not be meaningful to use error rates based on incident reports as an indicator of the quality of drug distribution in hospitals.[100]

Fear of disciplinary action is a deterrent to incident reporting.[96,101,102] Examples of punishments for medication administration errors include remedial education,[96] counseling,[96,103,104] sanctions,[105] suspension without pay,[103] and termination of employment.[103,106,107] Some authors advise against associating any type of discipline with incident reporting.[96,102,108] Disciplinary action for dispensing errors is also controversial, especially when one considers that the error could be due to a poor system design. Today the emphasis is on improving patient safety by learning from reported errors and near misses.

Critical Incident Technique

The critical incident technique is an event-sampling method that involves in-depth analyses of a large number of individual errors, with the goal of identifying common causal factors.[109-111] This method can involve direct observation of subjects or interviews of people who have committed an error. The sample size required for this type of research ranges from 100 to several thousand critical incidents and is based on the complexity of the behavior being evaluated. The minimum sample size is reached when no new behaviors are observed and there are at least three examples in each error cause category.[112] Categories are formed by identifying common characteristics among the circumstances surrounding each error. Solutions are then developed for each category of problems.

One limitation of the critical incident technique is that it entails interviewing subjects and is strongly dependent on their subjective memories. An advantage of the critical incident technique over observation is the consideration of subjective information obtained from the participants relative to the causes of the errors detected. Disadvantages of this method include the difficulty of interpreting the data and developing appropriate solutions.[112]

Chart Review

Chart review can be used to detect errors and adverse events related to medication ordering, transcribing, dispensing, administering, or monitoring. It is often used in research focusing on patient harm resulting from medication errors. The review is usually done by specially trained nurses who examine the medication orders, laboratory test results, physicians' progress notes, nursing notes, and MAR for clues that an error has occurred. They look for signs and symptoms typical of overdosage, underdosage, omission, and administration of unordered drugs. For example, an elevated blood glucose concentration might indicate an omitted insulin dose.[113] The administration of naloxone or flumazenil might suggest that a medication error has occurred.[114]

Chart review has been used in combination with self-report and review of medication records to detect errors and evaluate the number of ADEs occurring as a result of those errors; 5 of 530 errors (0.9%) appeared to result in ADEs.[115] In another study, chart review detected 24 medication administration errors, compared with 456 detected by direct observation of the same 2,557 doses.[99] When retrospective chart review was compared with self-reporting of medication errors in a psychiatric hospital, 2,194 errors over 1,448 patient-days were detected by chart review and 9 through self-reporting.[116]

Computerized Monitoring

Computerized monitoring can not only screen for orders and test results possibly associated with an error or ADE but can also alert hospital personnel that follow-up is needed to confirm the error and treat the patient if necessary.[117,118] When computerized monitoring of ADEs was compared with chart review and voluntary reporting, chart review identified the most ADEs (398 in 21,964 patient-days evaluated), followed by computerized monitoring (275), and voluntary reporting (23).[119] Sixty-seven of the ADEs were identified by both chart review and computerized monitoring; two were detected by voluntary reporting and computerized monitoring. In a retrospective computerized analysis of outpatient medication records, an ADE rate of 5.5 per 100 patients was detected.[120]

Observation

The direct observation technique, in which a trained observer accompanies the person giving medications and witnesses the preparation and administration of each dose, was developed by Barker and McConnell.[16] The observer writes down in detail what the subject does when preparing and administering the drug.[121] The notes are then compared with the prescriber's orders. An error is counted if the subject did not carry out the order accurately. The error rate is the percentage of doses administered in error, and the accuracy rate is the percentage of doses accurately administered. The observation is termed *disguised* if the subject is unaware of the precise goal of the study. Considerations in planning and conducting successful observations have been described.[121–123]

For studying medication administration errors, the observation method has several advantages.[99] It is not affected by lack of awareness of errors, lack of willingness to report errors, faulty memory, poor communication skills, or selective perception of the subject observed. Its reliability has been established through replication over many years. A large quantity of data can be accumulated at a rate 24 times that of chart review and 456 times that of incident reports. It can detect more errors and more types of error per unit of time than other methods, and it can identify clues about the causes so that future errors can be prevented.

The use of disguised observation to detect errors also has some disadvantages.[122] It is physically and mentally demanding of the observer. It is expensive because the observer must be a trained health professional with knowledge of medication names and appearances and the ability to read physician orders. Observers need training to correctly process what they see and to use the proper error category definitions. To minimize the effects of close observation upon the subjects, the observer must strive to remain unobtrusive and nonjudgmental.

Barker and colleagues[2] checked for the possible effect of the observer on the observed by monitoring individual nurse error rates for 5 consecutive days. The consistency of each subject's medication error rate indicated that the observers did not affect the rate over time. Concern that observers would make a subject more nervous (leading to more mistakes) or careful (preventing errors) seems unfounded. Dean and Barber[124] confirmed these findings. It has long been known that if observation is unobtrusive and nonjudgmental, the observed subject will quickly resume normal behavior.[125]

In the participant observer approach, an employee collects data while performing the normal tasks of the job, but co-workers are unaware that a study is taking place.[2,122] Mayo et al.[42] studied medication cart distribution errors using this technique. A pharmacy resident checked the cart contents against the MAR with a nurse and noted differences; an error was defined as any difference between what was found in the cart and what was on the MAR.

Detecting Dispensing Errors

The approaches used to study errors that occur before the medication is prepared for administration, such as pharmacy dispensing errors, are variations on methods for detecting administration errors. The critical incident method has been used to study possible causes of missing doses.[50] Double-checking medication carts against the MAR identified a communication problem. Solving the problem resulted in a significant decrease (from 0.93% to 0.33%) in missing doses.

Observers have been used to double-check the accuracy of medication cart filling,[41,43,126] filling new orders,[42] and filling prescriptions.[53–56,58,60] The observation method has advantages and disadvantages for double-checking. Consideration should be given to whether the data collection should be disguised and to whether reliability checks of the error detection process should be performed. For example, will the investigator perform the double check in the same location as the subjects? This could make the investigator vulnerable to the same stresses and environmental conditions as the subject and could result in missed errors. As long as the investigator does not have to fulfill any other duties and can concentrate on the task of inspection, it can be argued that accurate error detection is possible.

Self-reporting of dispensing errors and near misses in four prescription-filling operations in the United Kingdom has been described.[127] Data were collected in each pharmacy for 8 weeks; self-reporting of near misses yielded valuable information on error types, particularly incorrect drugs, strengths, dosages, and labels.

Choosing a Method

The objective of a study should dictate the most appropriate error detection technique. The observation technique is superior for studies of medication administration error rates and trends. Chart review and computerized monitoring are recommended for studies of patient harm resulting from errors. If the goal is to evaluate the root cause of an error, the critical incident and voluntary reporting methods are suitable.

REVIEW OF MEDICATION ERROR RESEARCH

This section provides an overview of more than 40 years of research on medication administration errors in inpatient settings. Table 2-1 summarizes the findings of many of these studies. Error rates are not directly comparable among these studies because of methodological issues discussed below. An evaluation of the validity of 16 medication error studies in hospitals was published in 1990.[69]

This section also describes studies of sterile product preparation errors, the impact of automated dispensing devices, and an observational study of errors in a pediatric emergency department.

The 1960s

In 1962, Barker and McConnell[16] became the first to show that medication errors occur much more frequently than anyone had suspected—at a rate of 16 errors per 100 doses. Two years later, Barker and colleagues[17] performed a pilot study at the University of Arkansas Medical Center in which they compared the center's existing drug distribution system with an experimental centralized unit dose dispensing system. After implementation of the unit dose system, the error rate (including wrong-time errors) decreased from 16% to 7%. The pilot study was later expanded to eight nursing units.[19] Across shifts (day and evening) and patient care services (medical, surgical, and pediatric), the expanded study showed a significantly lower error rate with the unit dose system. This experimental unit dose system featured on-line real-time processing of orders, medication cart exchanges every 2 hours, and unit dose packaging of all medications.

In 1966, Barker, Kimbrough, and Heller[2] studied medication errors in a large general hospital. They analyzed the effect of the observer on the subjects, the role of situational factors and of the psychological characteristics of nurses involved in errors, and comments of the observer about causes of the errors.

A study of administration errors and discrepancies at the University of Iowa Hospitals before and after implementation of decentralized unit dose dispensing[18] is noteworthy. Excluding left-at-bedside discrepancies and wrong-time errors, the error rate was less than 1% both before and after implementation. However, the denominator used to calculate the error rate was unclear. Also, the observers reviewed each patient's MAR before observation and were therefore in a position to prevent errors. From a researcher's perspective, this presents an ethical dilemma as well as a potential liability problem.

The 1970s

Hynniman et al.[3] compared the error rate for the unit dose system at the University of Kentucky Hospital with error rates in four hospitals with traditional methods of drug distribution (three used the prescription order system, one used floor stock). Observers did not witness administration of the dose to the patient, so they could not detect omission, wrong-route, wrong administration technique, and wrong administration rate errors.

At the Ohio State University Hospitals,[21] accuracy was compared between traditional medication administration by registered nurses and pharmacy-coordinated administration by technicians using the unit dose system. The error rate was significantly lower with the latter system; however, the study design (static group comparison[128]) does not rule out reasons for the lower error rate other than the pharmacy-coordinated program. This study was repeated 10 years later to determine whether the low technician error rates were maintained.[28,67] The error rate was still less than 5%, despite a change from four cart exchanges per day to once-daily exchange.

A study at the Johns Hopkins Hospital[22] tested the hypothesis that the error rate would be lower with a computer-based unit dose distribution system than with a multidose system. The results suggest that patients on the unit dose floor experienced fewer errors (this study used average error rates per patient instead of error rate per drug distribution system). However, the error rate on the nursing unit under study was not measured before implementation of the computer-based system.

Schnell[6] measured error rates in four Canadian hospitals before and after implementation of unit dose drug distribution. The results should be viewed cautiously because of the method used to detect omitted doses. Also, an unexpected increase in the error rate at one hospital after unit dose implementation may have been attributable to a rise in extra-dose errors because of lax pharmacy enforcement of automatic stop orders; if extra-dose and wrong-time errors had been omitted, the error rate decrease after implementation (from 8.5% to 5.8%) would have been significant.

The 1980s

Rosati and Nahata[129] conducted a study of drug administration technique errors involving pediatric patients, because pediatric doses can require manipulations that may increase the risk of error. They found 28 technique errors during 217 administrations (12.9% error rate); the rate was 5.5% when wrong-time errors were excluded. The study included only a limited number of error categories, and whether omissions were corrected was not specified. A problem with this study was that the observer told the subject he or she had committed an error immediately after administration of the drug. The effect of this feedback on the subject may have altered the error rate. Furthermore, the observer's knowledge that an error was about to be committed and failure to prevent it raise an ethical issue.

An interdisciplinary group led by Barker[15] analyzed the unit dose distribution system at a large hospital. The initial error rate was 9.0% (183 errors per 2,018 OE, excluding wrong-time errors), which was far higher than rates reported for some other unit dose systems. Fourteen recommendations were made for improving the unit dose system,[130] only two of which were fully implemented: the use of an MAR created in the pharmacy and an increase of pharmacy staff during peak workload periods. Four recommendations were partially implemented: dispensing a greater percentage of doses in unit dose packages, using dispensing envelopes, increasing the frequency of deliveries, and dispensing prn medications from the pharmacy upon request. Recommendations that were not implemented included computerized control and labeling of doses and redesign of the pharmacy's facilities. Two years after the recommendations were made, the error rate had not changed significantly. This suggests that all facets of the unit dose concept should be implemented in order to achieve the lowest possible error rate.[26] However, the results at this hospital may also reflect error-causing factors that are not affected by a change in drug distribution system, such as inadequate lighting and visual impairment of workers.[55]

Errors in an intensive care nursery and a pediatric intensive care unit were studied in an effort to justify an upgrade of pharmacy services in these settings.[5] The methods used to calculate the reported error rates had several limitations.[39] Table 2-1 includes recalculated error rates for this study. If wrong-time errors are excluded and the corrected ratios of errors to no errors are used, the chi-square analysis with McNemar's test for correlated proportions is not significant for either location. There were also problems with the error category definitions. The observer was aware of each patient's drug regimen prior to observation and was allowed to intervene in the event of an impending error but did not have occasion to do so.

Technology's Effect on Administration Errors

In the 1980s Barker and colleagues[27] studied the effect of an automated bedside dispensing system on errors. The system sounded an alert to the nurse when medications were due, and the dispensing machine allowed access to only the medications to be given at that time. The error rate in this observational study was significantly lower with the bedside dispensing system (10.6%) than with the previous unit dose system (15.9%). With the automated system, errors still occurred in all categories (i.e., errors of omission, unordered drug errors, extra-dose, wrong-dose, wrong-route, and wrong-time errors), but the error rates in most categories were lower than with the previous system.

Cooper and colleagues[30] compared the effects of three distribution systems on administration error rates in long-term care facilities: a blister card drug distribution system, the Baxter ATC-212 single unit dose packaging system, and the Baxter ATC Plus multidose packaging system. With the ATC Plus system, all oral solid doses to be given to a patient at the same time were placed in the same package in the patient's medication drawer. The packaging was done in a central location (typically the pharmacy), and a pharmacist inspected each package for accuracy before it was delivered to the nursing unit. No errors were detected with the multidose ATC Plus system. Error rates for the single unit dose package system and the blister card system were 2.5% and 8.0%, respectively.

Administration error rates were studied by observation on two nursing units using the Pyxis MedStation system.[33,131] The MedStation system allowed nurses to obtain any medication stored in the device for any patient. The system was not linked to a list of the patient's medications in the hospital's computer system, so any medication stored in the device could be removed for any patient. Examples of the errors with this device are shown in Table 2-3. The error rate without wrong-time errors was 6.9%. The error rate for all doses retrieved from the MedStation was 17% (21 errors per 123 OEs), compared with

TABLE 2-3   Errors Involving an Automated Medication-Dispensing Device at a U.S. Hospital[33]

Type of Error	No. Errors per 123 Opportunities for Error
Unordered Drug	
Ketorolac	1
Percocet	4
Unipen	1
Furosemide	1
Wrong Dose	
Lorazepam injection, 1 mg ordered, 2 mg given	1
Promethazine injection, 12.5 mg ordered, 25 mg given	12
Meperidine injection, 100 mg ordered, 50 mg given	1
Total no. errors	21

5% (43 errors per 796 OEs) for doses retrieved from patient medication drawers in a traditional unit dose cart.

Borel and Rascati[31] studied errors with the Pyxis MedStation Rx system. This device, linked to patient profiles in the hospital's computer system, was designed to give nurses access to only medications prescribed for the patient and approved by a pharmacist. It was possible to override the system (e.g., in an emergency) and obtain a medication without prior pharmacy approval of an order. Although the authors reported overrides during the study, they did not state whether any were associated with errors. The error rate after implementation of the MedStation Rx was 10.4% (97 errors in 929 OEs), compared with 16.9% (148 errors for 873 OEs) with the existing unit dose system, a significant difference. The new system reduced omission errors, but unauthorized-drug errors and wrong-dose errors were not affected and the rate of wrong-time errors increased. The authors did not observe any instances in which the device was refilled incorrectly.

More recent studies have used bar code technology to reduce errors. When a handwritten 7-day MAR was replaced with a computerized daily MAR with bar-code checking of medication administration at a 70-bed hospital, the administration accuracy rate as detected by observation increased significantly, from 90.2% (146 errors in 1,495 doses) to 94.3% (93 errors in 1,600 doses).[132] The greatest impact was on wrong-time and wrong-technique errors. With wrong-time errors excluded, the accuracy rate increased from 93.1% to 96.9%.

In another study of a bar-code medication administration system used on two nursing units, observed administration errors decreased 36%; with wrong-time errors excluded, the decrease was 54%.[133] The error rate on a control nursing unit did not change significantly. (The actual error rates were not reported.)

Best-practice recommendations for bar-code medication administration are available; they are based on studies in the Veterans Health Administration using observers with a human-factors background.[134]

The effects of computerized prescriber order entry systems on administration errors have been evaluated in two studies.[135,136] Since both of these studies used incident reports to detect errors, their usefulness is limited.

Errors in Sterile Product Preparation

An observational study of errors in IV admixture compounding at five large hospital pharmacies detected a 9% error rate (147 errors per 1,679 doses).[137] The rate of errors that were potentially clinically significant was 1.5%. Wrong-dose errors, defined as a deviation of 5% or more from the dose listed on the pharmacy label, were the most common type. The product type with the highest error rate was parenteral nutrition solutions (37% with manual preparation and 22% when some automation was used).

High error rates were found in a study of 184 acetylcysteine admixtures prepared by nurses and pharmacists.[37] Errors were detected by measuring drug concentration before and after administration. The rate of wrong-dose errors, defined as deviation of more than 10%, was 64%. The concentration in 17 bags (9%) differed by 50% or more from the intended concentration.

In a study of cytotoxic drug preparation errors in a centralized area, the overall preparation error rate was 0.45% in 30,819 preparations.[138] Errors were self-reported by the technicians preparing the admixtures or detected during the final inspection process. Daily workload, number of bottles, and volume of active solution (>50 mL) were identified as major risk factors.

Errors in preparing and administering injectable drugs on a hospital medical ward in the United Kingdom were studied.[139] There were 27 errors during 107 observations, for a 25.2% error rate (10.3% when wrong-time errors were excluded). Preparation errors were detected in technique and in the base solution used. Because more than one error could be counted for a single dose, the reported error rate may be higher than in studies that count only one error per dose.

Taxis and Barber[68] used disguised observation of the preparation and administration of intravenous doses at a hospital in the United Kingdom. One or more preparation or administration errors were detected in 212 of 430 doses, for an error rate of 49%. Most errors involved administration (36% error rate). Preparation errors were observed for 7% of the doses and both preparation and administration errors for 6% of the doses. The authors concluded that at a 400-bed hospital with 300 intravenous doses administered per day, at least one patient will experience a potentially serious error every day.

In a separate study, Taxis and Barber[140] used observation and interview to identify causes of intravenous medication errors. They observed the preparation of 483 doses and the administration of 447 doses; they detected 265 errors. The causes of the errors included deliberate violation of guidelines for the administration of an IV push dose, lack of perceived risk, poor role models, and inadequate design of technology.

Wirtz, Taxis, and Barber[36] used disguised observation to compare intravenous drug errors in the United Kingdom and Germany. Preparation error rates ranged from 22% to 31%, and administration error rates ranged from 22% to 49%. Most errors were judged to have the potential for moderate to severe patient harm.

In another study involving intravenous medications, prospective observation was used to detect ordering, preparation, and (mock) administration errors during simulated resuscitation in a pediatric emergency department. Wrong-dose errors occurred on 16% of 58 syringes analyzed.[141]

DISPENSING ERRORS IN PRESCRIPTION-FILLING OPERATIONS

In analyzing studies of prescription-filling operations, it is important to note the considerable differences in the definitions of dispensing error and in the error categories used. The error rates shown in Table 2-2 reflect only the error categories that all of those studies had in common.

The methods and procedures used should also be noted in evaluating studies of dispensing errors. For example, did technicians, pharmacists, or both fill the prescriptions? Were errors detected by disguised observation, incident reports, or retrospective analysis?[142] Were prescription errors corrected before being dispensed to the patient? If so, who made the correction (pharmacist who filled the prescription, or the observer)?

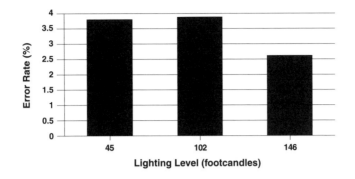

FIGURE 2-1   Relationship of lighting level to medication error rate.[55]

EFFECT OF WORK ENVIRONMENT AND WORKLOAD

Pharmacists and technicians can be affected by their work environment in ways that can increase or decrease the rate of dispensing errors. Kelly[143] has written an overview of pharmacy's contributions to ADEs and discussed procedural and systems problems and other sources of error in pharmacies. Grasha[144] outlined principles for identifying the causes of error and preventing human errors in complex systems. An evaluation of studies of the effect of work environment on patient safety has been published.[145] Research on the association of various factors with medication errors is summarized here.

Lighting

Buchanan and colleagues[55] studied the effect of lighting level on dispensing errors in a high-volume Army outpatient pharmacy. Three different lighting levels were analyzed: 45, 102, and 146 footcandles (fc). There was a significant decrease in the dispensing error rate only when the lighting level was increased from 102 to 146 fc (Figure 2-1).

Interruptions and Distractions

The effect of interruptions and distractions on errors in an ambulatory care pharmacy was studied.[57] The researcher inspected 5,072 prescriptions over 23 days. The average dispensing error rate was 3.23%. Two video cameras recorded the pharmacists' and technicians' work environment, and the tape was reviewed to count interruptions and distractions. The study methods controlled for prescription workload and pharmacist distractibility.

Interruptions were defined as cessation of productive activity because of an external stimulus before completion of a prescription-filling task. Distractions were counted if a pharmacist continued to work on prescription filling while responding to an external stimulus. A total of 2,022 interruptions were detected. Pharmacists were interrupted up to 17 times in a half-hour period; the average was 3 times per half-hour. The most frequent reasons for interruptions were questions from co-workers about prescriptions or procedures. The error rate for uninterrupted prescription sets was 5.67%, compared with 6.65% for interrupted sets.

In the same study, 2,547 distractions were detected. Pharmacists were distracted up to 16 times per half-hour; the average was 4 times per half-hour. The error rates were 5.64% for prescription sets without distractions and 6.55% with distraction. Figure 2-2 displays the relationship between the dispensing error rate and pharmacist distractibility as measured by the group embedded figures test for field dependence.[146]

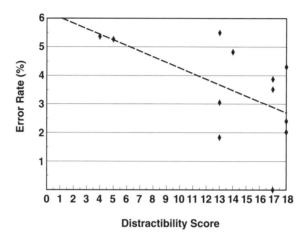

FIGURE 2-2 Relationship of distractibility score to medication error rate. A high score indicates lower distractibility.[57]

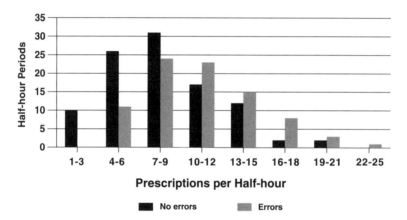

FIGURE 2-3 Relationship between prescription workload and risk of dispensing error.[148]

Noise

Certain types of noises and sounds have been found to decrease the occurrence of dispensing errors.[147] Unpredictable sounds, controllable sounds, and noise had a significant effect on pharmacists that resulted in a lower dispensing error rate. In this study the error rate increased up to a point as sounds became louder, but then it began to decrease. The results suggest that the quality of pharmacist prescription-filling accuracy is not adversely affected by ambient sound.

Workload

Do busy pharmacists make more errors? Studies have assessed the relationship between prescription workload and dispensing errors. In three studies, errors increased as prescription workload increased,[54,55,57] and one study[58] found no relationship. One study showed that the risk of error increases when a pharmacist fills more than 10 to 12 prescriptions per half-hour (Figure 2-3).[148] In another study, the percentage of hours with one or more errors increased as workload increased.[54]

Other Factors

In hospitals, significantly more wrong-time errors per OE occur during the day shift.[13] Oral liquids are the dosage form most often involved in errors. Most errors occur in routine orders (these are primarily wrong-time errors), rather than in stat or prn orders.

APPLICATIONS OF ERROR-MONITORING TECHNIQUES

Medication error detection by means of monthly observation has been used as part of a quality improvement effort in inpatient settings. Routine observation permits one to assess the impact of changes in a drug distribution system on the quality of service, using medication errors as an indicator. One use of this approach is to verify medication administration accuracy for drug distribution systems that have been automated.

The Centers for Medicare and Medicaid Services (CMS) continues to use observation-based medication error rates to assess long-term care facilities (LTCFs).[149] A facility does not qualify for Medicare reimbursement if its medication error rate exceeds 5%. In addition, the detection of a single error judged significant by the observer results in a deficiency report.[149] A survey found that 4,000 of 15,000 nursing homes participating in Medicare or Medicaid programs did not accurately carry out physicians' orders when administering medications.[150]

Quality assurance programs in prescription-filling operations have been described. Retrospective review was used to compare 16,000 original prescriptions with what was entered in the computer.[142] The program decreased the total error rate from 4.2% to 2%, with serious errors decreasing from 0.6% to 0.1%. Most errors were corrected by changing an entry in the computer so that refills would be dispensed correctly. Serious errors were corrected through follow-up contact with the patient.

RECOMMENDATIONS FOR ERROR PREVENTION

The research on medication errors has identified factors that can reduce error rates. The following features of automated medication systems help prevent errors in hospitals:[151]

1. *Comprehensiveness.* Control over the medication distribution system should start with entry of the order into the computer and continue through administration to the patient.
2. *Focus.* The system should accommodate dosage forms (e.g., specially prepared pediatric doses, oral liquids) that are often involved in errors.
3. *Unit dose dispensing.* Medications delivered to the nursing unit should not require further manipulation or preparation before administration.
4. *Signals.* To minimize omission and wrong-time errors, a signal should remind the nurse when a dose is due.
5. *Labeling.* A machine-printed label should be affixed to the medication container before it arrives on the patient care unit.
6. *Machine identification.* It should be possible to identify the dose, patient, and person administering the dose before the dose is administered. This can be done with bar codes or radio frequency tags.
7. *Controlled access.* Medications should be accessible only at the right place and right time according to the patient's medication profile, and only to approved personnel as verified by the dispensing device.
8. *Capture of dose administration.* Documentation of medication administration time and location should take place at the bedside via an electronic MAR.

9. *Drug-use information.* Information needed by the nurse for correct administration of the medication should be included on the package up to the point of administration.

10. *Controls.* Compromises or overrides of existing technology should trigger a visible or audible alarm. Overrides should be documented simultaneously and automatically.

In addition, changes in the work environment can prevent errors. Increasing the lighting in prescription-filling areas to 146 fc can significantly decrease dispensing error rates.[55] Changes in pharmacy facility design should be directed at preventing interruptions and distractions. The effects of workload on staff should be studied further and managed.

Patient counseling can help reduce dispensing errors.[152] A successful example is the Indian Health Service method, which involves verification of the patient's identity, dispensing from the chart (the original prescription order is used during counseling for a final check), and showing the medication to the patient.

FUTURE RESEARCH DIRECTIONS

Understanding the causes of errors is an important part of error prevention. Root cause analysis (RCA), described in Chapter 5, seeks to identify the system component that, if altered, changes the outcome. Failure mode and effects analysis (see Chapter 21) involves identification of processes most susceptible to failure. It is used prospectively, in contrast to RCA after an error occurs. RCA is time-consuming, and causation is seldom easy to prove.

Another approach to error prevention is illustrated by the development and implementation of unit dose distribution systems. This was the first important systems change to have an impact on medication errors. The pharmacists who developed these systems refined them as they observed "what worked." Today's pharmacy researchers can push for technological innovations by device manufacturers and monitor their effectiveness.

Research on systems changes to reduce errors should not be limited to serious, potentially harmful errors. All errors should be counted in analysis of a system so that all system defects can be identified and eliminated.

Data on near-errors should not be combined with or compared with data representing actual errors that have occurred. The frequency of near-errors does not reliably predict undesirable outcomes. Discovering near-errors can improve the vigilance and thus the performance of a human responsible for checking medications.

CONCLUSION

Research over 45 years has contributed to reducing medication errors. More research is needed as automated systems are improved and as computerized prescriber order entry is implemented.

REFERENCES

1. Bates DW, Cullen DJ, Laird N, et al. Incidence of adverse drug events and potential adverse drug events. implications for prevention. ADE Prevention Study Group. *JAMA.* 1995;274(1):29–34.
2. Barker KN, Kimbrough WW, Heller WM. *A Study of Medication Errors in a Hospital.* Fayetteville, Ark: University of Arkansas; 1966.
3. Hynniman CE, Conrad WF, Urch WA, et al. Comparison of medication errors under the University of Kentucky unit-dose system and traditional drug distribution systems in four hospitals. *Am J Hosp Pharm.* 1970;27(Oct):802–14.

4. Hall KW, Ebbeling P, Brown B, et al. Retrospective-prospective study of medication errors: basis for an ongoing monitoring program. *Can J Hosp Pharm.* 1985;38(Oct):141–3, 146.

5. Tisdale JE. Justifying a pediatric critical care satellite pharmacy by medication error reporting. *Am J Hosp Pharm.* 1986;43(Feb):368–71.

6. Schnell BR. Study of unit-dose drug distribution in Canadian hospitals. *Can J Hosp Pharm.* 1973;26(Nov–Dec):255–7.

7. Barker KN, Flynn EA, Pepper GA, et al. Medication errors observed in 36 health care facilities. *Arch Intern Med.* 2002;162(16):1897–903.

8. Schneider PJ, Gift MG, Lee YP, et al. Cost of medication-related problems at a university hospital. *Am J Health Syst Pharm.* 1995;52(Nov 1):2415–8.

9. Jones CD, Como JA, Kelly BD, et al. The Cost of Medication Errors at a University Hospital. Paper presented at American Society of Health-System Pharmacists Midyear Clinical Meeting; December 2002; Atlanta, Ga:P-238E.

10. Wou K. Costs associated with recurrent hypoglycemia caused by dispensing error. *Ann Pharmacother.* 1994;28(Jul–Aug):965–6.

11. Hynniman CE, Hyde GC, Parker PF. How costly is medication safety? *Hospitals.* 1971;45(Sep 16):73–85.

12. Summerfield MR. *Unit Dose Primer.* Bethesda, Md: American Society of Hospital Pharmacists; 1983:28–36.

13. Barker KN, Pearson, RE. Medication distribution systems. In: Brown T, Smith MC, eds. *Handbook of Institutional Pharmacy Practice.* 2nd ed. Baltimore: Williams & Wilkins; 1986:341–2.

14. *Medication Error Study.* Washington, DC: Physician Insurers Association of America; June 1993.

15. Barker KN, Harris JA, Webster DB, et al. Consultant evaluation of a hospital medication system: analysis of the existing system. *Am J Hosp Pharm.* 1984;41(Oct):2009–16.

16. Barker KN, McConnell WE. The problems of detecting medication errors in hospitals. *Am J Hosp Pharm.* 1962;19:360–9.

17. Barker KN, Heller WM, Brennan JJ, et al. The development of a centralized unit dose dispensing system. Part six: the pilot study—medication errors and drug losses. *Am J Hosp Pharm.* 1964;21:609–25.

18. *A Study of Patient Care Involving a Unit Dose System, Final Report.* Iowa City: University of Iowa; 1967. U.S. Public Health Service grant HM-00328-01.

19. Barker KN. The effects of an experimental medication system on medication errors and costs. I. Introduction and errors study. *Am J Hosp Pharm.* 1969;26(6):324–33.

20. Crawley HK III, Eckel FM, McLeod DC. Comparison of a traditional and unit dose drug distribution system in a nursing home. *Drug Intell Clin Pharm.* 1971;5(Jun):166–71.

21. Shultz SM, White SJ, Latiolais CJ. Medication errors reduced by unit-dose. *Hospitals.* 1973;47(6):106–12.

22. Means BJ, Derewicz HJ, Lamy PP. Medication errors in a multidose and a computer based unit-dose drug distribution system. *Am J Hosp Pharm.* 1975;32(Feb):186–91.

23. Brown WM, Blount CW, Harley GD. *Quality of Pharmaceutical Care in Small Hospitals.* Kansas City: Missouri Regional Medical Program; March 1976.

24. Barker KN, Mikeal RL, Pearson RE, et al. Medication errors in nursing homes and small hospitals. *Am J Hosp Pharm.* 1982;39(Jun):987–91.

25. Reitberg DP, Miller RJ, Bennes JF. Evaluation of two concurrent drug delivery systems in a skilled nursing facility. *Am J Hosp Pharm.* 1982;39:1316–20.

26. Barker KN, Harris JA, Webster DB, et al. Consultant evaluation of a hospital medication system: implementation and evaluation of the new system. *Am J Hosp Pharm.* 1984;41(Oct):2022–9.

27. Barker KN, Pearson RE, Hepler CD, et al. Effect of an automated bedside dispensing machine on medication errors. *Am J Hosp Pharm.* 1984;41(Jul):1352–8.

28. Jozefczyk KG, Schneider PJ, Pathak DS. Medication errors in a pharmacy-coordinated drug administration program. *Am J Hosp Pharm.* 1986;43(Oct):2464–7.

29. O'Brodovich M, Rappaport P. A study pre and post unit dose conversion in a pediatric hospital. *Can J Hosp Pharm.* 1991;44:5–15, 50.

30. Cooper S, Zaske D, Hadsall R, et al. Automated medication packaging for long-term care facilities: evaluation. *Consult Pharm.* 1994;9(Jan):58–70.

31. Borel JM, Rascati KL. Effect of an automated, nursing unit-based drug-dispensing device on medication errors. *Am J Health Syst Pharm.* 1995;52(17):1875–9.

32. Ruffin DM, Hodge FJ. Pharmacists' impact on medication administration errors in long-term care facilities. *Consult Pharm.* 1995;10:1025–32.

33. Barker KN, Allan EL. Research on drug-use-system errors. *Am J Health Syst Pharm.* 1995;52(4):400–3.

34. Wilson DG, McArtney RG, Newcombe RG, et al. Medication errors in paediatric practice: insights from a continuous quality improvement approach. *Eur J Pediatr.* 1998;157(9):769–74.

35. Tissot E, Cornette C, Demoly P, et al. Medication errors at the administration stage in an intensive care unit. *Intensive Care Med.* 1999;25(4):353–9.

36. Wirtz V, Taxis K, Barber ND. An observational study of intravenous medication errors in the United Kingdom and in Germany. *Pharm World Sci.* Jun 2003;25(3):104–11.
37. Anton C, Ferner RE. Medication errors detected in infusions. *Arch Intern Med.* 2003;163(8):982.
38. Croskerry PSM, Campbell S, LeBlanc C, et al. Profiles in patient safety: medication errors in the emergency department. *Acad Emerg Med.* 2004;11(Mar):289–99.
39. Douglas JB, Wheeler DS. Evaluation of Trained Pharmacy Technicians in Identifying Dispensing Errors. Paper presented at American Society of Health-System Pharmacists Midyear Clinical Meeting; December 1994:P-244(E).
40. Woller TW, Stuart J, Vrabel R, et al. Checking of unit dose cassettes by pharmacy technicians at three Minnesota hospitals: pilot project. *Am J Hosp Pharm.* 1991;48(Sep):1952–6.
41. Becker MD, Johnson MH, Longe RL. Errors remaining in unit-dose carts after checking by pharmacists versus pharmacy technicians. *Am J Hosp Pharm.* 1978;35(Apr):432–4.
42. Mayo CE, Kitchens RG, Reese L, et al. Distribution accuracy of a decentralized unit-dose system. *Am J Hosp Pharm.* 1975;32(Nov):1124–6.
43. Taylor J, Gaucher M. Medication selection errors made by pharmacy technicians in filling unit dose orders. *Can J Hosp Pharm.* 1986;39(Feb):9–12.
44. Hassall TH, Daniels CE. Evaluation of three types of control chart methods in unit dose error monitoring. *Am J Hosp Pharm.* 1983;40(Jun):970–5.
45. Hoffmann RP, Bartt KH, Berlin L, et al. Multidisciplinary quality assessment of a unit dose drug distribution system. *Hosp Pharm.* 1984;19(Mar):167–9, 173–4.
46. Cina J, McCrea M, Mitton P, et al. Detection of Medication Error Rates. Paper presented at American Society of Health-System Pharmacists Midyear Clinical Meeting; December 2003;MED-08.
47. Chi J. Tech-check-tech, as sanctioned practice, gaining in states. *Hosp Pharm Rep.* August 1994;8:14, 17.
48. Ness JE, Sullivan SD, Stergachis A. Accuracy of technicians and pharmacists in identifying dispensing errors. *Am J Hosp Pharm.* 1994;51(Feb 1):354–7.
49. Campbell GM, Facchinetti NJ. Using process control charts to monitor dispensing and checking errors. *Am J Health Syst Pharm.* 1998;55(9):946–52.
50. Pang F, Grant JA. Missing medications associated with centralized unit-dose dispensing. *Am J Hosp Pharm.* 1975;32(Nov):1121–3.
51. Flynn EA, Barker KN, Carnahan BJ. National observational study of prescription dispensing accuracy and safety in 50 pharmacies. *J Am Pharm Assoc.* 2003;43(2):191–200.
52. Wertheimer AI, Ritchko C, Dougherty DW. Prescription accuracy: room for improvement. *Med Care.* 1973 January–February;11(1):68–71.
53. McGhan WF, Smith WE, Adams DW. Randomized trial comparing pharmacists and technicians as dispensers of prescriptions for ambulatory patients. *Med Care.* 1983 April;21:445–53.
54. Guernsey BG, Ingrim NB, Hokanson JA, et al. Pharmacists' dispensing accuracy in a high volume outpatient pharmacy service: focus on risk management. *Drug Intell Clin Pharm.* 1983 October;17(10):742–6.
55. Buchanan TL, Barker KN, Gibson JT, et al. Illumination and errors in dispensing. *Am J Hosp Pharm.* 1991;48(10):2137–45.
56. Spader TJ, Hatfield GM, Hanson EC. Dispensing Errors and Detection at an Outpatient Pharmacy. Paper presented at American Society of Health-System Pharmacists Annual Meeting; December 1995:FGF-4.
57. Flynn EA, Barker KN, Gibson JT, et al. Impact of interruptions and distractions on dispensing errors in an ambulatory care pharmacy. *Am J Health Syst Pharm.* 1999;56(13):1319–25.
58. Kistner UA, Keith MR, Sergeant KA, et al. Accuracy of dispensing in a high-volume, hospital-based outpatient pharmacy. *Am J Hosp Pharm.* 1994;51(Nov 15):2793–7.
59. Allan EL, Barker KN, Malloy MJ, et al. Dispensing errors and counseling in community practice. *Am Pharm.* 1995;NS35(Dec):25–33.
60. Rolland P. Occurrence of dispensing errors and efforts to reduce medication errors at the Central Arkansas Veteran's Healthcare System. *Drug Saf.* 2004;27(4):271–82.
61. Carmenates J, Keith MR. Impact of automation on pharmacist interventions and medication errors in a correctional health care system. *Am J Health Syst Pharm.* 2001;58(May 1):779–83.
62. Manasse HR. Medication use in an imperfect world: drug misadventuring as an issue of public policy. Part 1. *Am J Hosp Pharm.* 1989;46(May):929–44.
63. Manasse HR. Medication use in an imperfect world: drug misadventuring as an issue of public policy. Part 2. *Am J Hosp Pharm.* 1989;46(Jun):1141–52.
64. Phillips J, Beam S, Brinker A, et al. Retrospective analysis of mortalities associated with medication errors. *Am J Health Syst Pharm.* 2001;58(Oct 1):1835–41.
65. Cullen DJ, Bates DW, Small SD, et al. The incident reporting system does not detect adverse drug events: a problem for quality improvement. *Jt Comm J Qual Improve.* 1995;21(10):541–8.
66. Allan B. Calculating medication error rates. *Am J Hosp Pharm.* 1987;44:1044, 1046.

67. Taxis K, Barber N. Ethnographic study of incidence and severity of intravenous drug errors. *BMJ.* 2003;326(7391):684–7.
68. Allan EL, Barker KN. Fundamentals of medication error research. *Am J Hosp Pharm.* 1990;47:555–71.
69. Andrews LB, Stocking C, Krizek T, et al. An alternative strategy for studying adverse events in medical care. *Lancet.* 1997;349(9048):309–13.
70. Goldstein MS, Cohen MR, Black M. A method for monitoring medication omission error rates. *Hosp Pharm.* 1982;17(6):310–2.
71. Gift MG, Mavko LE, Vanderpool WH. Evaluating returned doses as an approach to improving medication use. Paper presented at American Society of Health-System Pharmacists Midyear Clinical Meeting; December 1996:P-446E.
72. Ballinger BR, Simpson E, Stewart MJ. An evaluation of a drug administration system in a psychiatric hospital. *Br J Psychiatry.* 1974;125(0):202–7.
73. Phillips DP, Christenfeld N, Glynn LM. Increase in U.S. medication error deaths between 1983 and 1993. *Lancet.* 1998;351(Feb 28):643–4.
74. Baker HM. Rules outside the rules for administration of medication: a study in New South Wales, Australia. *Image—J Nurs Scholar.* 1997;29(2):155–8.
75. Cunningham MC, Basile SB, Timmons VL, et al. Categorizing Errors on the Medication Administration Record. Paper presented at American Society of Health-System Pharmacists Midyear Clinical Meeting; December 1996:P-216E.
76. Fontan JE, Maneglier V, Nguyen VX, et al. Medication errors in hospitals: computerized unit dose drug dispensing system versus ward stock distribution system. *Pharm World Sci.* 2003;25(3):112–7.
77. Shuttleworth TA, Ruelle S. Detecting Medication Errors with Automated Distribution. Paper presented at American Society of Health-System Pharmacists Midyear Clinical Meeting; December 1996:P-217R.
78. Oren E, Griffiths LP, Guglielmo BJ. Characteristics of antimicrobial overrides associated with automated dispensing machines. *Am J Health Syst Pharm.* 2002;59(15):1445–8.
79. Rudman WJ, Brown C, Hewitt CR, et al. The use of data mining tools in identifying medication error near misses and adverse drug events. *Top Health Inf Manage.* 2002;23(2):94–103.
80. Murff HJ, Patel VL, Hripcsak G, et al. Detecting adverse events for patient safety research: a review of current methodologies. *J Biomed Inform.* 2003;36(1-2):131–43.
81. Blegen MA, Vaughn T, Pepper G, et al. Patient and staff safety: voluntary reporting. *Am J Med Qual.* 2004;19(2):67–74.
82. Hartwig SC, Denger SD, Schneider PJ. Severity-indexed, incident report-based medication error-reporting program. *Am J Hosp Pharm.* 1991;48(Dec):2611–6.
83. Stump LS. Reengineering the medication error reporting process: removing the blame and improving the system. *Am J Health Syst Pharm.* 2000;57(Dec Suppl 4):S10–S17.
84. Phillips MA. Voluntary reporting of medication errors. *Am J Health Syst Pharm.* 2002;59(23):2326–8.
85. Chopra V, Bovill JG, Spierdijk J, et al. Reported significant observations during anaesthesia: a prospective analysis over an 18-month period. *Br J Anaesth.* 1992;68(1):13–7.
86. Currie M, Mackay P, Morgan C, et al. The "wrong drug" problem in anaesthesia: an analysis of 2000 incident reports. *Anaesth Intens Care.* 1993;21:596–601.
87. Wong IC, Ghaleb MA, Franklin BD, et al. Incidence and nature of dosing errors in paediatric medications—a systematic review. *Drug Saf.* 2004;27(9):661–70.
88. Ross LM, Wallace J, Paton JY. Medication errors in a paediatric teaching hospital in the UK: five years operational experience. *Arch Dis Child.* 2000;83(6):492–7.
89. Winterstein AG, Johns TE, Rosenberg EI, et al. Nature and causes of clinically significant medication errors in a tertiary care hospital. *Am J Health Syst Pharm.* 2004;61(18):1908–16.
90. Kennedy AG, Littenberg B. Medication error reporting by community pharmacists in Vermont. *J Am Pharm Assoc.* 2004;44(4):434–8.
91. Quinlan P, Ashcroft DM, Blenkinsopp A. Medication errors: a baseline survey of dispensing errors reported in community pharmacy. *Int J Pharm Pract.* 2002;10(suppl):R68.
92. Santell JP, Protzel MM, Cousins D. Medication errors in oncology practice. *US Pharm.* 2004;29(4, suppl). Available at: www.uspharmacist.com/index.asp?show=article&page=8_1259.htm.
93. Hicks RW, Cousins DD, Williams RL. Selected medication-error data from USP's MEDMARX program for 2002. *Am J Health Syst Pharm.* 2004;61(10):993–1000.
94. Forrey RA, Pedersen CA, Schneider PJ. Coding accuracy of USP MEDMARX users. Paper presented at American Society of Health-System Pharmacists Midyear Clinical Meeting; December 2004:P213E.
95. Tribble DA, Lamnin M, Garich JL. Ideas for action: reporting medication error rate by microcomputer. *Top Hosp Pharm Manage.* 1985;5(Nov):77–88.
96. Lunik M, Gaither M. Medication errors; new form aids in discovery, analysis, and prevention. *Hosp Form.* 1991;26:666–7, 671.

97. Shannon RC, DeMuth JE. Comparison of medication error detection methods in the long term care facility. *Consult Pharm.* 1987;2(Mar-Apr):148–51.
98. Brown GC. Medication errors: a case study. *Hospitals.* 1979;53(20):61–2, 65.
99. Flynn EA, Barker KN, Pepper GA, et al. Comparison of methods for detecting medication errors in 36 hospitals and skilled-nursing facilities. *Am J Health Syst Pharm.* 2002;59(5):436–46.
100. Van Leeuwen DH. Are medication error rates useful as comparative measures of organizational performance? *Jt Comm J Qual Improve.* 1994;20(Apr):192–9.
101. Cohen MR. Report or not to report: that is the question. *Hosp Pharm.* 1982;17(Mar):114–6.
102. Duran G. Positive use of incident reports. *Hospitals.* 1979;53(14):60.
103. Cobb MD. Evaluating medication errors. *Hosp Pharm.* 1986;21(Oct):925–7, 929.
104. Betz RP, Levy HB. An interdisciplinary method of classifying and monitoring medication errors. *Am J Hosp Pharm.* 1985;42(8):1724-32.
105. Landrie RM. A study of medication errors. *Wash State J Nurs.* Summer-Fall 1977;49(3):9–12.
106. Regan WA. Legal case briefs for nurses. IL: R.N.'s delayed medication: fatality; NY: Kidney disease: orders ignored. *Regan Rep Nurs Law.* 1980;21(4):3.
107. Regan WA. Medication mistakes: fire the nurse? Case in point: Edgewood Nursing Center v NLRB (581 F. 2d 373 - PA.). *Regan Rep Nurs Law.* May 1980;20(12):2.
108. Germaine A, Rinneard B. How effectively do you use your incident/accident report? *Hosp Admin Can.* 1976;18(8):24–6.
109. Safren MA, Chapanis A. A critical incident study of hospital medication errors: part one. *Hosp JAHA.* 1960;34:32–66.
110. Safren MA, Chapanis A. A critical incident study of hospital medication errors: part two. *Hosp JAHA.* 1960;34:53, 65, 66, 68.
111. Cooper JB, Newbower RS, Kitz RJ. An analysis of major errors and equipment failures in anesthesia management: considerations for prevention and detection. *Anesthesiology.* 1984;60(1):34–42.
112. Flanagan JC. The critical incident technique. *Psychol Bull.* 1954;51:327–58.
113. Kaushal R. Using chart review to screen for medication errors and adverse drug events. *Am J Health Syst Pharm.* 2002;59(23):2323–5.
114. Dalton-Bunnow MF, Halvachs FJ. Computer-assisted use of tracer antidote drugs to increase detection of adverse drug reactions: retrospective and concurrent trial. *Hosp Pharm.* 1993;28(Aug):746–9, 752–5.
115. Bates DW, Boyle DL, Vander Vliet MB, et al. Relationship between medication errors and adverse drug events. *J Gen Intern Med.* 1995;10(4):199–205.
116. Grasso BC, Genest R, Jordan CW, et al. Use of chart and record reviews to detect medication errors in a state psychiatric hospital. *Psychiatr Serv.* 2003;54(5):677–81.
117. Classen DC, Pestotnik SL, Evans RS, et al. Computerized surveillance of adverse drug events in hospital patients. *JAMA.* 1991;266(Nov 27):2847–51.
118. Bates DW. Using information technology to screen for adverse drug events. *Am J Health Syst Pharm.* 2002;59(23):2317–9.
119. Jha AK, Kuperman GJ, Teich JM, et al. Identifying adverse drug events: development of a computer-based monitor and comparison with chart review and stimulated voluntary report. *J Am Med Inform Assoc.* 1998;5(3):305–14.
120. Honigman B, Lee J, Rothschild J, et al. Using computerized data to identify adverse drug events in outpatients. *J Am Med Inform Assoc.* 2001;8(3):254–66.
121. Barker KN, Flynn EA, Pepper GA. Observation method of detecting medication errors. *Am J Health Syst Pharm.* 2002;59(23):2314–6.
122. Barker KN. Data collection techniques: observation. *Am J Hosp Pharm.* 1980;37(Feb):1235–43.
123. Mays N, Pope C. Qualitative research: observational methods in health care settings. *BMJ.* 1995;311(6998):182–4.
124. Dean B, Barber N. Validity and reliability of observational methods for studying medication administration errors. *Am J Health Syst Pharm.* 2001;58(1):54–9.
125. Kerlinger FN, Lee HB. *Foundations of Behavioral Research.* 4th ed. Fort Worth, Tex: Harcourt College Publishers; 2000:727–52.
126. Grogan JE, Hanna JA, Haight RA. Study of accuracy of pharmacy technicians working in a unit-dose system. *Hosp Pharm.* 1978;13(Apr):194–9.
127. Chua SS, Wong IC, Edmondson H, et al. A feasibility study for recording of dispensing errors and 'near misses' in four UK primary care pharmacies. *Drug Saf.* 2003;26(11):803–13.
128. Campbell DT, Stanley JC. *Experimental and Quasi-Experimental Designs for Research.* Boston: Houghton Mifflin Co; 1963:12–13.
129. Rosati JR, Nahata MC. Drug administration errors in pediatric patients. *Qual Rev Bull.* 1983;9(Jul):212–3.
130. Barker KN, Harris JA, Webster DB, et al. Consultant evaluation of a hospital medication system: synthesis of a new system. *Am J Hosp Pharm.* 1984;41(Oct):2016–21.

131. Dean BS, Allan EL, Barber ND, et al. Comparison of medication errors in an American and a British hospital. *Am J Health Syst Pharm.* 1995;52(22):2543–9.
132. Tuchel NW, Michel RA, Hurd D. Strategies and Challenges in Implementing Bar Code Technology. Paper presented at American Society of Health-System Pharmacists Midyear Clinical Meeting; December 2003; New Orleans, La.
133. Harry D, Howe R. Impact of an Electronic Medication Administration Record and Bar Code Scanning System on the Accuracy of Medication Administration in Hospitalized Patients. Paper presented at American Society of Health-System Pharmacists Midyear Clinical Meeting; December 2004:P310E.
134. Patterson ES, Rogers ML, Render ML. Fifteen best practice recommendations for bar-code medication administration in the Veterans Health Administration. *Jt Comm J Qual Safety.* 2004;30(Jul):355–65.
135. King WJ, Paice N, Rangrej J, et al. The effect of computerized physician order entry on medication errors and adverse drug events in pediatric inpatients. *Pediatrics.* 2003;112(3):506–9.
136. Spencer DC, Leininger A, Daniels R, et al. Effect of a computerized prescriber-order-entry system on reported medication errors. *Am J Health Syst Pharm.* 2005;62(4):416–9.
137. Flynn EA. Observational study of accuracy in compounding i.v. admixtures at five hospitals. *Am J Health Syst Pharm.* 1997;54(8):904–12. Erratum in: *Am J Health Syst Pharm.* 1997;54(9):1110.
138. Limat S, Drouhin JP, Demesmay K, et al. Incidence and risk factors of preparation errors in a centralized cytotoxic preparation unit. *Pharm World Sci.* 2001;23(3):102–6.
139. Bruce J, Wong I. Parenteral drug administration errors by nursing staff on an acute medical admissions ward during day duty. *Drug Saf.* 2001;24(11):855–62.
140. Taxis K, Barber N. Causes of intravenous medication errors: an ethnographic study. *Qual Saf Health Care.* 2003;12:343–8.
141. Kozer E, Seto W, Verjee Z, et al. Prospective observational study on the incidence of medication errors during simulated resuscitation in a paediatric emergency department. *BMJ.* 2004;329(7478):1321.
142. Boneberg RF, Kellick KA, Pudhorodsky TG, et al. Results of a Retrospective Outpatient Medication Error Prevention Program at a Department of Veterans Affairs Medical Center. Paper presented at American Society of Health-System Pharmacists Midyear Clinical Meeting; December 1991:P-325E.
143. Kelly WN. Pharmacy contributions to adverse medication events. *Am J Health Syst Pharm.* 1995;52(4):385–90.
144. Grasha AF. Into the abyss: seven principles for identifying the causes of and preventing human error in complex systems. *Am J Health Syst Pharm.* 2000;57(6):554–64.
145. Hickam DH, Severance S, Feldstein A, et al. *The Effect of Health Care Working Conditions on Patient Safety.* Evidence Report/Technology Assessment No. 74. (Prepared by Oregon Health Sciences University under contract 290-97-0018.) Rockville, Md: Agency for Healthcare Research and Quality; April 2003. AHRQ publication 03-031.
146. Oltman P, Raskin E, Witkin H. *Group Embedded Figures Test.* Palo Alto, Calif: Consulting Psychologists; 1971.
147. Flynn EA, Barker KN, Gibson JT, et al. Relationships between ambient sounds and the accuracy of pharmacists' prescription-filling performance. *Human Factors.* 1996;38(4):614–22.
148. Allan EL. *Relationships among Facility Design Variables and Medication Errors in a Pharmacy* [dissertation]. Auburn, Ala: Pharmacy, Auburn University; 1994.
149. Feinberg JL. *Med Pass Survey: A Continuous Quality Improvement Approach.* Alexandria, Va: American Society of Consultant Pharmacists; 1993.
150. Thousands of nursing homes do not follow drug orders, U.S. survey reveals [news]. *Am J Hosp Pharm.* 1989;46:426, 434.
151. Barker KN. Ensuring safety in the use of automated medication dispensing systems. *Am J Health Syst Pharm.* 1995;52(21):2445–7.
152. Kuyper AR. Patient counseling detects prescription errors. *Hosp Pharm.* 1993;28(Dec):1180–1, 1184–9.

CHAPTER 3

HEALTH CARE PROVIDERS' EXPERIENCES WITH MAKING FATAL MEDICATION ERRORS

Zane Robinson Wolf

First, do no harm.

This time-honored standard directs nurses, pharmacists, and physicians to the primary goal of health care: to act with and on behalf of patients to improve their health and well-being. Health care providers' fundamental priority is the welfare of the people they serve. As caregivers and healers, they are most fearful of causing harm, however inadvert or unintentional, rather than doing good.

Society expects that nurses, pharmacists, and physicians will devise systems for providing safe, competent care and that the professionals within the system will police themselves. Each year, the Joint Commission on Accreditation of Healthcare Organizations (JCAHO) sets National Patient Safety Goals. Some hospital administrators conduct patient safety rounds with frontline caregivers to emphasize the need for reporting safety issues and adverse events and instituting preventive measures.[1] State laws require health care organizations to engage in multidisciplinary patient safety efforts that involve members of the community. Patient safety is the minimum standard for all actions taken on behalf of the public seeking health care services.

When a nurse, physician, or pharmacist makes a medication error and causes harm to a patient, both the provider and the patient are violated. In current efforts to promote a "culture of safety," the importance of disclosing errors to patients and families has been recognized.[2–4] Little attention has been paid, however, to the feelings of health care professionals who make errors.

Much of the pain that a nurse, physician, or pharmacist feels after making an error is rooted in the standard of perfection instilled in health professionals[5–9] and the belief that error is prohibited.[7] Health professionals expect that if they are well educated and follow up-to-date policies, procedures, and guidelines, medication errors will not happen.

When policies and procedures fail them and errors occur, they are puzzled. They may have great difficulty admitting they have made a mistake. To admit to an error would be the same as confessing that they are "bad" caregivers. It would soil their image as perfect clinicians.

Yet mistakes are part of everyday clinical practice. Despite technology such as bar code medication administration and computerized prescriber order entry, adverse drug events will persist.[10] Seasoned clinicians may even make more medication errors than in the past, as technology enables their involvement with greater numbers of patients. The more medications they prescribe, dispense, or administer, the more chances they have to make a mistake. Tension over this heightened opportunity for error may put the caregiver at even greater risk of making a mistake.

Errors made by health care providers are viewed as more serious than errors in other occupations,[11] although the outcomes vary widely (from no effect to a patient's death). Nurses, physicians, and pharmacists involved in medication errors feel guilty and want to make amends.[12–14] They are fearful about the safety of their patients and about disciplinary actions and punishment for their mistakes. They fear malpractice lawsuits[15] and possible criminal charges if a mistake is fatal.[16,17] Some health care providers seek psychological counseling after an error; a few are anxious and depressed throughout their lives and may even commit suicide.[18]

The purpose of this chapter is to explore the responses of health care providers who make errors that have devastating results. The chapter describes interviews by the author with a nurse and a pharmacist whose errors resulted in patient deaths.

BACKGROUND RESEARCH

A review of published literature on serious errors by health care providers, including first-person reports by those involved in errors, established a framework for studying responses to fatal errors.

When health care providers make mistakes, they are panicked, horrified, and apprehensive.[5,19] For example, one physician described a patient whose negative pregnancy tests suggested she had had a "missed abortion" (i.e., that the fetus had died but was retained in utero).[5] The physician performed a dilatation and curettage and panicked when he saw that he had extracted "body parts that were recently alive." On the basis of this experience, he encouraged physicians to recognize their errors and the consequences and find ways to deal with their emotional responses. He suggested that when physicians are unable to admit their mistakes, they are deprived of their chance to heal.[19] He noted the emotional toll: physicians' high rates of alcoholism, drug addiction, and suicide after making an error.

Christensen, Levinson, and Dunn[20] described how prior beliefs and coping strategies influence physicians' responses to making mistakes. Eleven physicians participated in probing, open-ended interviews. Their errors, which led to deaths and other serious consequences, included missed diagnoses, medication errors, failure to monitor closely, failure to readmit a patient, an error in following procedures, inadequate supervision of a nurse practitioner, and lack of aggressiveness in patient work-up. The physicians' emotional responses included shock, agony, dysphoria, fear, anger, embarrassment, humiliation, and persistent guilt. Their ability to cope with their mistakes was influenced by their beliefs about the degree of control health care providers have over physiological events and the probability of error. Coping was of two types: problem-focused (processing the mistake intellectually and learning from it) and emotion-focused (dealing with feelings). The physicians feared disclosing their errors to patients, family members, and other physicians. Some physicians lost confidence after their errors. The investigators concluded that discussion of physicians' mistakes should be brought into the mainstream of medicine. They cautioned physicians against denying their mistakes and redefining them as technical errors.

Wu et al.[21] examined ethical and practical issues in disclosing medical mistakes to patients. They noted that the ethical principle of patient autonomy encourages disclosure of mistakes that seriously harm patients. They stated that such disclosure promotes patients' health and may help them achieve compensation for irreparable harm. They described how physicians can tell patients about mistakes and the actions taken to correct them.

Goldberg and colleagues[22] reviewed the literature on physician errors, with emphasis on affective responses. They suggested coping with mistakes by analyzing and learning from them. They noted the shift in medicine from an environment of nondisclosure to one of open acknowledgment of errors and analysis in keeping with ethical principles.

Dean et al.[23] prospectively identified 88 potentially serious errors in prescribing for hospital patients and interviewed 41 physicians who made 44 of the errors. They used critical incident technique during semistructured interviews, distributed questionnaires, and reviewed medical notes. Using the four-stage model in Reason's[24] human error theory, they noted that most of the mistakes were made because of slips in attention (actions in which there are failures in recognition or selection) or lapses (failure of memory or attention) or were rule-based mistakes (incorrect choice of objective or choice of an incorrect path to achieve it). Slips predominated; the subjects said they had been busy or interrupted during routine tasks. Only two violations (instances in which rules of correct behavior are consciously ignored) were discovered. Workload, staffing issues, and team factors (e.g., absent or poor communication) were cited as error producing. Errors were prevented by the thought processes of the physicians, by nurses, or by pharmacists. None of the errors reached patients.

Wolf and Cohen[25] performed a content analysis of literature on human error, including medication errors, to determine patterns in health care providers' responses to making errors. Nurses, pharmacists, and physicians understood that a serious mistake is possible whenever patient care is given. They believed errors would be prevented if correct procedures were followed, so they were puzzled when procedures failed and errors occurred. They feared discipline, litigation, and loss of reputation. Their confidence was shaken after a medication error; they were shocked and angry. When they admitted making an error, they blamed themselves, acknowledging their personal pain and their deep regret that patients were injured.

Wu et al.[26] reported that physicians were seriously affected by their errors. If the physicians felt angry with themselves and guilty, they were more likely to take responsibility for the error and take corrective action. If, however, they were angry with others and were concerned about consequences, their behavior tended to be defensive. The physicians tended to blame their errors on many factors, thus absolving themselves of guilt. Their healing took time, and there was little evidence that they sought psychotherapy to ease their personal pain after an error.

Mizrahi,[27] studying the impact of the socialization of graduate medical internists on physician–patient relationships, conducted in-depth interviews of house staff in an urban medical center. The physicians denied mistakes by redefining them as nonmistakes. They discounted errors by blaming the bureaucratic system outside medicine, and they blamed superiors, subordinates, colleagues, the disease, and the patient. They saw themselves as the sole judges of their mistakes and singularly responsible for their actions.

CONCEPTUAL PERSPECTIVES

Errors can be studied from different conceptual perspectives. Human-factors analysis focuses on the interaction between humans and their environment. It emphasizes the influence of cognitive, sociological, organizational, and contextual factors on individual performance.[28]

Error can also be studied in the context of human cognition. Reason[24] linked error with intention and defined it as planned actions that fail to achieve desired consequences. Reason classified error levels as behavioral, contextual (internal and external circumstances), and conceptual (cognitive mechanisms).

Paget[29] proposed that the meaning of mistakes, such as medication errors, is located in human consciousness. Paget said blame transforms the meaning of mistakes; it scorns the one who made the mistake. The inevitability of mistakes creates "the complex sorrow of medical work,"[29] characterized by "intellectualizations of action, situated in periods of reflections, between a multiplicity of other clinical acts, other patients, other problems, and other thoughts about the work and the problems of the work." Medication errors can be explained and analyzed in many ways, but health care providers experience their impact personally, socially, and culturally.

INTERVIEWS WITH CAREGIVERS

The author's colleagues suggested possible interviewees. The La Salle University institutional review board approved the study. Five health care providers who had made fatal errors were contacted by telephone, and two (a female nurse and a male pharmacist) agreed to be interviewed. Both were middle-aged, seasoned clinicians who were responsible for a medication error that had resulted in a patient's death.

The nurse and pharmacist gave consent for telephone interviews and for the use of notes from conversations with the Institute for Safe Medication Practices (ISMP) after their errors. Each interviewee was given a written description of the phenomenon of making his or her error and asked to mark any areas of disagreement and indicate changes.

In the interviews and follow-up with the caregivers, making a medication error resulting in a patient's death was treated as a phenomenon whose meaning would be explored qualitatively through the providers' recollected experiences. Phenomenology focuses on human existence and individuals' perception of everyday life experience in a complex world.[30] This approach holds that the essences and meaning of a phenomenon are depicted in a linguistic construction or a description of the phenomenon. The hope was that descriptions of the caregivers' experiences might help sensitize others to the consequences of errors and ways of dealing with them, since nursing, pharmacy, and medical students receive little education on how to deal with errors.[31]

During the interviews, the nurse and pharmacist were engaged in active dialogue to draw out their feelings and perceptions about the errors. They were asked to consider and respond to the following:

1. Please try to recall the personal experience that you had when you made a medication error that resulted in a patient's death. Try to describe how you felt in that situation.
2. How did the experience of making the medication error impress you?
3. If you ever discussed the situation of making the medication error with someone after you realized that you made the error, who was the person and what did you discuss?
4. How did you "talk to yourself" or relive the medication error experience after you made the medication error that was followed by a patient's death?
5. What differences did you detect within yourself after making the medication error?
6. Please describe the personal consequences of making the medication error.
7. Is there anything that you wish to add? Please continue until you feel that you have discussed your feelings as fully as possible.

The interviews were audiotaped and transcribed verbatim. To establish the study's credibility,[32] the interviewer reflected on the transcribed interviews and other documents. Another investigator (peer reviewer) reviewed and commented on the materials. The interviewer asked the nurse and pharmacist to review the accuracy of the resulting narratives. The themes discerned by the interviewer were believed to be consistent with the experiences of other caregivers who have made fatal errors. Dependability of the findings was established through independent review of the audit trail[33] (the field notes, documents, transcribed interviews, coding schemes, themes, indicators, and a narrative description of the phenomenon).

The interviewer was aware of herself in relation to the participants and the data—of her interpretation of the material and her sensitivity to the meanings and essences of the phenomenon.[34] The validity[35] of this research will likely be confirmed by others seeking to understand and prevent medication errors.

THE CLUB OF HURT AND PAIN

The narratives of the nurse's and pharmacist's experiences are presented in the following section, which uses the pseudonyms Emily and Brian. Emily is still practicing nursing. Brian has retired from pharmacy practice.

Nurse's Story

Emily, an experienced advanced-practice pediatric nurse, initially did not know the cause of cardiac and respiratory arrest in the newborn infant under her care. Team members had done all they could to resuscitate him, to no avail. Later, Emily realized that the nurses had given 10 times the amount of the ordered drug by the wrong administration route. In addition to the nurses, a pharmacist was implicated in the error. Emily had not "noticed that the pharmacist had sent up 10 times" the ordered dose, and another nurse had administered the medication.

When Emily realized the fatal error, she was devastated—"in total shock." She shared with friends "how hard it was and how bad I felt." She continues to feel overwhelmed by the event.

Emily and the pharmacist were fired from the hospital. Although Emily nearly left the nursing profession, she continues to work as an advanced-practice pediatric nurse. She no longer works with newborns, however.

Holidays, especially those focused on children, are difficult for Emily. It is painful for her to see children with their parents at those times, because she realizes she "deprived someone of the love of their child."

Criminal charges were brought against Emily. She felt humiliated. She needed support, not isolation from other nurses and health care providers. She still worries about the nurses and the pharmacist involved in the error, and she considers the isolation that follows such an event to be "just about the worst thing we in society can do to people." She hopes that others involved in serious errors will seek long-term psychological counseling. "When you have had that kind of trauma happen to you…it is just never going away."

Health care providers who have not been involved in a serious error have little insight into what it is like, Emily has learned. She asks them to avoid directing anger at those who make errors. Instead, "We have to sit down with them and try to go through that process of what happened, what went wrong that made this occur. Because so much of it is complex." Despite the blame that was directed at her, she has found support from patients and providers as she continues to tell her story.

She believes physicians do not understand how nurses feel about their patient care responsibilities. She is incredulous that physicians seem able to put serious outcomes, such as death of a patient, behind them, with the attitude that "the patient is gone; forget about it, but learn from it."

Emily is acutely aware that nurses practice on "the sharp end" of patient care. "We repeatedly hear there isn't time to do everything we have to do. Well, you have to take time." Living with the overwhelming consequences of one serious error, Emily cannot stress strongly enough that health care providers take the time to check medications.

An effect of the error on her current nursing practice is Emily's excessive checking, even when simple interventions are called for. This extends beyond medication administration and "can drive my co-workers crazy."

After Emily's trial, she was required to perform community service by telling other nurses her story of the perils of medication administration. She has voluntarily continued these talks despite the pain that comes back each time she revisits the infant's death, because she wants to protect others from such errors.

Emily is troubled that nurses and other health care providers "don't listen" to her message. She says the inability to change their thinking "hurts me more than anything....People are just scared to be accountable." She worries that those who do not acknowledge their errors have no one to talk with about their feelings. She says it is dangerous when providers ignore small problems and rationalize that "this is not a big deal, we'll just fix it." "It would be a wonderful feeling if I could ever know that I helped one person not make a mistake and saved a patient. To be able to make something better because of this horrible incident—that is why I keep lecturing."

Although Emily is realistic about her scope of influence, she is concerned when others ignore her message: "It could happen to you. Change your behavior to prevent future errors. Always be vigilant. Take time to check and double-check. You must be accountable."

Emily calls her sentence to community services "the most wonderful thing that happened." She is comforted when she discusses her errors with nurses, chiefly her friends. Their support sustains her. She has also been an adviser to other health care providers who have shared their medication error stories.

Emily is frustrated that providers lack information on administering medications safely to children. She points out the inaccuracy of some reference books and the inappropriateness of using manufacturers' product information (i.e., the *Physicians' Desk Reference*). She emphasizes the importance of balancing the demands of patient care with taking the time to consult pharmacists and other experts before administering medications that are in question.

Emily calls for careful review of the hospital's medication-use process after each error so that improvements can be made. As she grieves her patient's death, she regrets not having followed her usual practice of calling a pharmacist to ask questions. "Why, that day, I didn't, I have no idea. It has haunted me every day since. Why didn't I call him and say, 'This is what I am seeing; is this really OK?'"

Pharmacist's Story

Brian, a seasoned hospital pharmacist, learned of a deadly error after hearing about a cluster of "codes" in the intensive care unit. Four patients were involved, and two of them died. Several days later, Brian pieced together comments by other pharmacists about mixed-up IV bags and realized this had happened while he was the responsible pharmacist—that "those dosages would have gone out on my tour." Another pharmacist had moved "the plain, foil-wrapped bags that were covering the piggyback inside." The wrong label was on the IV bags dispensed from the pharmacy; look-alike bags had been stored next to one another. Since all the equipment had been discarded after the codes, no evidence was available to confirm what had happened. An autopsy showed that one of the two deaths was not attributable to the medication error.

Brian had missed the wrong label on the wrong drug and let the medication leave the pharmacy. He had to "live with the knowledge that I was responsible for people getting the wrong dose of drug that almost killed most of them and did kill one of them."

Brian's disbelief that this could happen to him was followed by shock and fear that exhausted him. His annual performance reviews had always described him as a pharmacist who did not make mistakes. He had dispensed medications carefully, double- or triple-checking them. Knowing he had made the mistake was humbling. The fatal error was "unusual" for Brian, but, as he said, "An accident is something that happens that shouldn't have happened."

It was a "terrible time" in Brian's life. The error challenged his self-confidence and self-worth. He believed he had "lost that edge and was just careless." Brian suffered long periods of insomnia. He joined a unique club of health care providers, the "club of hurt and pain"—"not a club I would recommend joining. But we understood each other. We knew the hurt and the pain, and we were all just trying to recover from it."

Brian had told the inpatient pharmacy supervisor what he suspected had happened. Up to that point, administrators had been trying to understand what caused the cluster of codes. After an investigation, Brian took an involuntary leave of absence. He was later fired, fought that action, and was eventually reinstated to his pharmacy job.

Some of Brian's colleagues avoided him. "I was concerned about how my peers looked at me. Maybe they didn't trust me anymore or thought I was dangerous and were afraid to associate with me, although most of the people were on my side." The other pharmacists feared being involved in a similar event, and some reacted by improving their own practice. One pharmacist supported Brian as he took responsibility for the error. This colleague investigated the medication profiles of the affected patients.

Brian was "terrified" of making another mistake. His fear led to extreme caution in his practice. He checked his work even more carefully than before. When he caught subtle mistakes or potential errors, he would "almost have a flashback." When a drug name was confused with another, similar-sounding name, Brian's knees would shake. He knew how easy it is to make an error and how devastating the outcome could be.

Working in hospital pharmacies after the error, Brian noted the stress associated with the many demands of dispensing medications. He noticed the near misses that happen when the staff is busy, stressed, and frequently interrupted. He was always vigilant, aware of the ever-present possibility of another serious error.

Like Emily, Brian gave speeches about his error. The sympathy of audiences who understood his story "did me a world of good." He also received crucial support and encouragement from his wife. Nevertheless, Brian was "dying of guilt." He sought counseling and gradually learned to accept and live with the mistake.

Brian was grateful that Michael Cohen of ISMP had testified on his behalf. Cohen said that the way the IV bags were stored in the pharmacy led to an error that was destined to happen.

DISCUSSION

Some of the worst medication errors involve some of the best, most experienced practitioners. The euphemism "medical misadventure" fails to acknowledge the tragedy of health care errors that result in serious outcomes such as the death of a patient. The pain felt by this nurse and pharmacist will never go away. When they speak about their experiences, the old wound is opened.

Charges of criminal negligence against health care providers involved in fatal errors are infrequent but troubling. Another concern, expressed by Emily, is that nurses may fail to report errors. Failure to report near misses is also alarming; a culture of safety in health care requires the reporting of errors that almost occurred.

Emily and Brian's stories show the influence of contextual factors[24]—factors emerging from external circumstances—on serious errors that occur. Both practitioners intended to do the best for their patients. Rule-based and other types of mistakes will continue to thwart the most vigilant providers. Because medication-use systems, patient situations, and the knowledge and skill required of health care providers are complex, errors can be expected.

These cases illustrate the "complex sorrow"[29] of health care providers whose patients die as a result of an error. They feel the impact in the context of their work, in interactions with professional colleagues, and in their private lives. When experienced practitioners like Emily and Brian choose to leave their professions, it is a great loss. Efforts to improve the safety of medication-use systems may help ensure against such loss of skilled health care professionals.

REFERENCES

1. ECRI. Patient safety rounds—A new tool for reducing medical errors. *Risk Manage Rep.* 2003;22(6):1,3–7.
2. Greely HT. Do physicians have a duty to disclose mistakes? *West J Med.* 1999;171:82–3.
3. Hobgood C, Peck CR, Gilbert B, et al. Medical errors—what and when: What do patients want to know? *Acad Emerg Med.* 2002;9(11):1156–61.
4. Witman AB, Park DM, Hardin SB. How do patients want physicians to handle mistakes? *Arch Intern Med.* 1996;156:2565–9.
5. Hilfiker D. Facing our mistakes. *New Engl J Med.* 1984;310(2):118–22.
6. Kennedy EM, Heard SR. Making mistakes in practice. *Aust Fam Phys.* 2001;30(3):295–9.
7. Newman MC. The emotional impact of mistakes on family physicians. *Arch Fam Med.* 1996;5:71–5.
8. Smith ML, Forster HP. Morally managing medical mistakes. *Cambridge Q Healthcare Ethics.* 2000;9:38–53.
9. Wolf ZR. *Medication Errors: The Nursing Experience.* Albany, NY: Delmar; 1994.
10. Patterson ES, Cook RI, Render ML. Improving patient safety by identifying side effects from introducing bar coding in medication administration. *J Am Med Inform Assoc.* 2002;9(5):540–53.
11. Hughes EC. Mistakes at work. *J Econom Pol Sci.* 1951;17:320–7.
12. Wolf ZR, Serembus JF, Smetzer J, et al. Responses and concerns of health care providers to medication errors. *Clin Nurse Spec.* 2000;14(6):278-90.
13. Wolf ZR, Serembus JF, Youngblood N. Consequences of fatal medication errors for health care providers: a secondary analysis study. *MEDSURG Nurs.* 2001;10(4):193–201.
14. Wolf ZR, Serembus JF. Reported actions of supervisors and administrators following disclosure of medication errors: a secondary analysis study. *Nurs Manage.* 2004;35(8):41–2,44–8.
15. Kapp MB. Legal anxieties and medical mistakes: barriers and pretexts. *J Gen Intern Med.* 1997;12(12):787–8.
16. Holbrook J. The criminalisation of fatal medical mistakes. *BMJ.* 2003;327:1118–9.
17. Smetzer JL, Cohen MR. Lessons from the Denver medication error/criminal negligence case: look beyond blaming individuals. *Hosp Pharm.* 1998;33:640–57.
18. Das. Personal communication. March 5, 2004.
19. Hilfiker D. *Healing the Wounds: A Physician Looks at His Work.* New York: Pantheon Books; 1985.
20. Christensen JF, Levinson W, Dunn PM. The heart of darkness: the impact of perceived mistakes on physicians. *J Gen Intern Med.* 1992;7:424–31.
21. Wu AW, Cavanaugh TA, McPhee SJ, et al. To tell the truth: ethical and practical issues in disclosing medical mistakes to patients. *J Gen Intern Med.* 1997;12:770–5.
22. Goldberg RM, Kuhn G, Andrew LB, et al. Coping with medical mistakes and errors in judgment. *Ann Emerg Med.* 2002;39(3):287–92.
23. Dean B, Schachter M, Vincent C, et al. Causes of prescribing errors in hospital inpatients: a prospective study. *Lancet.* 2002;359:1373–8.
24. Reason J. *Human Error.* Cambridge, UK: Cambridge University Press; 1990.
25. Wolf ZR, Cohen M. Caregivers' reactions to making medication errors. In Cohen M, ed. *Medication Errors.* Washington, DC: American Pharmaceutical Association; 1999: 7.1–7.10.
26. Wu AW, Folkman S, McPhee SJ, et al. Do house officers learn from their mistakes? *JAMA.* 1991;265:2089–94.
27. Mizrahi T. Managing medical mistakes: ideology, insularity and accountability among internists-in-training. *Soc Sci Med.* 1984;19(2):135–46.
28. Shortell S, O'Brien J, Carman J, et al. Assessing the impact of continuous quality improvement/total quality management: concept versus implementation. *Health Serv Res.* 1995;30(2):377–401.
29. Paget M. *The Unity of Mistakes: A Phenomenological Interpretation of Medical Work.* Philadelphia: Temple University Press; 1988.
30. Van Manen M. *Researching Lived Experience.* Albany: State University of New York Press; 1990.

31. Lape CP. Disclosing medical mistakes. *J Gen Intern Med*. 1998;13(4):283-4.
32. Lincoln YS, Guba E. *Naturalistic Inquiry*. Beverly Hills, Calif: Sage; 1985.
33. Wolf ZR. Exploring the audit trail for qualitative investigations. *Nurse Educ*. 2003;28(4):175–8.
34. Lipson JG. The use of self in ethnographic research. In: Morse JM, ed. *Qualitative Nursing Research*. Rockville, Md: Aspen; 1989:61–75.
35. Kahn DL. Ways of discussing validity in qualitative nursing research. *West J Nurs Res*. 1993;15(1):122–6.

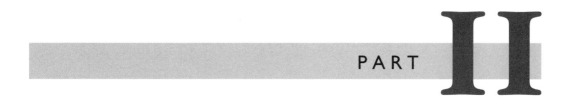

PART **II**

UNDERSTANDING THE CAUSES OF MEDICATION ERRORS

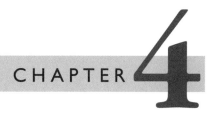
CAUSES OF MEDICATION ERRORS

Michael R. Cohen

Most health care professionals have learned the "five rights" of safe medication use: the right patient, right drug, right time, right dose, and right route of administration. Yet even when practitioners believe they have verified these "rights," errors, including fatal ones, occur.

One reason for such errors is that health professionals may have difficulty putting the five rights into practice. For example, how does a pharmacist identify the right patient when the patient's name and room number on an order copy are blurred and the physician's signature is illegible? Whom does he call for follow-up? How does a home care nurse identify the right patient in an assisted-living facility where name bracelets are not used? Can she rely on questioning the staff or residents, which can lead to errors if names are misheard or patients are confused? Without adequate systems to help practitioners achieve the goals of the five rights, errors are likely.

The five rights focus on individual performance and overlook crucial system components that contribute to errors. For example, poor lighting, inadequate staffing patterns, poorly designed medical devices, handwritten orders, doses with trailing zeroes, and ambiguous drug labels can prevent health care professionals from verifying the five rights, despite their best efforts. This chapter describes causes of medication errors in the context of key system elements identified by the Institute for Safe Medication Practices (ISMP).

A SYSTEMS APPROACH

Where medication errors are concerned, finding out who was involved is less important than learning what went wrong, how, and why.[1-6] This is the basis of the error-prevention approach promoted by ISMP. Through its involvement with the U.S. Pharmacopeia in the USP-ISMP Medication Errors Reporting Program (MERP) and with the Food and Drug Administration (FDA) MedWatch Program, ISMP has reviewed thousands of reports of medication errors and visited hundreds of sites after accidents have occurred. In all cases, the causes have been multifactorial, cutting across many processes, lines of responsibility, and organizationwide systems. At the same time, most medication errors involve similar circumstances.

In their landmark article on systems analysis of adverse drug events, Leape et al.[1] defined broad categories, or domains, where the underlying problems that result in medication errors may be found. They then identified the following "proximal causes" of medication errors:

- Lack of knowledge of the drug,
- Lack of information about the patient,
- Violations of rules,
- Slips and memory lapses,
- Transcription errors,
- Faulty identity checking,
- Faulty interaction with other services,
- Faulty dose checking,
- Infusion pump and parenteral delivery problems,
- Inadequate patient monitoring,
- Drug stocking and delivery problems,
- Preparation errors, and
- Lack of standardization.

Other authors have suggested different categorization systems. In many cases, the key differences lie primarily in the nomenclature.

SYSTEM ELEMENTS IMPLICATED IN ERRORS

The system-based causes of errors can best be uncovered through interdisciplinary efforts, since they stem from weaknesses in systems (defined in the sidebar) throughout an organization. For example, when a medication error occurs, organizationwide system weaknesses are often identified in

- How information is collected and communicated,
- How colleagues interact,
- How patients and staff are educated,
- How the organizational culture and physical environment are managed,
- How staff is provided to carry out patient care functions,
- How staff learns about system errors and their causes, and
- How patients are safeguarded from harm.

ISMP has identified 10 key system elements that have the greatest influence on medication use. System-based causes of medication errors can be directly traced to weaknesses or failures in these key elements.

1. Patient information. To guide appropriate drug therapy, health care providers need readily available demographic and clinical information (such as age, weight, allergies, diagnoses, and pregnancy status) and patient-monitoring information (such as laboratory values and vital signs) that gauge the effects of medications and the patient's underlying disease processes.

2. Drug information. To minimize the risk of error, the drug inventory must be controlled in some way, and up-to-date drug information must be readily accessible to health care providers through text references, protocols, order sets, computerized drug information systems, medication administration records and patient profiles, and regular clinical activities by pharmacists in patient care areas or the pharmacy.

3. Communication related to medications. Because failed communication is at the heart of many errors, health care organizations must enhance collaborative teamwork, eliminate communication barriers among health care providers, and standardize the way prescription orders and other drug information are communicated to avoid misinterpretation.

DEFINING "SYSTEMS"

A system is a perceived whole whose key elements hang together, continually affecting each other, as it moves toward a common purpose. Derived from the Greek word *sunistánai*, meaning "to cause to stand together," a system comprises a pattern of interrelationships that encompass everything from the ways in which decisions are made to the ways that processes flow.[6] The medication-use process is influenced by three large interconnecting systems that define the way information is managed, the environment is structured, and human resources are handled. Each of these systems is defined by key elements (Table 4-1) that continually overlap while moving toward a common purpose: safe and effective medication use.

4. Drug labeling, packaging, and nomenclature. To facilitate proper identification and use of drugs, product manufacturers, regulatory agencies, and health care organizations, especially pharmacies, should ensure that all drugs are provided in clearly labeled containers, including unit dose packages for institutional use, and should take steps to prevent errors with look-alike and sound-alike drug names, ambiguous drug packaging, and confusing or absent drug labels.

5. Drug standardization, storage, and distribution. Many errors can be prevented by minimizing the availability of medications (e.g., reducing hospital floor stock), restricting access to high-alert drugs and hazardous chemicals, and distributing or dispensing medications from the pharmacy in a timely fashion. Whenever possible, health care organizations should use commercially available products rather than compounding medications. In hospitals, the use of commercially prepared intravenous solutions and standard concentrations can minimize error-prone processes such as pharmacy IV admixture preparation and dose calculations.

6. Medication delivery device acquisition, use, and monitoring. The design of certain medication delivery devices facilitates, rather than precludes, medication errors. Health care organizations must assess a device's safety before purchase, ensure appropriate fail-safe protections (e.g., free-flow protection for IV lines used in conjunction with pumps, incompatible connections for various tubings and catheters), limit variety to promote familiarity, and require independent double checks of processes in which errors could cause serious patient harm (e.g., refilling automated dispensing equipment, setting patient-controlled analgesia pumps).

7. Environmental factors. Environmental factors such as poor lighting, cluttered work spaces, noise, interruptions, high patient acuity, and nonstop activity can contribute to errors if they hinder health care providers' ability to remain focused on medication use. The deficient staffing patterns and excessive workload in many of today's health care organizations create the potential for a broad range of errors.

8. Staff competency and education. Although staff education alone is an insufficient approach to error reduction, it can play an important role when combined with system-based error-reduction strategies. The most effective activities include ongoing assessment of health care providers' baseline competencies and education about new medications, nonformulary medications, high-alert medications, and error prevention.

9. Patient education. Patients can play a vital role in preventing errors if they have been educated about their medications and encouraged to ask questions and seek satisfactory answers. Patients who know the names and doses of their medications, the reason for taking each one, how they should be taken, what they look like, and how they work are in an excellent position to help minimize the chance of error. Health care providers should not only teach patients how to protect themselves from medication errors but also seek their input in quality improvement and safety initiatives.

10. Quality processes and risk management. Health care organizations, including community pharmacies, pharmacy benefit managers, and mail service pharmacies, need systems for identifying, reporting, analyzing, and reducing the risk of medication errors. A nonpunitive culture of safety must be cultivated to encourage frank disclosure of errors and near misses, stimulate productive discussions, and identify effective system-based solutions. Strategically placed quality control checks are necessary. Simple redundancies that support a system of independent double checks for high-alert medications and error-prone processes can promote the detection and correction of errors before they reach and harm patients.

On the basis of these key system elements, the causes of medication errors can be summarized as follows:

1. Lack of information about the patient,
2. Lack of information about the drug,
3. Communication and teamwork failures,
4. Unclear, absent, or look-alike drug labels and packages, and confusing or look-alike or sound-alike drug names,
5. Unsafe drug standardization, storage, and distribution,
6. Nonstandard, flawed, or unsafe medication delivery devices,
7. Environmental factors and staffing patterns that do not support safety,
8. Inadequate staff orientation, ongoing education, supervision, and competency validation,
9. Inadequate patient education about medications and medication errors, and
10. Lack of a supportive culture of safety, failure to learn from mistakes, and failed or absent error-reduction strategies, such as redundancies.

Table 4-1 lists the 10 key system elements, examples of weaknesses in these elements that put patients at risk for errors, and examples of safety strategies that are likely to reduce the risk of errors. The elements in the table can be used to evaluate medication use in two ways: proactively (before an error occurs) and retrospectively (after an error occurs). For example, a new infusion pump, a new medication, or parts of an existing process can be examined to identify the risk of error so that action can be taken to reduce the chance of serious patient harm. Most often, a process called failure mode and effects analysis (see Chapter 21) is used to help uncover these risks. As part of this process, the key system elements in Table 4-1 can be used to prompt discussion about the possible causes of error. After a serious error occurs, a root cause analysis (see Chapter 5) is often conducted. Again, the system elements in Table 4-1 can be used to identify breakdowns in the system that led to the error.

CONCLUSION

When an error occurs, it is tempting to blame individuals. Analyzing errors in an inter-disciplinary, systems-based context avoids this punitive approach. A systems-based approach does not remove individual accountability for medication safety; rather, it expands accountability to all who could potentially influence the medication-use process. In this approach, accountability lies not in perfect job performance but in identifying safety problems and implementing system-based solutions.

TABLE 4-1 ISMP Key System Elements of Medication Use

Element	Examples of Safety Problems	Examples of Safety Strategies
1. **Patient information** (e.g., age, sex, diagnoses, pregnancy, allergies, height, weight, lab values, diagnostic study results, vital signs, ability to pay for prescriptions, patient identity) *Essential patient information is obtained, readily available in useful form, and considered when prescribing, dispensing, and administering medications.*	▪ Untimely access to lab studies ▪ Failure to adjust doses for patients with hepatic or renal impairment ▪ Patient allergies unknown ▪ Teratogenic medication given to pregnant patient ▪ Failure to notice significant respiratory depression in patients receiving IV opioids ▪ Patient misidentified ▪ Patient unable to pay for prescriptions ▪ Patient weight unavailable for proper dosing	▪ Gain electronic access to lab values ▪ Communicate patient allergies to pharmacy before medications are dispensed and administered ▪ List allergies and diagnoses on order forms and medication administration records (MARs) ▪ Place allergy alert bracelets on hospitalized patients ▪ Use two unique identifiers (or bar coding) to confirm institutional patient identity ▪ Take MAR to the bedside during drug administration; consult patient drug profile prior to pharmacy dispensing ▪ Require special monitoring for high-risk patients (those with obesity, asthma, or sleep apnea) receiving IV opioids ▪ Assess patient's ability to pay for prescriptions and refer to case management/social services if problems are uncovered
2. **Drug information** (e.g., maximum dose, typical dose, route, precautions, contraindications, special warnings, drug interactions, cross-allergies) *Essential drug information is readily available in useful form to those ordering, dispensing, or administering medications.*	▪ Incomplete information about the patient's at-home medications ▪ Knowledge deficit leading to dispensing or administration of the wrong dose or use of the wrong route ▪ Lack of staff awareness of special precautions or special monitoring needed with new medication ▪ Computer warnings about unsafe doses overlooked or ignored ▪ Serious drug interaction unknown or overlooked	▪ Provide up-to-date, timely drug information (textbooks and online at all computer terminals) ▪ Have staff pharmacists in patient care units for consultation and education ▪ Provide readily accessible dosing charts, protocols, guidelines, and checklists for high-alert medications (Chapter 14) ▪ Establish maximum doses for high-alert medications; list applicable doses on preprinted orders; build alerts into computer systems to warn staff if doses exceed safe limits ▪ Have a pharmacist review all prescriptions and drug orders before administration (except in an emergency) ▪ Establish a reconciliation process for verifying patient's at-home medication list and verifying medication lists upon each transfer of care

TABLE 4-1 ISMP Key System Elements of Medication Use (continued)

Element	Examples of Safety Problems	Examples of Safety Strategies
3. **Communication** (e.g., communication dynamics among colleagues, team dynamics, communication of drug orders) *Methods of communicating drug orders and other drug information are standardized and automated to minimize the risk for error.*	■ Failure to question ambiguous or unclear orders or pursue safety concerns because of intimidation by prescriber ■ Illegible handwritten orders ■ Error-prone presentation of medication orders on MARs or patient profiles ■ Incomplete medication orders (missing dose or route, orders to resume same medication upon transfer or to take at-home medications upon admission) ■ Abbreviations misunderstood (e.g., U misread as a zero) ■ Spoken orders misheard ■ Failure to transmit all orders or prescriptions to the pharmacy	■ Use electronic prescribing systems that connect to the pharmacy computer and electronic MAR ■ Use carefully designed, standard preprinted orders ■ Prohibit error-prone abbreviations, symbols, and dose expressions on orders, MARs, labels, computer screens (see Chapter 8) ■ Discourage spoken (including telephone) orders except in emergencies, and prohibit them for cancer chemotherapy ■ Read back spoken orders to confirm understanding ■ Require complete, reconciled orders (not "resume" orders) upon admission, transfer, and discharge ■ Establish a procedure that specifies the steps practitioners should take when there is disagreement about the safety of an order ■ Send all orders to the pharmacy, even if the medication prescribed is available on the unit or the order does not contain a medication
4. **Drug names, labels, and packages** *Readable labels that clearly identify drugs and doses are on all medication containers, and drugs remain labeled up to the point of administration.* *Strategies are undertaken to minimize the possibility of errors with products that have similar or confusing labels, packages, or drug names.*	■ Product misidentification due to look-alike drug labels and packages or look-alike/sound-alike drug names ■ Confusing or ambiguous labels on medications ■ Unlabeled medications or syringes ■ Unlabeled solutions or syringes on a sterile field ■ Poorly positioned labels that obscure vital information ■ Doses dispensed in bulk supplies without patient-specific labels ■ Mislabeled medications	■ Consider the potential for look-alike appearance or label ambiguity of commercial containers ■ For institutional use, dispense medications in labeled, unit dose form ■ Label all containers, with drug name and strength most prominent ■ Within institutions, keep oral medications in original packaging until administered at the bedside ■ Store drugs with look-alike names or packages in separated areas or in separated drawers of automated dispensing equipment ■ Use warning labels to alert staff to unusual strengths and special precautions ■ Ensure that pharmacy labels are easy to read and understand ■ Require prescribers to include the indication for prn medications to differentiate them from drugs with look-alike names

5. **Drug standardization, storage, and distribution** (e.g., storage of unit stock medications and pharmacy-dispensed medications, preparation of IV medications, use of standard concentrations, pharmacy delivery services)

Intravenous solutions, drug concentrations, and administration times are standardized whenever possible.

Medications are provided to patient care units in a safe and secure manner and available for administration within a time frame that meets essential patient needs.

Unit-based floor stock is restricted.

- Multiple concentrations of IV solutions leading to potential use of the wrong concentration
- Nurse preparation of IV solutions
- Failure to properly dilute concentrated medications and electrolytes before administration
- Selection of the wrong drug or dose caused by unsafe storage of medications in the pharmacy or on patient care units
- Storage of hazardous chemicals, fixatives, and developers with medications, leading to mix-ups
- Missing medications because of problems with pharmacy distribution or nursing transmission of orders
- Nonstandard medication administration times
- Delay in therapy due to untimely delivery of new medications or failure of nursing transmission of the order
- Unsafe nursing access to pharmacy after hours

- Standardize concentrations of insulin, heparin, morphine, and vasopressor drips (adult and pediatric) to a single concentration
- Use commercially available premixed IV solutions whenever possible
- Limit nurse preparation of IV solutions to emergency situations
- Dispense medications from the pharmacy according to realistic time frames for stat, urgent, and routine medications
- Store high-alert drugs in the pharmacy until needed for a specific patient, or secure and restrict access if they are available on the unit
- Remove concentrated forms of electrolytes from patient care units
- Provide all stock medications in unit dose form (no bulk supplies)
- Remove discontinued medications from the unit in a timely manner
- Do not borrow medications from patient supplies
- Prohibit nursing access to the pharmacy after hours; establish a night cabinet with a restricted supply of medications for use when pharmacy is closed

6. **Medication delivery devices** (e.g., infusion pumps, implantable pumps, oral and parenteral syringes, glucose monitors)

The potential for human error is mitigated through careful procurement, maintenance, use, and standardization of devices used to prepare and deliver medications.

- Pump programming errors
- Accidental administration of an oral solution by the IV route via devices with Luer connections
- Rapid free-flow of solution when tubing is removed from the pump
- Failure to notice incorrect default setting on pump, leading to dosing errors
- Unfamiliarity with medication delivery devices, leading to misuse
- Line mix-ups (e.g., connecting an IV solution to an epidural line)
- Insufficient supply of infusion pumps to meet patient needs
- End users (often nurses) not involved in purchase decisions regarding medication delivery devices

- Examine new devices for the potential for errors before purchase and use
- Limit the variety of infusion pumps to promote staff proficiency
- Prohibit the use of infusion pumps without free-flow protection
- Train staff adequately about use of new devices and ensure competency before independent use
- Require one nurse to set up a pump and another to independently double-check the solution, settings, line attachment, and patient before infusing IV solutions that contain high-alert medications
- Label the distal ends of all tubing if patients are receiving solutions via multiple routes (e.g., IV, intra-arterial, enteral, epidural, bladder instillation)
- Use specially designed oral syringes to administer oral solutions to prevent inadvertent connection to an IV port
- Purchase and use pumps that offer technology that can intercept and prevent wrong-dose or infusion rate errors

TABLE 4-1 ISMP Key System Elements of Medication Use (continued)

Element	Examples of Safety Problems	Examples of Safety Strategies
7. **Environmental factors and staffing patterns** (e.g., physical surroundings, physical health of staff, organization of unit, lighting, noise, foot traffic, storage, ergonomics, workload, staffing patterns, work schedules) *Medications are prescribed, transcribed, prepared, and administered in a physical environment that offers adequate space and lighting and allows practitioners to remain focused on medication use.* *The complement of qualified, well-rested practitioners matches the clinical workload without compromising patient safety.*	■ Drug mix-ups due to lack of space or cluttered work spaces ■ Drug mix-ups due to crowded and disorganized storage of medications in refrigerators ■ Misinterpretation of spoken/telephone orders because of noise and distractions ■ Errors in preparation or drug mix-ups due to poorly lighted work spaces and drug storage cabinets ■ Interruptions during medication administration or preparation causing mental slips and other errors ■ Inadequate staffing patterns leading to task overload and rushed procedures ■ Staff member fatigue causing impaired judgment and flawed performance of job functions ■ Mental overload and error potential due to inadequate breaks ■ Lack of staffing contingency plans to cover illness and vacations ■ Human resources required for new services not fully considered	■ Ensure adequate space, storage, and lighting in stock medication areas, including automated dispensing cabinets ■ Provide work spaces that are free of distractions for transcription of medication orders ■ Arrange areas for IV and oral dose preparation so that they are isolated from noise, foot traffic, and other distractions ■ Make computer screens and patient monitors adjustable for staff comfort and safety during use ■ Purchase refrigerators that are of adequate size for organized storage of medications ■ Establish a realistic staffing plan to safely provide care to patients during staff illnesses, vacations, and fluctuations in patient acuity ■ Schedule adequate staffing to allow for staff meals and breaks ■ Manage and monitor individual staff schedules to allow adequate rest between shifts and to prohibit shifts longer than 12 hours ■ Minimize the use of transient agency staff ■ Communicate plans for new services to all involved staff, and carefully consider the resources necessary to handle additional work volume without compromising patient safety

8. **Staff competency and education** (e.g., orientation, in-service training, certifications, annual competencies, skills labs, simulation of events, off-site education)

Practitioners receive sufficient orientation to medication use and undergo baseline and annual competency evaluation of knowledge and skills related to safe medication practices.

Practitioners involved in medication use are provided with ongoing education about medication error prevention and the safe use of drugs that have the greatest potential to cause harm if misused.

- Delays and errors due to misunderstanding between nursing and pharmacy, stemming from lack of knowledge of each discipline's practice patterns and environments
- Inappropriate medication doses or errors in patient assessment and monitoring due to lack of knowledge about particular patient populations
- Errors related to task overload and rushed procedures for those with added responsibility of training new staff
- Medication errors by new or reassigned ("floated") staff who are required to perform unfamiliar tasks or give unfamiliar medications without proper orientation, education, or supervision
- Errors with new medications given to patients without full knowledge of the preparation, dose, route, action, or effects to anticipate
- Errors (including near misses) that are not reported, with consequent loss of knowledge about the causes of errors and their prevention

- Organize all orientation schedules according to individual learning needs and assessments
- Arrange staffing so that trainers have reduced workload to avoid overload of normal duties
- Require new nurses to spend time in the pharmacy to become familiar with drug dispensing processes
- Require new pharmacists to spend time on patient care units to become familiar with drug administration processes
- Provide staff education about new medications before they are used
- Require pharmacy to affix special alerts or provide nurses with other important information about nonformulary drugs when dispensing these medications
- Ensure that reassignment to other clinical areas ("floating") is not permitted until staff have undergone orientation and competency verification
- Provide staff with ongoing education about medication errors that have occurred within the organization and in other organizations, as well as strategies to prevent these errors
- Include in job descriptions and performance evaluations specific accountability standards for patient/medication safety that do not include the absence of errors or a numeric error threshold
- Provide staff with the necessary support and time to attend internal and external education programs related to medication use and error prevention

TABLE 4-1 ISMP Key System Elements of Medication Use (continued)

Element	Examples of Safety Problems	Examples of Safety Strategies
9. **Patient education** (e.g., drug information sheets, dosing schedules for complex medication regimens, discharge instructions, tips for avoiding errors, consumer representation in drug safety efforts) *Patients are included as active partners in their care through education about their medications and ways to avert errors.*	▪ Patients might feel uncomfortable reminding staff to verify their identity ▪ Patients might be reluctant to ask questions about the medications they are receiving ▪ Patients might not understand information given to them orally because of medical jargon or other language barriers ▪ Low health literacy or poor reading skills might prevent patients from understanding printed information or directions for using medications ▪ Patients often lack resources for questions about drug therapy after discharge ▪ Patients might not remember all the medications and doses they are taking, which increases the risk of errors in prescribing medications upon admission ▪ Patients lack information about the causes of medication errors and how to prevent them	▪ Teach patients how to actively participate in proper identification before accepting medication or undergoing procedures ▪ Provide patients/families with the brand and generic names of each medication administered, the general purpose, the prescribed dose, and important adverse effects ▪ Consult a pharmacist for assistance, especially if patients are, or will be, taking more than five medications at home ▪ Encourage patients to ask questions about their drug therapy ▪ Fully investigate and resolve all patient questions or concerns about drug therapy before drug administration ▪ Provide patients with written materials that use lay terminology (eighth-grade reading level or lower) for high-alert medications prescribed at discharge ▪ Instruct patients on when and whom to call with concerns or questions about their drug therapy after discharge ▪ Encourage patients to keep a written record of all their prescription and nonprescription medications, herbal products, and vitamins, and to show the list to health care providers during each inpatient and outpatient visit

10. **Quality process and risk management** (e.g., culture, leadership, error reporting, safety strategies, safety redundancies)

A nonpunitive, systems-based approach to error reduction is in place and supported by management, senior administration, and the board of trustees.

Practitioners are stimulated to detect and report errors, and interdisciplinary teams regularly analyze errors that have occurred within the organization and in other organizations for the purpose of redesigning systems to best support safe practitioner performance.

Simple redundancies that support a system of independent double checks or an automated verification process are used for vulnerable parts of the medication-use process to detect and correct errors before they reach patients.

- Lack of leadership and budgetary support for medication safety
- Disincentives (shame, blame, fear of disciplinary action, documentation of errors in personnel files) encourage underreporting of errors
- Culture of secrecy and blame prevents disclosure of errors to patients and families
- Inaccurate error rates determined by using error reports, with a counterproductive goal of reducing the number of error reports
- Ineffective error prevention strategies focused on individual performance improvement rather than system improvements
- Lack of understanding of medication administration as a system and ways to safeguard the system as a whole
- Lack of automated or manual double checks for critical steps in the medication-use process
- Failure of manual double checks, often because they are not performed independently
- Misplacement or misuse of double checks in place of system enhancements that would prevent error

- Clearly articulate patient/medication safety in the organization's mission/vision statements
- Train midlevel managers to effectively evaluate competency and handle difficult behavior without allowing the presence or absence of errors to be a factor
- Promote a culture where human error is anticipated and accountability for medication safety is shared among organizational leaders and professional staff without blame
- Promote and reward reporting of errors and hazardous conditions that could lead to errors, and expect a sustained, not reduced, error-reporting rate
- Disclose all errors that reach a patient
- Include discussions about errors and their prevention in all staff meetings as a standing agenda item
- Convene an interdisciplinary team to routinely review errors and other safety data to identify system-based causes and facilitate implementation of system-based enhancements
- Invite patients and community representatives to participate in medication safety discussions, and solicit their input
- Disseminate information regularly throughout the organization about errors and safety strategies
- Recalculate all doses for chemotherapy and pediatric medications to verify the prescriber's order
- Perform an independent double check (manual or automated) to verify the drug, dose, concentration, infusion rate, patient, route, and line attachment before administering selected high-alert medications such as IV insulin, IV chemotherapy, and IV opioids (including those used in patient-controlled analgesia)
- Use bar-coding technology during drug administration

REFERENCES

1. Leape LL, Bates DW, Cullen DJ, et al. Systems analysis of adverse drug events. *JAMA*. 1995;274:35–43.
2. Wieman TJ, Wieman EA. A systems approach to error prevention in medicine. *J Surg Oncol*. 2004;88(3): 115–21.
3. Cousins DD. Preventing medication errors. *US Pharm*. August 1995;20:70–5.
4. Davis NM, Cohen MR, Teplitsky B. Look-alike and sound-alike drug names: the problem and the solution. *Hosp Pharm*. 1992;27:95–110.
5. Perlstein PH, White CC, Barnes B, et al. Errors in drug computations during newborn intensive care. *Am J Dis Child*. 1979;133:376–9.
6. Senge PM, Kleiner A, Roberts C, et al. *The Fifth Discipline Fieldbook*. New York: Doubleday; 1994:90.

CHAPTER 5

ROOT CAUSE ANALYSIS OF MEDICATION ERRORS

Mary Burkhardt, Caryl Lee, Lesley Taylor, Rodney Williams, and James Bagian

Root cause analysis (RCA) is used to identify the critical underlying reasons for the occurrence of an adverse event or close call (near miss). This analytical approach has long been used by reliable organizations and industries to find out

- What happened? (What happened on that particular day?)
- Why did it happen? (What made that particular day different? What usually happens? What are the norms? What should have happened according to policy and procedure?)
- What will prevent it from happening again? (What actions need to be taken? How will outcomes be measured?)

Through evaluation of evidence and information supplied by people associated with the incident, contributory factors at the root of the event can be identified and noncontributory factors can be excluded. RCA offers safety, quality, and clinical managers an opportunity to implement more reliable and more cost-effective policies and improved processes that help prevent adverse events and near misses. Applying RCA to one individual event or to many events (aggregated RCA) can reduce or prevent harm to patients.

RCA is relatively easy to use. Any event has multiple root causes. Breaking the chain of events at any point, beginning with any of the root causes, can avoid the final breakdown. Successful RCA involves presenting the data clearly, generating practical recommendations, and developing appropriate corrective action. RCA not only provides specific, concrete ways of correcting the problem at hand but also establishes systemic controls to avoid recurrence.

A quick search of the Internet provides numerous RCA resources (www.apollorca.com, www.failsafe-network.com, www.jointcommission.org, www.patientsafety.gov, www.reliability.com, www.rootcause.com, www.rootcauseanalyst.com, www.taproot.com). Regardless of the specific approach used, RCA provides a structure for continually asking why things happen the way they do. It helps health care providers avoid jumping to conclusions about an event and choosing an inappropriate or suboptimal solution.

CONSIDER THE ENVIRONMENT

Before deciding which approach to RCA best fits an organization's needs, it is essential to consider the reporting environment (culture) in that particular workplace.[1] According to Leape et al.,[2] "The medical imperative is clear: To make health care safe we need to redesign our systems to make errors difficult to commit, and create a culture in which the existence of risk is acknowledged and injury prevention is recognized as everyone's responsibility." If people are accustomed to situations and unaware that they are unsafe, or if they fear punishment or repercussions for reporting an adverse event or close call, they will not speak up when things go wrong.

On the other hand, if an organization believes that everyone comes to work to do the best possible job, and fosters a culture where openness about errors is nonthreatening, then that organization can broaden and strengthen its focus on weaknesses or vulnerabilities in the systems that support every employee's performance. Clearly, this perspective facilitates RCA.

STEPS IN RCA

The following steps are common to all methods of conducting RCA.

1. Charter the team

- *People:* The most effective teams are cross-disciplinary; they include individuals who are versed on the processes in question but were not directly involved with the actual event or close call.
- *Places, tools, and time:* The team must have meeting space, computer access, and adequate time to devote to the effort.
- *Management support:* The team should brief management on what it is doing and obtain written consent for allocating assets to complete the RCA.

2. Document and research

- Write a description of the event based on the preliminary report.
- Collect data related to the event (i.e., existing policies, photographs, equipment involved).
- Interview key personnel (those actually involved in the event).
- Gather credible references that may aid in understanding the event; refer to these throughout the process.
- Rewrite the event description, adding the new information.

3. Identify root causes

- Diagram the flow of events (see examples in Figures 5-1 and 5-2).
  - Chart how events unfolded chronologically leading up to the adverse event or close call.
  - Examine the process to identify where vulnerabilities exist.
    - Be sure to capture what actually happened, not what was supposed to have happened.
    - Break down the event flow, asking "Why?" at each step to discover the causes.
    - Give RCA teams easy-to-use tools in order to increase the likelihood that all teams will be equally rigorous over time. The questions in Table 5-1[3] illustrate the many things a team must consider to discern what happened and how to prevent it from happening again.
  - Use fishbone or cause-and-effect diagramming[4] (see example in Figure 5-3) to provide a useful bridge from analysis to actions. Information on how to use these diagrams can be found in the literature.

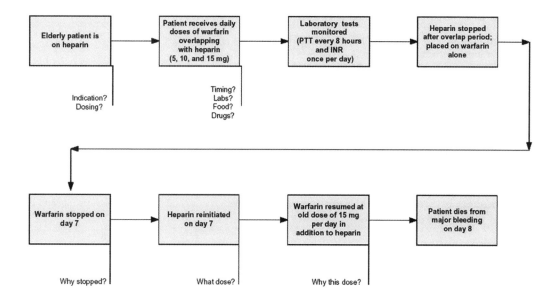

FIGURE 5-1 "Initial understanding" event flow diagram. The focus is on the facts and on identifying questions or gaps in the information. (PTT = partial thromboplastin time; INR = international normalized ratio)

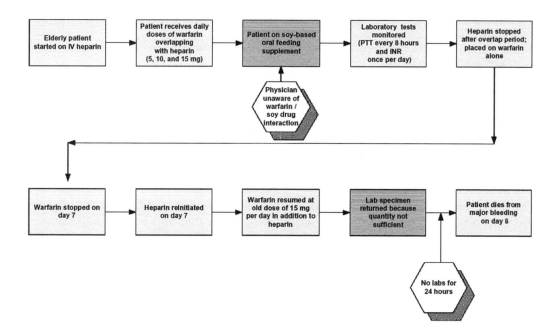

FIGURE 5-2 "Final understanding" event flow diagram. The focus is on presenting new information to complete the picture of why things happened the way they did. (PTT = partial thromboplastin time; INR = international normalized ratio).

TABLE 5-1 Questions for Assessing System-Level Vulnerabilities[3]

Communication
Was the patient correctly identified?
Was information from various patient assessments shared and used by members of the treatment team on a
    timely basis?
Was communication between management/supervisors and frontline staff adequate?
Was communication between frontline team members adequate?

Training
Was training provided prior to the start of the work process?
Were the results of training monitored over time?
Were training programs for staff designed up-front with the intent of helping staff perform their tasks without
    errors?
Had procedures and equipment been reviewed to ensure that there was a good match between people and the
    tasks they did, or people and the equipment they used?

Fatigue/Scheduling
Were the levels of vibration, noise, or other environmental conditions appropriate?
Did scheduling allow personnel adequate sleep?
Was the environment free of distractions?
Was there sufficient staff on hand for the workload at the time?

Environment/Equipment
Was the work area/environment designed to support the function it was being used for?
Had there been an environmental risk assessment (i.e., safety audit) of the area?
Were emergency provisions and backup systems available in case of equipment failure?
Were equipment displays and controls working properly and interpreted correctly?

Rules/Policies/Procedures
Did management have an audit or quality control system to inform them how key processes related to the
    adverse event were functioning?
Were the staff members involved in the adverse event or close call properly qualified and trained to perform
    their functions?
If policies and procedures were not used, what were the barriers to their usefulness to staff?
If policies and procedures were not used, what positive and negative incentives were absent?

Barriers
Were existing barriers designed to protect patients, staff, equipment, or environment?
Had these barriers and controls been evaluated for reliability?
Would the adverse event have been prevented if the existing barriers and controls had functioned correctly?
Were the systems or processes tested before they were implemented?

- ■ Develop statements of cause
  - – Using the causes found in the event-flow diagrams and cause-and-effect
    diagrams, write concise descriptions of the cause-and-effect relationship.
    Ensure that the team has not focused on the actions of individuals or in any
    way placed blame. To determine whether a statement is effective, ask, "If
    this is corrected, will it reduce the likelihood of another adverse event?" The
    answer should be yes.

4. Develop actions

- ■ The actions a team develops to address the root cause and contributing factors
  should be stated specifically and concretely so that they can be readily understood
  and implemented. If possible, the team should consider a trial or simulation of

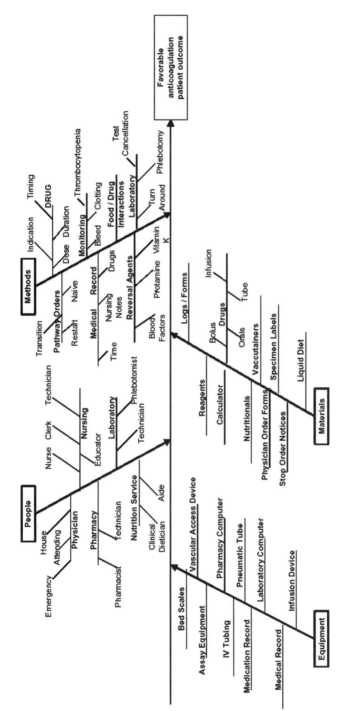

FIGURE 5-3 Fishbone diagram of anticoagulation events. The diagram shows the complexity of the process and where events may have occurred.

TABLE 5-2   Examples of Actions Proposed in Root Cause Analysis

- Make architectural or physical plant changes (e.g., provide cubicles for consulting with patients instead of conversing or relaying information in a busy, noisy hallway)
- Develop cognitive aids for complex or high-risk processes (e.g., pocket card for calculations, poster for indication/use of reversal agents)
- Use effective communication skills (e.g., read back stat orders, hold multidisciplinary briefings for total parenteral nutrition rounds)
- Separate products that look alike and whose names sound alike (e.g., physically separate IV solutions and irrigation solutions)
- Use forcing functions—designs to ensure that the right or ideal thing happens the first time and every time (e.g., a car can be started only when it is in "park," so it is impossible to drive sooner than the driver intends)
- Consider consultation with a human-factors engineer (e.g., invite a consultant to analyze and streamline work areas and processes or to evaluate the many different ways staff members use the same piece of equipment)
- Prevent fatigue (e.g., limit consecutive hours of work, do not assign complex tasks to staff working a double shift)
- Build in redundancy, double checks, and fail-safe features (e.g., designate a printer for producing hard copies of medication records on a regular basis, in case the computerized system goes down)
- Simplify and standardize processes and equipment (e.g., use the same protocols for treating patients undergoing detoxification regardless of treatment setting, use the same type and layout for crash carts in all treatment settings so staff can easily locate emergency equipment and medications)
- Test usability (before purchasing new equipment types or models, have frontline staff methodically test those items, and include their critique in the final purchase decision)

the actions prior to full implementation. The action statement should have buy-in from the process owners.

- Ideally, the actions a team proposes will prevent the same adverse event or close call from happening again, or at least minimize its occurrence. The strongest actions in this regard tend to be physical rather than procedural (e.g., install speed bumps in a busy parking lot, instead of relying on a speed limit sign to do the job) and permanent rather than temporary (e.g., remove and replace equipment that is known to malfunction in the hands of less experienced or "floating" staff, instead of gluing or taping warnings or additional instructions onto the machine). In general, the proposed actions should not burden people's memory (i.e., it is best to avoid unnecessary training or new policies—and not to ask providers to "pay more attention next time"). Table 5-2 gives examples of actions that can make a difference.

5. Establish outcome measures

- Include measures for evaluating whether your actions prevent future events. This helps ensure follow-up. See Chapter 23 for more on measuring medication safety.
- Outcome measures should
  - Measure the effectiveness of the action, not whether the action was completed.
  - Be quantifiable, with clear numerators and denominators (if appropriate).
  - Define strategies clearly, including the frequency and time frame for monitoring.
  - Include a threshold or goal, and ensure that it is realistic.

AGGREGATED ROOT CAUSE ANALYSIS

Some types of events (e.g., patient falls) occur fairly often but do not always result in serious harm. A facility may not have the resources for individual analysis of every event, and batch analysis of these events may be advantageous. At Veterans Health Administration (VHA) facilities, aggregated review is required for potentially serious events such as

TABLE 5-3 Veterans Health Administration Safety Assessment Matrix for Root Cause Analysis

Probability	Severity			
	Catastrophic	Major	Moderate	Minor
Frequent	3	3	2	1
Occasional	3	2	1	1
Uncommon	3	2	1	1
Remote	3	2	1	1

Source: www.patientsafety.gov.

patient falls, missing patients, parasuicidal events, and adverse drug events. If an event actually was severe according to the VHA safety assessment code (Table 5-3), individual RCA is still required. Key factors in determining severity include the extent of injury, length of stay, and level of care required for remediation. For potential adverse events, severity is assigned on the basis of the most likely worst-case systems-level scenario. Actual events with a score of 3 require RCA. Potential medication events with a score of 3 can be analyzed individually or in quarterly aggregate RCA. Details of this process are described on the Department of Veterans Affairs National Center for Patient Safety Web site (www.patientsafety.gov).

The process for aggregated review is the same as for individual RCA, except that a subset of events is selected for more intensive review and action planning. For example, for one quarter of the year, the team may review 100 reports and select the 15 ambulatory-care dispensing events for intensive review; the next quarter the team may review 85 reports and focus on the 20 dosing errors. Often, RCA teams members serve for 1 year. This provides for efficient resource use and consistency among analyses.

Aggregated review teams may use different approaches to the analysis, since there is no single event. It is important for teams to think creatively and try new approaches so that RCA does not become routine. Tools such as fishbone diagrams, floor plans, and bar charts can help the team members think in different ways about the set of events.

SYSTEM-LEVEL VULNERABILITIES

Every organization has system-level features that contribute to safety (e.g., leadership, professional and institutional beliefs and processes, teamwork, individual expertise, technology, policies and procedures), as well as features that can detract from safety (e.g., production pressures, distractions, insufficient training or communication, clumsy technology).[5] The primary task of the RCA team is to identify these system-level features and then shore up the systems or processes that contribute to safety and eliminate or control the systems or processes that make things more dangerous. Tools such as the diagram in Figure 5-1 can help RCA teams determine efficiently and comprehensively how events happened.

Once the RCA team knows which system-level vulnerabilities (root causes or contributing factors) need to be fixed, it is important to state those findings clearly and in enough detail that what to fix and how become obvious.[6] The following guidelines can be used in writing statements about root causes and contributing factors:

- Show cause and effect (e.g., "nearly identical packaging increased the likelihood that X and Y would be misidentified").
- Do not make negative statements about people or things (e.g., instead of "the medication package insert was poorly written," say "the use of 8-point type

and lack of photographs and diagrams decreased the likelihood that the insert would be used by pharmacy staff").

■ Focus on system-level problems, not individual performance (e.g., instead of "the nurse gave the wrong stat medication," say "absence of formal read-back confirmation of stat orders increased the likelihood that a stat order would be misunderstood").

■ Get to the norms behind procedure violations (e.g., instead of "the nurse on the night shift did not 'wand' the patient's identification band and medication before administration," say "lack of training on the computerized medication administration contingency plan, coupled with the 10 pm crash of the bar code medication administration system, increased the likelihood that the night shift would revert to previously approved methods of passing medications").

■ Remember that failure to act is causal only when there is a preexisting duty to act.

HUMAN-FACTORS ENGINEERING

After an RCA team understands how things happened and what features make things more and less safe, it can recommend actions to prevent or at least minimize the impact of similar events or close calls in the future. Ideally, these proposed actions should not require staff members to increase their vigilance or memorize new information. Instead, the actions should "design-in" safety by putting "knowledge in the world."[7]

Designing-in safety is a human-factors engineering approach. Broadly defined, human-factors engineering is the study of how people interact and work successfully with other people and things in their world, and how to increase success or improve human performance by designing-in physical or environmental cues or processes (e.g., instructions; alarms or warnings; incentives; visual displays; buttons, switches, or control panels; specific modes of communication).[8] Table 5-2 lists examples of actions that design-in safety. The sidebar on pages 75–77, contributed by the Institute for Safe Medication Practices (ISMP), illustrates how failure to consider human factors has led to device failures and errors.

ACTIONS AND OUTCOMES

Several obstacles can derail the work of an RCA team: lack of information about exactly why things happened the way they did, too broad a focus ("saving the world"), too narrow a focus (saving one particular patient), and frequently recurring events (things that may happen again before corrective action is implemented).

There are ways to work through these obstacles:

■ Collect additional information through interviews with a broad range of staff. Interview patients and families. Simulate the event.

■ Focus on the situation at hand (set clear boundaries for the scope of work).

■ Look at individual tragedy without staring (do not become hypnotized by the event; instead, focus on what can be done to prevent a similar situation).

■ Find out what others have done to address similar situations (talk with professional colleagues, check relevant Web sites, ask a librarian to do a tailored search).

The team's proposed actions are more likely to be successful if they are pilot tested, or at least simulated, in one or two units or care settings before being deployed across an entire facility. The team can seek out volunteers or champions who are willing to try the action for a few weeks and provide feedback on what worked so that adjustments can be made. Time for pilot testing should be built into the overall plan for implementing and evaluating actions.

NEED FOR FOCUS ON HUMAN FACTORS IN DEVICE DESIGN
Institute for Safe Medication Practices

Failure of device manufacturers to consider human-factors engineering principles can contribute to user error. When the design of medication delivery devices is flawed, adverse patient outcomes can result. For example, a design flaw in IV infusion pumps widely used several years ago allowed free-flow of solutions if the tubing was removed from the pump before the set's gravity flow control clamp was closed. There are numerous design flaws with other devices, from syringes and administration sets to complex infusion pumps. Typically, practitioners using these devices are blamed for errors. Yet ISMP continues to receive error reports suggesting that some manufacturers and regulatory authorities fail to pay attention to user needs and human factors. Examples of problems with administration devices are described below.

Examples

Abbott (now Hospira) Lifecare 4100 PCA Plus II Infuser. A fatality occurred after a practitioner misprogrammed the drug concentration for a loading dose of morphine. During programming, the pump defaults to its minimum setting of 0.1 mg/mL. If the practitioner fails to adjust the concentration and accepts the 0.1 mg/mL default value, the pump calculates a delivery volume that results in a 10-fold overdose if morphine syringes with a concentration of 1 mg/mL are used. A 50-fold overdose would occur with 5 mg/mL morphine syringes. Further, setting dose limits will not prevent overinfusions, because the pump "thinks" it is delivering the proper volume and dose based on the concentration selected during programming. Erroneous low-concentration settings pose the highest risk of patient harm during the administration of loading doses (typically larger doses than those self-administered) and when higher drug concentrations (5 mg/mL) are used. Other fatalities with this device have been described.[1] A newer version of the pump, the LifeCare PCA Infusion System with Hospira MedNet, is now marketed. The device addresses the human-factors issue by reading a bar code on prefilled drug syringes and automatically setting the proper concentration.

Baxter AP-II infusion pump. When the pump alarm sounded to signify that the total volume of a 250 mL epidural infusion of fentanyl and bupivacaine had finished, a nurse found that the bag currently hanging was still full. No solution had infused over the past 20 hours, but the pump had been running and recording the volume as infused without registering an "upstream" occlusion. The manufacturer intends to release a new model that will detect upstream occlusions, but current models still lack features to alert practitioners to this device failure.

Medfusion syringe pump model 2010. A physician asked a nurse to press the Prime button on a pump already delivering a continuous fentanyl infusion to a neonate. He wanted to give a bolus dose to manage pain before placing an additional venous line in the infant. Rather than ordering a specific dose, the physician erroneously used an unsafe method that delivers an unknown quantity of drug and solution. The pump's design should not allow the Prime button to be activated during infusion delivery. After 16 seconds, an alarm will sound, but if the button remains depressed, the fluid will continue to flow. In this case, the nurse accidentally pressed the Prime button on the wrong pump, which was delivering a potassium chloride infusion of 0.1 mEq/kg. The infant received an unknown amount of the concentrated electrolyte by IV bolus, but, luckily, did not sustain any harm.

Medtronic SynchroMed infusion pumps. The Food and Drug Administration (FDA) has received reports of fatal overdosages caused by accidental intrathecal injection of concentrated morphine during attempts to refill Medtronic SynchroMed infusion pumps (Figure 5-4).[2] The pump is a titanium device about the size of a hockey puck. It is surgically implanted under the skin of the abdomen or flank and has a catheter that resides in the intrathecal space. Centered on the front of the device is a small injection port leading to a drug reservoir. This port is used to replenish the drug supply via passage of a thin needle through the skin. A template to help locate this reservoir (Figure 5-5, left) is included in the pump's refill kit. However, there is also

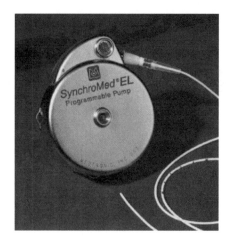

FIGURE 5-4   SynchroMed implantable infusion pump.

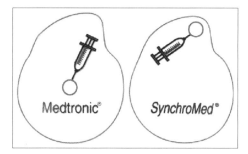

FIGURE 5-5   SynchroMed templates. These clear plastic overlays are placed over the palpated pump to help locate the correct port. The refill kit template (left) allows only reservoir access. The catheter access kit template (right) allows only catheter access; accidental use of this template for pump refilling has led to fatalities. (Newer design lists "SynchroMed" on all templates.)

a catheter access kit for this device that has a similar-looking template (Figure 5-5, right), but this template is for finding a side port that allows direct intrathecal access. Both kits look identical.

CADD-Prizm PCS Pain Control System pumps.   Patients have died or been injured after an unseen default to a prior setting occurred during programming of a CADD-Prizm PCS Pain Control System pump (model 6101). During programming, the pump will automatically revert to a prior setting if the current setting is not confirmed by pressing Enter within a short period of time. In these cases, fentanyl in a 50 mcg/mL concentration was used and initially programmed into the pump, but a default setting to 1 mcg/mL occurred when the nurses did not press the Enter key within the allotted time.[3]

Hospira's ADD-Vantage system, Baxter's Minibag Plus system, dual-chambered IV containers.   Errors of omission are frequently reported when nurses forget to activate and mix drugs administered intermittently via the ADD-Vantage or Minibag Plus system. Until 1996, heparin was available in a dual-chamber bag that required users to break a seal between the drug and 5% dextrose injection diluent to provide the final admixture. However, staff working on busy medical–surgical units either did not know that mixing was required or forgot to activate the container. In one case, after staff twice neglected to activate the container, a patient's leg had to be amputated because of impaired circulation from deep vein thrombosis. The patient received only dextrose from the bottom chamber; he received no heparin. Similarly designed bags of amino acids and dextrose are still marketed and are likewise occasionally misused.

High-alert drug concentrates in IV additive syringes—Lidocaine concentrate syringes. Before 1993, lidocaine concentrate syringes to facilitate admixture preparation were available from three manufacturers. However, the syringe needle also fit the Y site of IV administration sets. Before the products were discontinued, there were at least 70 deaths or brain injuries from direct IV injection of the drug concentrate. When ISMP became aware of a manufacturer that was considering a similar syringe design for packaging another concentrated cardiac medication, concern was expressed to FDA. This packaging apparently is no longer being considered.

Epi-Pen syringes designed to deliver epinephrine for emergency treatment of allergic reactions. A 1998 study showed that 10% of patients and family members did not know to remove the syringe cap before injection; 62% did not know to hold the syringe in place for at least 10 seconds; and 46% did not know that it could be used without removing clothing.[4] In one reported case, a nurse held the pen upside down and pushed her thumb against the black tip that houses the needle, believing this would uncap the device. Since the black tip is supposed to be placed against the thigh for injection, the spring-loaded needle automatically injected the nurse's thumb instead of the patient's thigh.

Recommendations

These examples show that careful application of human factors and user testing during device design are necessary to identify and correct device attributes that increase the potential for human error. Until FDA demands better-designed devices and forces redesign or removal of unsafe devices currently on the market, implementing the following recommendations can enhance safety:

❑ Use patient-controlled analgesia (PCA) pumps that read bar codes to automatically set the concentration or default to a high concentration or zero setting. Strive to use a single concentration of analgesics. Avoid stocking and using multiple concentrations of the same drug that differ by a factor of 10 (e.g., 0.5 mg/mL and 5 mg/mL of morphine).

❑ Carefully position syringe labels so that important drug information can be seen readily during pump setup and infusion.

❑ Monitor patients frequently and have antidotes readily available.

❑ Consider using oximetry and capnography for PCA patients and those on continuous narcotic infusions so that errors can be detected more rapidly and consequences can be minimized.

❑ Avoid using pumps with a priming function that can deliver a bolus during infusions.

❑ When new devices are purchased, use failure mode and effects analysis (ask what could possibly go wrong) to identify design flaws and all points at which user error might occur so that proactive safety measures can be taken.

❑ Establish a system of independent double checks when high-alert medications (Chapter 14) are administered. For example, have one practitioner program a pump and have another independently check the drug, concentration, rate of infusion, and other pump settings. Verify identification of the patient and use of the correct route and attachment to the appropriate line. Making practitioners aware of poor device design and the potential for user error can encourage the practice of independent verification before administration.

❑ If patients or family members will be using medication delivery devices, provide them with clear spoken and written instructions. Alert them to potential user error with the devices. Require return demonstrations with sufficient practice to ensure competency.

❑ Report drug-related device failure and user error to the USP-ISMP Medication Errors Reporting Program and to FDA so that timely action can be taken to alert others to problems.

1. ECRI. Hazard Report. Abbott PCA Plus II—Patient controlled analgesic pumps prone to misprogramming, resulting in narcotic overinfusions. *Health Devices.* 1997;26:389–91.

2. Template for disaster? Fatal injection into wrong port of implanted infusion pump. *ISMP Medication Safety Alert!* January 15, 2004;9(1):1–2.

3. Safety issues with patient controlled analgesia. Part I: How errors occur. *ISMP Nurse Advise-ERR.* 2005;3(1):1–3.

4. Huang S. A survey of Epi-PEN use in patients with a history of anaphylaxis. *J Allergy Clin Immunol.* 1998;102:525–6.

Once an action has been implemented, it is essential to find out whether (and how much) it has made things better or worse. The strongest outcome measures use a realistic time frame for evaluation and take into account the urgency of the correction. For example, outcome measures for an event that "must never happen again" would be different from measures with a less urgent time frame.

In addition, the measure itself must be clearly defined and quantifiable. A description of how the measurement will be done should be included (e.g., through record review, observation/walk-around, competency testing, questionnaires/surveys, reduction in the frequency of the adverse event or close call, reduction in the severity of the adverse event, increase in the desired activity/behavior). Indirect measures might include increases in teamwork, or reductions in lost time from injuries, staff turnover, equipment breakage or malfunction, and patient and staff complaints. A target population should be described, as well as a sample size and threshold for success (with numerators and denominators).

The best way to craft an outcome measure to fit a particular action is to ask people knowledgeable about the adverse event or close call, "What do you think would prevent this situation from ever happening again?" "How would you know whether or not that action made a difference?" "How would you measure the effect of the action?"

UTILITY OF RCA IN THE MEDICATION-USE PROCESS

The following examples illustrate the applications and benefits of RCA.

- A patient received a large dose of phenytoin suspension, resulting in mild toxicity. The immediate reaction was to blame the nurse for giving the dose. Instead, the RCA team found that system-level issues existed. The resident ordering the drug was confused about how to express the dose in the order entry software. The pharmacist finishing the electronic order was distracted. The medication was supplied to the nurse in bulk bottles, not unit dose packaging. These system-level issues affect more than one patient and one nurse; fixing them yields larger benefits.
- A team looked at an event related to the use of floor-stock IV solutions. It would have been easy to blame the nurse for selecting the wrong IV solution. Instead, the RCA team looked into how the products were replenished and the process for oversight of the items in automated dispensing machines. As a result, system-level improvements were implemented, such as dispensing IV solutions with additives through the pharmacy only. This action benefited many patients, and nurses were freed from some materials management activity.
- Figures 5-1 and 5-2 depict the initial and final understanding of an anticoagulation event. A hospitalized patient was treated with heparin and warfarin. His therapy was changed and restarted and eventually he experienced fatal bleeding. Through the RCA interviews, the team uncovered several processes that contributed to the high level of anticoagulation. The final understanding diagram (Figure 5-2) contains information that was discovered through investigation of system-level causes.
- Figure 5-3 shows an Ishakawa fishbone diagram used in aggregated RCA of anticoagulation-related events. Notations on various branches indicate the portions of the process associated with an adverse event.
- The sidebar on pages 79–80, contributed by ISMP, describes system-based causes of a medication error and strategies for error reduction identified through RCA.
- An appendix contributed by ISMP describes an investigation of root causes and system failures after a fatal error.

TRACING SYSTEM-LEVEL VULNERABILITIES
Institute for Safe Medication Practices

Case Report

A report of a medication error that reached a 4-year-old child demonstrates that errors are almost never caused by the failure of single element in the system. More often, multiple underlying system failures lead to an error. Many of them can be identified through root cause analysis (RCA).

Partial patient identifier. An order for carbamazepine 400 mg twice daily was handwritten for an adult patient with a history of seizures. After receiving the order, a pharmacist retrieved the patient profile by typing the last name only and inadvertently entered the medication into the profile of a 4-year-old child with the same last name.

Computer system weaknesses. During order entry, the pharmacist did not recognize that the dose of carbamazepine would be an overdosage for a small child. In fact, he failed to notice that the patient was a child; patient age was not in a prominent location on the order entry screen. Patients' diagnoses and comorbid conditions were not usually listed on the pharmacy profiles, so the pharmacist was unable to match the prescribed medication to the patient's medical condition. The pharmacy computer did not require entry of a weight for pediatric patients; even if a weight had been entered, there were no functional dose alerts in the system.

Nonstandard MAR checks. A medication administration record (MAR) generated by the pharmacy computer system was delivered to the patient care unit that night, but the nurse did not notice that carbamazepine was listed in error for the child. MAR verification was not standardized in the hospital; it was done in various ways by different nurses—if it was performed at all. There was no official policy requiring MAR verification and no written procedure to refer to, and the process was not covered during nursing orientation.

Adult dose and dosage form for a child. The next morning, after crushing the tablets, a nurse gave the child the first erroneous 400 mg dose of carbamazepine, as listed on the MAR. She failed to recognize that the dose was too high for a child. She did not question why the pharmacy had sent oral tablets for a 4-year-old child or ask whether there was a more suitable dosage form (the drug is available in chewable tablets and as a liquid suspension).

Unverified patient history. The nurse who administered the first dose of carbamazepine assumed that the child was receiving the medication because he had a history of seizures. However, the nurse did not verify this by checking the patient's medical record. Although the child did not have a history of seizures, the nurse passed that erroneous information on to nurses on the next shift, who passed it on in turn. Thus, the child received three doses in error, from three different nurses, all of whom believed the child had a history of seizures.

Language barrier. The child's parents were present when one of the erroneous doses was administered. The nurse had attempted to tell the parents that the medication was used to control seizures. However, the parents, like the child, had a limited understanding of English and were unable to intervene to correct the erroneous seizure history.

Poor physician access to MAR. The child's physician did not detect the error right away during routine rounds. The nursing MAR was not readily accessible for review, and there was no electronic or pharmacy computer-generated summary of prescribed therapy on the chart. Thus, the physician did not notice that his patient was receiving a medication that he had not prescribed.

The error was finally detected after the child became lethargic and developed nausea and vomiting. At that point, one of the nurses suspected a problem with the carbamazepine dose and contacted the physician, who stated that the medication had never been prescribed for the patient. At the time of discovery, the child's carbamazepine level was 18 mcg/mL (normal therapeutic range is 4–12 mcg/mL). This error delayed the child's discharge, although he recovered without further problems.

Discussion

It can be discouraging to see how many things have gone wrong when a medication error reaches a patient. However, RCA clearly demonstrates that there are many ways to avoid similar errors. Had any one of the following system enhancements been present, the error probably would have been prevented or corrected before it reached the child, or at least detected before the child sustained any harm.

❑ Use two patient identifiers (e.g., full name, identification number, date of birth) to verify patient identity when entering orders. Although this is not required by the Joint Commission on Accreditation of Healthcare Organizations, ISMP highly recommends it.

❑ Ask the pharmacy system vendor to build "look-alike patient name" alerts into the order entry system for activation when more than one patient has the same last name.

❑ Use a computerized prescriber order entry system that is interfaced with the pharmacy computer system to eliminate the need for pharmacy order entry.

❑ Standardize, document, and require the use of an MAR verification process whenever new MARs are distributed (or rewritten). Orient new nurses to the required process. Also ask nurses to compare the pharmacy label (on dispensed medications) with the initial MAR entry before the first dose is administered to ensure that the pharmacist's and nurse's interpretation and transcription of a medication order is correct.

❑ Require documentation of medical history (including comorbid conditions) on order entry screens, MARs, and other records used during change-of-shift reports. Establish an effective method for communicating this information to pharmacy so that nurses and pharmacists can always match the prescribed drug therapy to a verified medical condition.

❑ Require recalculation of all doses of pediatric medications before the drug is dispensed (pharmacists) and during initial order transcription/verification onto the MAR (nurses) to ensure that the dose is appropriate.

❑ Require the entry of weight in computer systems before orders for pediatric patients can be processed, and establish a process for timely communication of accurate patient weights from nursing to the pharmacy.

❑ Build and test maximum and subtherapeutic dose alerts in the order entry system (based on patient age and weight when applicable).

❑ Encourage nurses to investigate the possibility of an error if drugs for pediatric patients are dispensed in adult dosage forms.

❑ Post a daily electronic or computer-generated summary of prescribed medications on each patient's chart and educate physicians about its value in detecting inaccuracies.

❑ Provide translators for teaching patients and families about diagnoses, treatment plans, and newly prescribed medications. Offer written drug information sheets (8th grade level or lower) to patients in their primary language. Ask the patient or family to demonstrate their understanding of the written and spoken information provided.

❑ Establish a process for thoroughly investigating all "missing" medications before asking nurses to resend an order or before dispensing the medication again. In this case, carbamazepine had not been dispensed for the intended patient. Thus, nurses likely called the pharmacy for the "missing" medication. When the drug could not be found on the correct patient profile, if a pharmacist had located the initial order and noticed that it had been processed, perhaps further investigation would have resulted in earlier discovery of the error.

CONCLUSION

RCA can show organizations what changes are needed to improve patient safety. However, unless the recommended actions are implemented, the best RCA will not help subsequent patients. An organization should choose a method for RCA that meets its needs. In effective RCA the recommended actions are based on human-factors engineering principles and reduce the burden of memory on staff. Standardized tools and good examples make the work of RCA teams easier and more uniform over time.

REFERENCES

1. Weeks WB, Bagian JP. Developing a culture of safety in the Veterans Health Administration. *Eff Clin Pract.* 2000; 3(Nov–Dec):270–6.
2. Leape LL, Woods DD, Hatlie MJ, et al. Promoting patient safety by preventing medical error [editorial]. *JAMA.* 1998;280:1444–7.
3. Department of Veterans Affairs, National Center for Patient Safety. *NCPS Triage Cards for Root Cause Analysis.* October 2001.
4. Gano D. *Apollo Root Cause Analysis: Effective Solutions to Everyday Problems Every Time.* 2nd ed. Yakima, Wash: Apollonian Publishers; 2003.
5. Reason J. *Human Error.* Cambridge, England: Cambridge University Press; 1990.
6. Marx D. Maintenance Error Causation. Prepared under contract for Office of Aviation Medicine. AAM-240. June 9, 1999.
7. Norman D. *The Design of Everyday Things* (reprint, originally published: *The Psychology of Everyday Things*; 1988). New York: Basic Books; 2002.
8. Gosbee L, Burkhardt M. Application of human factors engineering in process and equipment design. In Manasse H, Thompson K, eds. *Medication Safety: A Guide for Health Care Facilities.* Bethesda, Md: American Society of Health-System Pharmacists; 2005.

APPENDIX

LESSON FROM DENVER: LOOK BEYOND BLAMING INDIVIDUALS

Institute for Safe Medication Practices

In October 1996, a medication error at a Denver area hospital resulted in the death of a newborn infant. The error involved IV administration of a large dose of penicillin G benzathine, a medication that is insoluble and must not be injected intravenously. Since nurses are charged with the responsibility of knowing about the potential dangers of the drugs they administer, many who learned about the incident were quick to blame the death solely on the nurses. The district attorney of Adams County, Colorado, brought this case before a grand jury. Three nurses who were involved in the infant's care were eventually indicted for criminally negligent homicide. In preparation for the trial that followed, a systems analysis was performed by ISMP on behalf of the defense team. The analysis revealed more than 50 latent failures in the system that contributed to the tragedy and allowed the accident to occur.

Latent failures are weaknesses in the structure of an organization, such as faulty information management or ineffective personnel training. These weaknesses are the result of both good and ill-conceived decisions made by upper management.[1] Even the best strategic decision in an organization carries with it both risks and benefits, as well as a certain degree of compromise. Individual winners and losers can be easily identified once a decision is made. However, the far-reaching effects of these decisions often go undetected. This is especially apparent when strategic decisions involve solutions that shift a problem from one part of a system to another and those solving the problem are different from those who ultimately inherit the new problem.[2]

Because it is not possible to immediately recognize all problems associated with management decisions, latent failures are inevitable in all organizations. They lie dormant in the system—hence the term *latent* failures. By themselves, they are often subtle and may cause no problems. Their consequences are hidden, becoming apparent only when they occur in proper sequence with each other and combine with the active failures of individuals to penetrate or bypass the system's safety nets.

Active failures are errors committed by individuals, such as physicians, nurses, or pharmacists, who are in direct contact with vulnerabilities and weaknesses in the structure of an organization. When individuals fall victim to these weaknesses, mistakes are made. Often, it is these points of human fallibility on which we focus our attention.[3] Although it may seem easier to concentrate on the human contribution to errors, the root causes of problems can be traced to latent failures in the systems inherited by individuals in the work force, which often go unnoticed until an error occurs. Therefore, the only effective way to decrease the likelihood of medication errors is to strengthen the system's resistance to chance combinations of latent and active failures.[3]

The Denver case was riddled with both latent and active failures (Table 5-4). Examining that case, described briefly here and in more detail elsewhere,[4] is a useful exercise in identifying failures that may be present in an institution. Any failures discovered through such an exercise should be evaluated by the institution's pharmacy and therapeutics committee.

The mother of this infant had a history of syphilis. Despite incomplete information about her past treatment and the current status of both mother and child, a decision was made to treat the infant for congenital syphilis. (It was later learned that the mother had previously given birth to two healthy children after her disease was successfully treated; her laboratory tests confirmed effective treatment.) After telephone consultation with infectious disease specialists and the health department, an order was written for one dose of "Benzathine Pen G 150,000 U IM" (Figure 5-6).

The physicians, nurses, and pharmacists were unfamiliar with the treatment of congenital syphilis. Furthermore, they had limited knowledge about this nonformulary drug. The pharmacist consulted the infant's progress notes and *Drug Facts and Comparisons* to determine the usual dose of penicillin G benzathine for an infant. However, she misread the dose in both sources as 500,000 units/kg—a typical adult dose—instead of 50,000 units/kg. Consequently, the pharmacist also incorrectly read the "U" for units as two additional zeros and prepared the order as 1,500,000 units, a 10-fold overdose. The pharmacy lacked a consistent procedure for independent double-checking, and the error was not detected. Because a unit dose system was not used in the nursery, the pharmacy dispensed the 10-fold overdose in a plastic bag containing two full syringes of Permapen 1.2 million units/2 mL each, with green stickers on the plungers that warned to "Note Dosage Strength." A pharmacy label on the bag indicated that 2.5 mL of medication was to be administered intramuscularly, to equal a dose of 1,500,000 units.

After glancing at the medication sent from the pharmacy, the infant's primary care nurse expressed concern to her colleagues about the number of injections required to give the infant the medication. (The maximum volume of an IM injection for an infant is 0.5 mL, so the dose would require five injections.) Wanting to prevent unnecessary pain for the infant, two colleagues—an advanced-level nursery staff registered nurse and a neonatal nurse practitioner (NP)—decided to investigate the possibility of administering the medication IV instead of IM. They did not think to call a pharmacist, because pharmacists were rarely on the unit to offer their clinical expertise to the nurses.

Instead, they used references available on the unit, including *Neofax '95*. The Neofax monograph on penicillin G noted the use of aqueous crystalline penicillin G by slow IV push or penicillin G procaine IM for the treatment of congenital syphilis. Nowhere in the two-page monograph was penicillin G benzathine mentioned. No warnings were present about administering penicillin G procaine and penicillin G benzathine by the IM route only.

Unfamiliar with the various forms of penicillin G, the NP believed that "benzathine" was a brand name for penicillin G. This misconception was reinforced by the physician's method of writing the drug order—with "Benzathine" capitalized and placed on a line above "Pen G" rather than after it on the same line (Figure 5-6). Many texts use ambiguous synonyms for the various forms of penicillin; for example, penicillin G benzathine is

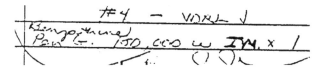

FIGURE 5-6 A misconception that benzathine was a brand name for penicillin G was reinforced by the prescriber's method of writing this order—with Benzathine capitalized and placed above penicillin G, rather than after it on the same line.

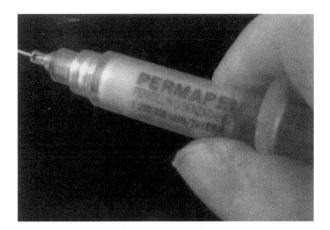

FIGURE 5-7 Although this syringe is labeled "IM use only," the warning is not visible unless the syringe is rotated 180 degrees away from the drug name; furthermore, a right-handed user's thumb can hide the warning.

frequently associated with the terms "crystalline penicillin" and "aqueous suspension." Believing that aqueous crystalline penicillin G and penicillin G benzathine were the same drug, the NP concluded that the drug could be safely administered intravenously. Although the nurses had been taught that only clear liquids can be injected intravenously, they knew that certain milky-white substances, such as lipid-based products, are given IV. Therefore, they did not know that penicillin G benzathine, a milky-white substance, could not be given IV.

Hospital policies and practices did not clearly define the prescribing authority of nonphysicians. In making the decision to administer the drug intravenously, the NP assumed that she was operating under Colorado licensure and a national protocol that allows neonatal NPs to plan, direct, implement, and change drug therapy, as she had done many times before. The infant's primary-care nurse, not certified to administer IV medications to infants, transferred the care of the infant to the advanced-level nurse and the NP.

While preparing to administer the drug, neither the nurse nor the NP noticed the 10-fold overdose or the manufacturer's label on the syringe stating "IM Use Only." The manufacturer's warning is visible only when the syringe is rotated 180 degrees away from the drug name (Figure 5-7). The nurses began to administer the first syringe of Permapen by slow IV push. After about 1.8 mL had been administered, the infant became unresponsive, and resuscitation efforts were unsuccessful.

Medication errors are almost never caused by the failure of a single element or the fault of a single practitioner. Rather, a catastrophic event such as this is the result of the combined effects of latent failures in the system and active failures by individuals (Figure 5-8).[1] Had even one of these failures not occurred, either the accident would not have

TABLE 5-4 Summary of Active and Latent Failures

Key System Elements	Latent Failures	Active Failures
Prescribing Phase		
Patient information	Incomplete clinical information on prior treatment and current status of mother for syphilis Incomplete clinical information on current status of infant for congenital syphilis Lack of systemic method of communicating mother's prenatal care to infant's physician	Decision to treat infant for congenital syphilis
Patient education	Inefficient education of parents about the possibility of congenital syphilis in infant and options for treatment	Decision to treat infant prior to discharge from hospital
Drug information	Insufficient drug information (rarely used in practice or in the hospital)	No active failures: called expert in field for consultation
Communication	Lack of efficient means of communicating with parents when language barrier exists Incomplete communication of drug information Nonstandard method of communicating drug order	Health department recommendation documented in progress notes only as penicillin G, not penicillin G benzathine; route of administration not documented Order for drug written with "Benzathine" capitalized and placed above penicillin G; "IM" appeared written over; "U" used to denote units
Order Processing Phase		
Drug information	Insufficient drug information (rarely used in practice or in the hospital)	Misreading of both health department recommendation and drug resource used to determine units/kg for infant
Staff education and staffing patterns	Lack of specialized training/education in neonatal/pediatric pharmacy Failure to staff pharmacy with neonatal/pediatric pharmacist in a hospital providing these services	Misreading of "U" for units as extra zeros, causing misinterpretation of the order as 10-fold overdose
Quality control	Lack of maximum dose warning system on the pharmacy computer	10-fold overdose not detected
Drug Dispensing Phase		
Quality control	Inconsistent pharmacy procedure for independent double check of drugs before dispensing	10-fold overdose prepared and dispensed without detection of error
Labeling, packaging, and nomenclature of the drug	Lack of unit dose system for dispensing medications to neonatal unit Communication of dose on label in millions numerically instead of phonically	Two syringes, each labeled "1,200,000 units" (instead of 1.2 million units), dispensed in bag with label instructing nurse to give 1,500,000 units (instead of 1.5 million units); "Note Dosage Strength" sticker on plungers Pharmacy label and syringes lacked auxiliary label warning, "For IM Use Only"
Staff education	No procedure for educating staff before dispensing an infrequently used drug	Rarely used drug dispensed without education of staff responsible for administering it

TABLE 5-4 Summary of Active and Latent Failures (continued)

Key System Elements	Latent Failures	Active Failures
Drug information	Insufficient information on volume of medication that can be safely administered IM to neonates (maximum of 0.5 mL per injection) Insufficient information on serious effects of several IM injections of drug in neonates	Medication dispensed with directions to administer 2.5 mL of drug IM to neonate, requiring five separate injections with a 1½ inch needle

Drug Administration Phase

Drug information	Insufficient information about various forms of penicillin G (never used penicillin G benzathine before in practice; rarely used drug) Inadequate drug references; penicillin G benzathine frequently referred to by the ambiguous synonym "crystalline penicillin" or "aqueous suspension" Inadequate drug reference: Neofax '95 does not mention penicillin G benzathine in the monograph but notes that aqueous crystalline penicillin G IV push is used to treat congenital syphilis; no specific warnings that penicillin G benzathine (or procaine) can be administered only IM Inadequate drug reference: NICU Medication Administration does not mention penicillin G benzathine in monograph for penicillin G Conflicting information about IV use of milky-white substances Lack of Food and Drug Administration requirement for "black box" or other vivid warning about IV administration of penicillin G benzathine in drug monographs Pharmacists were not well known by nurses; little face-to-face contact	Benzathine misunderstood as brand name for aqueous penicillin G (reinforced by physician's order with "Benzathine" capitalized and placed above "penicillin G") Incorrectly thought that "aqueous penicillin" was penicillin G benzathine; consequently, problem with IV administration went unrecognized Decision to administer drug IV to avoid pain from multiple IM injections
Competency	Hospital had unclear definition of prescribing authority for nonphysicians	Nurse practitioner assumed authority to change route of administration on basis of current licensure, national protocol, and current practice in hospital
Labeling, packaging, and nomenclature of the drug	Manufacturer's warning for "IM Use Only" not prominently placed on syringe; cannot be seen unless syringe is rotated 180 degrees away from the drug name When syringe plunger is depressed, black ring obscures the warning and other black print Manufacturer states dose in all numerals (1,200,000 units, not 1.2 million units), which leads to errors when comma is misread	Warning on syringe for "IM Use Only" not seen 10-fold overdose not recognized Penicillin G benzathine administered intravenously

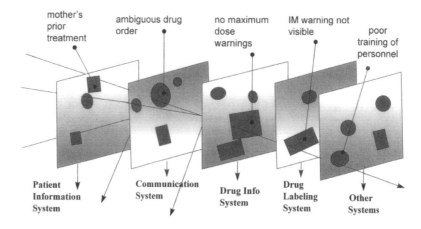

FIGURE 5-8   Medication errors are almost never caused by the failure of a single element; rather, they result from the combined effects of latent failures in the system and active failures by individuals.

happened or the error would have been detected and corrected before reaching the infant. The actions of individuals are largely governed by systems, and the causes of errors often are not within the control of individuals, despite their best efforts.

After hearing the evidence in this case, the jury found the nurses not guilty. This verdict delivered an important message to health care providers: We must look beyond blaming individuals and focus on the multiple underlying systems failures that shape individual behavior and create the conditions under which medication errors occur.

1. Reason H. The contribution of latent human failures to the breakdown of complex systems. *Philos Trans R Soc Lond B Biol Sci.* 1990;327, 475–84.
2. Senge PM, Kleiner A, Roberts C, et al. *The Fifth Discipline Fieldbook: Strategies and Tools for Building a Learning Organization.* New York: Currency Doubleday; 1994: 91–4.
3. Reason J. Foreword. In: Bogner MS, ed. *Human Error in Medicine.* Hillsdale, NJ: Erlbaum; 1994: vii–xv.
4. Smetzer JL, Cohen MR. Lesson from the Denver medication error/criminal negligence case: look beyond blaming individuals. *Hosp Pharm.* 1998;33:640–57.

CHAPTER 6

THE ROLE OF DRUG NAMES IN MEDICATION ERRORS

Michael R. Cohen, George Di Domizio, and Robert E. Lee, Jr.

Trademarks (brand names) for drug products are intended to be unique and memorable—to provide a simple and convenient way to identify products and distinguish one manufacturer's product from its competitors. However, as noted in the Institute of Medicine (IOM) report *To Err Is Human: Building a Safer Health System*[1] and the 2006 IOM report *Preventing Medication Errors*,[2] pharmaceutical trademarks that look or sound alike have a major role in medication errors. Confusion related to product names is one of the most common causes of medication errors reported to the U.S. Pharmacopeia (USP), the Food and Drug Administration (FDA), and the Institute for Safe Medication Practices (ISMP).[3]

Why do drug name mix-ups occur? Some would say that pharmaceutical manufacturers should be more careful in developing and adopting trademarks.[4] Others would say prescribers are too careless when they write or phone in orders and too slow to adopt computerized prescribing. When names are blurred on handwritten prescriptions or slurred in spoken orders, medication errors are more likely, as illustrated by the examples in this and other chapters. Busy pharmacists may not have time to make phone calls to clarify or verify orders, or to implement error-prevention practices such as computerized reminders of problem name pairs. Health care institutions may not have adequate safety protocols. FDA and other regulatory organizations are often criticized for not doing more to prevent problem-prone names from entering the market and for reacting too slowly when problems surface.

As we seek to create an environment with fewer medication errors, it is helpful to examine the sources of trademark-related errors. It is also helpful to review what FDA, manufacturers, and practitioners have learned in recent years and what they are doing to minimize medication errors.

PREVENTING ERRORS INVOLVING SIMILAR DRUG NAMES

Which names look or sound alike is subjective. Little research on the topic is available, but regulators and industry have begun discussing what level of similarity leads to confusion and error.

In June 2003, FDA, ISMP, and the Pharmaceutical Research and Manufacturers of America (PhRMA) sponsored a public meeting to explore methods of evaluating the error potential of proposed new trademarks.[4] There was broad agreement among experts that the current processes lacked a validated standard, were not objective, and could not be relied on to produce repeatable results. The development of good naming practices for product sponsors was proposed.

In December 2003, the FDA Drug Safety and Risk Management Advisory Committee (DSaRM) concluded that research is needed to determine the role of trademarks as a contributing factor to medication errors.[5] The committee recommended that FDA, PhRMA, and other interested parties meet to agree on causation research and prevention methods and then report back to the committee.

The *ISMP Medication Safety Alert!* newsletter has published many examples of errors related to handwriting and drug nomenclature, with recommendations for prevention, such as the following.

- *Daptomycin (Cubicin) and dactinomycin (Cosmegen):* Similarity of the generic names led to a mix-up between the antibiotic daptomycin and the cancer drug dactinomycin. Both agents are given once daily, supplied as lyophilized powders, and reconstituted to a yellowish solution, but because of differences in dosing, the error was detected before it reached the patient. ISMP recommends building name alert warnings into the pharmacy computer system, verifying the indication before dispensing either drug, and using shelf stickers to alert staff to these look-alike names.
- *Mucomyst (acetylcysteine) and Mucinex (guaifenesin):* Two patients received the wrong medication because of mix-ups between this pair. Neither patient was harmed, but serious injury could occur if Mucomyst was inadvertently not administered to treat an acetaminophen overdose or prevent contrast media–induced nephrotoxicity. ISMP recommends confirming the indication before dispensing and administering any medication.
- *Purinethol (mercaptopurine) and propylthiouracil:* A child with leukemia missed 6 months of chemotherapy because propylthiouracil, an antithyroid agent, was dispensed instead of the antimetabolite Purinethol. Mix-ups in which Purinethol was dispensed instead of propylthiouracil have also been reported. Propylthiouracil doses are often several hundred milligrams a day, and mistakes that result in giving Purinethol at these high doses could cause harm. ISMP recommends that the two drugs not be stored near each other, and that warnings posted on storage bins and alerts in computer systems be used to remind staff about the potential for confusion between the pair. Prescribers should list both brand and generic names on orders for Purinethol. In outpatient pharmacy dispensing, the National Drug Code number should be matched against the one listed in the computer database.

An extensive list of look-alike and sound-alike medication names that have been involved in errors described in the *ISMP Medication Safety Alert!* is available at www.ismp. org/Tools/confuseddrugnames.pdf. The following scenarios involving names that look or sound similar further illustrate the problem and suggest error-prevention strategies.

Name Changes

Some trademarks have been changed in response to serious medication errors. A patient for whom the thyroid preparation Levoxine had been prescribed received Lanoxin (digoxin) after a pharmacist misread the prescription (Figure 6-1).[6] In addition to having similar brand names, these medications have the same dosage form (tablet), route of administration (oral), and frequency of administration (daily) and share an uncommon tablet strength (0.125 mg). After similar errors involving this trademark pair were reported, ISMP and FDA advocated a name change, and the manufacturer of Levoxine changed the product name to Levoxyl.

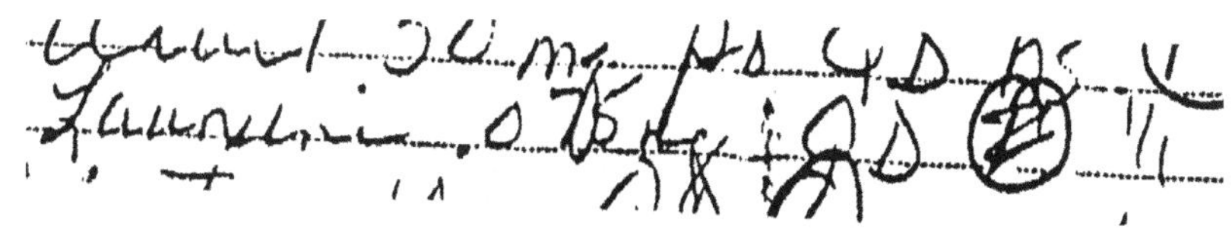

FIGURE 6-1 Levoxine (lower line) was read as Lanoxin.

In 1990, some patients who were supposed to receive Losec (omeprazole) accidentally received Lasix (furosemide), a diuretic. Since each product was prescribed at 20 mg and the names appeared quite similar when written in cursive script, practitioners confused the two drugs. Merck, which licensed Losec in the United States, changed the product trademark to Prilosec after the company received several reports of errors, near misses, and practitioner concerns from both the hospital and retail sectors.

More recently, Janssen changed the trademark for Reminyl (galantamine), its drug for Alzheimer's disease, to Razadyne because of several reports of confusion with Amaryl, a drug used to lower blood sugar in patients with diabetes. Both medications were available in a 4 mg oral dosage form. Accidental administration of Amaryl poses great danger to any patient, especially an older patient with Alzheimer's who may be more sensitive to its hypoglycemic effect. Practitioners were alerted to the potential for serious error by ISMP and FDA, as well as through Dear Doctor and Dear Pharmacist letters from the company.

Another recent name change involved two cholesterol-lowering agents. This case highlights FDA's concern about medication errors and a sponsor's legal concerns about infringement. Kos Pharmaceuticals received FDA approval in February 2002 to market Advicor, a combination product containing niacin and lovastatin. Andrx received FDA approval in May 2002 to market Altocor, its extended-release formulation of lovastatin. Although FDA reviewed and approved both of these names, Kos did not believe the names should coexist. Kos instituted an infringement action in court against Andrx. At about that time, when medication errors surfaced, FDA also requested a name change from Andrx, and the company changed the name from Altocor to Altoprev.

Use of Tall-Man Letters

Changing a name is not the only way to manage risks associated with similar name pairs. After reports of mix-ups between Zyprexa (olanzapine), an antipsychotic from Lilly, and Zyrtec (cetirizine), an antihistamine from Pfizer, the *ISMP Medication Safety Alert!* newsletter suggested using "tall-man" (mixed-case or enlarged) letters to emphasize the differing portions of the two names.[7] Research has shown that this approach can effectively differentiate names.[8–10]

Tall-man letters have been used successfully to alert health professionals to the potential for error with several generic name pairs. For example, hydroxyzine and hydralazine look like hydrOXYzine and hydrALAZINE. FDA now requires that tall-man letters be used in 16 generic name pairs that are associated with errors (Table 6-1).

Lilly voluntarily modified its package label in November 2002 and took other actions to help clinicians avoid dispensing mix-ups between Zyprexa and Zyrtec (Figure 6-2, left). As shown in Figure 6-2 (right), the use of tall-man letters puts the visual emphasis on PREXA, the portion of the trademark that is different from RTEC in Zyrtec.

Similarly, GlaxoSmithKline modified the labeling of its antiepileptic drug Lamictal (lamotrigine). The company changed the package label to reduce the potential for errors due to confusion with Lamisil (terbinafine), a Novartis product (Figure 6-3, left). The new label (Figure 6-3, right) highlights the ICTAL part of the name by italicizing it and placing it on a yellow background with red letters. In addition, the front label panel states,

TABLE 6-1   FDA Recommended Revisions
in Generic Name Pairs

Drug Product	Recommended Revisions
acetohexamide	acetoHEXAMIDE
acetazolamide	acetaZOLAMIDE
bupropion	buPROPion
buspirone	busPIRone
chlorpromazine	chlorproMAZINE
chlorpropamide	chlorproPAMIDE
clomiphene	clomiPHENE
clomipramine	clomiPRAMINE
cyclosporine	cycloSPORINE
cycloserine	cycloSERINE
daunorubicin	DAUNOrubicin
doxorubicin	DOXOrubicin
dimenhydrinate	dimenhyDRINATE
diphenhydramine	diphenhydrAMINE
dobutamine	DOBUTamine
dopamine	DOPamine
glipizide	glipiZIDE
glyburide	glyBURIDE
hydralazine	hydrALAZINE
hydroxyzine	hydrOXYzine
medroxyprogesterone	medroxyPROGESTERone
methylprednisolone	methylPREDNISolone
methyltestosterone	methylTESTOSTERone
nicardipine	niCARdipine
nifedipine	NIFEdipine
prednisone	predniSONE
prednisolone	prednisoLONE
sulfadiazine	sulfADIAZINE
sulfisoxazole	sulfiSOXAZOLE
tolazamide	TOLAZamide
tolbutamide	TOLBUTamide
vinblastine	vinBLAStine
vincristine	vinCRIStine

"CAUTION: Verify Product Dispensed," and the company conducted an educational campaign about the problem and resulting label changes.

LISTS OF SIMILAR NAME PAIRS

USP periodically publishes a list of look-alike and sound-alike drug names (www.usp. org/patientSafety/newsletters/qualityReview/qr792004-04-01.html). Name pairs that have been included in medication error reports are listed alphabetically. The list can be used to

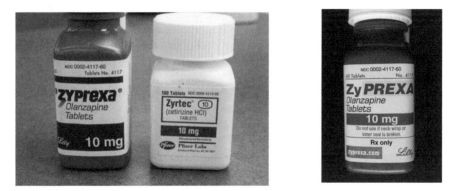

FIGURE 6-2 Former Zyprexa label (left) next to Zyrtec label. New Zyprexa label is at right.

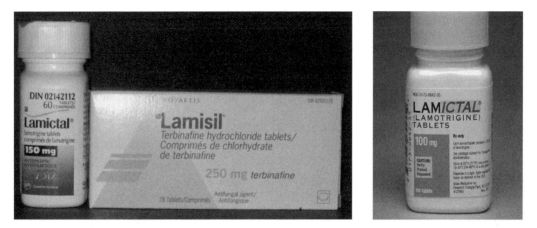

FIGURE 6-3 The Lamictal label (left) has changed to help prevent confusion with Lamisil. The new Lamictal label is at right.

identify products for which reminders such as auxiliary labeling or computerized alerts may be appropriate. However, the USP compilation has limited usefulness, for several reasons:

- With nearly 1,000 name pairs, the list is too long for practitioners to remember. Also, for such a compilation to be useful during drug dispensing, a practitioner would need to recognize that a prescription is unclear. However, confirmation bias (seeing that which is most familiar while overlooking any evidence to the contrary) sometimes causes pharmacists or nurses to automatically "recognize" a familiar name instead of the unfamiliar actual name. (They have no reason to check the list, because they truly believe they have identified the correct drug.)
- Some name pairs with little or no trademark similarity may be on the list because of packaging or other problems.
- There is no easy way to distinguish name pairs that are listed because of a single practitioner's report of a possible problem from pairs that have been involved in multiple actual errors with serious consequences.

More practical lists of potentially problematic drug names have been developed for the Joint Commission on Accreditation of Healthcare Organizations (JCAHO) by ISMP in collaboration with FDA, USP, and a peer review panel established for this purpose by ISMP. These lists (Tables 6-2 through 6-4) were posted on JCAHO's Web site with instructions for addressing a 2005 JCAHO National Patient Safety Goal (NPSG): at least annually, review a list of look-alike and sound-alike drug names and take action to prevent mix-ups. Each health care organization was asked to choose five items from Table 6-2 or Table 6-3, as appropriate, and five more from any of these three tables.

The panel of medication safety experts selected these sets of drug names as those with the greatest potential to cause confusion and result in serious errors. Although JCAHO's NPSG requires organizations to address just 10 of these name pairs, all practitioners and facilities that provide patient care, including nonaccredited sites, would benefit from learning about the problems noted in the tables and following the recommendations. In addition to the specific safety strategies suggested in the tables, the JCAHO site includes general recommendations for preventing drug name mix-ups, prepared in collaboration with ISMP (sidebar, pages 100–101).[11,12]

GENERIC NAME MIX-UPS

It is important to understand the ways in which both trademarks and nonproprietary drug names are selected.[13] Most drugs have the same nonproprietary (generic) name throughout the world. This facilitates global scientific discourse, and many academic institutions encourage preferential use of generic names. The World Health Organization (WHO) International Nonproprietary Names (INN) committee works to develop generic drug names that will be accepted worldwide. In the United States, the U.S. Adopted Names (USAN) Council, a group with representatives from medical, pharmaceutical, and regulatory organizations, assigns generic drug names. The USAN Council designates a name only after the WHO INN committee has approved a name for the drug.

During this process, only cursory measures are taken to ensure that proposed nonproprietary names do not conflict with existing trademarks (brand names) or generic names. Although the USAN expert committee performs internal analysis before assigning or approving generic names, no study or testing of names for similarity with other drug names is undertaken. In contrast, many pharmaceutical companies base their final choice of a trademark on protocols that engage frontline practitioners, expert panels, and computer-assisted searching to help predict whether the proposed name could contribute to look-alike or sound-alike errors or other confusion. The need for such assessment was highlighted in recent FDA guidance for industry.[14]

It is apparent from the list of drug names selected for the JCAHO NPSG that generic name mix-ups can contribute to medication errors. Nine of the 10 sets of potentially problematic names on the hospital list (Table 6-2) include generic names. Also, the USAN may differ from the INN, and this can add an element of confusion. For example, acetaminophen is known as paracetamol outside the United States, and glyburide is glibenclamide.

A resolution encouraging practice settings to use only generic names for new, single-active-ingredient products marketed after January 1, 2006, was adopted at USP's 2005 convention. The resolution was intended to improve safety. However, if only generic names were used, many physicians, pharmacists, nurses, and others could have so much difficulty recalling and properly spelling those names that errors would increase. Or, practitioners could resort to the use of abbreviations, with the same result.

TABLE 6-2 Look-Alike and Sound-Alike Drug Choices—Critical Access Hospital, Hospital, and Office-Based Surgery[a,b]

Potentially Problematic Names[c]	Brand and Generic Names[c]	Potential Errors and Consequences	Safety Strategies
cisplatin and carboplatin	Platinol (cisplatin) Paraplatin (carboplatin)	Similarity in names can lead to confusion between these two products. Doses appropriate for carboplatin usually exceed the maximum safe dose of cisplatin. Severe toxicity and death have been associated with accidental cisplatin overdoses.	Install maximum-dose warnings in computer systems. A boxed warning notes that cisplatin doses greater than 100 mg/m^2 once every 3 to 4 weeks are rarely used and that the package insert should be consulted for further information. Use safe-handling recommendations and safety stickers for cisplatin as provided by manufacturer. Do not store these two agents next to each other. Use generic names when prescribing and not chemical names or abbreviations.
Concentrated liquid morphine products versus conventional liquid morphine concentrations	Concentrated: Roxanol, MSIR Conventional: morphine oral liquid	Concentrated forms of oral morphine solution (20 mg/mL) have often been confused with the standard concentration (listed as 10 mg/ 5 mL or 20 mg/5 mL), leading to serious errors. Accidental selection of the wrong concentration, and prescribing/labeling the product by volume, not milligrams, contributes to these errors, some of which have been fatal. For example, "10 mg" has been confused with "10 mL." If concentrated product is used, this represents a 20-fold overdose.	Dispense concentrated oral morphine solutions only when ordered for a specific patient (not as unit stock). Segregate the concentrated solution from the other concentrations wherever it is stored. Purchase and dispense concentrated solutions in dropper bottles (available from at least two manufacturers) to help prevent dose measurement errors and differentiate the concentrated product from the conventional products. Verify that patients and caregivers understand how to measure the proper dose for self-administration at home. For inpatients, dispense concentrated solutions in unit doses.
ephedrine and epinephrine	Adrenalin (epinephrine) ephedrine	The names of these two medications look very similar, and their clinical uses make storage near each other likely, especially in obstetrical areas. Both products are available in similar packaging (1 mL amber ampuls and vials).	See general recommendations (sidebar, pages 100–101).
fentanyl and sufentanil	Sublimaze (fentanyl) Sufenta (sufentanil)	The products are not interchangeable. Confusion has resulted in episodes of respiratory arrest due to potency differences between these drugs. Some errors occurred when sufentanil was used during shortages of fentanyl.	Do not stock sufentanil in patient care units outside OR/PACU[d] settings. Do not store these agents near one another if both products are available (e.g., pharmacy anesthesia supplies).

TABLE 6-2   Look-Alike and Sound-Alike Drug Choices—Critical Access Hospital, Hospital, and Office-Based Surgery[a,b] (continued)

Potentially Problematic Names[c]	Brand and Generic Names[c]	Potential Errors and Consequences	Safety Strategies
hydromorphone injection and morphine injection	Dilaudid (hydromorphone) Astramorph, Duramorph, Infumorph (morphine)	Some health care providers have mistakenly believed that hydromorphone is the generic equivalent of morphine. However, these products are not interchangeable. Fatal errors have occurred when hydromorphone was confused with morphine; based on equianalgesic dose conversion, this may represent significant overdose, leading to serious adverse events. Storage of the two medications in close proximity and in similar concentrations may contribute to such errors. Confusion has resulted in episodes of respiratory arrest due to potency differences between these drugs.	Stock specific strengths for each product that are dissimilar. For example, stock units with hydromorphone 1 mg unit dose cartridges, and morphine in 2 mg unit dose cartridges. Ensure that health care providers are aware that these two products are not interchangeable.
Insulin products: Lantus and Lente Humalog and Humulin Novolog and Novolin Humulin and Novolin Humalog and Novolog Novolin 70/30 and Novolog Mix 70/30	Lantus (insulin glargine) Lente (insulin zinc suspension) Humulin (human insulin products) Humalog (insulin lispro) Novolin (human insulin products) Novolog (human insulin aspart) Novolin 70/30 (70% isophane insulin [NPH] and 30% insulin injection [regular]) Novlog Mix 70/30 (70% insulin aspart protamine suspension and 30% insulin aspart)	Similar names, strengths, and concentration ratios of some products (e.g., 70/30) have contributed to medication errors. Mix-ups have also occurred between the 100 units/mL and 500 units/mL insulin concentrations.	Limit the use of insulin analog 70/30 mixtures to just a single product. Limit the variety of insulin products stored in patient care units, and remove patient-specific insulin vials from stock upon discharge. For drug selection screens, emphasize the word "mixture" or "mix" along with the name of the insulin product mixtures. Consider auxiliary labels for newer products to differentiate them from the established products. Also apply bold labels on atypical insulin concentrations.

Lipid-based daunorubicin and doxorubicin products versus conventional forms of daunorubicin and doxorubicin	Lipid-based: Doxil (doxorubicin liposomal) Daunoxome (daunorubicin citrate liposomal) Conventional: Cerubidine (daunorubicin, conventional) Adriamycin, Rubex (doxorubicin, conventional)	Many drugs now come in liposomal formulations indicated for special patient populations. Confusion may occur between the liposomal and the conventional formulation because of name similarity. The products are not interchangeable. Lipid-based formulation dosing guidelines differ significantly from conventional dosing. For example, a standard dose of doxorubicin liposomal is 20 mg/m^2 given at 21-day intervals, compared with doses of 50 to 75 mg/m^2 every 21 days for conventional drug. Doses of liposomal daunorubicin are typically 40 mg/m^2 repeated every 2 weeks, while doses of conventional daunorubicin vary greatly and may be administered more frequently. Accidental administration of the liposomal form instead of the conventional form has resulted in severe side effects and death.	Staff involved in handling these products should be aware of the differences between conventional and lipid-based formulations. Encourage staff to refer to the lipid-based products by their brand names and not just their generic names. Stop and verify that the correct drug is being used if staff, patients, or family members notice a change in the solution's appearance from previous infusions. Lipid-based products may be seen as cloudy rather than a clear solution. Storage of lipid-based products in patient care areas and automated dispensing cabinets is highly discouraged. Include specific method of administration for these products.
Lipid-based amphotericin products versus conventional forms of amphotericin	Lipid-based: Ambisome (amphotericin B liposomal) Abelcet (amphotericin B lipid complex) Amphotec (amphotericin B cholesteryl sulfate complex for injection) Conventional: Amphocin, Fungizone Intravenous (amphotericin B desoxycholate)	Many drugs now come in liposomal formulations indicated for special patient populations. Confusion may occur between the liposomal and the conventional formulations because of name similarity. The products are not interchangeable. Lipid-based formulation dosing guidelines differ significantly from conventional dosing. Conventional amphotercin B desoxycholate doses should not exceed 1.5 mg/kg/day. Doses of the lipid-based products are higher, but vary from product to product. If conventional amphotericin B is given at a dose appropriate for a lipid-based product, a severe adverse event is likely. Confusion between these products has resulted in episodes of respiratory arrest and other dangerous, sometimes fatal outcomes due to potency differences between these drugs.	Staff involved in handling these products should be aware of the differences between conventional and lipid-based formulations. Encourage staff to refer to the lipid-based products by their brand names and not just their generic names. Stop and verify that the correct drug is being used if staff, patients, or family members notice a change in the solution's appearance from previous infusions. Lipid-based products may be seen as cloudy rather than a clear solution. Storage of lipid-based products in patient care areas and automated dispensing cabinets is highly discouraged. To reduce potential for confusion, consider limiting lipid-based amphotericin B products to one specific brand.

TABLE 6-2 Look-Alike and Sound-Alike Drug Choices—Critical Access Hospital, Hospital, and Office-Based Surgery[a,b] (continued)

Potentially Problematic Names[c]	Brand and Generic Names[c]	Potential Errors and Consequences	Safety Strategies
Taxol and Taxotere	Taxol (paclitaxel) Taxotere (docetaxel)	Confusion between these two drugs can result in serious adverse outcomes since they have different dosing recommendations and use in various types of cancer.	Install maximum-dose warnings in computer systems to alert staff to name mix-ups during order entry. Do not store these agents near one another.
vinblastine and vincristine	Velban (vinblastine) Oncovin (vincristine)	Fatal errors have occurred, often because of name similarity, when patients were erroneously given vincristine intravenously, but at the higher vinblastine dose. A typical vincristine dose is usually capped at around 1.4 mg/m^2 weekly. The vinblastine dose is variable but, for most adults, the weekly dosage range is 5.5 to 7.4 mg/m^2.	Install maximum-dose warnings in computer systems to alert staff to name mix-ups during order entry. Do not store these agents near one another. Staff involved in handling these products should be aware of the differences. Use brand names or brand and generic names when prescribing and do not use abbreviations for these drug names.

[a] A 2005 National Patient Safety Goal set by the Joint Commission on Accreditation of Healthcare Organizations was for organizations to, at least annually, review a list of look-alike and sound-alike drug names and take action to prevent mix-ups. Each health care organization in this category was to choose five items from this table (Table 6-2) and five more from Tables 6-2 through 6-4.

[b] The names on this list were selected after review of error reports received by the Institute for Safe Medication Practices, the United States Pharmacopeia, and the U.S. Food and Drug Administration and of previously published listings of sound-alike and look-alike drug names. Ratings based on judgments of severity and likelihood of confusion in the clinical setting were then provided by outside experts using a modified Delphi process.

[c] Names beginning with capital letters are brand names; names beginning with lowercase letters are generic names.

[d] OR = operating room; PACU = postanesthesia care unit.

TABLE 6-3 Look-Alike and Sound-Alike Drug Choices—Ambulatory Care, Assisted Living, Behavioral Health Care, Disease-Specific Care, Home Care, and Long-Term Care[a,b]

Potentially Problematic Names[c]	Brand and Generic Names[c]	Potential Errors and Consequences	Safety Strategies
Amaryl and Reminyl	Amaryl (glimepiride) Reminyl (galantamine hydrobromide)	Handwritten orders for Amaryl (used for type 2 diabetes) and Reminyl[d] (used for Alzheimer's disease) can look similar. Patients receiving Amaryl in error would not be provided with blood glucose monitoring, which could lead to a serious error.	See general recommendations (sidebar, pages 100–101).
Avandia and Coumadin	Avandia (rosiglitazone) Coumadin (warfarin)	Poorly handwritten orders for Avandia (used for type 2 diabetes) have been misread as Coumadin (used to prevent blood clot formation), leading to potentially serious adverse events. Mix-ups originally occurred because of unfamiliarity with Avandia; staff read the order as the more familiar Coumadin. However, mix-ups between these two products continue to occur. Neither medication is safe without appropriate monitoring that is specific to the drug.	See general recommendations (sidebar, pages 100–101).
Celebrex and Celexa and Cerebyx	Celebrex (celecoxib) Celexa (citalopram hydrobromide) Cerebyx (fosphenytoin)	Patients affected by a mix-up between these drugs may experience a decline in mental status, lack of pain or seizure control, or other serious adverse events.	See general recommendations (sidebar, pages 100–101).
clonidine and clonazepam (Klonopin)	Catapres (clonidine) Klonopin (clonazepam)	The generic name clonidine can easily be confused with the trade or generic name for clonazepam.	See general recommendations (sidebar, pages 100–101).
Concentrated liquid morphine products versus conventional liquid morphine concentrations	Concentrated: Roxanol, MSIR Conventional: morphine oral liquid	Concentrated forms of oral morphine solution (20 mg/mL) have often been confused with the standard concentration (listed as 10 mg/5 mL or 20 mg/5 mL), leading to serious errors. Accidental selection of the wrong concentration, and prescribing/labeling the product by volume, not milligrams, contributes to these errors, some of which have been fatal. For example, "10 mg" has been confused with "10 mL." If concentrated product is used, this represents a 20-fold overdose.	Dispense concentrated oral morphine solutions only when ordered for a specific patient (not as unit stock). Segregate the concentrated solution from the other concentrations wherever it is stored. Purchase and dispense concentrated solutions in dropper bottles (available from at least two manufacturers) to help prevent dose measurement errors and to differentiate the concentrated product from conventional products. Verify that patients and caregivers understand how to measure the proper dose for self-administration at home. Dispense concentrated solutions in unit doses if possible for residents in long-term care facilities.

TABLE 6-3 Look-Alike and Sound-Alike Drug Choices—Ambulatory Care, Assisted Living, Behavioral Health Care, Disease-Specific Care, Home Care, and Long-Term Care[a,b] (continued)

Potentially Problematic Names[c]	Brand and Generic Names[c]	Potential Errors and Consequences	Safety Strategies
hydromorphone injection and morphine injection	Dilaudid (hydromorphone) Astramorph, Duramorph, Infumorph (morphine)	Some health care providers have mistakenly believed that hydromorphone is the generic equivalent of morphine. However, these products are not interchangeable. Fatal errors have occurred when hydromorphone was confused with morphine. Based on equianalgesic dose conversion, this may represent significant overdose, leading to serious adverse events. Storage of the two medications in close proximity and in similar concentrations may contribute to such errors. Confusion has resulted in episodes of respiratory arrest due to potency differences between these drugs.	Stock specific strengths for each product that are dissimilar. For example, stock units with hydromorphone 1 mg unit dose cartridges, and morphine in 2 mg unit dose cartridges. Ensure that health care providers are aware that these two products are not interchangeable.
Insulin products: Lantus and Lente Humalog and Humulin Novolog and Novolin Humulin and Novolin Humalog and Novolog Novolin 70/30 and Novolog Mix 70/30	Lantus (insulin glargine) Lente (insulin zinc suspension) Humulin (human insulin products) Humalog (insulin lispro) Novolin (human insulin products) Novolog (human insulin aspart) Novolin 70/30 (70% isophane insulin [NPH] and 30% insulin injection [regular]) Novolog Mix 70/30 (70% insulin aspart protamine suspension and 30% insulin aspart)	Similar names, strengths, and concentration ratios of some products (e.g., 70/30) have contributed to medication errors. Mix-ups have also occurred between the 100 units/mL and 500 units/mL insulin concentrations.	For drug selection screens, emphasize the word "mixture" or "mix" along with the name of the insulin product mixtures. Consider auxiliary labels for newer products to differentiate them from the established products. Also apply bold labels on atypical insulin concentrations.
Lamisil and Lamictal	Lamisil (terbinafine hydrochloride) Lamictal (lamotrigine)	Patients with epilepsy who do not receive Lamictal because of an error would be inadequately treated and could experience serious consequences. Conversely, patients erroneously receiving Lamictal would be unnecessarily subjected to a risk of potential adverse effects (including serious rash) and would miss important antifungal therapy.	See general recommendations (sidebar, pages 100–101).

| Serzone and Seroquel | Serzone (nefazodone)
Seroquel (quetiapine) | Beyond name similarity, these medications are both available in 100 mg and 200 mg strengths; both have similar instructions and dosage ranges; and both are used in similar clinical settings. Sedation or dizziness has occurred when Seroquel was dispensed instead of Serzone. Decompensation of mental status has occurred when Serzone was given instead of Seroquel. Further, there are many potentially dangerous drug interactions with Serzone. For example, there are reports of serious, sometimes fatal, reactions when patients receiving monoamine oxidase inhibitors are given drugs with pharmacologic properties similar to nefazodone. | See general recommendations (sidebar, pages 100–101). |
| Zyprexa and Zyrtec | Zyprexa (olanzapine)
Zyrtec (cetirizine) | Name similarity has resulted in frequent mix-ups between Zyrtec, an antihistamine, and Zyprexa, an antipsychotic. Patients who receive Zyprexa in error have reported dizziness, sometimes leading to injury from a fall. Patients on Zyprexa for a mental illness have relapsed when given Zyrtec in error. | See general recommendations (sidebar, pages 100–101). |

---

a A 2005 National Patient Safety Goal set by the Joint Commission on Accreditation of Healthcare Organizations was for organizations to, at least annually, review a list of look-alike and sound-alike drug names and take action to prevent mix-ups. Each health care organization in this category was to choose five items from this table (Table 6-3) and five more from Tables 6-2 through 6-4.

b The names on this list were selected after review of error reports received by the Institute for Safe Medication Practices, the United States Pharmacopeia, and the U.S. Food and Drug Administration and of previously published listings of sound-alike and look-alike drug names. Ratings based on judgments of severity and likelihood of confusion in the clinical setting were then provided by outside experts using a modified Delphi process.

c Names beginning with capital letters are brand names; names beginning with lowercase letters are generic names.

d Reminyl was changed to Razadyne in 2005.

TABLE 6-4   Additional Name Sets for Use in Meeting National Patient Safety Goal[a,b]

---

acetohexamide, acetazolamide
Advicor, Advair
Avinza, Evista
bretylium, Brevibloc
chlorpropamide, chlorpromazine
Diabeta, Zebeta
Diflucan, Diprivan
folic acid, leucovorin calcium ("folinic acid")
heparin, Hespan
idarubicin, doxorubicin, daunorubicin
lamivudine, lamotrigine
Leukeran, leucovorin calcium
opium tincture, paregoric (camphorated opium tincture)
Prilosec, Prozac
Primacor, Primaxin
Retrovir, Ritonavir
tizanidine, tiagabine
Wellbutrin SR, Wellbutrin XL
Zantac, Xanax
Zantac, Zyrtec

---

[a] A 2005 National Patient Safety Goal set by the Joint Commission on Accreditation of Healthcare Organizations was for organizations to, at least annually, review a list of look-alike and sound-alike drug names and take action to prevent mix-ups. Each health care organization was to select five items from Table 6-2 or 6-3 as appropriate and an additional five from Tables 6-2 through 6-4. The supplemental sets in Table 6-4 were rated or suggested by experts.
[b] Names beginning with capital letters are brand names; names beginning with lowercase letters are generic names.

RECOMMENDATIONS FOR PREVENTING DRUG NAME MIX-UPS[11,12]
What Prescribers Can Do

❑ Maintain awareness of look-alike and sound-alike drug names as published by various safety agencies.
❑ Clearly specify the dosage form, drug strength, and complete directions on prescriptions. These variables may help staff differentiate products.
❑ With name pairs known to be problematic, reduce the potential for confusion by writing prescriptions using both the brand and generic name.
❑ Include the purpose of medication on prescriptions. In most cases, drugs with names that sound or look similar are used for different purposes.
❑ Alert patients to the potential for mix-ups, especially with known problematic drug names. Advise ambulatory care patients to insist on pharmacy counseling when picking up prescriptions, and to verify that the medication and directions match what the prescriber has told them.
❑ Encourage inpatients to question nurses about medications that are unfamiliar or look or sound different than expected.
❑ Give spoken orders (including telephone orders) only when truly necessary, and never for chemotherapeutic agents. Include the drug's intended purpose to ensure clarity. Encourage staff to read back all orders, spell the product name, and state its indication.

What Organizations and Practitioners Can Do

❑ Maintain awareness of look-alike and sound-alike drug names identified by various safety agencies. Regularly provide information to professional staff.

❑ Whenever possible, determine the purpose of a medication before dispensing or administering it. Most products with look-alike or sound-alike names are used for different purposes.

❑ Accept spoken orders (including telephone orders) only when truly necessary, and never for chemotherapeutic agents. Encourage staff to read back all orders, spell the product name, and state its indication.

❑ Consider the possibility of name confusion when adding a new product to the formulary. Review information previously published by safety agencies.

❑ Computerize prescribing. Use preprinted orders or prescriptions as appropriate. If possible, print out current medications daily from the pharmacy computer system and have physicians review the list for accuracy.

❑ When possible, list brand and generic names on medication administration records (MARs) and automated dispensing cabinet (ADC) computer screens. Such redundancy could help identify an error.

❑ Change the appearance of look-alike product names on computer screens, pharmacy and nursing unit shelf labels and bins (including ADCs), pharmacy product labels, and MARs by highlighting, through boldface, color, or tall-man letters, the parts of the names that are different (e.g., hydrOXYzine, hydrALAzine).

❑ Install and use computerized alerts to remind providers about potential problems during prescription processing.

❑ Configure computer selection screens and ADC screens to prevent the two potentially confused drugs from appearing consecutively.

❑ Affix name alert stickers (available from pharmacy label manufacturers) to areas where look-alike or sound-alike products are stored.

❑ Store products with look-alike or sound-alike names in different locations in pharmacies, patient care units, and other settings, including patient homes. When applicable, use a shelf sticker to help locate the product that has been moved.

❑ Continue to use independent double checks in the dispensing process (one person interprets and enters the prescription into the computer and another reviews the printed label against the original prescription and the product prior to dispensing).

❑ Encourage reporting of errors and potentially hazardous conditions with look-alike and sound-alike product names, and use the information to establish priorities for error reduction. Also maintain awareness of problematic product names and error prevention recommendations provided by ISMP (www.ismp.org), FDA (www.fda.gov), and USP (www.usp.org).

JCAHO and ISMP encourage prescribers to use both the brand (trademark) and generic name, especially in the case of a problematic name pair. Eliminating brand names would remove the safety net of redundancy. One of the most important causes of medication errors related to name mix-ups is the continued use of pen, paper, and telephone to communicate medical orders, and the practice of using a single name, whether brand or generic, fails to address this.

TRADEMARK SUFFIXES

Many errors with brand name products have involved confusion and misinterpretation of letter or number suffixes used to designate specific properties of a drug or dosage form.[13,15] For example, when the trademark Percocet-5 was coined to indicate that a tablet contained 5 mg of oxycodone, some nurses thought the dose was supposed to be five tablets, and overdosages resulted. The manufacturer soon dropped the numeric suffix.

FDA requires that each new formulation be distinguished by a separate suffix. Errors involving suffixes are more likely to be a problem just after the launch of a product, when health professionals may not yet know the meaning of the newly coined suffix and may confuse it with a prescription abbreviation or other medical term. Some such problems are persistent, however.[16,17]

The same suffix may suggest different things in different product names. For example, the antidepressant Wellbutrin (bupropion) has been marketed in several formulations; Wellbutrin SR is a twice-a-day formulation and Wellbutrin XL is a once-a-day formulation. Whereas Wellbutrin SR (for "sustained-release") is given twice a day, another SR product, Dilatrate SR (isosorbide dinitrate) is given once a day. Furthermore, the bupropion product Budeprion SR, generically equivalent to the twice-a-day Wellbutrin SR, is labeled extended-release. If drug name suffixes must be used, then FDA and drug companies need to avoid the adoption of suffixes whose meanings are inconsistent with the way USP defines dosage formulations for modified-release tablets. According to the 2005 edition of *The United States Pharmacopeia and The National Formulary,*

- *Extended-release* tablets are formulated so that the active ingredient is available over an extended period of time after ingestion. Although terms including "prolonged-action," "repeat action," and "sustained-release" have been used for such dosage forms, USP uses the term extended-release. Individual USP monographs typically specify requirements for drug release.
- *Delayed-release* tablets have enteric coatings intended to delay release of the active ingredient until the tablet has passed through the stomach.

AD HOC ABBREVIATIONS

A physician treating a patient for a urinary tract infection intended to prescribe the antimicrobial Noroxin (norfloxacin).[18] On the prescription he wrote "norflox," his abbreviation for the generic name. The community pharmacist interpreted the order as Norflex, a brand name for the muscle relaxant orphenadrine citrate. The patient received Norflex, and the error was discovered when his spouse called the pharmacy to report that the patient felt weak and was hallucinating.

In this case, using an unapproved abbreviation increased the probability for error. No one knows how often this kind of prescription shorthand is used, but it occurs frequently enough to cause significant concern. An informal survey of 41 hospital-based physicians conducted in 1992 at the University of Michigan revealed that about half of them routinely used "norflox" as an abbreviation for norfloxacin on prescriptions.

ISMP has published a list of abbreviations, symbols, and dose designations to be avoided (Table 8-3). Examples of generic name abbreviations associated with medication errors include the following:

- AZT for zidovudine (formerly azidothymidine) has been mistaken for azathioprine and aztreonam.
- HCT for hydrocortisone has been mistaken for hydrochlorothiazide.
- MTX for methotrexate has been mistaken for mitoxantrone.

Using drug name stems can also lead to errors. For example, Adria (for Adriamycin, a brand of doxorubicin) has been misread as Aredia in handwritten orders.

BRAND-NAME EXTENSIONS

Manufacturers of nonprescription drugs sometimes use a slight variation of a popular trademark to name a new product with different active ingredients.[19] Federal regulations

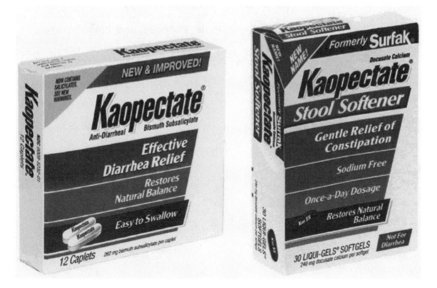

FIGURE 6-4 Kaopectate products with different active ingredients.

do not prevent companies from marketing nonprescription products without specific FDA approval of the product names.[20] A new drug application or abbreviated new drug application does not have to be filed, and companies can capitalize on the well-known and trusted brand name and use it for another product, even one with entirely different ingredients and uses.

For example, the Kaopectate brand name has been used for an antidiarrheal product for years, despite several formulation changes. However, a new Kaopectate product acts as a stool softener; the brand name has replaced another well-known brand name, Surfak, for a docusate calcium product (Figure 6-4). Thus, the same brand name is used for products with opposing indications.

Similarly, physicians, office staff, nurses, and pharmacists may be unaware that there are several nonprescription products using the brand name Dulcolax. One has bisacodyl, a laxative, as its main ingredient; another contains docusate sodium, a stool softener. An example of a mix-up between these products is described in Chapter 13.

These and other examples involving extension of brand names (e.g., Tucks, Neosporin) show the need for regulatory change to give FDA the opportunity to ensure safety in naming nonprescription products.[20] ISMP takes the position that brand name extensions for nonprescription products should not be allowed unless at least one ingredient from the original product is present in the new or modified product.

FOREIGN DRUG NAMES AND IMPACT OF REIMPORTATION

A company planning to market a drug only in the United States might not perform a worldwide search to ensure that the proposed brand name is not used elsewhere. Because there is interest in using a single brand name for a product worldwide, companies planning to sell their products outside the United States perform searches in their major markets. Still, a proposed brand name might not be evaluated in every market.

Whereas the WHO INN system attempts to harmonize generic names worldwide, there is no such system for brand names. Once a brand is marketed, there is no universal monitoring system to prevent the same brand name from being used in other countries

TABLE 6-5 U.S. Brand Names with Different Ingredients in Europe

| Brand Name | Active Ingredients, Purpose, and Manufacturer | |
	U.S. Manufacturers	**European Manufacturers**
Dilacor	Diltiazem Angina, hypertension Watson Labs	Digoxin (Serbia) Congestive heart failure, arrhythmia Zdravlje
Flomax	Tamsulosin Benign prostatic hyperplasia Boehringer Ingelheim	Morniflumate (Italy) Inflammation, pain, fever Chiesi
Naqua	Trichlormethiazide Diuretic Schering	Furosemide (Portugal) Diuretic Bial
Norpramin	Desipramine Depression Aventis	Omeprazole (Spain) Peptic ulcer, gastroesophageal reflux CEPA
Sominex	Diphenhydramine Insomnia SmithKline Beecham Consumer	Promethazine (United Kingdom) Insomnia Thornton & Ross
Trexan	Naltrexone Opioid dependence DuPont	Methotrexate (Finland, Hungary) Malignant neoplasm, psoriasis, rheumatoid arthritis Orion
Vivelle	Estradiol Estrogen deficiency, menopausal disorders, osteoporosis Novartis	Ethinyl estradiol, norgestimate (Austria) Acne, triphasic oral contraceptive Janssen-Cilag

for different products. When a brand name represents different active ingredients than those intended by the prescriber, the consequences can be serious. The wrong drug can be dispensed without the patient's knowledge. Health care providers may not know what their patients are really taking.

For example, a patient traveling in Serbia ran out of Dilacor XR (diltiazem extended release), marketed by Watson Labs in the United States. A Serbian pharmacist filled the prescription with digoxin 0.25 mg. In Serbia, Dilacor is a brand name for digoxin. The patient took digoxin without realizing it and was hospitalized with life-threatening toxicity after his return to the United States.

Table 6-5 provides a few examples of U.S. medication trademarks that are used in Europe for products containing different ingredients. Many other examples are listed in the Index Nominum database and in *Martindale: The Complete Drug Reference* (available by subscription through Micromedex). Multiple, dissimilar products in other countries may use the same name as a U.S. trademark. For example, while Dilacor is a brand name for diltiazem in the United States and digoxin in Serbia, it is also a brand name for barnidipine in Argentina and verapamil in Brazil.

FDA recently advised consumers who fill U.S. prescriptions abroad, either while traveling or when shopping at foreign Internet pharmacies, to use caution because of foreign drugs with names similar to U.S. products.[21] The advisory lists products with names identical and similar to U.S. brand names but with different active ingredients.

The safety risk posed by use of the same name for different products is of particular concern in light of the growing interest in drug reimportation to lower consumer costs. Although U.S. laws and regulations prohibit reimportation, several states are actively pursuing it, and even operating state-run Web sites that refer citizens to Canadian pharmacies. Now, with Canada threatening regulatory change to make it difficult or impossible to fill prescriptions for U.S. patients, some states are looking to import medications from

Europe. As with the patient who took the wrong Dilacor, the opportunity for error is substantial—unless good naming practices endorsed by global health authorities are adopted to minimize or prevent use of the same brand name for different products. Unlike some other dangers in importing drugs (e.g., counterfeiting, lax drug approval processes in some countries), this drug name problem has not been widely recognized.

Two additional problems with reimportation also come to mind. The lack of standardization of suffixes (e.g., CD, CR, ER, LA, SA, SR, TD, XL) for various dosage forms has led to medication errors in the United States. The European Agency for Evaluation of Medicinal Products discourages the use of suffixes for drug names used in European countries. However, it is possible that a U.S. patient could receive an imported product with a different suffix in the name, even when the foreign product has the same active ingredient as the branded U.S. product. Another possible source of error is look-alike and sound-alike brand names in spoken orders for drugs being imported, although such orders are unlikely. For example, Ambyen is one branded amiodarone product in the United Kingdom. Receiving a supply of Amyben in place of Ambien (zolpidem tartrate) could have disastrous results.

Failure mode and effects analysis of drug importation should be undertaken before further consideration of this seemingly cost-effective alternative. In addition to carrying an adequate supply of their U.S. medications, patients traveling abroad should take a list of their medications by both generic and brand name in order to confirm that they receive the correct drug if their supply runs out.

ROLE OF FDA

Premarketing Review of Proposed Trademarks

The FDA Office of Drug Safety, Division of Medication Errors and Technical Support (DMETS), reviews all trademarks. FDA bases its authority to evaluate the error potential of proposed trademarks on a federal regulation that disallows "designation of a drug or ingredient by a proprietary name that, because of similarity in spelling or pronunciation, may be confused with the proprietary name or the established name of a different drug or ingredient."[22]

The FDA Center for Drug Evaluation and Research (CDER) has made substantial organizational changes that reflect changes in its approach to trademark evaluation. Before 1990, medication errors related to trademarks were hardly a consideration. Then, around 1990, the Labeling and Nomenclature Committee (LNC) began to evaluate proposed proprietary and established names and make recommendations to CDER's reviewing divisions about the acceptability of new proprietary names. The LNC was reconfigured in 1999 to make way for the Office of Postmarketing Drug Risk Assessment (OPDRA), one of three units in the newly created Office of Drug Safety (ODS). Whereas the LNC was a voluntary group of FDA staffers with broad experience in health care and the regulatory area, OPDRA was staffed with individuals devoted full-time to its mission, which included proprietary name evaluation. In 2002 the ODS underwent another organizational change that included the creation of DMETS as successor to OPDRA.

Although a trademark may be evaluated at the investigational new drug stage, about 90% of requests for trademark review are submitted at the new drug application (NDA) stage. DMETS does not approve proprietary or established names; rather, its responsibility is to evaluate these names and submit a recommendation on their acceptability to the reviewing division where the final decision is made. There are two levels of trademark approval. The first is provisional approval, subject to change if FDA first grants final approval for a new product with a trademark that is unacceptably similar to the one with

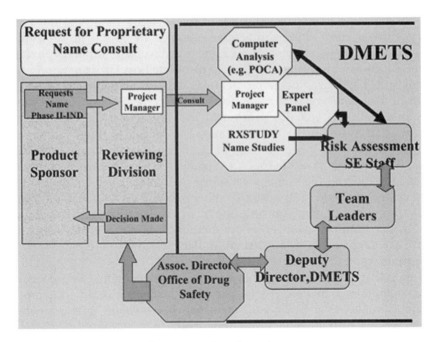

FIGURE 6-5   FDA review process for proposed trademarks.

provisional approval. The second trademark approval occurs 90 days from the target date for product approval set under the Prescription Drug User Fee Act. This final trademark approval is based on a review of all trademarks associated with FDA product approvals since the date of the provisional approval.

A sponsor can submit one or two trademarks as early as Phase II clinical trials. The request for trademark review is made to the reviewing division responsible for the application for which the submitted trademark is intended (Figure 6-5). The reviewing division forwards the name to the project manager of a group within DMETS for safety evaluation. The group looks at references to identify existing or recently approved drug names that raise concerns about the proposed trademark.

In the late 1990s, Lambert[23] worked with FDA on the development of a computerized method of calculating measures of similarity between medication names. A program known as Phonetic and Orthographic Computer Analysis (POCA) uses algorithms to select a list of names from a database that have some similarity to the trademark being evaluated. Although DMETS is using POCA as one tool in trademark evaluation, the program has not been validated and is not available to sponsors or the public. It is left to human judgment to determine which names are likely to contribute to confusion based on similarities in sight or sound.

As part of the DMETS evaluation, simulated written and spoken prescriptions are given to about 100 FDA volunteers to obtain data on what the volunteers think they see or hear. To act as a control, the prescription includes orders for two existing products whose names the volunteers should recognize.

The DMETS group considers all the retrieved information (identified as potential problems) and comes to a decision on the safety of the product name. A detailed consultation is written and forwarded to the reviewing division, which makes the final determination and informs the applicant of the findings. The sponsor has an opportunity to rebut a negative DMETS consultation by providing clarifying information to the reviewing division to remove or mitigate concerns.

DMETS has recommended disapproval of trademarks for the following reasons:

- Names that are too similar to existing names when in print, handwritten, or spoken
- Misleading, incorrect, or unsafe elements encoded into a name
- Claims that are not supported by clinical data
- Prefixes or suffixes that may be confused with a common medical abbreviation
- Inclusion of a dosage form or regimen in the proprietary name
- Suggestion of an unapproved use
- Similarities in storage environment (Two products with similar names will cause the committee less concern if they are physically separated in pharmacy storage areas and will always remain so—for example, if one is a topical product and the other an oral solution.)
- Unacceptable similarity between the generic and brand names (The USAN Council discourages the use of large portions of a USAN in a trademark; therefore, DMETS generally does not approve names that contain too much of the USAN or of the USAN stem in the "stem" position, or the wrong stem for that product.)

DMETS has been working on external guidance and an internal manual of policies and procedures that will describe in detail the procedures for trademark evaluation and timely approval.

Postmarketing Surveillance and Risk Management

A recent FDA effort to promote safe use of approved products was development of the Phase IV Medication Error Monitoring Program that can be part of the NDA approval letter. Information is collected from internal and external sources to determine the number and seriousness of medication errors that have some element of trademark involvement.

For example, trademark review revealed a theoretical risk of confusion between Astra-Zeneca's Faslodex trademark for fulvestrant (used for breast cancer) and three other trademarks: Casodex (bicalutamide) for prostate cancer, Zoladex (goserelin acetate) for various oncologic problems, and Fosamax (alendronate) for osteoporosis. Negotiations between AstraZeneca and FDA led to a timely product approval contingent on a 2-year postmarketing commitment to monitor medication errors, with quarterly reports beginning in April 2002. The commitment was fulfilled in July 2004, and monitoring data showed that the theoretical risk of potential confusion between Faslodex and the other products did not materialize in the marketplace.

ROLE OF THE PHARMACEUTICAL INDUSTRY

Pharmaceutical companies invest a great deal of time and money finding and protecting globally available trademarks for their products. An effective trademark

- Distinguishes a seller's product from competitors' products;
- Identifies a common source of goods, thereby unifying brand preference;
- Conveys an image of consistent product quality; and
- Generates brand loyalty.

The development of a trademark begins as early as 5 or 6 years before the expected product launch. To be successful, a trademark must be legally clear of infringement (i.e., the new trademark must not be likely to cause confusion with existing trademarks), free of bad meanings or connotations, relatively easy to pronounce, memorable, and in compliance with all regulatory requirements. It must meet marketing needs, and most important, support safe use of the product. This is a demanding process when conducted in a single country. Meeting all of these criteria in all the countries where the product will be sold is extremely difficult.

To ensure that a proposed trademark is not confusingly similar to previously approved product names, professional searchers use a variety of techniques and linguistic algorithms. Next, linguistic and cultural checks are performed. When a trademark survives the legal evaluation, many companies conduct an analysis of potential error, assisted by private-sector services. Such services, described below, may seek input from health care professionals—mainly practicing pharmacists—who will encounter the trademark.

Then, the surviving globally available trademarks (as few as two or three) are ranked in order of preference in market studies. Available trademarks are filed in trademark offices in the United States and around the world, where trademark examiners conduct their own evaluations. In the United States and many other countries, proposed trademarks are published so that they may be contested by competitors and the public.

To encourage sponsors to follow best practices in developing and clearing trademarks, PhRMA's Trademark and Copyright Focus Group is developing a set of good naming practices, built upon the robust processes for legal clearance and medication error prevention analysis that are currently used by many pharmaceutical companies.

Private-sector services that analyze trademarks for error potential share some features of the DMETS process and offer customized elements to meet client needs. In addition to simulating handwritten prescriptions and spoken orders to elicit the reactions of pharmacists and nurses (i.e., to detect visual and phonetic similarities to marketed products), services evaluate proposed trademarks for other factors associated with medication errors, such as similar dosages, dosage strengths, dosage forms, dosage regimens, clinical indications, storage requirements, and trade packaging. To test for potential problems, attempts may be made to simulate the way a product will be used in clinical settings. Organizations that offer trademark evaluation include Med-E.R.R.S., a subsidiary of ISMP; Drug Safety Institute, a subsidiary of Brand Institute; and RxMARK, a subsidiary of Interbrand Wood Healthcare.

Although none of the trademark evaluation methods used by industry or FDA have been scientifically validated, such proactive evaluation is helpful in detecting potential problems prior to marketing.

ROLE OF PRACTITIONERS AND ORGANIZATIONS

To reduce the chance of medication errors caused by products with similar names, practitioners and organizations can follow the recommendations in the sidebar on pages 100–101. Computerized prescriber order entry can reduce the chance for misreading or mishearing drug names. Handwritten prescriptions should be legible and complete, and spoken orders should be given slowly and clearly.[11,12,24] Spoken orders, including telephone orders, should be accepted only when it is truly necessary. The person receiving such an order should transcribe it and then read it back to the person giving the order. This ensures that the correct name has been heard and that the transcription is correct.

When a new product is added to the formulary, the possibility of name confusion should be considered. To determine whether the new product's name might look or sound like any other product name or medical term, frontline nurses, pharmacists, technicians, unit secretaries, and physicians can be asked to view samples of the handwritten product name and directions as they might appear in a typical order and then to pronounce the name. If potential for confusion with other products is determined, steps can be taken to avoid errors, as described below and in the sidebar on pages 100–101.

Computers can be programmed to display a "clinical flag" or "formulary note" on the monitor that alerts the user to potential mix-ups.[25] Like a road sign that warns about a dangerous intersection ahead, this can alert the person entering the order when a look-alike or sound-alike danger is present. For the most serious confusing name pairs, the alert should be generated when either of the drugs is selected. The alert should appear on automated dispensing cabinet screens as well as during prescription entry. If possible, both visual and auditory reminders should be used.

Pharmacists and nurses must read prescription orders carefully. Considering medication orders in the context of patients' diagnoses can help prevent errors. Being knowledgeable about new products can help pharmacists and nurses to recognize errors in interpretation.

Pharmacies should have adequate and easily accessible shelf space, ample lighting, sound amplifiers on telephone speakers, prescription holders, and magnifiers near computer displays. Pharmacists' workload should be monitored; they should have time to be sure that prescriptions are clear and unambiguous. Products with look-alike or sound-alike names should be stored in different locations, and both products should not be stored in the fast-mover area.

Physicians can contribute to error reduction by printing the product name and including the purpose of each medication on the prescription. This helps ensure accurate identification of the medication and facilitates patient education.

States are beginning to pass laws to ensure safe prescription writing. For example, as of July 1, 2003, prescriptions written by Florida practitioners must be legibly printed or typed, the quantity of the drug prescribed must appear in both text and numeric formats [e.g., ten (10)], and the prescription must be dated with the month spelled out (e.g., October 5, 2003, not 10/5/03).[26] The law is intended to encourage clear communication and set the stage for computerized prescribing. However, it could encourage physicians to delegate some responsibility for prescription writing to office staff who may not have the requisite training and supervision. If the physician failed to review the prescription before it was given to a patient, this could open a new pathway for medication errors. Also, such laws could force pharmacists to reject all cursive prescriptions, thus delaying treatment for sick patients and placing stress on physician–pharmacist–patient relationships. The Florida law does not require prescribers to include the drug's purpose on the prescription, although knowing the purpose helps pharmacists identify the desired medication.

Physicians should educate patients or family members about the names and purposes of all their medications, and nurses and pharmacists should reinforce this information. A patient who knows what to expect is better prepared to question a misinterpreted order. The pharmacist or nurse can open the prescription bottle or unit dose package in front of the patient to confirm the expected appearance and review the indication. If a patient questions the appearance or name of a prescribed medication, the pharmacist or nurse should take time to fully investigate. Patients should be cautioned about error potential when taking products that are known to have a look-alike or sound-alike counterpart.

CONCLUSION

Patient safety clearly requires improved methods for naming pharmaceutical products. The 2006 IOM report[2] calls for renewed effort in this regard, noting that FDA, the federal Agency for Healthcare Research and Quality, the pharmaceutical industry, USP, ISMP, and others need to collaborate on a guidance document for product naming. Such guidance should propose a common nomenclature with standardized abbreviations, acronyms, and terms. Although there is no single or simple answer to reducing medication errors, a new coordinated effort by FDA, USP, ISMP, and the pharmaceutical industry to research problems associated with drug naming should lead to a plan of action that produces timely and measurable results.

REFERENCES

1. Kohn LT, Corrigan JM, Donaldson MS, eds. *To Err Is Human: Building a Safer Health System.* Washington, DC: National Academies Press; 2000.
2. Committee on Identifying and Preventing Medication Errors; Aspden P, Wolcott J, Bootman JL, et al., eds. *Preventing Medication Errors.* Washington, DC: National Academies Press; 2006. Prepublication copy available at http://darwin.nap.edu/books/0309101476/html/R2.html. Accessed July 21, 2006.
3. Starr CH. When drug names spell trouble. *Drug Top.* May 15, 2000;144(10):49–58
4. Zwillich T. FDA and industry puzzle over drug-name fixes. *Drug Top.* July 21, 2003;147:38.
5. Glaser M. Are drug names taking too much blame for Rx mixups? *Drug Top.* January 12, 2004;148:68.
6. Cohen MR. Medication error reports: Levoxine could be read as Lanoxin. *Hosp Pharm.* 1992;27:906–7.
7. Institute for Safe Medication Practices. Action needed to prevent dangerous Zyrtec–Zyprexa mix-ups. *ISMP Medication Safety Alert!* 2001;6(22):2.
8. Filik R, Purdy KJ, Gale AG, et al. Drug name confusion: evaluating the effectiveness of capital ("Tall Man") letters using eye movement data. *Soc Sci Med.* 2004; 59(12): 2597–601.
9. Filik R, Purdy KJ, Gale AG, et al. Investigating medication errors caused by confusable drug names. In: Schmalhofer F, Young RM, Katz G, eds. *Proc EuroCogSci 03.* London: Lawrence Erlbaum Associates; 2003:383.
10. Hoffman JM, Proulx SM. Medication errors caused by confusion of drug names. *Drug Saf.* 2003;26(7):445–52.
11. Institute for Safe Medication Practices. What's in a name? Ways to prevent dispensing errors linked to name confusion. *ISMP Medication Safety Alert!* June 12, 2002.
12. Joint Commission on Accreditation of Healthcare Organizations. *Sentinel Event Alert.* May 2001(19).
13. Cohen MR. Medication error reports: naming drug products is a serious business. *Hosp Pharm.* 1990;25:747–8.
14. Food and Drug Administration. Guidance for Industry. Premarketing Risk Assessment. March 2005. Available at: www.fda.gov/cder/guidance/6357fnl.htm. Accessed July 26, 2005.
15. Cohen MR. Medication error reports: name "Procardia XL" is problem for pharmacists. *Hosp Pharm.* 1990;25:403–4.
16. Institute for Safe Medication Practices. FDA and the pharmaceutical industry must be more responsive for a safer healthcare system. *ISMP Medication Safety Alert!* November 4, 2004.
17. Institute for Safe Medication Practices. Still SR and XL confusion. *ISMP Medication Safety Alert!* December 4, 2004.
18. Pincus JM, Ike RW. Norflox or Norflex? [letter]. *N Engl J Med.* 1992;326:15.
19. Rupp MT, Parker JM. Drug names: when marketing and safety collide. *Am Pharm.* 1993;NS33:39–42.
20. Institute for Safe Medication Practices. Caution: Dulcolax brand name extensions. *ISMP Medication Safety Alert!* 2004; 9(7):1–2.
21. Food and Drug Administration. *Consumers Filling U.S. Prescriptions Abroad May Get the Wrong Active Ingredient Because of Confusing Drug Names.* Public Health Advisory, January 2006. Available at: www.fda.gov/oc/opacom/reports/confusingnames.html.
22. 21 CFR 201.10(c)(5). Available at: www.accessdata.fda.gov/scripts/cdrh/cfdocs/cfcfr/CFRSearch.cfm. Accessed July 26, 2005.
23. Lambert BL. Predicting look-alike and sound-alike medication errors. *Am J Health Syst Pharm.* 1997;54: 1161–71.
24. Davis NM. Drug names that look and sound alike. *Hosp Pharm.* 1999;34:1160–78.
25. Institute for Safe Medication Practices. A novel way to prevent medication errors associated with drug mix-ups. *ISMP Medication Safety Alert!* 1996;1(15):1.
26. Institute for Safe Medication Practices. A weak link in the chain. *ISMP Medication Safety Alert!* 2003;8(14): 1–2.

CHAPTER 7

THE ROLE OF DRUG PACKAGING AND LABELING IN MEDICATION ERRORS

Michael R. Cohen

Both consumers and health care practitioners use product packaging and labeling to select the correct medication and dose. Health care professionals are taught to read labels at least three times: when obtaining a drug package, when using it, and when returning it to stock or discarding an empty package. Most claim to do this routinely, but there is much evidence to the contrary. Although proper training and increased vigilance are undeniably important, attention to the design of drug packaging and labeling is also essential. Poor labeling and packaging frequently contribute to medication errors.

The Food and Drug Administration (FDA) and the pharmaceutical industry have made advances in this regard since the first edition of *Medication Errors.* Some of the problems that led to errors described in this new edition have been remedied,[1-3] but errors rooted in labeling and packaging continue to be reported to the U.S. Pharmacopeia (USP)–Institute for Safe Medication Practices (ISMP) Medication Errors Reporting Program (MERP). Errors may occur when key information appears in an inconspicuous place on the label, is presented in an ambiguous manner, or is overshadowed by less important information. The print may be less than optimal in size, boldness, or contrast. Highly stylized graphics, superiorly positioned corporate names, or logos may distract from the primary purpose of the label: to permit the user (pharmacist, nurse, physician, or patient) to identify the name(s), dosage form, and strength of the product. Complicating the situation is that labels are often read under less-than-ideal conditions (e.g., in a patient's room at night when lights are dimmed, or by paramedics working on an accident victim).

This chapter examines medication errors associated with labeling and packaging and suggests techniques for preventing them. Such errors are not made because label information is incorrect, but carefully planned and tested label design may help prevent them. The chapter briefly addresses the influence of unsafe designations in drug product advertising and the role of product shortages in medication errors.

HUMAN FACTORS AND CONFIRMATION BIAS

Before examining the features of product labels and packages, it is helpful to consider human and environmental factors in safe medication use.[4-6] Efforts to ensure the availability of trained individuals and improve the way people work within their environment can reduce the likelihood of error. For example, visual problems that contribute to the misreading of labels can be detected through regular employee eye examinations. Intensifying light, using magnifying lenses, and printing information in exaggerated, nonconventional type fonts can help individuals read labels more accurately.

PARIS
IN THE
THE SPRING

FIGURE 7-1   Confirmation bias causes most readers to overlook the error in this phrase.

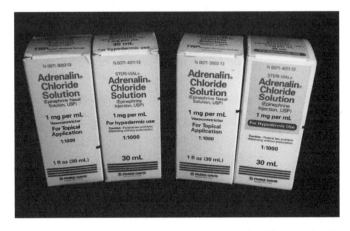

FIGURE 7-2 (also in color section following page 120)   Look-alike packaging (left) of these topical and injectable Adrenalin products was redesigned (right) to prevent errors.

Confirmation bias plays a role in product mix-ups. Errors are often induced by familiarity with procedures and materials, coupled with the innate tendency of humans to perceive confirming evidence more readily than disconfirming evidence.[6] People tend to see what is familiar or what they want to see, rather than what is actually there. For example, if asked to glance at the words in Figure 7-1, most people would see "Paris in the spring," because it is a familiar phrase. Close reading, however, reveals that the word *the* appears twice.

Recent pharmacy graduates, not yet familiar with many medications, read labels carefully. After a while, they can picture a sought-after item in their mind's eye, and they are no longer as careful. If a drug has very distinctive packaging, the potential for mix-ups is slight. If several products have similar packaging, or if labeling is hard to read, the potential for error involving confirmation bias increases. Especially in suboptimal working conditions, drug look-alikes can cause health professionals to overlook important information.

An example of how a product label can contribute to confirmation bias appears in Figure 7-2. The original packaging (left) was changed after reports of delays in treatment because of the similarity in packaging between topical Adrenalin, used to stop bleeding, and injectable Adrenalin, used in emergencies such as cardiac arrest and asthma attacks. Medical personnel had unknowingly stocked their emergency box with the topical agent; when they opened the box for emergency treatment, they did not have the product they needed. The staff replenishing the emergency supply boxes had exhibited confirmation bias. They wanted the injectable form, but they identified the item by its appearance: the title (Adrenalin Chloride Solution), the distinctive white and dark-red design, the shape of the box, the horizontal bands at the bottom of the label, and the "1:1000" concentration. The distinguishing words (i.e., "Nasal Solution" and "Topical Application," versus "Injection" and "Hypodermic Use") were relatively small and were not seen. The redesigned packaging (right) is distinguished by a sharp color contrast. The words "For Hypodermic Use" appear in white letters in a red box. Since this packaging was introduced, no mix-ups of these products have been reported to MERP.

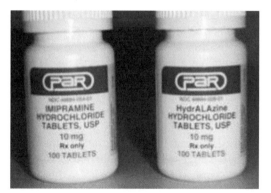

FIGURE 7-3 (also in color section following page 120) Look-alike packaging of imipramine (left) and hydralazine.

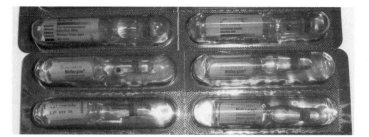

FIGURE 7-4 (also in color section following page 120) Look-alike ampuls of Brethine (top row) and Methergine (middle and bottom rows).

It is not enough to caution health care providers to be more careful. It is human nature to identify items by color, shape, type font, symbols used, and other such characteristics. The health care community, especially pharmaceutical purchasers, regulators, and the pharmaceutical industry, must recognize poorly designed product labeling that may contribute to mix-ups.

To a drug company, its name and corporate identity may be the most important information on the label, but most important to practitioners is clear identification of the product name and strength. On the containers shown in Figure 7-3, the company logo is the most prominent feature. It appears in a highly stylized font within an oval, dark-blue bar, above the drug name. The salt name "hydrochloride," common to both products, is spelled in full, not abbreviated as HCl, in the same size as the active moiety. Another similarity is the red type used to designate both 10 mg and 100 mg tablets. The user's eyes are drawn everywhere except toward the name of the active drug, and the result could be a dispensing error.

Another example of how poor packaging and labeling can increase error potential appears in Figure 7-4. Soon after Novartis introduced new packaging for Methergine (methylergonovine maleate) injection and Brethine (terbutaline sulfate) injection, ISMP learned about a serious look-alike problem. The external cartons were well labeled and easily distinguishable, but in clinical locations the products are usually removed from the cartons for storage. Inside the cartons of both products, 1 mL ampuls were packaged in an amber plastic tub covered by a foil label with the name in tiny print. Both ampuls had similar-colored ring markings on the necks that could be seen through the plastic, adding to the similarity of their appearance.

Both of these drugs are used in labor and delivery settings, but for very different clinical reasons. Terbutaline is used to treat preterm labor, and methylergonovine is used primarily after delivery of the placenta to treat uterine atony, subinvolution, or hemorrhage. Since methylergonovine has abortifacient properties, it is absolutely contraindicated in pregnancy and would be especially dangerous to a patient in preterm labor. Interchanging these two drugs could result in serious adverse outcomes for the mother and baby. In one reported case, the administration of four doses of Methergine to a patient in preterm labor was believed to contribute to fetal death.

Methergine ampuls should be refrigerated, which helps separate the products. As an additional precaution, ISMP suggested that pharmacists apply reminder labels to the ampuls prior to dispensing to prevent mix-ups. Despite the submission of numerous error reports and ISMP's telephone calls to company representatives, the packaging was not changed for several years. The company responded that practitioners should be more careful when reading the labels. After yet another reported error resulting from the look-alike ampul packaging, the *ISMP Medication Safety Alert* newsletter (October 21, 2004) called for health care providers at hospitals and birthing centers to immediately replace Brethine ampuls with vials, which had recently become available. (Brethine was acquired from Novartis by aaiPharma in 2001 and later became available in vials from this and other generic vendors of terbutaline.)

Look-alike packaging has contributed to mix-ups between tetanus toxoid and other immunologic products. Between September 2000 and December 2005, ISMP received many reports of errors in which tetanus toxoid or tetanus and diphtheria toxoids was inadvertently injected intradermally in response to orders for purified protein derivative (PPD, tuberculin for skin testing). Some patients had localized responses that were interpreted as positive PPD tests, which resulted in unnecessary treatment for tuberculosis with isoniazid, a drug with a black box warning about liver toxicity. The Centers for Disease Control and Prevention (CDC)[7] reported in 2004 that 100 patients in 21 states had been identified as receiving a tetanus toxoid vaccine product instead of PPD; one patient developed cellulitis and may have suffered permanent scarring. No adverse reactions to isoniazid were reported in the patients involved in these errors.

Most of these errors were discovered when staff noticed that vials had been mixed up or when clusters of what appeared to be positive PPD skin tests occurred. The lot numbers on products thought to be PPD showed that they were tetanus toxoid products, underscoring the importance of recording vaccine lot numbers in patient records.

The reporters of these errors with vaccine products have noted that similar packaging contributed. The manufacturer's biological products are all available in stylized, colorful cartons, as shown in Figures 18-4 and 18-5 (see color section following page 120). The colors differ from product to product, but practitioners may be distracted by the style itself and not read the label carefully. The cartons are the same size, regardless of the volume of the enclosed vial. The number "5" appears in a circle on the carton front panel and the vial label, designating 5 TU [tuberculin units] for PPD but 5 mL for the vaccine products. The products are stored in the refrigerator and may be located side by side. Tetanus–diphtheria toxoids is not available in single-dose syringes, which forces providers to purchase multiple- dose vials, further contributing to the problem.

ISMP contacted the company (Aventis Pasteur) to suggest a restyled label, and FDA has also been alerted to the problem. In January 2006 the company informed ISMP that FDA had approved packaging and labeling changes including a color change for the Tubersol (PPD) package, a reduction in the container label text on tetanus toxoid products and an increase in the type size for essential text, inclusion of the route of administration on all container labels, and generic abbreviations on the labels (PPD on the Tubersol label, TTOX on the tetanus toxoid label, FLU on the influenza vaccine label). Also, preservative-

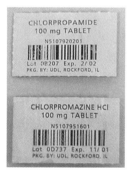

FIGURE 7-5   Similar-appearing unit dose packages of chlorpropamide and chlorpromazine.

free tetanus toxoid adsorbed will now be packaged as 10×1 mL single-dose vials, labeled "preservative-free" on both the carton and vial, which should help differentiate the product from other vaccines available in multiple-dose vials.

The use of tall-man letters on packaging can help practitioners differentiate products. In this lettering style, now referred to by USP as "mixed-case" lettering, distinguishing letters in similar name pairs are enlarged or capitalized. A pharmacist reported incidents involving mix-ups between similar unit dose packages of the oral hypoglycemic chlorpropamide 100 mg and the antipsychotic chlorpromazine 100 mg (Figure 7-5). Because the storage bins for the two drugs were near each other, a pharmacy technician pulled the wrong drug. A pharmacist missed the error during a routine check, and chlorpropamide, rather than chlorpromazine, was placed in an automated drug distribution module. Nurses did not notice the error, and two patients each received four or five doses of the drug. These patients suffered no serious harm, but other such errors have resulted in central nervous system impairment or death because of hypoglycemia from the chlorpropamide. ISMP asked the manufacturer to consider enlarging the unique letters in this look-alike drug name pair (chlorproMAZINE and chlorproPAMIDE). FDA's Division of Generic Drugs has asked generic manufacturers to differentiate similar name pairs (Table 6-1) in this way. Pharmacists may wish to make such changes in their own labels, preprinted order forms, computer screens and printouts, and drug storage location labels.

READABILITY OF LABELS AND PACKAGES

Manufacturers can improve the readability of drug labeling and packaging in a number of ways[8,9]; some of the most important are discussed in the following sections.

Three premature infants died in a hospital nursery after receiving erroneously prepared heparin flushes through umbilical-line catheters.[10] The problem began in the pharmacy, where heparin for catheter flushes was normally prepared by adding 250 units of heparin to 250 mL of 5% dextrose injection. Syringes of heparin 2.5 mL, 1 unit/mL, were prepared from the admixture, labeled, and sent to the neonatal intensive care unit (ICU). The fatal errors occurred because an employee pulled a 250 mL container of 15% (2 mEq/mL) potassium chloride concentrate that had been placed in the bin intended to hold 250 mL containers of 5% dextrose injection. The heparin was diluted with the potassium chloride instead of dextrose. Each infant received about 5 mEq of potassium by IV push.

The potassium chloride container was correctly labeled. Had it been properly read, the error would not have occurred. The problem was linked to similarities in appearance between the containers of 5% dextrose and 15% potassium chloride. Dextrose 5% injection is used directly for IV infusion and as a vehicle for other drugs, whereas 15% potassium chloride 250 mL is a pharmacy bulk package intended only for use in preparing IV

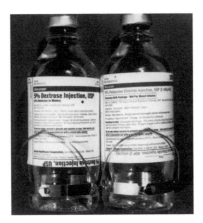

FIGURE 7-6 5% Dextrose injection (left) and 15% potassium chloride for injection.

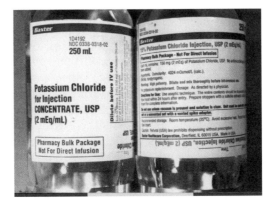

FIGURE 7-7 Redesigned (left) and old labels for potassium chloride for injection.

admixtures (in which the potassium is diluted). The packaging of the two products was nearly identical (Figure 7-6). Both had the same shape, contained equal volumes of clear liquid, and had the same aluminum bail for hanging the bottle on an IV pole. For years, pharmacy employees had gone to the same bin for dextrose. They had correctly prepared thousands of syringes. This time, the potassium bottle rested in a bin labeled "Dextrose," and its label was partially obscured because the container was turned on its side. The name of the drug, printed in red, was not visible.

After this error occurred, the manufacturer redesigned the packaging for potassium chloride (Figure 7-7). The name is now more prominent, and it appears on a side panel as well as on the front. It is more evident that the product is a pharmacy bulk package meant for dilution before use. The peel-off cap and bottle ferrule have been modified. The statement "Dilute before IV Use" appears in contrasting print.

Many words commonly used on prescription drug labels (e.g., "Brand of," "Preparation of," "Mix-O-Vial") serve the manufacturer more than the user and therefore should be eliminated. Figure 7-7 illustrates how label clutter can be reduced. Essential information should appear in a prominent position on the front label. This includes the brand and generic names, strength or concentration, and warnings, if any (sidebar, page 117). Less important information, including the manufacturer's name and logo, National Drug Code

---

ISMP RECOMMENDED HIERARCHY OF INFORMATION ON FRONT PANEL (PRINCIPAL DISPLAY) OF U.S. PRESCRIPTION DRUG LABELS

The drug name and strength are the most important pieces of information and should appear close to one another in the same field of view. Color may be used to help differentiate products with similar names or strengths. The appearance of other marketed products must be considered.

Brand name. Use bold, sans-serif typeface.
—Consider tall-man lettering to prevent confusion with other drug names.

Generic name (in parentheses immediately under brand name at one-half the type size used for brand name). Use bold, sans-serif typeface.
—Use tall-man lettering when suggested by the Food and Drug Administration.
  (Do not contrive non-FDA-approved methods of using tall-man lettering.)

Dosage form (e.g., tablet, capsule, suspension)

Strength of medication (use metric system only; use no trailing zeros)
  Individual tablet or capsule strength
  —Tablet or capsule count
  Concentration of liquid
  —Include within same border or background:
    Strength per container volume (e.g., 500 mg/10 mL)
    Strength per mL (e.g., 50 mg per mL)

Suggested route(s) of administration

Warnings and dose preparation information if space allows; otherwise, note where important information can be found.

Single-use, single-dose, multiple-dose, or pharmacy bulk package container, if injectable product.

Manufacturer, distributor, packager information (never place at top of container). Logos and highly stylistic label designs distract from user readability and should be avoided.

"Rx only" statement and other federal requirements. (The Code of Federal Regulations spells out additional information that may be required on the principal display panel and how it should be displayed.)

(NDC) number, package size, USP designation, control number, expiration date, bar code, and needle length and size (or needleless designation), is best placed on the side panel or in the package insert, unless noted otherwise in the U.S. Code of Federal Regulations (21 CFR 201 10).

In 1992, the Committee to Reduce Medication Errors of the Pharmaceutical Manufacturers Association (PhRMA, now the Pharmaceutical Research and Manufacturers of America) submitted recommendations to USP and FDA for the design of labels for small-volume injectable products. The committee recommended eliminating the words "sterile," "nonpyrogenic," and "pyrogen-free," as well as the phrases "May be habit forming," "Federal law prohibits dispensing without prescription," and "For usual dose, see accompanying package insert" (or other words to that effect). A USP-FDA advisory panel on label simplification adopted these recommendations and added some of its own, including the elimination of controlled-substance designators (e.g., "C-II") and of lists of storage requirements when an article can be stored at room temperature in normal light.[11] The implementation of some of these recommendations required changes in federal law. The FDA Modernization Act of 1997 authorized replacement of the federal legend statement ("Federal law prohibits dispensing without prescription") with an "Rx only" symbol. In

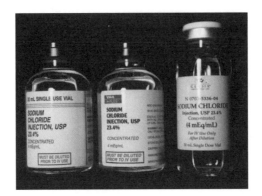

FIGURE 7-8 (also in color section following page 120) Red warnings that the products must be diluted.

addition, the phrase "Warning: May be habit forming" may be eliminated from certain controlled substances. FDA has the authority to make other changes called for in the label simplification project.

USES OF COLOR

Color has been used in several ways on drug packaging and labeling. For example, manufacturers may use red to draw attention to warnings on the product label. The three sodium chloride concentrate products shown in Figure 7-8 have warnings in red print that the product must be diluted. Some industrial engineers believe red provides an especially vivid warning (perhaps because it looks like blood), but this has not been proved. At the practice level, a yellow highlighter can be used to draw attention to important label information such as the drug concentration or the total volume in a vial.

Color coding is the systematic application of color to aid in classification and identification. A color-coding system enables users to associate a color with a function. Such a system is used for ophthalmic medications in the United States; the caps and labels are color-coded according to their pharmacologic class. Practitioners who know the system can assume that a manufacturer's vial with a yellow label means the product is a beta-blocker, while a tan label means the product is an anti-infective. The effectiveness of color-coding systems depends on users' ability to remember what each color means. As noted in Chapter 1, excessive reliance on memory increases the likelihood of mistakes. Labels and charts accompanying a color-coding system make users less dependent on memory.

Color is also used to make certain elements stand out, as in Figure 7-8, or to help distinguish one item from another; this is *color differentiation*. A vaccine product for adults may be packaged in an orange box, while the company's pediatric formulation is packaged in a light blue box. In contrast to color coding, the color is not used as a standard code for classifying and identifying products. Although color differentiation has not been proven to prevent medication errors, practitioners believe it helps reduce the risk of selecting the wrong product from within a manufacturer's line. The idea is that color helps the user efficiently find and select a medication—before carefully reading the label for verification. The problem is that users may *not* read the label carefully.

Color matching, also different from color coding, has been used to reduce the risk of error. A medical device may have a blue plug that attaches to a blue receptacle and a yellow plug that attaches to a yellow receptacle, but the colors have no special meaning beyond matching one item with another. The Broselow tape (Figure 17-3) uses colors keyed

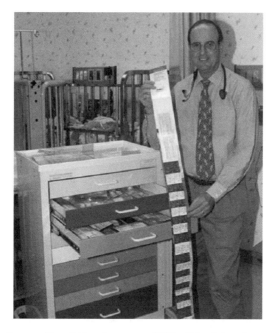

FIGURE 7-9 (also in color section following page 120) Physician James Broselow displays the Broselow tape, which uses colors keyed to a child's height to help practitioners select drug doses and equipment in pediatric emergencies; the color on the tape is matched to the appropriate crash cart drawer.

to a child's height to help practitioners quickly estimate drug doses and resuscitation equipment sizes in pediatric emergencies. The color on the tape matches the color of the correct drawer on a crash cart (Figure 7-9). Thus, if a child's length is in the red range on the tape, the red drawer contains emergency equipment appropriate for that child's size.

PROBLEMS WITH USES OF COLOR

Health care practitioners need to recognize the problems associated with the use of color in drug product packaging and labeling. Color should not draw attention away from the name and strength of the drug. Although color may be an effective means of distinguishing products, other variables such as the type font and layout of labeling must be considered.

Color coding of pharmaceutical products should be used with extreme caution. The variety of discernible colors available for commercial use is limited. Color-coding research in other industries[12,13] has shown that subtle distinctions in color are poorly discernible unless products are adjacent to each other. Contrast with background or surrounding colors can be problematic if a certain color must be used for product identification. Furthermore, clinicians or patients with colorblindness may misidentify color-coded products. Colorblind people have difficulty recognizing certain ranges of colors.[14] One in 12 Caucasian (8%), 1 in 20 Asian (5%), and 1 in 25 African (4%) males have red–green colorblindness. In addition, medications can alter one's visual perception or ability to differentiate between colors.[15] (Colorblindness may not be a significant disadvantage as it relates to color code schemes used in labeling.[16] Some people are able to adapt to color deficiencies and properly use color-coding schemes.[17])

A single variable such as color should never be relied upon to prevent error.[18] Factors such as the amount and size of text on a product label, the corporate dress, the shape and size of fonts and logos, and the background can make containers look similar and distract from label

TABLE 7-1   Colors Denoting Drug Class of Ophthalmic Products

Class	Color	Pantone Number
Anti-infectives	Tan	467
Anti-inflammatories/steroids	Pink	197
Mydriatics and cycloplegics	Red	1797
Nonsteroidal anti-inflammatories	Gray	4
Miotics	Dark green	348
Beta-blockers	Yellow	Yellow C
Beta-blocker combinations	Dark blue	281
Adrenergic agonists	Purple	2583
Carbonic anhydrase inhibitors	Orange	1585
Prostaglandin analogs	Turquoise	326

reading. The American Society of Health-System Pharmacists (ASHP),[19] ISMP, FDA and many in industry oppose the use of color to identify drug products. The American Medical Association recommends that color coding of pharmaceutical products for the purpose of preventing medication errors be considered cautiously on a case-by-case basis.[20] Participants in an industrywide public hearing conducted by FDA in March 2005 voiced little support for color coding and called for additional research before it is used.[21]

Color coding can contribute to errors that would not happen without it. The color coding of ophthalmic products by pharmacologic category has led to numerous errors involving products within the same class. In 1996, the American Academy of Ophthalmology (AAO) urged manufacturers to convert to a uniform color-coding system, based on therapeutic class, for eye solutions and ointments; FDA and manufacturers of these products later agreed to this (Table 7-1).[22] The color-coding system reportedly helps ophthalmologists and patients quickly differentiate medications. Although it is intended to be an actual color-code system as defined above, in reality it is more likely that practitioners use the colors to differentiate products rather than to identify products by pharmacologic class. The system may contribute to errors if nurses and pharmacists confuse similar-appearing products in the same class. Color-coding may work well in an office setting or in the patient's home, but when similar corporate logos, fonts, and package sizes are also factored in, it may not be safe in pharmacies or on nursing units where larger numbers of medications are stored.

The products in Figure 7-10, all beta-blockers with yellow on the packaging, were found together in the same storage location, even though they should have been stored alphabetically by generic name. A pharmacy technician confused these while putting away an order from the wholesaler.[23] ISMP has also received reports of mix-ups between cyclopentolate hydrochloride 1% solution and tropicamide 1% solution, mydriatic/cycloplegics packaged in almost identical red-and-white cartons and similar containers inside the cartons. It takes four times longer to recover from the effects of cyclopentolate than tropicamide, so a mix-up could be significant. All of these ophthalmics are marketed by Falcon Pharmaceuticals, an affiliate of Alcon Laboratories. Figure 7-11 shows the similar packaging of Bausch and Lomb products, which use colored backgrounds for the labeling (and on the caps) to indicate drug class.

ISMP has contacted FDA, AAO, and various manufacturers about mix-ups of ophthalmic products within the same class but has received no indication that the situation will change. To reduce similarities and prevent errors, ISMP recommends purchasing ophthalmic products in the same class from different vendors. In many pharmacies, topical products are separated from other inventory and stored by brand, which means look-alike ophthalmic products from the same vendor would be stored next to each other.

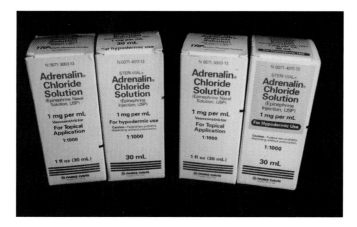

FIGURE 7-2 Look-alike packaging (left) of these topical and injectable Adrenalin products was redesigned (right) to prevent errors.

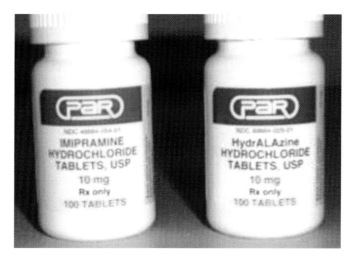

FIGURE 7-3 Look-alike packaging of imipramine (left) and hydralazine.

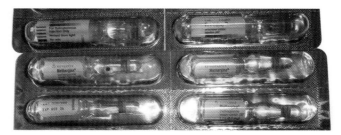

FIGURE 7-4 Look-alike ampuls of Brethine (top row) and Methergine (middle and bottom rows).

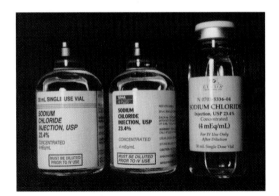

FIGURE 7-8 Red warnings that the products must be diluted.

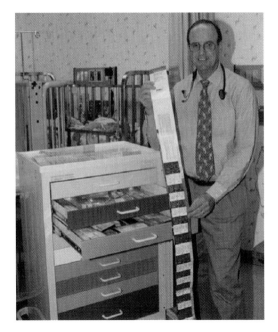

FIGURE 7-9 Physician James Broselow displays the Broselow tape, which uses colors keyed to a child's height to help practitioners select drug doses and equipment in pediatric emergencies; the color on the tape is matched to the appropriate crash cart drawer.

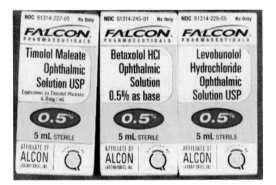

FIGURE 7-10 Ophthalmic solutions of timolol, betaxolol, and levobunolol incorrectly stored together.

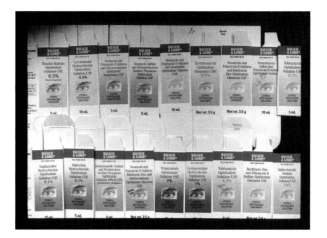

FIGURE 7-11 Using color to indicate drug class of ophthalmic products does not eliminate look-alike packaging of products within a class. Furthermore, there is too much similarity between some of the colors used.

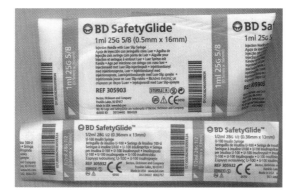

FIGURE 7-12 The color orange, traditionally associated with insulin syringes (below) is now mandated for safety-engineered syringes with 25 gauge needles (above).

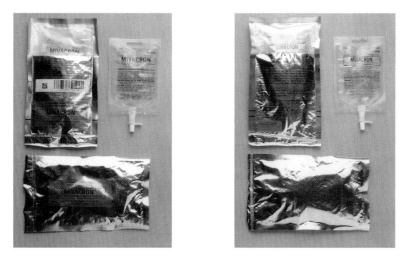

FIGURE 7-13 Improved packaging of Mivacron (left), with label on back of the overwrap and more prominent label on the front. The previous packaging (right) had led to errors.

Phenytoin 150-200 mg | Naloxone 1.0 mg | *ATROP 0.20 mg 2.0 ml
Max Rate = 10 mg per min. | DEFIB | BICARB 10 meq 10 ml
Lorazepam 1 mg | 20 J, 40 J if reqd | CALC 200 mg 2 ml
| | *LIDO 10 mg 0.5 ml

9 kg

SEIZURE	ICP	RESUSCITATION
Diazepam	Mannitol 9 gm	EPI 1st dose (1:10,000)
I.V. 0.9-2.7 mg q 5 min.	Furosemide 9 mg	0.09 mg 0.9 ml
Rectal 4.5 mg	OVERDOSE	*EPI 2+ doses (1:1,000)
Phenobarbitol 135-180 mg	D5W 18 ml	0.9-1.8 mg 0.9-1.8 ml
Phenytoin 135-180 mg	Naloxone 0.9 mg	*ATROP 0.18 mg 1.8 ml
Max Rate = 9 mg per min.	DEFIB	BICARB 9 meq 9 ml
Lorazepam 0.9 mg	18 J, 36 J if reqd	CALC 180 mg 1.8 ml
		*LIDO 9 mg 0.45 ml

8 kg

SEIZURE	ICP	RESUSCITATION
Diazepam	Mannitol 8 gm	EPI 1st dose (1:10,000)
I.V. 0.8-2.4 mg q 5 min.	Furosemide 8 mg	0.08 mg 0.8 ml
Rectal 4 mg	OVERDOSE	*EPI 2+ doses (1:1,000)
Phenobarbitol 120-160 mg	D5W 16 ml	0.8-1.6 mg 0.8-1.6 ml
Phenytoin 120-160 mg	Naloxone 0.8 mg	*ATROP 0.16 mg 1.6 ml
Max Rate = 8 mg per min.	DEFIB	BICARB 8 meq 8 ml
Lorazepam 0.8 mg	16 J, 32 J if reqd	CALC 160 mg 1.6 ml
		*LIDO 8 mg 0.4 ml

7 kg

SEIZURE	ICP	RESUSCITATION
Diazepam	Mannitol 7 gm	EPI 1st dose (1:10,000)
I.V. 0.7-2.1 mg q 5 min.	Furosemide 7 mg	0.07 mg 0.7 ml
Rectal 3.5 mg	OVERDOSE	*EPI 2+ doses (1:1,000)
Phenobarbitol 105-140 mg	D5W 14 ml	0.7-1.4 mg 0.7-1.4 ml
Phenytoin 105-140 mg	Naloxone 0.7 mg	*ATROP 0.14 mg 1.4 ml
Max Rate = 7 mg per min.	DEFIB	BICARB 7 meq 7 ml
Lorazepam 0.7 mg	14 J, 28 J if reqd	CALC 140 mg 1.4 ml
		*LIDO 7 mg 0.35 ml

6 kg

SEIZURE	ICP	RESUSCITATION
Diazepam	Mannitol 6 gm	EPI 1st dose (1:10,000)
I.V. 0.6-1.8 mg q 5 min.	Furosemide 6 mg	0.06 mg 0.6 ml
Rectal 3 mg	OVERDOSE	*EPI 2+ doses (1:1,000)
Phenobarbitol 90-120 mg	D5W 12 ml	0.6-1.2 mg 0.6-1.2 ml
Phenytoin 90-120 mg	Naloxone 0.6 mg	*ATROP 0.12 mg 1.2 ml
Max Rate = 6 mg per min.	DEFIB	BICARB 6 meq 6 ml
Lorazepam 0.6 mg	12 J, 24 J if reqd	CALC 120 mg 1.2 ml
		*LIDO 6 mg 0.3 ml

5 kg

SEIZURE	ICP	RESUSCITATION
Diazepam	Mannitol 5 gm	EPI 1st dose (1:10,000)
I.V. 0.5-1.5 mg q 5 min.	Furosemide 5 mg	0.05 mg 0.5 ml
Rectal 2.5 mg	OVERDOSE	*EPI 2+ doses (1:1,000)
Phenobarbitol 75-100 mg	D5W 10 ml	0.5-1.0 mg 0.5-1.0 ml
Phenytoin 75-100 mg	Naloxone 0.5 mg	*ATROP 0.10 mg 1.0 ml
Max Rate = 5 mg per min.	DEFIB	BICARB 5 meq 5 ml
Lorazepam 0.5 mg	10 J, 20 J if reqd	CALC 100 mg 1 ml
		*LIDO 5 mg 0.25 ml

4 kg

SEIZURE	ICP	RESUSCITATION
Diazepam	Mannitol 4 gm	EPI 1st dose (1:10,000)
I.V. 0.4-1.2 mg q 5 min.	Furosemide 4 mg	0.04 mg 0.4 ml
Rectal 2 mg	OVERDOSE	*EPI 2+ doses (1:1,000)
Phenobarbitol 60-80 mg	D5W 8 ml	0.4-0.8 mg 0.4-0.8 ml
Phenytoin 60-80 mg	Naloxone 0.4 mg	*ATROP 0.10 mg 1.0 ml
Max Rate = 4 mg per min.	DEFIB	BICARB 4 meq 4 ml
Lorazepam 0.4 mg	8 J, 16 J if reqd	CALC 80 mg 0.8 ml
		*LIDO 4 mg 0.2 ml

3 kg

SEIZURE	ICP	RESUSCITATION
Diazepam	Mannitol 3 gm	EPI 1st dose (1:10,000)
I.V. 0.3-0.9 mg q 5 min.	Furosemide 3 mg	0.03 mg 0.3 ml
Rectal 1.5 mg	OVERDOSE	*EPI 2+ doses (1:1,000)
Phenobarbitol 45-60 mg	D5W 6 ml	0.3-0.6 mg 0.3-0.6 ml
Phenytoin 45-60 mg	Naloxone 0.3 mg	*ATROP 0.10 mg 1.0 ml
Max Rate = 3 mg per min.	DEFIB	BICARB 3 meq 3 ml
Lorazepam 0.3 mg	6 J, 12 J if reqd	CALC 60 mg 0.6 ml
		*LIDO 3 mg 0.15 ml

RED
VASCULAR ACCESS: 22-24 Catheter, 23-25 Butterfly, Intraosseous Needle
N.G. TUBE 6F
URINARY CATHETER 8F
CHEST TUBE Newborn/Infant

PINK
E.T. TUBE Infant/Small Child
E.T. Tube at lip Infant
STYLET Newborn
SUCTION CATHETER 1 Straight
B.P. CUFF

3.5 mm uncuffed
10-10.5 cm

ORAL AIRWAY
B.V.M.
O. MASK
LARYNGOSCOPE

SMALL INFANT 3.5 E.T. TUBE
(SEE PINK-RED ZONE FOR COMPLETE EQUIPMENT LIST)

FIGURE 17-3 Section of the Broselow Pediatric Emergency Tape.

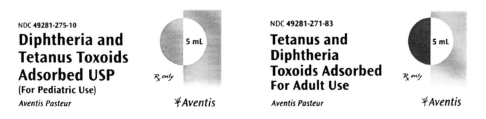

FIGURE 18-1 The package labels make adult and pediatric vaccines difficult to differentiate.

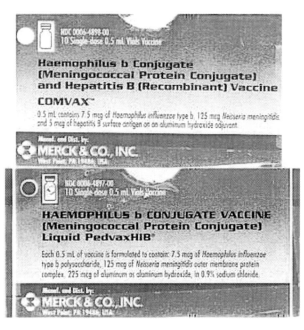

FIGURE 18-3 PedvaxHIB (Haemophilus b conjugate vaccine) and Comvax (Haemophilus b conjugate and hepatitis B recombinant vaccine) packages.

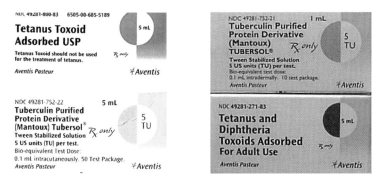

FIGURE 18-4 All of these products are stored in the refrigerator and may be located side by side. Limited availability of Td in single-dose syringes forces providers to purchase multidose vials, further contributing to the problem.

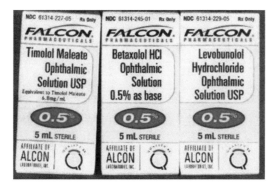

FIGURE 7-10 (also in color section following page 120) Ophthalmic solutions of timolol, betaxolol, and levobunolol incorrectly stored together.

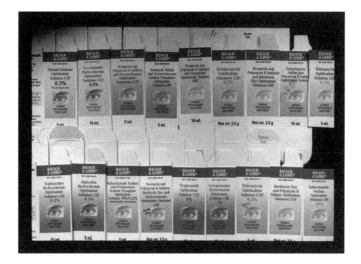

FIGURE 7-11 (also in color section following page 120) Using color to indicate drug class of ophthalmic products does not eliminate look-alike packaging of products within a class. Furthermore, there is too much similarity between some of the colors used.

A recent change in color used to identify needle gauges on disposable syringes further illustrates problems with color coding. The International Organization for Standardization (ISO) mandated orange color coding for all safety-engineered syringes with 25 gauge needles. Several 10-fold insulin overdoses have been associated with the color orange on the packaging (Figure 7-12), syringe cap, and hub of 25 gauge needles of tuberculin syringes. Traditionally, orange has been associated with insulin syringes and insulin vial caps, whereas 25 gauge needles, typically used for subcutaneous injections, have had a blue hub. Mistaking a safety-engineered tuberculin syringe and needle for an insulin syringe, a nurse gave a patient 50 units of insulin instead of the prescribed 5 units. (In addition to choosing the wrong syringe, the nurse read the ".5" mark on the syringe scale as 5 units instead of 0.5 mL.)

ISMP has been unable to learn why ISO made this change. Manufacturers must conform in order to export and import their products globally. According to a major syringe manufacturer, Becton, Dickinson and Company, the change affects only safety-engineered products, not the core hypodermic product line. ISMP recommends that hospitals switch to 26 gauge needles (brown) on tuberculin syringes so that the only orange syringe caps

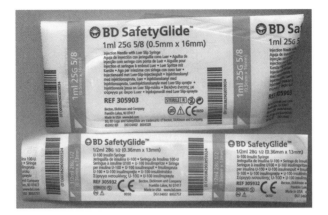

FIGURE 7-12 (also in color section following page 120) The color orange, traditionally associated with insulin syringes (below) is now mandated for safety-engineered syringes with 25 gauge needles (above).

will be on insulin syringes. Hospitals may also be able to substitute a 27 gauge needle (gray).

Inconsistent application across the industry or within a manufacturer's product line can add to the problems with color coding. One company used a product-specific color-coding scheme for the labels on some of its products, and blue-and-yellow labeling for the remainder of its products. Practitioners occasionally mixed up products with blue-and-yellow labels because they failed to recognize that the blue-and-yellow labels were not a product-specific color code.

Problems can also occur with color code schemes to be applied by users, such as the American Society for Testing and Materials (ASTM) standard for user-applied syringe labels in anesthesiology (Table 7-2).[24] Some of the label colors reflect characteristics of the drug class.[25] For example, a neon red-orange used for neuromuscular blockers indicates "danger." Blue signifies cyanosis of opiate-related respiratory depression. Labels for some antagonists are linked by color to the specific agonist (e.g., naloxone shares the color of opiates) but have diagonal lines printed along the border of the label. Drug names are printed on the labels, which are on rolls mounted alongside one another on a dowel so that anesthesia personnel can easily retrieve the required label.

Although these label colors identify a drug category, they do not identify a specific drug, strength, or dose contained in a syringe. Anyone other than the person who prepared the syringe does not know its content and thus could administer the wrong drug or dose. If the system is used as intended—to quickly distinguish the different drug classes—the ASTM color scheme has merit.[26] However, the user should add the drug name (if it is not already printed on the label) and strength.

ISMP supports the use of color-coded, user-applied labels in areas such as the operating room (OR), where a small number of drugs are used in an enclosed environment by a small number of individuals who are well trained and familiar with the ASTM system. However, extension of the ASTM user-applied label standard to labels of commercial injectable products has been suggested. Color codes on commercial vials and ampuls of high-alert drugs would be dangerous. As has occurred with topical ophthalmic products, color-coding by multiple manufacturers across product lines could lead to mix-ups of look-alike products and confusion between dosage strengths. Errors with high-alert drugs would likely be more serious. The challenge of ensuring that all practitioners knew the meaning of the label colors would be insurmountable.

TABLE 7-2　Specifications for User-Applied Drug Labels in Anesthesiology[24]

Drug Class[a]	Examples	Pantone Color, All Uncoated
1. Induction agents	Thiopental, methohexital, thiamylal, etomidate, ketamine	Yellow
2. Tranquilizers	Diazepam, midazolam	Orange 151
3. Muscle relaxants	Succinylcholine,[b] curare, mivacurium, vecuronium, pancuronium, atracurium	Fluorescent red 805
3a. Relaxant antagonists	Neostigmine, edrophonium, pyridostigmine	Fluorescent red 805 or warm red[c] and white diagonal stripes
4. Narcotics	Morphine, fentanyl, meperidine	Blue 297
4a. Narcotic antagonists	Levallorphan, naloxone	Blue 297 and white diagonal stripes
5. Major tranquilizers	Droperidol, chlorpromazine	Salmon 156
5b. Combinations of narcotics and major tranquilizers	Innovar (fentanyl–droperidol combination)	Blue 297 and salmon 156 longitudinal stripes
6. Vasopressors	Epinephrine,[b] ephedrine, phenylephrine	Violet 256
6a. Hypotensive agents	Trimethaphan, nitroprusside, nitroglycerin, phentolamine	Violet 256 and white diagonal stripes
7. Local anesthetics	Bupivacaine, lidocaine	Gray 401
8. Anticholinergic agents	Atropine, glycopyrrolate	Green 367

[a] Drugs that do not fit into these classes should be labeled with black printing on a white background.
[b] All printing is to be in black bold type, with the exception that "succinylcholine" and "epinephrine" shall be printed against the background color as reversed plate letters within a black bar running from edge to edge of the label.
[c] Warm red may be used if the printing of 805 fluorescent red stripes presents insurmountable difficulties.

If all products had identical black-and-white labels and were packaged in the same size and shape, careful reading of the labels would be the only way to differentiate them. That is not likely to happen, but perhaps it would reduce error potential. The Baxter ATC-212 dispenser and similar automated packaging and dispensing machines produce identically labeled unit dose packages of the same size and shape for all products. No errors have been associated with this approach; the only way to identify products is to read the labels. Even if practitioners misread or misunderstand the labeling, mix-ups of products stored together should be less likely since FDA now requires bar coding of prescription and nonprescription products used in hospitals and some products are identifiable through radio frequency methods.

TWO-SIDED LABELING

Practitioners' inability to see the front panel label has led to use of the wrong premixed IV product, with sometimes fatal results. Manufacturer labeling on both the front and back panels of containers can prevent such errors. Baxter Laboratories and Hospira package many of their premixed IV products with two-sided labeling on the foil overwraps of plastic minibags.

In one reported error, premixed Mivacron (mivacurium chloride, a neuromuscular blocker) was confused with Zantac injection; in another, Mivacron was confused with IV metronidazole. The minibags were impossible to differentiate from one another when stored face down, and the products were sometimes accidentally stored near one another. In addition, their foil outer wraps did not list the contents prominently (Figure 7-13).

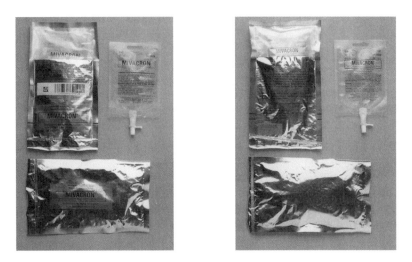

FIGURE 7-13 (also in color section following page 120) Improved packaging of Mivacron (left), with label on back of the overwrap and more prominent label on the front. The previous packaging (right) had led to errors.

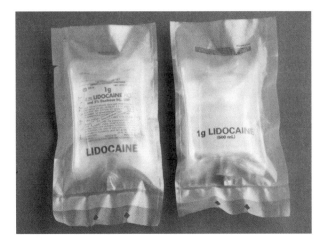

FIGURE 7-14 Premixed lidocaine from Abbott is labeled on both front and back of the plastic IV container and its overwrap.

Containers of IV lidocaine from all major manufacturers have been confused with containers of other premixed products, including heparin. In response to requests from ISMP, Hospira now uses two-sided labeling on both the immediate container of its pre-mixed lidocaine and the overwrap (Figure 7-14). Labeling products with crucial information on both the front and the back enables users to identify them no matter how the container is positioned.[27]

CONTRAST

Lack of contrast in labeling is especially problematic on small items. An ASTM standard[28] requires manufacturers to provide contrast between the type used for the proprietary and established names of the drug and the amount of drug per unit and either the immediate drug container or an opaque background. The standard also prescribes a legibility test requir-

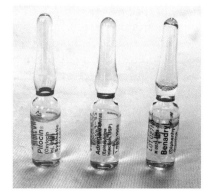

FIGURE 7-15 (also in color section following page 120) Patients have inadvertently received Adrenalin (center) rather than Pitocin (left) when the ampuls were mixed up; mix-ups between Pitocin and Benadryl (right) have also occurred.

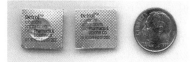

FIGURE 7-16 Detrol unit dose packaging.

ing that the name and amount of the drug be legible in 20 footcandles of light at a distance of about 20 inches (500 mm) by a person with 20/20 unaided or corrected vision. However, some manufacturers of products in ampuls outside the United States use ceramic print on clear glass, which has no contrasting background. Depending on the color of the print, the background, and lighting conditions, a label may be virtually illegible. In the past, ampuls of the Parke-Davis products Pitocin, Adrenalin, and Benadryl (Figure 7-15) were frequently mixed up when read against a dark background, sometimes with fatal consequences.[29]

Labeling on aluminum foil-wrapped unit dose products can be difficult to read because of the shininess. For example, 1 mg and 2 mg unit dose Detrol (tolterodine tartrate) tablets (Figure 7-16) were in dime-sized packages imprinted with tiny black characters on shiny foil. The drug name and strength overlapped the area where the foil is sealed to the plastic tray that holds the tablet and were almost impossible to read, especially in reflected room light. It took only one phone call from a practitioner to prompt Pharmacia to revise this poor labeling, making the strength more prominent through the use of bold type in a larger size, centered on a line of its own, and repositioning other text. However, the overall package is still dime size, with no room for a bar code, and how much the change improves readability is questionable. Manufacturers that use foil packaging should consider the effects of glare from reflected light on readability. Only nonreflective materials providing good contrast with printed information should be used for unit dose blister packaging.

Another example of poor contrast is the labeling of low-density polyethylene (LDPE) ampuls of respiratory therapy medications (Figure 13-3). This is one of the more frequent product problems reported to MERP. Many products from various manufacturers (Astra-Zeneca, Dey Labs, Genentech, Nephron, Roxane, Sepracor, Zenith-Goldline, and others) are packaged in look-alike plastic ampuls with little difference in shape or color. The drug name(s), strength, lot number, and expiration date are embossed into the plastic in transparent, raised letters and are virtually impossible to read. FDA was forced to exempt LDPE packaging from bar-code requirements because an embossed bar code cannot be scanned electronically.

Practitioners have reported confusion between plastic ampuls of ipratropium (Atrovent), albuterol (Proventil), levalbuterol (Xopenex), budesonide (Pulmicort Respules), dornase alfa (Pulmozym), and cromolyn (Intal). Some products in plastic ampuls (e.g., Pulmicort, Xopenex, and Accuneb [albuterol]) are available in multiple dosage strengths that are difficult to distinguish because of the poorly visible labels. The risk of a mix-up is heightened if staff keep various respiratory medications in their lab coat pockets or mixed together in a "respiratory bin" in a refrigerator.

The potential for error is even greater since some manufacturers (AstraZeneca, Avitro, Vital Signs) have introduced injectable products packaged in LDPE ampuls with the same type of labeling, such as heparin for IV flush use and Naropin (AstraZeneca's ropivacaine product), a local anesthetic. A hospital recently reported a near miss with look-alike vials of different strengths of Naropin. A pharmacy technician mistakenly placed vials of Naropin 1% (10 mg/mL) instead of 0.2% (2 mg/mL) in an automated dispensing cabinet on the labor and delivery unit. A resident removed a vial of Naropin 1% to prepare an epidural for a patient in labor, but the attending anesthesiologist caught the error before the drug was administered. AstraZeneca also manufactures Naropin in various strengths (2 mg/mL, 7.5 mg/mL, and 10 mg/mL) in prefilled, Polyamp DuoFit polypropylene containers. Lidocaine is available in this packaging, as well. These containers, which all look similar, can be mistaken for respiratory medications. It is difficult to see the small, black print placed directly on the clear plastic containers, especially when the container is held against a dark background.

Respiratory products in LDPE containers have been confused with clear, single-dose LDPE containers of eye drops. A nurse in a long-term care facility was about to administer what she thought was Hypotears PF (polyvinyl alcohol, preservative-free) drops to a resident. She had picked up a container of albuterol inhalation solution, which had been mistakenly placed in the resident's medication cart drawer. The nurse noticed the error and did not place albuterol into the resident's eyes.

FDA has allowed manufacturers to continue producing plastic ampuls with embossed labeling because of evidence that chemicals used in other types of labeling (e.g., paper labels with ink) can contaminate the products. LDPE is permeable to volatile chemicals that exist in the immediate packaging environment. In FDA studies, samples have tested positive for volatile chemicals whose presumed source was packaging and labeling materials such as adhesives, varnishes, inks, and solvents. Inhaled products can have irritant as well as toxic effects on patients with respiratory conditions. Patients with severe asthma, for example, might react to very low doses of inhaled chemical irritants, and adverse effects (e.g., bronchospasm) might not be recognized because they mimic disease symptoms. For these reasons, an FDA draft guidance for industry in 2002 ("Inhalation Drug Products Packaged in Semipermeable Container Closure Systems") recommended measures for limiting chemical contamination, including embossed labels as an alternative to paper labels and inks. Manufacturers have followed that recommendation, despite the many reports of problems. Suggestions considered in 2004 by the FDA Drug Safety and Risk Management Committee included the use of large, easy-to-read fonts in embossing and the use of aluminum foil overwraps. One company suggested using the product's initial (e.g., A = Atropine) in a large font on the flashing (the part of the ampul that does not touch the drug itself). This would not prevent errors, however, since Atrovent is also on the market in LDPE packaging.

Only the pharmacy staff, not respiratory or central supply staff, should order respiratory medications. Manufacturers should be asked to ship the products (including different strengths) separately in well-marked boxes to promote accurate placement into storage. Plastic ampuls should be placed in an outer package that can be labeled more clearly. Respiratory medications should never be stored together in a single bin or in lab coat pockets.

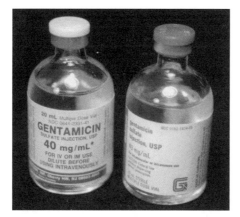

FIGURE 7-17 Prominent display of the gentamicin concentration (container at left) has led users to mistake it for the total contents of the container.

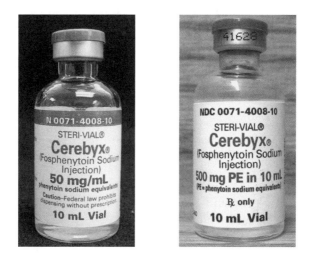

FIGURE 7-18 After errors in which the prominent "50 mg/mL" on the old Cerebyx label (left) was mistaken for the total amount of drug in the vial, the manufacturer redesigned the label (right).

EXPRESSIONS OF CONCENTRATION AND STRENGTH

The way in which a manufacturer denotes the strength of a drug can be confusing and may lead to errors. For example, a number of errors have been reported in which the entire contents of a 20 mL, 40 mg/mL gentamicin container were injected instead of the correct dose of 40 mg. Because the concentration (40 mg/mL) is listed so prominently on the original container (Figure 7-17 left), inexperienced users have thought the entire container held 40 mg. They failed to read additional important label information, including the volume of the vial.

Vials of Cerebyx (fosphenytoin) list the volume in one position and the strength in another position. On the old product label (Figure 7-18 left), the strength in milligrams of phenytoin sodium equivalent units [PE]) per milliliter ("50 mg/mL") could be misread as the total volume of the vial. In one case reported to ISMP, Cerebyx 150 mg IV (100 mg PE) was ordered in an emergency department (ED) for a 2-year-old child with seizures. A pharmacy technician misread the Cerebyx label and delivered three 10 mL vials (total of 1,500 mg PE) to the ED. A nurse

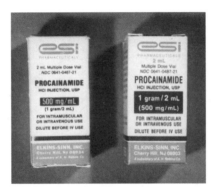

FIGURE 7-19   Old (left) and new labeling of procainamide; the new labeling gives equal prominence to the concentration and the total vial content.

also misread the label, assuming that 50 mg was in each vial. She drew up 30 mL (1,500 mg PE) instead of 150 mg of Cerebyx (100 mg PE) and handed it to another nurse, who administered the drug. Assuming that the proper dose had been diluted, the second nurse did not question the 30 mL volume. The patient died soon after the injection, and excessive amounts of phenytoin (fosphenytoin is a phenytoin prodrug) were found in the child's blood. Because of the confusing labeling, some hospitals placed restrictions on the prescribing and dispensing of this drug soon after it was marketed. In February 1999, after another child's death, FDA asked Parke-Davis to redesign the label to better reflect its 50 mg PE/mL (500 mg PE/10 mL) contents (Figure 7-18 right).

Similar problems have been reported with other products. At one time, Pronestyl and generic procainamide injections listed the concentration per milliliter in a prominent position on the packaging. The volume appeared elsewhere (Figure 7-19 left). Users repeatedly mistook the concentration per milliliter as the amount in the vial. After several error reports, ISMP asked that FDA require manufacturers to express both the concentration per milliliter and the total contents together on the front label panel (Figure 7-19 right). No further errors have been reported since this labeling change.

Several errors reports have involved labeling of unit dose liquid packets of the immunosuppressant Rapamune (sirolimus). The label identifies the concentration of the liquid as 1 mg/mL, but the 1, 2, and 5 mL packets (bottom to top in Figure 7-20) do not clearly display the total volume, which is in small type in the colored band at the top. At least two patients at one hospital received the wrong dose because of this packaging. The hospital now puts auxiliary labels on the products. In another hospital, a 5 mg dose of Rapamune was ordered, but the pharmacy was asked to dispense 1 mg packets to allow dose adjustment. The nurse instructed the patient's mother to give five (1 mg) packets to start, but the pharmacy dispensed 5 mg packets. The patient received two doses of 25 mg each. Another patient was to receive 4 mg of Rapamune oral solution. The pharmacy sent four packets labeled as 1 mg/mL, but each packet contained 2 mL (2 mg). The nurse administered 8 mg, double the dose ordered. Until the manufacturer changes the label, pharmacy-applied auxiliary labeling is probably the best way to prevent errors.

A practitioner reported in 1999 that the package label on Bentyl (dicyclomine) injection 2 mL ampuls listed only the drug concentration, 10 mg/mL, and did not indicate that the total volume of each ampul contained 20 mg (Figure 7-21), making accidental overdosage likely. In response, ISMP contacted FDA and the manufacturer (then Hoechst Marion Roussel, now Aventis) to urge a label correction. Eventually, the company revised the label, but a report reached ISMP 2 years later about a shipment of Bentyl with the old labeling. The manufacturer was continuing to ship its inventory of product with the old

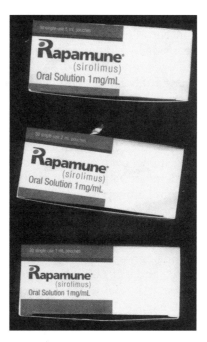

FIGURE 7-20   Unit dose packets of Rapamune oral liquid clearly display the 1 mg/mL concentration but not the volume in milliliters.

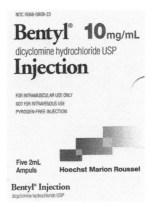

FIGURE 7-21   Old Bentyl package labeling.

labeling until the supply was exhausted. The company sent no advisory letter to its customers, and FDA issued no warnings. Patients who receive an overdose of this drug may suffer anticholinergic effects such as dry mouth, urinary retention, hallucinations, tachycardia, and blurred vision. Pharmacists should add a cautionary note to each ampul to remind users of the total contents (20 mg/2 mL).

FDA has not published specific guidance on how a drug's concentration or strength should be conveyed on package labels, but normally the agency has not allowed total content labeling of multiple-dose vials greater than 2 mL because of concern that someone might mistake the total content listed on the label as an appropriate single dose. The agency plans to publish a new guidance statement on labeling and packaging in 2006. Inconsistencies in company labeling practices and the FDA approval process allow the risk of serious error to continue. ISMP believes product labels should prominently display the total contents. Both the concentration per milliliter and the total volume and amount in metric weight should appear side by side or one just above the other, within the same border or shaded background, even on multiple-dose vials.

The expression of drug concentrations in pharmaceutical labeling as a percentage or ratio of weight to volume has been problematic. For most injectable products, the concentration is expressed in milligrams or micrograms per milliliter, but the concentration of a few drugs is expressed as a dilution ratio or percentage (e.g., epinephrine 1:1,000 [Figure 7-2], lidocaine 1%). Studies have shown that knowledge about concentrations expressed as a ratio or percentage is inadequate, even among physicians and emergency medicine residents.[30–32] These poorly understood expressions are particularly prevalent for drugs used in resuscitation (e.g., calcium, epinephrine, lidocaine, magnesium sulfate, neostigmine, sodium bicarbonate). An inappropriate dose or life-threatening delay in treatment is quite possible if these drugs are prescribed in milligrams (which requires knowledge of ratio or percent concentrations and calculations) or milliliters (a problem if multiple concentrations exist). For example, an epinephrine dose in milliliters was ordered in a neonatal emergency. Both 1:1,000 and 1:10,000 dilutions were available on the code cart. Despite initial confusion, a pharmacist who was present was able to provide guidance on the proper dose for the patient. Neonatal nurses and physicians had assumed that only the 1:10,000 dilution was available on the code cart.

Several incidents have been reported in which undiluted epinephrine 1:1,000 (1 mg/mL) was given IV to patients instead of the 1:10,000 (0.1 mg/mL) concentration. In each case, the more dilute epinephrine (1:10,000) was available, but staff members who did not understand the ratio expression inadvertently prescribed or selected the 1:1,000 concentration. One error occurred in an outpatient radiology unit where the nurse on duty rarely administered medications. The patient had an adverse reaction to a contrast agent, with hives and respiratory distress. The physician prescribed 3 mL of epinephrine 1:10,000 IV, but 3 mL of the 1:1,000 concentration was administered in error. Contributing to the error was the challenge of differentiating the labeling of the two concentrations. Depending on the typography and the available label space, 1:1,000 can look like 1:10,000, especially without a comma separating the zeros. In another case, a physician's assistant ordered the incorrect concentration for a patient in an urgent care clinic, and the nurse administered it without recognizing the problem. Some brands of epinephrine do not have a warning anywhere on the ampuls to dilute the 1:1,000 concentration before IV administration. These two errors caused rapid heart rates and increased blood pressure, necessitating overnight hospital stays for the patients.

Because not all health care practitioners are familiar with percent or ratio expressions of concentrations, or adept at calculating doses of drugs whose concentrations are expressed in this manner, it is helpful for hospitals to create a dose conversion chart reflecting concentrations available in the facility. The chart can be posted on code carts and in other areas where emergency medications may be prepared. Since an independent double check by another clinician may not be feasible in emergency situations, staff should refer to the dose chart before administration of these products. Many of the emergency medications with concentrations expressed in ratios or percentages date back before the 1938 Food, Drug and Cosmetic Act and thus are exempt from current FDA labeling standards. Concentrations expressed as a ratio or percent may be less dangerous for topical products and local anesthetics, but for systemic dosing they do not serve practitioners well. ISMP asked both FDA and USP to address the serious issue of epinephrine dose expression (since epinephrine is a USP listed drug). The petition to USP (www.ismp.org/Newsletters/acutecare/articles/20040812.asp) asked for the elimination of ratio expressions on labels of epinephrine injection. It stressed that the drug concentration should be

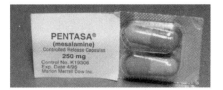

FIGURE 7-22   It is not clear to users whether the entire unit dose package or each capsule contains 250 mg.

expressed only in milligrams, except when epinephrine is mixed with local anesthetics such as lidocaine to prolong their duration.

The labeling of oral solid dosage forms in unit dose packaging sometimes expresses the amount of drug in a misleading way. For example, UDL Laboratories at one time distributed acetaminophen 650 mg (two 325 mg tablets) in a unit dose package labeled "325 mg." Pentasa (mesalamine) 250 mg capsules have been packaged in a two-capsule unit dose package labeled "250 mg" (Figure 7-22). It is not clear to users whether the entire package or each capsule contains 250 mg. Manufacturers should stipulate the amount per tablet as well as per package (e.g., Pentasa 500 mg [2 × 250 mg capsules]). A similar example, described in Chapter 13, is the original packaging and labeling of Children's Tylenol Meltaways.

LABELING OF BLISTER STRIPS

On some nonprescription medications packaged in blister strips, the product name and strength appears only once or randomly over the blister strip. Regardless of a product's prescription or nonprescription status, the name and exact strength should be present on each pocket of the blister strip. Whether or not the manufacturer intends this, many nonprescription drugs are used in institutions as part of a unit dose dispensing system. Therefore, a bar code is required by FDA regulations. The blisters can be cut and separated from one another, or the drug name may be torn, making identification impossible and contributing to subsequent errors if the product is relabeled extemporaneously.

COMPANY NAME, LOGO, AND CORPORATE DRESS

Logos and other designs can interfere with product identification, as illustrated by an error that led to an outbreak of severe, unexplained illness on a neonatal ward in a hospital in Canada.[33] Patients were initially thought to have sepsis, but investigation revealed that the illnesses resulted from repeated administration of racemic epinephrine to patients who were supposed to receive vitamin E. The packaging of the two products, both manufactured by the same company, was nearly indistinguishable (Figure 7-23). Both 15 mL screw-cap bottles were amber and bore a label with black print on angled blue and green bands, the label style used for the company's entire product line. Features such as lines, bars, and stripes contribute to mix-ups by interfering with readability.

Even the company name may get in the way of the drug name. ISMP recommends that the manufacturer's name always be placed at the bottom of the label and that the most prominent information on the label be the name and strength (or concentration) of the product (sidebar, page 117). Ideally, these two pieces of information should appear within the same background or border.

SYMBOLS

Symbols increase the risk of medication errors because they can be misinterpreted by the user. For example, the Roman numeral four (IV) is used in the name of Becton Dickinson's

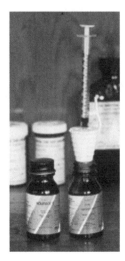

FIGURE 7-23 (also in color section following page 120)   Epinephrine and vitamin E in look-alike vials.

Micro-Fine IV needle for insulin. A hospital pharmacist expressed concern to ISMP that the "IV" could be misinterpreted as "intravenous." Someone giving insulin might, if not fully concentrating on the task, administer insulin intravenously instead of subcutaneously. Becton Dickinson told ISMP that it has received calls about this. The company makes an alternative product (Ultra-Fine) that does not use the "IV." FDA should recognize that the use of Roman numerals is a potential problem.

Similarly, misinterpretation of the Drug Enforcement Administration (DEA) symbol for schedule 4 controlled substances ("C-IV") has led to errors. In one case, someone crushed diazepam tablets, dissolved them, and gave them intravenously.[34] ISMP received a report about an ER patient for whom Phenergan VC with Codeine Syrup (promethazine, phenylephrine, and codeine) was ordered as a take-home prescription. A nurse located a bottle of generic promethazine with codeine syrup (without phenylephrine), which had a large C encircling a V on the front label panel. The nurse thought this was Promethazine VC with Codeine Syrup, but the "C-V" symbol indicated that the product contained a schedule 5 controlled substance. Federal regulations allows companies to use Arabic instead of Roman numerals on package labeling to decrease the chance of error.

Patients may misinterpret symbols that health care professionals would understand, such as the symbol warning that a product is teratogenic (a slash through a circle depicting a pregnant woman). However, CDC has reported that many uncounseled women did not understand this symbol, used on the labeling of Accutane (isotretinoin), Cytotec (misoprostol), and other teratogenic drugs. Some women thought it meant the product was a birth control pill. Some became pregnant while taking Accutane, despite the symbol and the manufacturer's efforts to warn against pregnancy. Health care providers should renew their efforts to ensure that patients who take teratogenic drugs know about the associated risks and understand the need for negative pregnancy tests, appropriate birth control, proper drug storage, and avoidance of sharing these medications with others. Companies need to employ communication experts to ensure that any symbols used on labels are well understood. Table 8-3 lists additional error-prone symbols.

STANDARDIZATION OF TERMINOLOGY

USP and FDA should standardize the terminology used on labels. Both "single-use" and "single-dose" have been used on container labels to mean the same thing: that the pharmacist

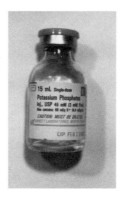

FIGURE 7-24 "Single-dose" as used on this label has been misinterpreted to mean the container holds one dose of medication.

or nurse should discard the container after withdrawing one dose for a patient, or the doses for several patients at the same time, or the amount needed to prepare an admixture for infusion. "Single-dose" on a vial is not intended to mean that the contents are to be given as a single dose. However, some users have interpreted it that way. A nurse gave a patient an entire 15 mL (45 mmol) "single-dose" vial of potassium phosphates injection (Figure 7-24), when the correct dose was 1 mL (3 mmol).[35] The USP-FDA advisory panel on label simplification preferred "single-use" rather than "single-dose."[11]

Package labeling for magnesium sulfate injection offers another example of lack of standardization. Six unit-of-measure designations are used: percent (%), milligram (mg), gram (g), milliliter (mL), milliequivalent (mEq), and milliosmole (mOsm). To add to the confusion, some prescribers order the drug in terms of the number of vials or ampuls. Because there are so many dosing expressions, it is difficult for practitioners to recognize excessive doses.

Cerebyx (fosphenytoin sodium injection) presents a unique example of nonstandard dose expression. This prodrug was brought to market to replace phenytoin sodium injection. FDA and the manufacturer agreed on labeling that calls for fosphenytoin to be prescribed in terms of its phenytoin equivalent (PE). Fosphenytoin sodium 75 mg is equivalent to phenytoin sodium 50 mg; thus, the equivalent of a 100 mg dose of IV phenytoin should be ordered as "fosphenytoin 100 mg PE," not as "fosphenytoin 150 mg." Asking practitioners to order one drug while referring to the dose of another is unprecedented, and it creates opportunity for error. The "PE" designation often is accidentally omitted in the ordering, transcribing, or dispensing (practitioner labeling) of this drug. Some prescribers dose the drug by its actual strength, while others follow the suggested method. Underdoses and overdoses have been the result.

LABEL REMINDERS AND WARNINGS

In some cases, the best way to reduce the potential for error is to add a warning to the label. In 1988, after learning of numerous deaths caused by the administration of undiluted potassium chloride injection instead of 0.9% sodium chloride injection, bacteriostatic water, or sterile water for injection, ISMP organized a meeting of practitioners, regulatory authorities, and manufacturers. The group brainstormed methods for preventing the recurrence of this error. As a result, USP eventually imposed new requirements for the nomenclature and packaging of potassium chloride.[36,37] The name was changed to "potassium chloride for injection concentrate," and a boxed warning that reinforces the need for

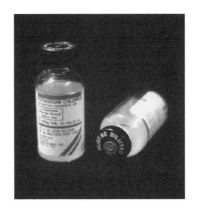

FIGURE 7-25   Vials of concentrated potassium chloride injection must carry a boxed warning that the product must be diluted.

dilution was added to the label (Figure 7-25). Black caps and a ferrule that seals the rubber stopper to the vial are now required. The phrase "Must be diluted" appears in contrasting color on the cap and ferrule. Although potassium chloride injection accidents still occur, no cases involving substitution for sodium chloride traced to misreading the label have been reported since these actions were taken. Restricting the availability of potassium chloride in clinical areas was proposed as the best way to eliminate this problem and is now required by the Joint Commission on Accreditation of Healthcare Organizations (JCAHO).[38]

Warning statements on vincristine have also helped reduce errors. After a number of reports of fatal intrathecal injections of the drug, which is intended for IV use only, modifications in the labeling and packaging were requested[39] and USP established a new dispensing standard for the drug.[39,40] The new standard requires health care workers to package vincristine in syringes or vials with a labeled overwrap that states, "Do not remove covering until moment of injection. Fatal if given intrathecally. For intravenous use only." All vincristine containers now carry this warning. Since 1995, FDA has also required manufacturers to include warning stickers and overwraps in the package for application by practitioners; this change was made at the request of ISMP.

Since the vincristine label standard went into effect in 1991, inadvertent intrathecal injection has continued to occur in the United States and elsewhere. In 1994, the World Health Organization informed regulatory authorities worldwide of the U.S. experience. The USP dispensing standard is not always followed in U.S. hospitals. In a 2005 survey by ISMP, about 25% of respondents said their acute care facilities were not using the overwrap, and 7% did not label the syringe with the appropriate warning.[41]

There may be value in a hierarchy of signal words for label warnings, such as, in decreasing order of seriousness, "danger," "warning," "caution," and "notice." Highlighting the warning with large or bold type, a box, or color may be effective. A brief description of the hazard and connection to consequences may be useful. An Environmental Protection Agency project on consumer product labeling provides further suggestions for enhancing understanding of label information.[42]

TYPEFACE

Clarity can be enhanced by the appropriate use of type elements such as serif or sans-serif and uppercase or lowercase letters.[43] Serifs are the short extenders attached to the tops and bottoms of letters in certain typefaces. Sans-serif (without serifs) type is plainer

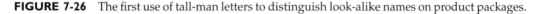

FIGURE 7-26   The first use of tall-man letters to distinguish look-alike names on product packages.

than serif type and generally works best for conveying short pieces of information such as that on product labels. Letters with serifs take up more space than sans-serif letters, and uppercase letters consume more space than lowercase letters. Lowercase letters have characteristics such as ascending and descending strokes that make them easier to read than uppercase letters, which are all the same height. Sans-serif typefaces such as Arial and Helvetica may provide a bolder warning than others because of their clarity and legibility.[8]

Manufacturers have used enlarged letters to enhance distinctive portions of look-alike names on look-alike packaging. Wyeth-Ayerst (now Wyeth) was the first to do this, with its Tubex line of prefilled syringe cartridges. After mix-ups between Tubex cartridges of dimenhydrinate and diphenhydramine, the company began labeling them diPHENhydraMINE and diMENhydriNATE (Figure 7-26). Fewer mix-ups were reported to the company and ISMP after the change. ISMP began referring to this method of differentiation as tall-man lettering in 1999,[44] and it has been used to differentiate the names of both generic and branded products.

Small ampuls and vials present particular problems because the print must be very small. Manufacturers should consider using partially filled ampuls or unit dose blister-packs to allow space for printing essential information in a legible size. To enhance legibility of essential information on small ampuls, FDA may allow manufacturers to omit some of the information that is normally required on packages and labels.

EXPRESSING PRODUCT EXPIRATION DATES

Federal regulations set forth conditions for listing expiration dates on drug product labels. With few exceptions, companies must list an expiration date on the immediate container and on any outer package if the date is not legible through the outer packaging. When single-use ("single-dose") containers are packed in individual cartons, the expiration date may appear on the carton instead of the immediate container. The regulations do not specify how expiration dates must be expressed, and confusion can occur. Axcan Scandipharm listed JN05 as the expiration date on a Canasa (mesalamine) suppository package label, which could have meant January or June. Lactaid Original, distributed by McNeil Nutritionals, uses an atypical abbreviation for April; thus, AL 05 meant April 2005. The Aventis Pasteur poliovirus vaccine (inactivated) listed an expiration date of 06 MAR 04; practitioners were not sure whether this meant March 6, 2004, or March 4, 2006.

Occasional medication errors have resulted from misinterpreted expiration dates. For example, a night nurse thought that vials of magnesium sulfate had expired. The expiration date was listed as 1-06, but the product lot number, 2002, appeared just before the expiration date. Because the nurse thought the drug expired on January 6, 2002, treatment was delayed. Similar problems may occur with nonprescription (over-the-counter [OTC]) products. Enforcement of expiration dates for nonprescription products is not required if the product labeling does not bear dosage limitations, and if the product is stable for at least 3 years. When they do appear, expiration dates on nonprescription products may be difficult to decipher. For example, Resource Benecalorie, a medical food supplement from Novartis Nutrition, does not list an expiration date, but it uses a 4-digit code for the month and year of production (e.g., 0504 for May 2004), which has been misinterpreted as an expiration date. The user is supposed to determine the expiration date by adding 270 days to the production date.

The 2005 edition of *USP-NF* (*U.S. Pharmacopeia, 29th Revision* and *National Formulary, 24th Edition*) addresses expiration dating in a way that may help FDA clarify ambiguous dating. On General Notices page 11, *USP-NF* states: "The label of an official drug product or nutritional or dietary supplement product shall bear an expiration date. All articles shall display the expiration date so that an ordinary individual under customary conditions of purchase and use can read it. The expiration date shall be prominently displayed in high contrast to the background or be sharply embossed, and easily understood (e.g., EXP 6/09," "Exp. June 09," or "Expires 6/09")."

The Consumer Healthcare Products Association's *Voluntary Codes and Guidelines of the OTC Medicines Industry* addresses the display, location, and legibility of expiration dates; expiration statements that are understandable to consumers (e.g., "Exp 6/09," "Expires 6/09"); the avoidance of packaging features that might interfere with legibility (e.g., end seals on shrink-wraps); and emerging technologies for the application of expiration dating (e.g., improved debossing techniques, advances in ink printing).

The International Organization for Standardization (ISO) has a standard for expression of dates (see www.cl.cam.ac.uk/~mgk25/iso-time.html), although it is not specifically designed for pharmaceutical labeling. The Canadian government, as well as many provincial governments and large corporations, is adopting the ISO standard for expressing dates in general, not just expiration dates. The ISO format calls for YYYY-MM-DD, YYYYMMDD, or YYYY MM DD (e.g., 2005 08 11). It moves from the longest to shortest time frame (year, month, day); the only variation is the separator. A hyphen, unlike a slash mark (/), is less likely to be mistaken for a 1 when handwritten. Hence, a hyphen, a space, or no separator is used. USP does not specify a format for expiration dating, although the United States has approved the ISO format for general uses; USP plans to evaluate this.

USE OF UNSAFE ABBREVIATIONS AND DOSE DESIGNATIONS

Numerous patient injuries have resulted from confusion about the meaning of abbreviations (e.g., U for units, QD for daily) and of dose designations that exclude a zero before the decimal point or include an unnecessary decimal point and a "trailing" zero after a whole number. Chapter 8 describes many such errors. A JCAHO National Patient Safety Goal now prohibits practitioners' use of abbreviations and dose designations recognized as dangerous (Table 8-1), and progress has been made toward changing prescribing habits to exclude these unsafe designations.

Drug companies have used these dangerous designations in official product labeling and packaging and in advertising (Figure 7-27). In addition, companies have abbreviated the drug name itself. An advertisement for methotrexate used the abbreviation MTX, which has been confused with mitoxantrone, another cancer drug with an overlapping

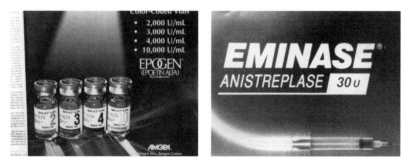

FIGURE 7-27 The abbreviation "U" for units in the Epogen ad (now changed) and Eminase label can be misread as a zero, leading to 10-fold overdosage.

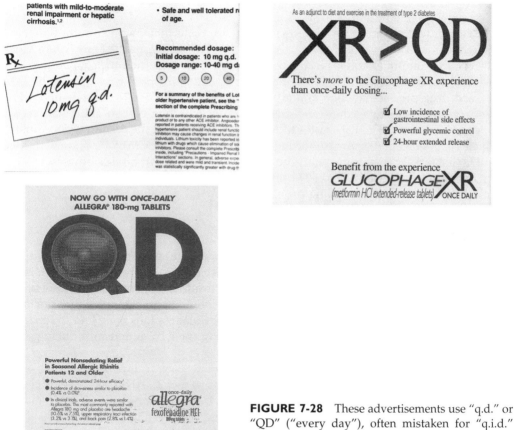

FIGURE 7-28 These advertisements use "q.d." or "QD" ("every day"), often mistaken for "q.i.d." ("four times a day").

dose. Although some ads with dangerous designations have been changed, others (Figure 7-28) continue to appear in medical journals and elsewhere.

The trailing zero, prohibited by USP, appears in product labeling. The packaging of Hectorol (doxercalciferol) ampuls uses not only a trailing zero but also the Greek letter mu (μ) in the abbreviation for micrograms (μg) (Figure 7-29). Neither is acceptable to ISMP or JCAHO.

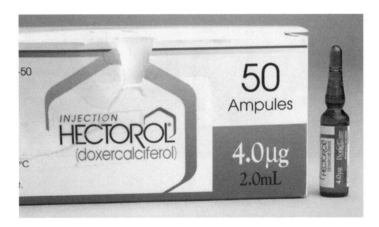

FIGURE 7-29   This advertisement uses trailing zeros and a Greek mu, both dangerous designations.

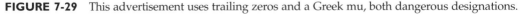

More than 50 medical organizations represented at a 2005 JCAHO summit agreed that health care providers should be held to a standard that calls for avoidance of the dangerous abbreviations and dose designations listed in JCAHO's National Patient Safety Goals. However, the summit attendees recognized the difficulty of gaining the cooperation of all providers, especially when the error-prone designations continue to appear in FDA-approved drug product labeling and advertising. Since the 1990s, ISMP has urged FDA to issue guidance to companies and advertisers on avoiding certain abbreviations and dose expressions. In 1996, FDA and PhRMA, both members of the National Coordinating Council for Medication Error Reporting and Prevention (NCCMERP), endorsed NCC-MERP's list of abbreviations that should never be used in prescribing (www.ncc-merp.org/council/council1996-09-04.html). In 2005, FDA and PhRMA committed to work with ISMP to address this ongoing problem.

BAR CODES

Bar code technology has long been used in many industries to improve productivity and accuracy. Bar code applications in the medication-use process are relatively recent, in part because the pharmaceutical industry has been slow to adopt a universal bar code standard and consistently apply bar codes to the immediate container of all medications, including unit dose packages. Hospitals and other health care organizations have had to repackage medications in order to apply bar codes—increasing their costs and introducing a new opportunity for error.

Hypothetically, if 1 million patients in U.S. hospitals each receive 16 doses of medication in a given day, and the error rate is a very conservative 2%, then 320,000 errors occur daily. Applying estimates by Leape and colleagues[45] that 38% of medication errors occur during the administration process and 11% during dispensing, more than 100,000 errors each day occur during medication administration and 35,000 during dispensing. The use of machine-readable code could prevent most of these errors, including some that cause death or permanent injury.

Recognizing the potential of bar coding to improve patient safety, FDA now requires bar codes, in a linear format, on the immediate package of most products.[46] The bar code must contain the NDC number, but the expiration date and lot number are optional. Reduced-size symbology may be used if it is linear. Composite bar codes are acceptable only for lot numbers and expiration dates. The FDA rule, issued in 2004, required all new products coming to market to comply; products already on the market were to comply

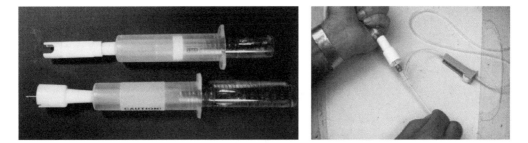

FIGURE 7-30 Prefilled syringes of lidocaine 100 mg for direct injection in emergencies (top left) and syringes of lidocaine 1 or 2 g for IV admixture preparation (bottom left) looked almost identical. More than 40 deaths occurred when the syringe of concentrated lidocaine was used for injection into patients' IV lines (right).

by April 2006. The rule allowed exceptions for a few products, including oral contraceptive dial packs, LDPE containers, radiopharmaceuticals, drug sample packages, and medical gases (www.fda.gov/OHRMS/DOCKETS/98fr/2002n-0204-nfr0001.pdf). Despite concern that manufacturers might procrastinate or decrease the availability of products in unit dose packaging,[47] bar coding is used in the medication process at a growing number of hospitals.

CONTAINER DESIGN

The design of the immediate container should make it difficult for users to administer products incorrectly. Several serious errors[48] led to withdrawal from the market in 1993 of lidocaine 10% and 20% packaged in syringes for IV admixture preparation.[49,50] More than 40 deaths and many serious accidents had occurred during the decade after introduction of these products when practitioners used the syringes of 1 or 2 g of lidocaine, intended for dilution in 5% dextrose injection, for direct injection into the Y-sites of patients' IV lines (Figure 7-30). Three pharmaceutical companies manufactured syringes of lidocaine 100 mg with an attached needle for use in cardiac emergencies; the usual loading dose for patients with ventricular arrhythmia is 75 mg to 100 mg. The 100 mg syringes for direct injection and the products for admixture preparation looked nearly identical. Because the 100 mg syringes contained 2% lidocaine, a "2" was prominent on the labeling. But the 2 g additive syringe also bore a large 2, and practitioners occasionally confused it with the 100 mg syringe and administered massive overdoses of lidocaine. Had the additive syringe been designed so that its needle would fit only the injection port of an IV bag, this could not have occurred.

Years later, a company asked ISMP to test nearly identical packaging for injectable diltiazem (a syringe of concentrated drug meant for addition to an IV container for infusion). The delivery system was rejected—as any similar packaging should be in the future.

Manufacturers' containers that require manual activation by a practitioner before drug administration have been involved in errors. One example was a Baxter dual-chamber container for IV administration of heparin in dextrose injection (Figure 7-31), which was withdrawn from the market in 1995. The user needed to fracture a plastic cannula to mix the heparin from the upper chamber with the diluent in the lower chamber. (Compatibility problems precluded premixing by the manufacturer.) When users failed to fracture the cannula, patients received the diluent without heparin, which presented a serious patient safety problem. The manufacturer could have equipped the product with a fail-safe mechanism that prevented administration until the solution had been mixed.

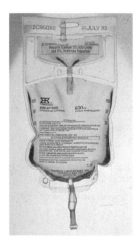

FIGURE 7-31 Dual-chamber container of heparin plus diluent.

A serious error occurred with a Baxter dual-chambered IV bag with amino acids in the lower chamber and 50% dextrose in the upper chamber, used for total parenteral nutrition (TPN). A seal separating the chambers must be broken by the user to mix the TPN base solution. Normally, pharmacy staff mixes the contents of the two chambers before injecting the additives. In a case reported to ISMP, a pharmacist injected electrolytes and insulin into a dual-chamber bag and sent it to the nursing unit without realizing that the two chambers had never been mixed. The nurse did not recognize the problem before administering the product. Since the IV administration set attaches directly to the lower chamber, where the solution had not been diluted with fluid from the upper chamber, the patient received the TPN additives, including electrolytes and insulin, in twice the intended concentration. The patient's condition declined a few hours after the solution was started. A nurse then noticed that the two chambers were not mixed, stopped the TPN, and called the pharmacy. The patient's blood glucose concentration dropped to 18 mg/dL at one point; he suffered no permanent harm but had to stay an extra day in the ICU. Because this was the second time a bag had left the pharmacy unmixed, the product was removed from the pharmacy inventory.

Premixed amino acid–dextrose products cannot be manufactured because heat sterilization will caramelize the solution. Dual-chamber containers are convenient in facilities that would ordinarily use a gravity method for mixing solutions from separate containers of amino acids and dextrose, and where the number of preparations does not warrant an automated IV compounder. Unmixed bags should not leave the pharmacy, but that can happen. Failure to recognize an unmixed bag is more likely when multivitamins have not been added, because the amino acid (light straw color) and dextrose (colorless) chambers look similar. Hospira manufactures similar combinations in dual-chamber containers but uses a different method to seal the chambers. With the Baxter bag, pressure is applied to the upper chamber to break a seal between the two chambers. A red plastic clip separates the two chambers of the Hospira bag; although the clip is a visual reminder, staff can still forget to activate the container.

Where dual-chamber bags must be used, pharmacists should consider adding multivitamins (i.e., a portion of the day's dose) to each bag to help ensure recognition of inactivated bags. In addition, mixing the solution could be included as a step on quality control checklists for TPN, and independent double checks of the admixture could be

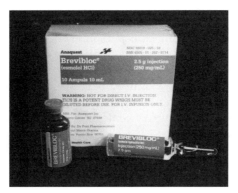

FIGURE 7-32 Overdoses of Brevibloc have been given when the 2.5 g ampul (right) was used instead of the 100 mg vial.

performed before products leave the pharmacy. Nurses should know to ensure that bags are properly mixed before hanging them.

At least 22 cases of Brevibloc (esmolol) overdosage were reported after the product became available in the late 1980s.[51] The overdoses occurred in part because a 2.5 g ampul intended for dilution and subsequent infusion, rather than a 100 mg vial, was used to prepare a loading dose (Figure 7-32). Ampuls, which are always single-dose (single-use) containers, normally are used for loading doses; vials most often are used for multiple doses. The packaging of this product, however, was the opposite. The manufacturer did not take into account that loading doses often are ordered in terms of number of ampuls. Although the company placed a warning flag on the ampul neck to underscore the need for dilution, another accident happened soon after this change. The manufacturer subsequently made the drug available in a ready-to-use form that eliminates the need for an ampul and thus improves safety.

Products not intended for ophthalmic use are error prone when packaged in bottles or tubes that look like containers of eye drops or ointment (Figure 11-4); such products should not be stored in bathrooms or other areas where they might be mistaken for ophthalmic products. Cases have been reported in which visually impaired people instilled cyanoacrylate cement ("super glue") instead of their eye drops. In addition, irrigation containers have been mixed up with IV solution containers,[52] and topical nitroglycerin packaged in tubes has been used sublingually and as a dentifrice.[53,54]

In a case reported to ISMP, a man with poor eyesight, intending to take a capsule of his heart medication, nearly asphyxiated when he gagged on a desiccant capsule left in the medication bottle.[55] Other such cases have also been reported; some of the patients required surgery. When dispensing an original manufacturer's container, pharmacy staff should warn the patient about desiccants. If possible, the desiccant should be removed prior to dispensing.

Tactile cues can be an important way of differentiating product containers. Because of the extreme consequences of a mix-up, some neuromuscular blocking agents, including Mivacron (mivacurium) and Tracrium (atracurium), are packaged in vials with hexagonal necks. In the past, insulin vials had a distinct shape related to the insulin type (i.e., regular insulin was packaged in round vials, NPH in a square vial, and Lente in a hexagonal vial). The system was discontinued when U-100 insulin products were introduced, even though patients found it helpful.[56]

PROTECTIVE OVERWRAPS

Hospital workers and other health care personnel need to realize the importance of keeping commercially premixed plastic IV containers in their protective overwraps during storage. Premixed minibags of medications have been removed from their overwraps months before they are needed, and unused bags have been returned to the pharmacy and restocked. Without the overwrap, fluid from the bag evaporates; as the fluid volume in the container decreases, the drug concentration increases, and patients are likely to receive more than the prescribed dose. If a 1 hour infusion of potassium chloride 40 mEq in 100 mL was prescribed and an infusion pump was set to deliver 100 mL over 1 hour, a premixed minibag exposed to room air for several weeks would contain a more concentrated potassium solution that would be infused in much less time than intended. One patient was to receive a 100 mL drug infusion over 1 hour, but the bag was empty in 30 minutes. The volume of another 100 mL minibag that also had been removed from its overwrap was measured; it contained only 85 mL.[57]

Evaporation from plastic containers depends on environmental factors (e.g., humidity, temperature) and the type of material used by the manufacturer. Many drugs are packaged in polyvinyl chloride (PVC) bags, but some are in less permeable plastics that have different rates of moisture transmission. Various manufacturers use different packaging materials. Hospira uses PVC or nonplasticized thermoplastic copolyester (CR3). The company recommends using PVC containers of premixed drugs in volumes greater than 25 mL within 30 days of storage at room temperature after removal from the overwrap. The CR3 material, which has greater clarity, has a shorter shelf life after removal from the overwrap. Five percent dextrose solutions with heparin or dopamine are good for only 7 days, but dobutamine is good for 14 days. Baxter recommends discarding minibags of 50 mL or less after 15 days out of the overwrap, while containers of 100 mL or more can be used for up to 30 days. Since drug stability depends on light sensitivity and other factors, it is difficult to recommend safe storage standards after removal from the overwrap. Baxter uses polyolefin, which is less permeable to water vapor, for some premixed minibags. B. Braun Medical products are packaged in a proprietary layered plastic that uses polyolefin as the solution contact layer. This allows longer storage without the plastic overwrap, so products of 250 mL or less are good for 2 months and 500 mL and 1000 mL products last for 3 months.

Products such as premixed antibiotics have high turnover and may never reach the expiration date after removal from the overwrap. For less frequently used products, clinicians may be tempted to mark IV bags with the expiration date. Practitioners should not write directly on IV bags (or LDPE plastic vials), especially with felt-tip markers. Commercial inks on IV bag labels have undergone rigorous testing to demonstrate their suitability for use, but the inks in markers and other writing tools have not been tested for safe use on IV bags. Volatile chemicals from the ink may reach the solution. Practitioners should indicate the expiration date by placing a label on a portion of the bag that does not come into contact with solution.

EXTERNAL CARTON LABELS

Sometimes the immediate container label on a product clearly expresses its contents but the carton holding several containers is not labeled clearly. ISMP Canada reported that two patients died after a technician made an error in compounding a batch of dialysis solution for continuous renal replacement therapy for several ICU patients. One of the additives required was sodium chloride injection 340 mEq for each 3 L bag of dialysis fluid. The technician determined that he needed to add 85 mL of 23.4% sodium chloride

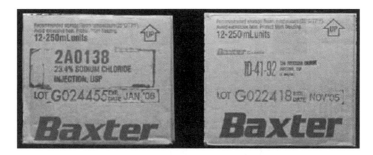

FIGURE 7-33   Lids of shipping cartons of sodium chloride (left) and potassium chloride 250 mL bottles.

injection (4 mEq/mL) to each of 35 bags. Therefore, an entire carton of 12 bottles, 250 mL each, was needed. But the technician picked up a carton of 12 bottles of concentrated potassium chloride (2 mEq/mL) instead of the intended sodium chloride bottles. The cardboard boxes, both from Baxter, were stored on shelves across from each other and looked very similar (Figure 7-33). The drug names on the cartons were in much smaller print than the product identification number and the manufacturer's name. Another pharmacy technician checked the items selected for preparation but did not detect the error. The glass bottles were identical in shape and size. The potassium chloride bottles had black caps, but the technician was unaware that black caps are reserved for potassium chloride. The technician used 85 mL (170 mEq) of potassium chloride in each 3 L bag. A third technician checked the completed batch but did not notice the error. When a dialysis patient suddenly died, the solution was immediately tested, revealing the error. The hospital recalled the remaining bags, but not before a second patient had died. Manufacturers must remember that the purpose of all labeling is to identify the container's contents. Labeling practices should take into account the needs of end users and those responsible for inventory control.

PROMOTIONAL ITEMS AND ADVERTISEMENTS

Pharmaceutical companies use promotional items such as pens and prescription pads as a constant reminder of their products. Errors can occur when manufacturers use promotional items that look like the product itself. For example, FDA received a report that Janssen Pharmaceuticals was distributing an antibacterial hand washing gel packaged in a white bottle that was labeled "Antibacterial Gel" but prominently displayed the proprietary name, Risperdal, of the company's risperidone product. Practitioners might have thought the bottle contained Risperdal oral solution. A pharmacist discovered several bottles in hospital medication rooms. Furthermore, the label did not state the active and inactive ingredients of the gel, which could be problematic if a user were allergic to an ingredient. FDA recommended that hospitals inspect patient care areas and remove this item from medication storage areas, and the manufacturer stopped distributing it.

In another case a dermatologist gave what he thought was a sample 30 g tube of Protopic (tacrolimus) ointment 0.1% to a 17-year-old patient, telling her to apply it for treatment of facial contact dermatitis and eczema. As directed, the patient applied the product to her rash, only to discover that the contents was purple ink from a felt-tip pen used for product promotion (Figure 7-34 bottom). The patient went to an ER and was prescribed a topical corticosteroid for a local reaction to the ink. Reportedly, the manufacturer has ceased distribution of the promotional marker mimicking its product.

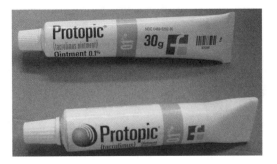

FIGURE 7-34   A physician, intending to give a patient a medication sample (top), mistakenly gave her a felt-tip pen used for product promotion (bottom).

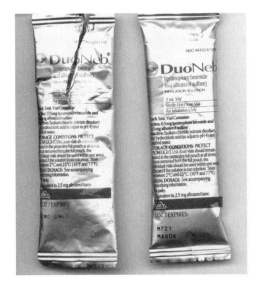

FIGURE 7-35   The package on the left is a demonstration item containing saline solution. It is distinguished only by the words "demo only" where the lot number and expiration date appear on the actual product.

Dey Laboratories manufactures Duoneb (ipratropium/albuterol) in 3 mL prediluted LDPE vials in individual foil overwraps. The company also made a demonstration product in a foil overwrap for use by sales representatives; it was labeled as DuoNeb and looked identical to the drug product package (Figure 7-35) but contained only saline solution. The saline package was distinguished only by the words "Demo Only" in small type at the bottom of the labeling below the heading for a lot number and expiration date. The demonstration package could have found its way into the drug distribution chain and caused harm to an asthmatic patient who received saline instead of active drug. Dey stopped using the item after ISMP expressed concern.

Some drug product advertisements use dose designations and abbreviations that violate practice standards or USP standards, as noted above, or omit important prescription information. Such poor practices in advertising may lead to bad habits on the part of practitioners and potential medication errors. The Hismanal advertisement in Figure 7-36 does not state a dose. "As directed" in the ad for Glynase Prestab 3 mg in Figure 7-36 is not an appropriate direction for use of the product. Practitioner review before approval of the ads could have prevented the use of these inappropriate expressions.

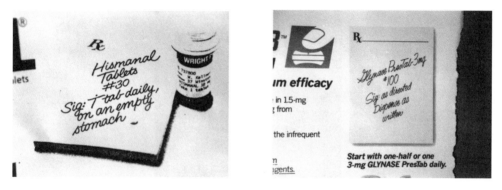

FIGURE 7-36   The mock prescription in the Hismanal ad does not state a strength, and the Glynase mock prescription gives inadequate directions for use ("as directed").

BRAND NAME EXTENSIONS FOR NONPRESCRIPTION DRUGS

Many of the patient safety issues associated with brand name extensions involve labeling and packaging. Strong brand names can help companies promote new or modified products, but the use of a familiar name can have unintended consequences if the product contains totally different ingredients. A few products that use familiar names but have different ingredients are described below; other examples are in Chapter 6.

- Neo-Synephrine, a well-known brand name for phenylephrine, is also used for oxymetazoline 0.05% spray.
- Afrin, a brand name for oxymetazoline, is also used for some products that contain only saline.
- Anacin may or may not contain aspirin.
- Betadine is used for one product with iodine and two without. Betadine povidone–iodine has been used for 40 years, but the name is also used for a topical antibiotic combination product, Betadine First Aid Antibiotics + Moisturizer, which contains bacitracin and polymyxin B. The third product, Betadine First Aid Antibiotics + Pain Reliever, contains bacitracin, polymyxin B, and pramoxine. The packaging of all three products in ointment form has a large blue H (suggesting that Betadine is the number 1 brand in hospitals), which makes them look alike. At one hospital, the pharmacy ordered a Betadine product that turned out to be bacitracin and polymyxin. A technician distributed it to the OR, and a nurse noticed that it was not the intended povidone–iodine product.
- The Maalox brand name is associated with several products, not all of which contain aluminum–magnesium hydroxide and simethicone. The bottle of Maalox Total Stomach Relief looks similar to regular Maalox (Figure 7-37) but contains only bismuth subsalicylate. All the products are packaged in white plastic containers of the same size and shape and prominently bear the Maalox name on the front label panel. The bismuth subsalicylate content is stated less prominently on the Maalox Total Stomach Relief bottle, and a banner in the upper corner proclaims, "Great new look. Same great Maalox," which is likely to mislead consumers. The back label panel contains warnings related to use by children or teens with flu symptoms, patients receiving oral anticoagulants, and patients allergic to aspirin, and lists noteworthy side effects (e.g., black stools and tongue). A pharmacist's grandfather noted black stools after she had suggested he use Maalox for stomach upset; this caused concern because he

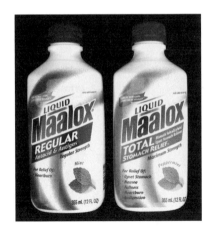

FIGURE 7-37   Banner at top left of both labels says "Same great Maalox," but the active ingredients are different.

had been receiving low molecular weight heparin and aspirin since recent orthopedic surgery. The pharmacist's mother had unknowingly bought the Total Stomach Relief formula with bismuth subsalicylate for the grandfather.

Brand name extension should not be allowed unless at least one main ingredient from the original product is present in the new or modified product. The mix-up with Betadine products highlights the importance of reading active ingredients on drug labels. It also makes a case for bar coding, especially since pharmacists may not consistently check all floor stock before it leaves the pharmacy. Furthermore, in a case such as the nonprescription Betadine products, a patient with allergies to any of the ingredients used in the product line might use an unintended product.

DRUG SHORTAGES

In addition to problematic packaging and labeling, shortages of drug products can disrupt the medication-use process and lead to errors. The pharmaceutical industry and regulatory authorities must do everything possible to avoid shortages and, when they do occur, to communicate better with practitioners about the reason for and expected duration of the shortage.

In 2001 ISMP surveyed hospital pharmacists about drug product shortages.[58] The pharmacists said a wholesaler's failure to deliver a product was often their first warning of a shortage. One respondent noted, "We rarely find out about shortages from manufacturers and find them unwilling to supply letters to answer physicians' questions about the projected length and rationale for the shortage."

The respondents cited the increased risk of dosing errors by practitioners unfamiliar with substitute products (e.g., errors when sufentanil, which has a much lower dose, was substituted during a fentanyl shortage), adverse reactions to higher-potency opiates, ineffective pain control, and contamination and drug diversion when multidose vials were used or single-dose vials were reused to prevent waste.

ISMP and others have recommended actions for dealing with shortages.[59,60] ASHP, in cooperation with the University of Utah and the group purchasing organization Novation, maintains a Web site (www.ashp.org/shortage/) on current drug shortages, the reasons, and the estimated resupply dates. Practitioners should report shortages to FDA (www.fda.gov/cder/drug/shortages).

INTERNATIONAL EFFORTS

ISMP encourages international communication about medication errors. U.S. practitioners' reports of errors to USP, ISMP, and FDA have led to the resolution of many problems related to commercial labeling, packaging, and nomenclature. Too often, however, the pharmaceutical industry has failed to apply in other countries the lessons learned in the United States, as shown in the following examples:

- USP bans the abbreviation "U" for units and the decimal point before a trailing zero in U.S. product labels, recognizing the error potential of these designations, yet a Canadian manufacturer's container of insulin cartridges expresses the concentration as "100U/mL, 3.0 mL cartridges."
- USP and FDA require U.S. manufacturers to package potassium chloride concentrate vials with a black cap and to place the warning "Must Be Diluted" on the cap and vial ferrule and in a box on the front label panel. Canada does not have these labeling requirements. There, a plastic ampul of the concentrate contains only a small black mark on the snap-off portion.
- In Canada, vials of the neuromuscular blocking agent Quelicin (succinylcholine) are devoid of warning that the drug is a paralyzing agent that causes respiratory arrest (and therefore can be used only when the patient is mechanically ventilated). In the United States, the vial cap and ferrule state, "Warning: Paralyzing Agent," and similar warnings appear on the front label panel.
- The U.S. trademark Losec (omeprazole) was changed to Prilosec because the names Losec and Lasix (furosemide) were often confused, yet Losec remains the brand name in other parts of the world; in Canada, for example, it is still being confused with Lasix.

The USP and FDA labeling requirements for preventing intrathecal administration of vincristine, discussed earlier in this chapter, have not been adopted in most other countries. The exception is the United Kingdom. Several deaths associated with intrathecal vincristine administration occurred in that country,[61] and more than 50 have been reported worldwide. Vincristine warning labels in the United Kingdom are now required to state, "For Intravenous Use Only." Only the approved administration route is mentioned, because U.K. authorities feared that a statement such as "Not for Intrathecal Use" might be misread as "For Intrathecal Use." The U.K. National Patient Safety Agency has taken steps to ensure that companies comply with this labeling change.

U.S. health care facilities sometimes use foreign-manufactured drug products, and errors can occur if practitioners are not familiar with dosing and administration methods used in the source country. For example, the foreign-manufactured oral syringe (referred to as a pipette) that accompanies Risperdal (risperidone) oral solution has a volumetric scale imprinted on the plunger, not the barrel (Figure 7-38). Also, the markings run in the opposite direction of conventional markings on U.S. syringes. The volume of liquid in the syringe is indicated on the portion of the plunger that is outside the barrel when the syringe is assembled, rather than on the portion inside the barrel. A nurse who intended to withdraw 0.25 mg (0.25 mL) of risperidone liquid drew up 2.75 mL instead. To avoid this problem, Risperdal tablets should be used whenever possible, or the pharmacy should prepare doses in U.S.-manufactured oral syringes.

Manufacturers and regulators worldwide need to put in practice the lessons learned in the global market. For example, U.S. authorities might consider the U.K. approach to vincristine labeling. Although many product improvement efforts have been reactive rather than proactive, FDA and U.S. pharmaceutical manufacturers now routinely analyze

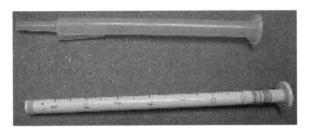

FIGURE 7-38 On this foreign-manufactured syringe for Risperdal (risperidone) oral solution, the markings are on the plunger, not the barrel, and they run in the opposite direction of conventional markings on U.S. syringes.

proposed brand names, labels, and packages to determine error potential before product approval.

Global pharmaceutical industry leaders need to support improvement efforts implemented everywhere their products are used. Along with its counterpart organizations in Canada and Spain, ISMP is working with the pharmaceutical industry and regulatory agencies in those countries to address identified product problems. Pharmaceutical labeling and packaging speak a universal language that must be clear to all pharmacists, physicians, nurses, and patients who make decisions based on the information presented.

PROSPECTIVE ANALYSIS TO PREVENT LABELING AND PACKAGING PROBLEMS

Labeling and packaging problems might occur less frequently if practitioners' input were considered in label and package design. Labeling often is reviewed on two-dimensional proofs several times the size of the actual label. Nurses, physicians, and pharmacists looking at the actual package in their work environment would be far more likely to discover problems than would designers sitting at desks.

Pharmaceutical and medical device manufacturers should use failure mode and effects analysis (FMEA) (Chapter 21) to anticipate errors. This would entail practitioner review of labeling, packaging, and nomenclature.[62,63] ASHP recommended in 1990 that FDA require manufacturers to include practitioners in industry discussions concerning drug labeling, packaging, and naming.

An example involving Bristol-Myers Squibb Oncology's Platinol-AQ (cisplatin injection) illustrates the application of FMEA.[64] After the launch of cisplatin injection in the 1980s, overdoses occurred because providers confused daily doses with the total dose for a course of therapy. Moreover, the drug was confused with Paraplatin (carboplatin) because of similarities in product names. Doses appropriate for carboplatin usually exceed the maximum dose of cisplatin. Severe toxicity and death were associated with cisplatin overdose.

The company decided to use FMEA to resolve this problem and, in conjunction with ISMP, appointed an advisory panel of oncology specialists in pharmacy, medicine, and nursing. An FMEA model developed by ISMP was used. Factors such as visibility of brand and generic names; strength, concentration, and volume; differentiation of strengths, forms, and sizes of the same product; presence, prominence, and visibility of required warnings, special instructions, and other label information; and method(s) of assembly and potential for proper use of the package were individually analyzed and collectively scored. The potential for confusion of Platinol with Paraplatin was discussed, as was the fact that practitioners failed to recognize that the dose they were using was excessive.

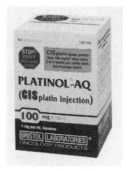

FIGURE 7-39 (also in color section following page 120)   Platinol-AQ labeling and packaging were changed to prevent mix-ups with Paraplatin.

As a result, labeling and packaging changes (Figure 7-39) were proposed, accepted by the company, and approved by FDA, as follows:

- The tall-man letters "CIS" appear in bold, red characters to differentiate this product from carboplatin.
- The word "Stop!" appears within an octagonal red stop sign, warning users to verify the drug name and dose.
- A boxed warning notes that cisplatin doses of greater than 100 mg/m^2 once every 3 to 4 weeks are rare and advises the user to consult the package insert for further information.
- Information appears on more than one side of the box. No matter how the product is placed on the shelf, the warnings are visible.
- The vial seal and closure call attention to the maximum dose of cisplatin.
- Stickers enclosed in the carton certify that cisplatin has been prepared at the proper dosage.

The company conducted an extensive advertising campaign to educate health professionals about the changes and proper drug dose. Since the change was implemented, no mix-ups between the two products have been reported to MERP.

Lyophilized cisplatin was eventually removed from market and is now available on special notice for chemo-embolism procedures. Only Platinol-AQ, a solubilized product, remains. This also helps differentiate cisplatin from carboplatin, which is now available only in powder form as a lyophilized product.

ISMP believes all labeling and packaging should undergo prototype testing by practitioners (and consumers, as appropriate) in their own environments using FMEA. Testing should take into account the human factors described earlier in this chapter. FDA should require FMEA by companies; the following criteria should be considered: the ordering and inventory process, drug storage and delivery, drug name and strength, and total amount in the container. As noted in Chapter 6, a number of proprietary consulting organizations exist to help companies determine the likelihood that a proposed trademark, label, or package would be vulnerable to user error.

CONCLUSION

Labeling, packaging, and nomenclature issues play a role in about half of all reported medication errors, but FDA and the pharmaceutical industry can be slow to respond when such problems are identified. The 2000 Institute of Medicine report *To Err Is Human: Building a Safer Health System*[65] asked FDA to (1) develop and enforce standards for the design of drug packaging and labeling to maximize safety; (2) require pharmaceutical testing of proposed drug names; and (3) establish an appropriate response to problems identified through postmarketing surveillance, especially those that are perceived to require immediate response to protect the safety of patients. To date, the agency has not established standard requirements for testing proposed drug names nor issued new guidance to industry on labeling and packaging. In 2006 a related IOM report, *Preventing Medication Errors*,[66] asked FDA to collaborate with the pharmaceutical industry, the Agency for Healthcare Research and Quality, USP, ISMP, and other appropriate parties to (1) develop a guidance document for industry on the methods of applying FMEA to labeling and packaging, (2) carry out additional studies of optimum designs for all drug labeling and information sheets that reflect human and cognitive factors, and (3) evaluate different methods of presenting unit-of-use packaging and designs that best support consumers in their medication self-management. FDA may need greater authority to require action on the part of the pharmaceutical industry.

REFERENCES

1. Kenagy JW, Stein GC. Naming, labeling, and packaging of pharmaceuticals. *Am J Health Syst Pharm.* 2001;58:2033–41.
2. Berman A. Reducing medication errors through naming, labeling, and packaging. *J Med Syst.* 2004;28:9–29.
3. Phillips J, Beam S, Brinker A, et al. Retrospective analysis of mortalities associated with medication errors. *Am J Health Syst Pharm.* 2001;58:1835–41.
4. Grasha A. A cognitive systems perspective on human performance in the pharmacy: implications for accuracy, effectiveness and job satisfaction. Executive Summary Report. Alexandria, Va: National Association of Chain Drug Stores; 2000 Oct. Report No. 062100.
5. Institute for Safe Medication Practices. Insights into people will improve our safety systems. *ISMP Medication Safety Alert!* June 27, 2001(6):1–2.
6. Senders J. Theory and analysis of typical errors in a medical setting. *Hosp Pharm.* 1993;28:505–8.
7. Centers for Disease Control and Prevention. Inadvertent intradermal administration of tetanus toxoid-containing vaccines instead of tuberculosis skin tests, *MMWR.* 2004;53(29):662–4. Available at: www.cdc.gov/mmwr/preview/mmwrhtml/mm5329a5.htm. Accessed March 17, 2006.
8. Swayne T. *Information Design for Patient Safety.* London: National Patient Safety Agency (United Kingdom) and Helen Hamlyn Research Center; 2005. Available at: www.hhrc.rca.ac.uk/resources/publications/IDPS.pdf. Accessed January 2006.
9. Canadian Standards Association. Standard Z264.2-99. Labelling of drug ampoules, vials, and prefilled syringes. General Instruction No. 1 and No. 2. January and October 1999.
10. Cohen MR. Potassium chloride injection mix-up [letter]. *Am J Hosp Pharm.* 1990;47:2457–8.
11. Stimuli to the revision process. Report and recommendations of the USP–FDA Advisory Panel on Simplification and Improvement of Injection Labeling. *Pharmacopeial Forum.* 1994;20:7885–8.
12. Christ RE. Review and analysis of color-coding research for visual displays. *Human Factors.* 1975;17:542–70.
13. American National Standards Institute, Association for the Advancement of Medical Instrumentation. Human factors engineering guidelines and preferred practices for the design of medical devices (ANSI/AAMI HE-48). Arlington, Va: Association for the Advancement of Medical Instrumentation; 1993:41.
14. Okabe M, Ito K. How to make figures and presentations that are friendly to color blind people. Available at: http://jfly.iam.u-tokyo.ac.jp/html/color_blind/. Accessed November 1, 2005.
15. Baker DE. Use of color on pharmaceutical labels and packaging [editorial]. *Hosp Pharm.* 2005;40:296–7.
16. Foster P. Drug syringe labeling. *Anesthesia.* 2003;58:99–100.
17. Cumberland P, Rahi JS, Peckham CS. Impact of congenital color vision deficiency on education and unintentional injuries: findings from the 1958 British birth cohort. *BMJ.* 2004;329:1074–5.
18. Van der Waarde K. An information design approach to labeling. A response to the FDA request for comments about the "Use of color on pharmaceutical product labels, labeling and packaging" (Docket No. 2005N-O036). Available at: www.fda.gov/cder/meeting/part15_3_2005/Transcript.pdf.
19. American Society of Health-System Pharmacists Council on Professional Affairs. Use of color to identify drug products. *Am J Health Syst Pharm.* 1996;53:1805.

20. American Medical Association. Report 5 of the Council on Scientific Affairs (A04). The role of color coding in medication error reduction. Available at: www.ama-assn.org/ama/pub/category/13662.html. Accessed November 1, 2005.

21. Food and Drug Administration. Center for Drug Evaluation and Research. Use of Color on Pharmaceutical Labeling and Packaging Part 15 Hearing. March 7, 2005. Available at: www.fda.gov/cder/meeting/part15_3_2005/Transcript.pdf.

22. American Academy of Ophthalmology. Policy statement: color codes for topical ocular medications. www.aao.org/aao/member/policy/color.cfm. Accessed December 1, 2005.

23. Cohen MR. An example of how color coding can contribute to medication errors. *Hosp Pharm*. 2003;38:905.

24. Standard specifications for user applied drug labels in anesthesiology. Standard No. D 4774-94 (2000). West Conshohocken, Pa: American Society for Testing and Materials.

25. Foster P. Labeling history reviewed and future explored. *Anesthesia Patient Safety Foundation Newsletter*. 2006;20:86–7.

26. Christie IW, Hill MR. Standardized colour coding for syringe labels: a national survey. *Anaesthesia*. 2002;57:793–8.

27. Cohen MR. Comments on pharmacy labeling practices. *Hosp Pharm*. 1993;28:1039–43.

28. Standard specification for labels for small-volume (100 mL or less) parenteral drug containers. ASTM D4267-95 (2001). West Conshohocken, Pa: American Society for Testing and Materials.

29. Cohen MR. Dangerous ampul mix-up. *Hosp Pharm*. 1988;23:91.

30. Rolfe S, Harper NJ. Ability of hospital doctors to calculate drug doses. *BMJ*. 1995;310:1173–4.

31. Jones SJ, Cohen AM. Confusing drug concentrations. *Anaesthesia*. 2001;56:195–6.

32. Nelson LS, Gordon PE, Simmons MD, et al. The benefit of houseofficer education on proper medication dose calculation and ordering. *Acad Emerg Med*. 2000;7:1311–6.

33. Solomon SL, Wallace EM, Ford-Jones EL, et al. Medication errors with inhalant epinephrine mimicking an epidemic of neonatal sepsis. *N Engl J Med*. 1984; 310:166–70.

34. Cohen MR. C-IV symbol continues to be misinterpreted. *Hosp Pharm*. 1988;23:1024.

35. McClure M. Human error—a professional dilemma. *J Prof Nurs*. 1991;7:207.

36. Cohen MR. Vials of potassium chloride injection. *Hosp Pharm*. 1990; 5:191–3.

37. Heller W. USP: of, by, and for the professions. *Am J Hosp Pharm*. 1989;46:2522.

38. Joint Commission on Accreditation of Healthcare Organizations. Medication error prevention—potassium chloride. *Sentinel Event Alert*. Issue 1. February 27, 1998.

39. Cohen MR. Hazard warning: deaths due to accidental intrathecal injection of vincristine. *Hosp Pharm*. 1989; 24:694.

40. Joint Commission on Accreditation of Healthcare Organizations. Preventing vincristine administration errors *Sentinel Event Alert*. Issue 34. July 14, 2005.

41. Institute for Safe Medication Practices. IV vincristine survey shows safety improvements needed. *ISMP Medication Safety Alert!* February 23, 2006;11:1–2. Available at: www.ismp.org/Newsletters/acutecare/articles/20060223.asp.

42. Environmental Protection Agency. Consumer labeling initiative. Phase II report. www.epa.gov/opptintr/labeling/cliphase2/html/Execsum.html. Accessed January 2006.

43. Nunn DS. Ampoule labeling—the way forward. *Pharmaceutical J*. March 14, 1992.

44. Institute for Safe Medication Practices. HESPAN and heparin mix-ups—reduce the risk by using generic name and product. *ISMP Medication Safety Alert!* September 8, 1999. Available at: www.ismp.org/Newsletters/acutecare/articles/19990908.asp.

45. Leape LL, Bates DW, Cullen DJ, et al. Systems analysis of adverse drug events. ADE Prevention Study Group. *JAMA*. 1995;274:35–43.

46. Food and Drug Administration. FDA issues bar code rule. Available at: www.fda.gov/oc/initiatives/barcode-sadr/fs-barcode.html. Accessed November 1, 2005.

47. Neuenschwander M, Cohen MR, Vaida AJ, et al. Practical guide to bar coding for patient medication safety *Am J Health Syst Pharm*. 2003;60:768–79.

48. Burlington B, Freed C. Massive overdose and death from prophylactic lidocaine. *JAMA*. 1980;243:1036–7.

49. Cohen MR. Medication errors: check carefully before administering a prefilled lidocaine syringe. *Nursing*. 1982;12:28, 30.

50. Lidocaine errors. How can they be prevented? *Hosp Pharm Rep*. July 1990:1.

51. O'Brien J. Confusing packaging blamed for deaths. *Post-Standard* (Syracuse, NY). May 12, 1997.

52. Cohen MR. Hazard warning! Renacidin for irrigation in IV look-alike packaging. *Hosp Pharm*. 1991; 26:373,376.

53. Cohen MR. Sublingual nitroglycerin ointment. *Hosp Pharm*. 1981;16:351.

54. Cohen MR. Nitroglycerin toothpaste. *Hosp Pharm*. 1987;22:195.

55. Institute for Safe Medication Practices. Safety briefs. *ISMP Medication Safety Alert!* November 29, 2000;5:1.

56. Cohen MR. Tactile cues for identifying insulin. *Hosp Pharm*. 1996;31:87–8.

57. Institute for Safe Medication Practices. Removing premixed IV drugs from protective pouch may increase drug concentration. *ISMP Medication Safety Alert!* May 29, 2002;7.

58. Institute for Safe Medication Practices. Part I. National survey on drug shortages reveals high level of frustration, low regard for safety. *ISMP Medication Safety Alert!* March 21, 2001;6.

59. Institute for Safe Medication Practices. Part II of our national survey on drug shortages: proactive guidelines to safely manage scarce supplies. *ISMP Medication Safety Alert!* April 4, 2001;6.

60. Schrand LM, Troester TS, Ballis ZK, et al. Preparing for drug shortages: one teaching hospital's approach to the IVIG shortage. *Formulary.* 2001;36:52–9.

61. Berwick DM. Not again! *BMJ.* 2001;322:247–.8

62. Cohen MR, Senders J, Davis NM. Failure mode and effects analysis: a novel approach to avoiding dangerous medication errors and accidents. *Hosp Pharm.* 1994;29:319–28, 330.

63. Vecchione A. War on errors. FDA targets problem names, labeling. *Hosp Pharm Report.* 1996;10:1, 8.

64. Clark C. Strategies for error-proofing drug labelling, packaging and nomenclature. *Hosp Pharm* (UK). 1998;5:117–21.

65. Kohn LT, Corrigan JM, Donaldson MS, eds. *To Err Is Human: Building a Safer Health System.* Washington, DC: National Academies Press; 2000.

66. Committee on Identifying and Preventing Medication Errors; Aspden P, Wolcott J, Bootman JL, et al., eds. *Preventing Medication Errors.* Washington, DC: National Academies Press; 2006. Prepublication copy available at http://darwin.nap.edu/books/0309101476/html/R2.html. Accessed July 21, 2006.

CHAPTER 8

ERROR-PRONE ABBREVIATIONS AND DOSE EXPRESSIONS

Michael J. Gaunt and Michael R. Cohen

The case of Wm. Galloway against C. F. Richards et al., in the Fourth District Court, was brought to a close yesterday evening, the jury, after two hours' absence, returning a verdict for four hundred dollars in favor of the plaintiff. The action was brought to recover damages laid at two thousand five hundred dollars, from defendants, who are druggists, for putting up a prescription in a wrongful manner, thereby causing a temporary injury to plaintiff's health. The verdict took some, who had heard the evidence throughout, by surprise; and a motion will be made on behalf of defendants for a new trial. The truth of the matter is, that in ninety-nine cases out of a hundred of these mistakes in putting up prescriptions, the whole blame lies with the prescribing physicians, who, like a majority of lawyers, and many preachers, write a most abominable scrawl, which might be deciphered by a dozen experts as many different ways, and each one sustain his version by the manuscript. When a physician writes the abbreviation of "pulverized cinchona" in such a manner that nine out of ten among experienced pharmacists would, without hesitancy, read it "pulverized cantharides," and damage results from it, if the apothecary is culpable at all, the physician certainly ought to come in for a share of blame. It would be a good thing for the world at large, however unpro-fessional it might be, if medical men were required by law to write out in full the ingredients named in their prescriptions. Let them adhere to the Latin, or Fejee, if they choose, but discard abbreviations, and form their letters as if they had been to school one day in their lives, so as to avoid the possibility of mistakes on that account.[1]

Mark Twain, October 1, 1864

Mark Twain's call to "discard abbreviations" could not ring more true in today's world. Except for the recent movement away from assigning blame to individual practitioners, not much has changed since 1864. Health care practitioners are still trying, often without success, to decipher the meaning of abbreviations and symbols.

The consequences of misinterpreting abbreviations, symbols, and dose expressions are many and sometimes fatal. An abbreviation may have more than one meaning. Practition-ers may be unfamiliar with the intended meaning. Poor handwriting can contribute to mistaken interpretations of drug doses, drug names, and routes of administration. Prac-titioners may see abbreviation use as a shortcut, but an unclear abbreviation can delay the start of therapy. Educating practitioners on the dangers of abbreviations places an additional demand on scarce health care resources.

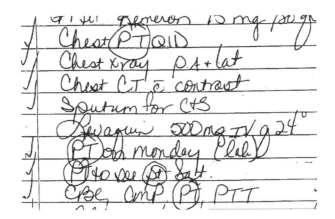

FIGURE 8-1   What does PT mean?

This chapter provides examples of abbreviations, symbols, and dose designations with great potential for harm. Although most of the examples involve handwritten communication, the same principles apply to machine-printed and electronic forms of communication, including orders, medication administration records (MARs), labels, and computer screens.

NEED FOR STANDARDS

There are no standards for many of the abbreviations used in health care.[2] For example, in the set of orders depicted in Figure 8-1, the abbreviation "PT" is used five times with four different meanings: percussion therapy, physical therapy, patient, and prothrombin time. In a 2004 Institute for Safe Medication Practices (ISMP) and Med-E.R.R.S. survey of pharmacists, the dosing frequency "daily" was expressed by 17 different abbreviations in the United States alone.[3]

Davis[2] has called for a controlled vocabulary, similar to those used in aviation and the military, where accurate communication is critical. All pilots and air traffic controllers use a standard nomenclature when repeating back the letters in a word; they say "alpha," "bravo," and "charlie" (for A, B, and C), not "apple," "beef," and "candy." Also, for the number 270, they say "two seven zero," not "two seventy," which can sound like "two seventeen."

Most health care facilities and practitioners maintain lists of "approved" abbreviations, symbols, and dose designations, and even health care education programs teach "standard" abbreviations. However, variations among practitioners and places can nullify any intended standardization.

A more effective way to standardize vocabulary and nomenclature is to maintain a list of prohibited abbreviations, which, when misinterpreted, can cause significant harm to patients. The Joint Commission on Accreditation of Healthcare Organizations (JCAHO) and ISMP are using this approach. A JCAHO 2004 National Patient Safety Goal (NPSG) to improve communication established the initial minimum requirements of a "do not use" list.[4] These requirements, continued in the 2005 and 2006 NPSGs (Table 8-1), apply to all orders and other medication-related documentation, including preprinted forms, but not to all patient-specific documentation.[5,6] One hundred percent compliance is expected for preprinted forms, and 90% is expected for handwritten documentation. Additional items considered for addition to the JCAHO do-not-use list are shown in Table 8-2.

TABLE 8-1   Abbreviations and Expressions on JCAHO "Do Not Use" List[4,a]

Do Not Use	Potential Problem	Use Instead
U (unit)	Mistaken for 0 (zero), the number 4 (four), or "cc"	Write "unit"
IU (International Unit)	Mistaken for IV (intravenous) or the number 10 (ten)	Write "International Unit"
Q.D., QD, q.d., qd (daily)	Mistaken for each other	Write "daily"
Q.O.D., QOD, q.o.d., qod (every other day)	Period after the Q mistaken for "I" and the "O" mistaken for "I"	Write "every other day"
Trailing zero (X.0 mg)[b]	Decimal point is missed	Write "X mg"
Lack of leading zero (.X mg)	Decimal point is missed	Write "0.X mg"
MS	Can mean morphine sulfate or magnesium sulfate	Write "morphine sulfate"
MSO_4 and $MgSO_4$	Confused for one another	Write "magnesium sulfate"

JCAHO = Joint Commission on Accreditation of Healthcare Organizations.

[a] Applies to all orders and all medication-related documentation that is handwritten (including free-text computer entry) or on preprinted forms.

[b] Exception: A "trailing zero" may be used only where required to demonstrate the level of precision of the value being reported, such as for laboratory results, imaging studies that report size of lesions, or catheter or tube sizes. It may not be used in medication orders or other medication-related documentation.

TABLE 8-2   Items for Possible Inclusion in JCAHO "Do Not Use" List[4]

Do Not Use	Potential Problem	Use Instead
> (greater than) and < (less than)	Misinterpreted as the number 7 (seven) or the letter L; confused for one another	Write "greater than" and "less than"
Abbreviations for drug names	Misinterpreted because of similar abbreviations for multiple drugs	Write drug names in full
Apothecary units	Unfamiliar to many practitioners; confused with metric units	Use metric units
@	Mistaken for the number 2 (two)	Write "at"
cc	Mistaken for U (units) when poorly written	Write "mL" or "milliliters"
μg	Mistaken for mg (milligrams), resulting in 1,000-fold overdosage	Write "mcg" or "micrograms"

JCAHO = Joint Commission on Accreditation of Healthcare Organizations.

ISMP offers a more extensive list of abbreviations, symbols, and dose designations that have led to medication errors (Table 8-3). Items in the table have been reported to the U.S. Pharmacopeia (USP)–ISMP Medication Errors Reporting Program as being frequently misinterpreted and involved in harmful medication errors. ISMP believes practitioners should go beyond the minimum JCAHO requirements and avoid all items in Table 8-3, in all forms of communicating medical information, including internal communications, spoken prescriptions (including telephone orders), computer-generated labels, labels for drug storage bins, MARs, and pharmacy and prescriber computer order entry screens.

BREAKING HABITS

Despite the benefits of controlling abbreviation use, implementing a do-not-use list can be difficult. Health care professionals rarely receive academic instruction on the potential

TABLE 8-3 ISMP List of Error-Prone Abbreviations, Symbols, and Dose Designations[a]

Abbreviation, Designation, or Symbol	Intended Meaning	Misinterpretation	Correction
Error-Prone Abbreviations			
μg	microgram	Mistaken as "mg"	Use "mcg"
AD, AS, AU	right ear, left ear, each ear	Mistaken as OD, OS, OU (right eye, left eye, each eye)	Use "right ear," "left ear," or "each ear"
OD, OS, OU	right eye, left eye, each eye	Mistaken as AD, AS, AU (right ear, left ear, each ear)	Use "right eye," "left eye," or "each eye"
BT	bedtime	Mistaken as "b.i.d." (twice daily)	Use "bedtime"
cc	cubic centimeters	Mistaken as "u" (units)	Use "mL"
D/C	discharge or discontinue	Premature discontinuation of medications if D/C (intended to mean "discharge") has been misinterpreted as "discontinued" when followed by a list of discharge medications	Use "discharge" and "discontinue"
IJ	injection	Mistaken as "IV" or "intrajugular"	Use "injection"
IN	intranasal	Mistaken as "IM" or "IV"	Use "intranasal" or "NAS"
HS	half-strength	Mistaken as bedtime	Use "half-strength" or "bedtime"
hs	at bedtime, hour of sleep	Mistaken as half-strength	Use "half-strength" or "bedtime"
IU**	international unit	Mistaken as IV (intravenous) or 10 (ten)	Use "units"
o.d. or OD	once daily	Mistaken as "right eye" (OD, *oculus dexter*); oral liquid medications might be administered in the eye	Use "daily"
OJ	orange juice	Mistaken as OD or OS (right or left eye); drugs meant to be diluted in orange juice might be given in the eye	Use "orange juice"
Per os	by mouth, orally	The "os" can be mistaken as "left eye" (OS, *oculus sinister*)	Use "PO," "by mouth," or "orally"
q.d. or QD**	every day	Mistaken as q.i.d., especially if period after the "q" or tail of the "q" is misunderstood as an "i"	Use "daily"
qhs	at bedtime	Mistaken as "qhr" or every hour	Use "at bedtime"
qn	nightly	Mistaken as "qh" (every hour)	Use "nightly"
q.o.d. or QOD**	every other day	Mistaken as "q.d." (daily) or "q.i.d. (four times daily) if the "o" is poorly written	Use "every other day"
q1d	daily	Mistaken as "q.i.d." (four times daily)	Use "daily"
q6PM, etc.	every evening at 6 pm	Mistaken as every 6 hours	Use "6 PM nightly" or "6 PM daily"

Abbreviation	Intended Meaning	Misinterpretation	Correction
SC, SQ, sub q	subcutaneous	SC mistaken as SL (sublingual); SQ mistaken as "5 every;" the "q" in "sub q" has been mistaken as "every" (e.g., a heparin dose ordered "sub q 2 hours before surgery" misunderstood as every 2 hours before surgery)	Use "subcut" or "subcutaneously"
ss	sliding-scale (insulin) or ½ (apothecary)	Mistaken as "55"	Spell out "sliding scale"; use "one-half" or "½"
SSRI	sliding-scale regular insulin	Mistaken as selective serotonin-reuptake inhibitor	Spell out "sliding scale (insulin)"
SSI	sliding-scale insulin	Mistaken as strong solution of iodine (Lugol's)	Spell out "sliding scale (insulin)"
1/d	one daily	Mistaken as "t.i.d."	Use "1 daily"
TIW or tiw	3 times a week	Mistaken as "3 times a day" or "twice in a week"	Use "3 times weekly"
U or u**	unit	Mistaken as the number 0 or 4, causing a 10-fold overdose or greater (e.g., 4U seen as "40" or 4u seen as "44"); mistaken as "cc" so dose given in volume instead of units (e.g., 4u seen as 4cc)	Use "unit"

Error-Prone Dose Designations

Dose Designation	Intended Meaning	Misinterpretation	Correction
Trailing zero after decimal point (e.g., 1.0 mg)**	1 mg	Mistaken as 10 mg if the decimal point is not seen	Do not use trailing zeros for doses expressed in whole numbers
No leading zero before a decimal dose (e.g., .5 mg)	0.5 mg	Mistaken as 5 mg if the decimal point is not seen	Use zero before a decimal point when the dose is less than a whole unit
Drug name and dose run together (especially problematic for drug names that end in "L" such as Inderal40 mg; Tegretol300 mg)	Inderal 40 mg; Tegretol 300 mg	Mistaken as Inderal 140 mg; Mistaken as Tegretol 1300 mg	Place adequate space between the drug name, dose, and unit of measure
Numerical dose and unit of measure run together (e.g., 10mg, 100mL)	10 mg; 100 mL	The "m" is sometimes mistaken as a zero or two zeros, risking a 10- to 100-fold overdose	Place adequate space between the dose and unit of measure
Abbreviations such as mg. or mL. with a period following the abbreviation	mg; mL	The period is unnecessary and could be mistaken as the number 1 if written poorly	Use mg, mL, etc., without a terminal period
Large doses without properly placed commas (e.g., 100000 units; 1000000 units)	100,000 units; 1,000,000 units	100000 has been mistaken as 10,000 or 1,000,000; 1000000 has been mistaken as 100,000	Use commas for dosing units at or above 1,000, or use words such as 100 "thousand" or 1 "million" to improve readability

TABLE 8-3 ISMP List of Error-Prone Abbreviations, Symbols, and Dose Designations[a] (continued)

Abbreviation, Designation, or Symbol	Intended Meaning	Misinterpretation	Correction
Error-Prone Drug Name Abbreviations			
ARA A	vidarabine	Mistaken as cytarabine (ARA C)	Use complete drug name
AZT	zidovudine (Retrovir)	Mistaken as azathioprine or aztreonam	Use complete drug name
CPZ	Compazine (prochlorperazine)	Mistaken as chlorpromazine	Use complete drug name
DPT	Demerol-Phenergan-Thorazine	Mistaken as diphtheria-pertussis-tetanus (vaccine)	Use complete drug name
DTO	diluted tincture of opium, or deodorized tincture of opium (Paregoric)	Mistaken as tincture of opium	Use complete drug name
HCl	hydrochloric acid or hydrochloride	Mistaken as potassium chloride ("H" is misinterpreted as "K")	Use complete drug name unless expressed as salt of a drug
HCT	hydrocortisone	Mistaken as hydrochlorothiazide	Use complete drug name
HCTZ	hydrochlorothiazide	Mistaken as hydrocortisone (seen as HCT250 mg)	Use complete drug name
MgSO4**	magnesium sulfate	Mistaken as morphine sulfate	Use complete drug name
MS, MSO4**	morphine sulfate	Mistaken as magnesium sulfate	Use complete drug name
MTX	methotrexate	Mistaken as mitoxantrone	Use complete drug name
PCA	procainamide	Mistaken as patient-controlled analgesia	Use complete drug name
PTU	propylthiouracil	Mistaken as mercaptopurine	Use complete drug name
T3	Tylenol with codeine No. 3	Mistaken as liothyronine	Use complete drug name
TAC	triamcinolone	Mistaken as tetracaine, Adrenalin, cocaine	Use complete drug name
TNK	TNKase	Mistaken as "TPA"	Use complete drug name
ZnSO4	zinc sulfate	Mistaken as morphine sulfate	Use complete drug name
Error-Prone Drug Stems			
"Nitro" drip	nitroglycerin infusion	Mistaken as sodium nitroprusside infusion	Use complete drug name
"Norflox"	norfloxacin	Mistaken as Norflex	Use complete drug name
"IV Vanc"	intravenous vancomycin	Mistaken as Invanz	Use complete drug name

Error-Prone Symbols

Symbol	Meaning	Potential Problem	Correction
ʒ	dram	Symbol for dram mistaken as "3"	Use the metric system
♏	minim	Symbol for minim mistaken as "mL"	Use the metric system
x3d	for three days	Mistaken as "3 doses"	Use "for three days"
> and <	greater than and less than	Mistaken as opposite of intended; mistaken use of incorrect symbol; "<10" mistaken as "40"	Use "greater than" or "less than"
/ (slash mark)	separates two doses or indicates "per"	Mistaken as the number 1 (e.g., "25 units/10 units" misread as "25 units and 110" units)	Use "per" rather than a slash mark to separate doses
@	at	Mistaken as "2"	Use "at"
&	and	Mistaken as "2"	Use "and"
+	plus or and	Mistaken as "4"	Use "and"
°	hour	Mistaken as a zero (e.g., q2° seen as q 20)	Use "hr," "h," or "hour"
"	seconds	Mistaken as "cc"	Use "seconds"

ISMP = Institute for Safe Medication Practices.

[a] Double asterisk indicates items included on the do-not-use list established as part of a National Patient Safety Goal by the Joint Commission on Accreditation of Healthcare Organizations.

danger of abbreviations. They learn bad habits early, in residencies and internships, and those bad habits are hard to break. Even when they see tragic outcomes of abbreviation use—such as brain injury after a nurse misinterpreted a "U," intended to mean "units," as a zero—practitioners are reluctant to change their habits.

Most of JCAHO's tips for compliance with the NPSGs (see www.jointcommission.org) focus on educating, advocating, and reminding staff. Only one of the tips addresses enforcement: "Direct pharmacy not to accept any of the prohibited abbreviations. Orders with dangerous abbreviations or illegible handwriting must be corrected before being dispensed."[7] A corollary to that is enlisting nurses to help notify physicians. An unfortunate outcome of this safety strategy has been increased workload (telephone calls to correct orders) and strained relationships between the medical staff and nurses and pharmacists.

A midsized hospital reported that in April through June 2004, pharmacists had made 519 calls to physicians for just one abbreviation, "QD."[8] Additional calls had been made for other prohibited abbreviations. In many facilities, pages to prescribers go unanswered or are returned only after significant delays—impeding patient care. This is an organizational problem that requires peer-to-peer interaction along with full support from hospital and medical staff leadership.

Hospitals report that the most effective way to enforce physician compliance is to make it a physician-owned process.[9,10] Since educational efforts alone failed to produce significant change, hospitals initially pursued operational changes, such as preprinted orders, targeted pages, and e-mail reminders. After enacting a zero tolerance policy, medical staff leaders interacted with physicians who were noncompliant. Pharmacists and nurses still played a role in data collection and notification of noncompliance, but shared accountability, with medical staff participation and leadership, was eventually achieved.

To help increase compliance, in January 2005 JCAHO surveyors were instructed to score prescribers' use on a patient's chart of any abbreviation on the NPSG "dangerous—do not use" list as noncompliance.[11] Facilities are no longer considered compliant if pharmacists or nurses call a prescriber for clarification of the abbreviation and document the intended meaning. The goal is to place responsibility for prescriber compliance on the medical and administrative staff instead of on nurses and pharmacists.

MISINTERPRETATIONS AND MULTIPLE MEANINGS

Among the abbreviations that most often lead to trouble are "U" for "units" in expressions of dosage and "Q" for "every" in expressions of dose frequency. Pennsylvania implemented a mandatory statewide error-reporting system (Pennsylvania Patient Safety Reporting System, or PA-PSRS) in 2004. In more than 200 selected reports of medication errors involving misinterpretation of abbreviations between June 2004 and February 2005, the abbreviations most commonly misinterpreted were

- "U" for unit,
- "QD" for daily,
- "QID" for four times daily,
- "QOD" for every other day,
- "D/C" for discontinue,
- "AU" for both ears, and
- "OU" for both eyes.[12]

U for Units

The abbreviation "U" for units is on JCAHO's do-not-use list. Insulin and heparin, both high-alert medications with great potential for patient harm from overdoses, are ordered

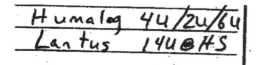

FIGURE 8-2   U for "units" in this patient history documentation looks like a 4.

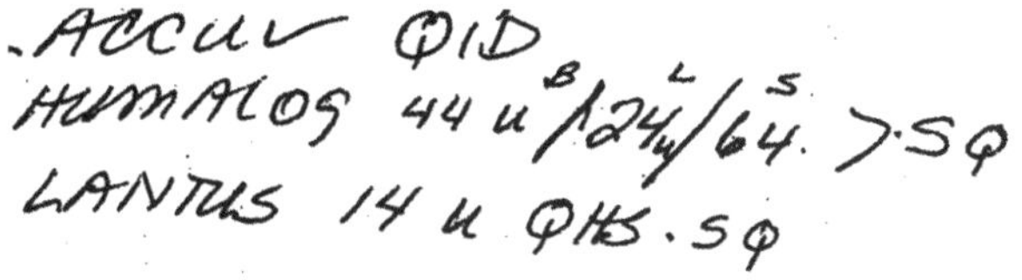

.ACCU✓ QID
HUMALOG 44 u [B]/24[L]/64.[S] ˃SQ
LANTUS 14 u QHS.SQ

FIGURE 8-3   When ordering Humalog, the physician misread U on the patient history as 4.

in units. The abbreviation has been read as a zero (0), which results in 10-fold overdosage, and as the number four (4). In one example, an order was written as "5U Humalog." The patient erroneously received 50 units of Humalog (insulin lispro recombinant) on two occasions and was later found in respiratory distress that progressed to cardiopulmonary arrest. He remained on mechanical ventilation until he died a week later.[12] In another case, an order written for "150000U" of penicillin G potassium for an infant was misinterpreted as 1,500,000 (1.5 million) units. Each million units of penicillin G potassium contains 1.7 mEq of potassium. The unintended bolus of 2.5 mEq of potassium led to cardiac arrest.

Another error occurred when a nurse who was taking a patient's history recorded the insulin dose using the letter U instead of the word unit (Figure 8-2). The physician misread the U as a 4 and wrote orders for doses dramatically different from what the patient had been taking (Figure 8-3). Although the physician also used the abbreviation U, it fortunately was not misread. The patient received a single overdose of insulin but was not harmed. Further overdoses were averted when the nurse said to the patient, "Here's your insulin, 44 units." The patient responded, "44 units? I take 4 units!"

Orders may include some variation of units, such as "IU" for international units. In an order for "Vitamin E 100 IU daily," IU was misinterpreted as IV (intravenous). As a result, capsule contents were drawn into a syringe for administration. Fortunately, the person preparing the injection contacted a pharmacist before administering the drug. The error could have been prevented by spelling the word units instead of using U and by including the route of administration with the order.

Habits such as the use of U for units may be hard to change. Educational efforts need to extend beyond JCAHO-accredited facilities. For example, a nursing student documented a sliding-scale dose of regular insulin as "12 units" on the MAR only to have it "corrected" by an instructor to "12 U." Even after a pharmacist explained that the dangerous abbreviation can lead to a 10-fold overdose, the instructor still insisted on use of the abbreviation.

Because U has been commonly used for units, this abbreviation can be "read" in an unclear order even when the prescriber did not intend to use it. In a hospital using a standard heparin infusion concentration of 20 thousand units per 500 mL (40 units per mL), a physician wrote an order for 1,000 units per hour by prescribing a rate of "25 cc/hr" (Figure 8-4). His handwriting made "cc" look more like a "u," so nurses and pharmacists initially interpreted the infusion rate as 25 units per hour, or only 2.5% of the actual prescribed dose. The rate in milliliters per hour was so low that the mistake was quickly recognized. However, if a concentration of insulin 100 units per 500 mL is prepared for

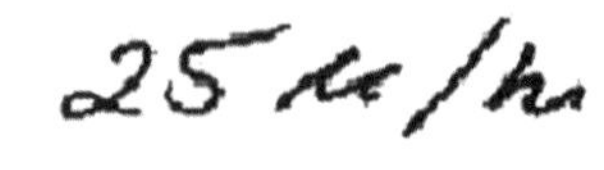

25 u /hr

FIGURE 8-4   25 u or 25 cc per hour?

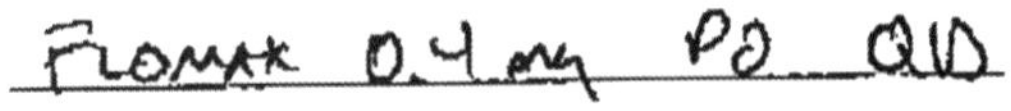

Flomax 0.4 mg PO QD

FIGURE 8-5   QD mistaken for QID.

infusion, misreading "15 cc/hr" (3 units per hour) as 15 units per hour could lead to severe hypoglycemia. Conversely, misreading "15 u/hr" as "15 cc/hr" could result in a subtherapeutic dose and contribute to ketoacidosis.

ISMP recommends avoiding the use of "cc" to indicate volume. Only "mL," which is unambiguous, should be used in handwritten, preprinted, and electronic prescriptions. It is the appropriate metric unit and is recognized in the *United States Pharmacopeia* as well as by the Food and Drug Administration (FDA) and the pharmaceutical industry. The uppercase L recommended by USP should always be used; it reduces the potential for confusion between "ml" and "mg" in handwriting.

QD and Variations

Q for "every," as well as other abbreviations with this letter (QD, QID, and QOD; or qd, qid, and qod), is often involved in medication errors. QD for "daily" can result in fourfold overdosages if seen as QID (q.i.d.) for "four times daily," or subtherapeutic doses if seen as QOD for "every other day." QD is prohibited by JCAHO, but an unexpected result has been the use of "Q day" In one case, a pharmacist misread an order for "phytonadione 10 mg PO today" as "Q day." The nurse verifying the electronic MAR did not notice the error. The patient received phytonadione 10 mg daily for 4 days before the physician noticed the mistake. The patient suffered no ill effects from the error.

Figure 8-5 illustrates how easily QD can become QID. Fortunately, the potential error was recognized before patient harm occurred. However, a newspaper article described a similar error that put a patient at risk for significant harm.[13] It reported that a prescription was written for a 1-month supply of Avinza (morphine sulfate extended-release capsules) 30 mg QD for a man with severe back pain. The pharmacist misinterpreted the QD and dispensed the prescription with the instructions "Take one capsule four times daily." The patient followed the instructions on the bottle and experienced excessive drowsiness and sedation but continued to work (as a construction inspector) and drive (often with his 7-year-old daughter in the car). The error was not discovered until the patient contacted his physician for a refill after only 1 week.

Errors associated with QD and QOD have been reported to PA-PSRS.[12] In one case, an order for Zithromax (azithromycin) 500 mg written as QD was misinterpreted as QID. The patient was not harmed, despite receiving the medication four times daily. In another report, an order was written for digoxin 0.125 mg po QOD (every other day), but the medication was given QD (every day). The patient received two extra doses before the error was discovered.

QID and QOD are not the only misinterpretations of QD. A prescriber intended a patient to receive Lovenox (enoxaparin sodium) 40 mg daily (Figure 8-6). A nurse misinterpreted the QD for "daily" in his order as "Q8" hours, even though the medication is typically administered daily or every 12 hours.

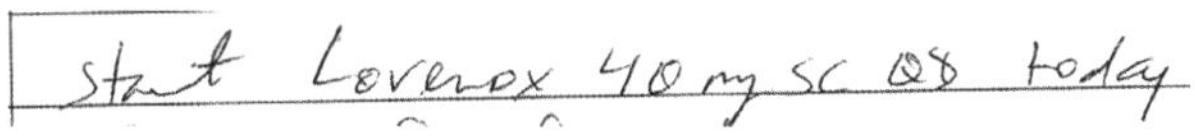

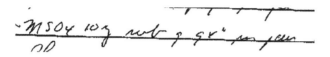

FIGURE 8-6 QD or Q8?

FIGURE 8-7 This order was misread as morphine by "neb," not "sub q."

In another example, a computerized prescription for "penicillin VK 500 mg Q1D X 7D" led a pharmacy technician to type a label as the directions implied: "Take 1 tab p.o. daily for 7 days." A pharmacist realized that penicillin for this patient was supposed to be taken four times a day, not once a day. The physician had erroneously typed Q1D (q one day) into the order entry system instead of QID. The report of this error did not explain why the physician needed to free-type the entry for frequency; some systems provide a forced-choice pick list with predetermined selections. The abbreviation "D" for day in "7D" was interpreted correctly in this case but can be misunderstood as "7 doses."

Other Dangerous Abbreviations

Misinterpretation is also possible with abbreviations not specifically targeted by JCAHO. When the abbreviation "PC" (after meals) was used to signify that a daily dose of colchicine 0.6 mg should be given after one meal each day (colchicine 0.6 mg daily pc), the order was interpreted to mean that the medication should be given three times daily after meals, and the patient received two extra doses. Although "daily" instructions had been included in the order, the nurse followed standard directions for PC and transcribed the order as t.i.d. (after meals). The pharmacy profiled the order as the physician intended and dispensed a single daily dose. The two additional doses were obtained by asking pharmacy to dispense each "missing" dose. The need for the extra doses was not questioned until the next day, when the error was discovered. To avoid such confusion, prescribers should state, for example, "Take after breakfast."

Abbreviations used for "subcutaneous" have been involved in errors. An order for morphine to be given "sc" was misread as "sl," and the drug was given sublingually. When "sq" or "sub q" is used, the letter "q" can look like an abbreviation for "every" followed by a number. One patient's surgery had to be postponed after an order for "heparin 5,000 units sub q 2 hours before surgery" was misread as "... q 2 hours before surgery." The patient had received injections every 2 hours. In another case, a patient was given morphine 10 mg by nebulizer instead of subcutaneously when "sub" in "sub q" was seen as "neb" (Figure 8-7). The patient's pain was not relieved, since intrapulmonary morphine is not appreciably absorbed. If an abbreviation for subcutaneous must be used, "subcut" is preferable.

AD is sometimes used as an abbreviation for right ear (*aura dexter*). A handwritten lowercase "a" can easily look like an "o." Thus, an otic medication may be instilled into a patient's right eye (OD, for *oculus dexter*) instead of the right ear. In a recently reported error, the physician had ordered Auralgan (antipyrine, benzocaine, glycerin) two drops AD for an emergency room patient, but the nurse administered the drops into the patient's right eye. When the error was discovered, the eye was flushed, and the patient suffered no permanent harm. Using AS for left ear or AU for each ear could cause similar problems. In addition, AD has been misread as QD (if the tail of a handwritten lowercase "a" looks

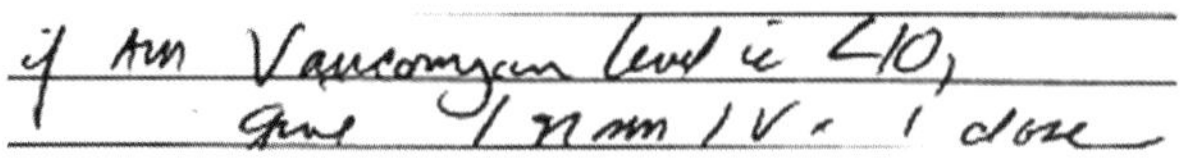

FIGURE 8-8   Vancomycin level of <10 or 40?

likes a "q") and PO (when poorly handwritten). In 1975, in one of ISMP's earliest error reports, a patient nearly received ear drops by mouth.[14] Another type of error has surfaced with the abbreviation AD. Tired of writing out "as directed" while transcribing prescriptions received by telephone, a pharmacist began to abbreviate that term as AD. Later, a pharmacy technician misinterpreted the directions for an oral liquid prescription transcribed as "5 mL t.i.d. AD" and typed the directions as "one teaspoonful three times a day in right ear."

Facilities should choose entries for their do-not-use lists carefully. Some abbreviations are less prone to serious errors than others. For example, some hospitals prohibit the use of QID (four times daily). This abbreviation can be dangerous if QD or QOD is misread as QID and the patient receives extra doses. However, mistaking QID for QD or QOD results in underdosage, which may be less harmful. Rather than banning the use of QID, it is more effective to prohibit QD and QOD so that they cannot be misread as QID. Similarly, the abbreviations for right/left/both ears (AD, AS, AU) are sometimes misread as the abbreviations for right/left/both eyes (OD, OS, OU). Eliminating the use of one set of abbreviations, preferably the less used AD, AS, and AU, should be enough to prevent confusion between ears and eyes. A facility that prohibits QID and all abbreviations for eyes and ears will only make it harder to succeed in eliminating the more dangerous abbreviations.

SYMBOLS

The use of symbols can be a quick way to communicate information without writing letters or words. However, a symbol such as > (greater than) can easily be confused with < (less than). These symbols can also be misread as other letters or numbers.

An elderly patient with an international normalized ratio (INR) of 2.8 mistakenly received a Coumadin (warfarin) dose that should have been withheld.[12] The order stated to give Coumadin if INR < 2.5 (less than 2.5). However, the "<" (less than) symbol was misinterpreted as the ">" (greater than) symbol, and the drug was administered.

Vasotec (enalaprilat) 1.25 mg IV was given to another elderly patient when the patient's blood pressure was less than 180 mmHg.[12] The order stated to hold the medication if the patient's "SBP<180." However, the "<" and ">" signs were confused, and the medication was administered when the patient's systolic blood pressure measured only 140 mmHg.

Other misinterpretations of the "<" symbol are possible. For example, in Figure 8-8, the physician intended to have the nurse administer another 1 g dose of vancomycin intravenously if the patient's serum drug level the next morning was "<10." However, the symbol for less than was written in a way that made the nurse interpret the number 10 as the number 40. The error was recognized after the nurse called the pharmacy to ask if a trough level of 35 mcg/mL was close enough that the next dose could be administered.

Many health care practitioners use up and down arrows to indicate "increase" and "decrease." These symbols can be confused for numbers or letters. For example, a pharmacist received a call from a nursing unit requesting a patient's "missing" trazodone dose. When he could not find an order on the patient's computer profile or among the most recent orders received that day, the pharmacist asked the nurse for a copy of the order. The faxed copy was recognized immediately as an order received in the pharmacy earlier

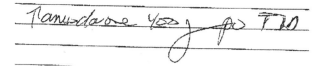

FIGURE 8-9 Here, "↑ amiodarone" was misread as trazodone.

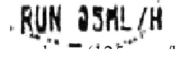

FIGURE 8-10 @ becomes 2.

in the day and interpreted as an order to increase amiodarone. The prescriber had used an up arrow to signify the word "increase," but it looked like a "T" (Figure 8-9). After the pharmacist explained that trazodone would not be given in a dose above 600 mg per day, the nurse looked more closely and realized it was indeed an order to increase amiodarone. At least two nurses had looked at this order and believed it was for trazodone.

Another order was written with an up arrow to indicate an increase in Diovan (valsartan) to 80 mg b.i.d.[12] The arrow was misread as the number 1. The pharmacy interpreted the order as Diovan 160 mg b.i.d., and one dose of Diovan 160 mg was administered. The patient suffered no harm from this overdose.

Another common error-prone symbol is the "at" sign, @. A physician ordered an octreotide infusion as 25 mcg/hour IV for 48 hours. The pharmacy prepared the solution and affixed a label to the bag with the directions to "run @5ML/H over 20 hours" (Figure 8-10). The "at" symbol printed on the label was misinterpreted as the number 2, and the infusion rate was set at 25 mL per hour (125 mcg/hour) instead of the intended 5 mL/hour (25 mcg/hour). A similar error happened with a handwritten "at" symbol. In this case, an order for an infusion with sodium bicarbonate to run "@50 cc/h" was misread as 250 mL per hour. Maintaining a space between the "at" symbol and the numerical dose might have averted the first of these errors. However, it is safest to avoid any use of the "at" symbol.

NUMBERS

Error-prone methods of expressing doses have also contributed to patient harm. More than once, fatal errors have occurred as a result of failure to include a zero before the decimal point for doses less than a whole unit (.1 instead of 0.1). In addition, the inclusion of an unnecessary decimal point and zero for whole number doses (1.0 instead of 1) has resulted in 10-fold overdoses.

One tragic case involved a 10-fold overdose of morphine in an infant. The order was written as ".5 mg;" however, it was misinterpreted and 5 mg was administered. The infant could not be resuscitated.

In another example, an elderly patient was ordered Dilaudid (hydromorphone); however, the order was written without the use of leading zeroes (.2–.4 mg).[12] The order was misread as 2–4 mg instead of the intended 0.2–0.4 mg. The nurse recognized the error after giving the initial dose. The patient was not harmed.

"Trailing zeros" (a whole number followed by a decimal point and a zero) should never be used. A prescriber, using a trailing zero, ordered Ativan (lorazepam) 1.0 mg. The order was misread and Ativan 10 mg was administered. The patient experienced heavy sedation and somnolence. If trailing zeros are used in orders for high-alert medications, the harm may be much greater. When prescriptions have been written for Coumadin 1.0 mg, patients have received 10 mg in error, placing them at risk of severe bleeding. A prescription for hydromorphone 1.0 mg could easily be misread as hydromorphone 10 mg, leading to respiratory distress.

Some medications are ordered in doses that require many sequential digits to be correctly seen and interpreted. It is safest to express such doses by using a combination of numbers and words. For example, the words "million" and "thousand" have nearly the same number of digits as their numerical expressions, but they are rarely confused because they contain different, distinguishable characters. In comparison, the pairs 100,000/1,000,000 and 100000/1000000 look very similar, especially when commas are omitted or misplaced.

Furthermore, abbreviations should not be used for "million" or "thousand." MM has been used to abbreviate million ($1,000 \times 1,000$), but it can be misunderstood. The letter M has often been used for millions in expressions such as MU for "million units," but M is also the Roman numeral for 1,000 and has been used to represent thousand. If M for thousand were misunderstood to represent million, a 1,000-fold error could occur. The letter K (for kilo) is also popular as an abbreviation for thousand (as in "10K race"). It too could be misinterpreted—for example, as potassium or vitamin K.

DRUG NAME ABBREVIATIONS AND COINED NAMES

Despite JCAHO's stance on abbreviations, errors related to abbreviated and coined drug names continue to be a significant problem, as demonstrated in reports to Pennsylvania's PA-PSRS.[12] Many mix-ups between morphine sulfate and magnesium sulfate have been reported. One physician wrote an IV order to "Increase Mg to 1.5 grams per liter" in an elderly patient. The physician intended magnesium sulfate, but a nurse misread Mg as MS and added morphine to the IV. The patient became hypotensive and apneic and was resuscitated and moved to the intensive care unit (ICU) for respiratory support. Since the reason for the patient's condition was unknown, staff administered Narcan (naloxone) to see if it would help, and it did.

A prescriber in another hospital wrote "MgSo4 2g IV × 1 dose" for a 45-year-old woman.[12] The unit clerk and the nurse misinterpreted the order as morphine sulfate 2 (mg) IV × 1 dose, which the patient received. Because the patient was in pain, an order for morphine seemed reasonable. The prescriber was notified, and magnesium was administered to the patient.

A dermatology consultant recommended "TAC 0.1%, apply t.i.d. to affected areas" for a hospitalized patient with a skin disorder. The patient's physician misinterpreted the recommendation as TAC (tetracaine/adrenalin/cocaine) and submitted a nonformulary drug request to obtain the medication. The pharmacist intervened and clarified the order with the prescribing dermatologist as triamcinolone cream 0.1%. A few months later, a hospitalized nursing home patient was referred to the same dermatologist for a rash unresponsive to hydrocortisone cream. This time, a different physician misinterpreted the dermatologist's "TAC" prescription as tacrolimus 0.1% and again submitted a nonformulary drug request. The pharmacist realized the similarity to the previous request and called the dermatologist, who again verified that the intended medication was triamcinolone 0.1%. Contacting prescribers is always the most direct way to clarify an uncertain medication order, and clarification takes more time than the prescriber may have saved by using an abbreviation.

Coined names can be confused with other medical terms, procedures, or tests. T3 is used occasionally as an abbreviation for both Tylenol with Codeine No. 3 (acetaminophen and codeine) and liothyronine (e.g., Cytomel). An order to "give patient T3" might also be misunderstood as a request for a lab test for triiodothyronine level. Again, workflow must be interrupted to clarify a nonstandard abbreviation.

A hospital reported several medication errors related to physicians' use of coined abbreviations:

- One physician group used DCN to abbreviate Darvocet-N 100 (propoxyphene and acetaminophen), while another used DCN for doxycycline.
- One physician used PROXL for Procardia XL (nifedipine extended-release), but a pharmacist misread the handwritten order as Paxil (paroxetine).
- One physician used DPH for diphenhydramine (Benadryl), while another used the same abbreviation for phenytoin (Dilantin), formerly called diphenylhydantoin. This led to an error while the order was being clarified. The pharmacist was not sure if the physician had prescribed DPH 50 mg or DPH 300 mg. She called to see if the order was for Dilantin 300 mg or Benadryl 50 mg. In the meantime, the unit secretary had transcribed this order as Benadryl 300 mg at HS. The nurse took Benadryl out of an automated dispensing cabinet (which, at the time, was not interfaced with the pharmacy computer) and gave it to the patient before the pharmacist had time to clarify the order. The patient was extremely sleepy for 24 hours but had no lingering effects. The physicians involved were made aware of the risk in using abbreviations and advised to use proper generic and brand names.

When coined names are used for thrombolytics, there is a high risk of patient harm from bleeding. Activase (alteplase) is commonly referred to as t-PA, and TNKase (tenecteplase) is sometimes called TNK or TNK-t-PA. These abbreviations can lead to confusion and to overdosages if TNKase is given in place of Activase. In one case, a nurse asked a physician who had prescribed "t-PA" if "TNK" was the same thing. Believing the nurse was asking if both were thrombolytics, the physician answered yes. The nurse obtained TNKase from an emergency department (ED) supply and gave the patient a dose that was appropriate for Activase.

In another case, an ED physician had prescribed "t-PA 8 mg IV" followed by 73 mg IV over 1 hour for a patient with cerebrovascular accident (CVA). The unit's thrombolytic box contained both Activase and TNKase, which is used for acute myocardial infarction (AMI) but not CVA. An inexperienced nurse assumed that both were the same product and gave 8 mg of TNKase to the patient. The nurse did not notice the order for the 1-hour infusion and transferred the patient to the ICU before administering the follow-up dose. A neurologist detected the errors, which may have contributed to the patient's poor recovery. ISMP continues to receive similar reports.

Given differences in the dosing methods for thrombolytics and the risk of hemorrhage even at therapeutic dosages, the potential for harm from errors is obvious. Sometimes, hospitals with several cardiology and neurology groups on staff have difficulty agreeing on specific agents for use in AMI and CVA; having multiple agents on the formulary only adds to the risk of error. One hospital restricted thrombolytics in the ED to Activase (for CVA) and Retavase (for AMI).

Additional measures to prevent errors include design of specific CVA and AMI preprinted order sets with both brand and generic names listed for all drugs. Also, warnings about the potential for mix-ups can be displayed on automated dispensing cabinet screens.

In one hospital, the pharmacy prints stickers that describe how to dose Activase in CVA patients. The pharmacy technician who receives the medications places these stickers over the opening of each carton as a seal. Staff education, while important, may not prevent all errors; other measures such as these are needed.

HIGH-RISK ABBREVIATION USE

From thousands of error reports involving the use of abbreviations, ISMP has identified particular hazards when abbreviations are used with certain medications. This was of great concern with the hydromorphone extended-release product Palladone, which came in 12, 16, 24, and 32 mg capsules for once-daily administration. The product had four to eight times the potency of morphine on a milligram for milligram basis; it was recommended for use only in patients already receiving opioid therapy who required a total daily dose of at least 12 mg of oral hydromorphone or its equivalent. If an order for this drug "QD" had been misread as QID, the fourfold overdosage could have been fatal for some patients. Palladone has been removed from the market for reasons unrelated to this concern, but the same problem could occur with another once-a-day narcotic, Avinza (morphine sulfate extended-release capsules). Such products should never be kept as floor stock. Not only should practitioners avoid abbreviations such as QD and QOD, but manufacturers should avoid them in advertising and packaging.

As another example, the intranasal route of administration has been used for a number of drugs, including corticosteroids, vasopressin, and, more recently, a nasal mist influenza vaccine (Flumist). Other intranasal drugs are under investigation. In the medical literature, authors have occasionally used "IN" as an abbreviation for intranasal. A new type of medication error can be expected if "IN" is used in clinical practice. A handwritten abbreviation could be seen as IV or IM, or "IN" could be misheard as IM in spoken orders. Such errors could be tragic. Even if no error occurred, misunderstanding this abbreviation could delay the start of therapy. "IN" should be considered for an organization's list of dangerous abbreviations. If "intranasal" cannot be used because the computer system limits the route field to three digits, consider NAS as a better alternative. Handwritten or computer-generated MARs and handwritten orders should spell out "intranasal."

DISCUSSION

Despite the steady flow of error reports involving misinterpreted abbreviations, symbols, and dose expressions, many practitioners continue to question whether evidence supports prohibiting their use in medical communications. Failure to substantially eliminate abbreviations on JCAHO's do-not-use list from medication orders is one of the most frequently cited findings during JCAHO surveys.[4] We are unaware of studies demonstrating the degree of risk incurred by using these abbreviations, or the effectiveness of avoiding them in preventing medication errors. Such research would be difficult to conduct, and it is doubtful that an institutional review board would approve a study with a control group, for obvious ethical reasons. We can affirm, however, that the abbreviations we have reported to be dangerous have been involved in harmful, even fatal, medication errors (visit www.ismp.org/newsletters/acutecare/articles/20010502.asp).

Even without studies, it is obvious that avoiding abbreviations helps prevent errors. No scientific validation is needed for the argument that removing potassium chloride concentrate vials from patient care areas and providing timely pharmacy distribution of solutions will prevent potassium from being given IV push. Similarly, it is obvious that using U for units has led to countless 10-fold overdosages of insulin, heparin, and penicillin G (including an infant death from hyperkalemia).

In discussing the dilemma between obvious patient safety strategies and evidence-based medicine, Leape, Berwick, and Bates[15] noted that "A common theme…is that they make sense. To a layperson, and to most physicians, these sound like obvious things to do. That is basically how aviation and anesthesia made progress: They did what seemed to be the obvious right thing to do (although we must also always keep in mind the potential for negative consequences, even when a safety measure seems obvious)."

ISMP and JCAHO are not the only patient safety organizations that suggest avoiding abbreviations and dose expressions that have led to serious medication errors. In 1997, the National Coordinating Council for Medication Error Reporting and Prevention (www.NCCMERP.org), which comprises 20 nationally recognized organizations, published a list of dangerous abbreviations. Several health care standards organizations have eliminated these abbreviations from their style manuals or, in the case of USP, from its official compendium. FDA is moving toward prohibiting their use in drug package labeling. The National Quality Forum Safe Practices Steering Committee (www.qualityforum.org) also recommends avoiding abbreviations and dose expressions deemed to be dangerous.

On November 23, 2004, JCAHO hosted the National Summit on Medical Abbreviations, in conjunction with the American College of Physicians, American College of Surgeons, American Hospital Association, American Medical Association, American Society of Health-System Pharmacists, USP, and ISMP. In all, 50 professional societies and associations and interest groups participated, discussing medical errors related to the misuse and misinterpretation of abbreviations, acronyms, and symbols. The objective was to reach consensus on the scope and implications of this serious and complex problem and to find reasonable solutions, using all the evidence at hand.

Conclusions of the summit were posted on JCAHO's Web site for public comment. During the 4-week comment period, JCAHO received 5,227 responses, including 15,485 comments. More than 80% of the respondents supported the creation and adoption of a do-not-use list. However, the responses from the public supported discontinuation of a previous stipulation that each health care organization identify an additional three organization-specific do-not-use abbreviations; attendees at the summit had supported organization-specific additions. Ultimately, JCAHO's Sentinel Event Advisory Group recommended that the requirement for three additional organization-specific do-not-use abbreviations be discontinued and that no additions be made to the 2006 do-not-use list. However, it was agreed that the symbols >, <, and @; the abbreviations cc and μg; apothecary units; and all drug name abbreviations (Table 8-2) should be reviewed annually for possible inclusion on the do-not-use list as part of the development of future JCAHO NPSGs. In May 2005 the list was confirmed by the professional organizations in attendance at the November 2004 meeting.[4] Action by JCAHO is pending.

Endorsement of a do-not-use list by ISMP, JCAHO, and professional organizations will not, by itself, stop the use of dangerous abbreviations in medical communications. Error-prone abbreviations need to be eliminated throughout organizations and externally. Practitioners cannot be expected to eliminate the use of specific abbreviations if those abbreviations continue to appear on computer screens, drug labels, MARs, and preprinted orders and in other forms of communication about drug therapy. Professional journals, academic facilities, medical device and computer software vendors, and the pharmaceutical industry need to give priority to eliminating error-prone abbreviations.

Some health care providers, pharmaceutical companies, publishers, and information system vendors believe handwritten materials present unique problems of illegibility that do not affect printed or electronic materials. Except in handwriting, they believe there is no reason to avoid using widely accepted abbreviations, including those known to be dangerous, such as U for units. Standard publishing guidelines often dictate the format of printed material, even when that format promotes dangerous methods of expressing doses. For example, style might dictate that if warfarin 1.5 mg is mentioned, then warfarin 2 mg must be carried out to the same number of decimal places and listed as 2.0 mg for consistency. There are many more such examples of dangerous expressions in professional literature, drug advertisements, preprinted prescriber order forms, computer screens, and computer-generated materials.

With the current emphasis on patient safety, such style guidelines need to be reconsidered. It is true that the type used in printed materials and on computer screens is clearer than handwriting. But even widely accepted abbreviations may not be interpreted as intended. Even if a practitioner can clearly read MTX on a screen, does that guarantee that it will be interpreted as methotrexate, as intended? Why not mitoxantrone? In print and electronic formats, some fonts, type colors, and spacing make it difficult to differentiate between 100U and 1000, or between 1.0 and 10. It is also a fact that practitioners mimic what they see every day in print and electronic formats. Allowing the use of abbreviations and dose expressions known to be dangerous in electronic and print formats but forbidding their use in handwriting reflects a double standard.

Publishers must redesign their style manuals and follow the example of the American Diabetes Association, which no longer allows the abbreviation U to be used in publications, and the *American Journal of Nursing*, which has incorporated the JCAHO do-not-use list into its editorial style. Information system vendors need to set a good example by avoiding the use of dangerous abbreviations and dose expressions in electronic forms of medical information. As purchasers of these products, health care providers need to stand firm on demands that vendors prohibit the use of knowingly dangerous abbreviations and dose expressions. Likewise, health care providers need to make sure that abbreviations and dangerous dose expressions are not used in printed materials (e.g., order forms, protocols, care maps, computer-generated MARs, prescription labels, in-house newsletters).

FDA should enforce prohibition of error-prone expressions in product advertising as well as in packaging and labeling, and the pharmaceutical industry needs to follow FDA requirements in designing ads, packages, and labels. In June 2006, FDA and ISMP launched a nationwide education campaign to reduce the use of unclear abbreviations, symbols, and dose expressions. The aim is to eliminate the use of potentially confusing abbreviations by health care professionals, medical students, medical writers, the pharmaceutical industry, and FDA staff. The campaign addresses the use of mistake-prone abbreviations in all forms of medical communication, including written medication orders, computer-generated labels, MARs, pharmacy or prescriber computer order entry screens, and commercial medication labeling, packaging, and advertising. More information is available at www.fda.gov/bbs/topics/NEWS/2006/NEW01390.html.

Regardless of the medium, there is no excuse for using abbreviations or expressing doses in a manner that may cause confusion. Error-prone abbreviations, symbols, and dose designations must never be used in communicating medical and drug information.

REFERENCES

1. Twain M. Damages awarded. *The San Francisco Daily Morning Call*. October 1, 1864. Available at: www.twainquotes.com/18641001.html. Accessed May 31, 2005.
2. Davis, NM. *Medical Abbreviations: 26,000 Conveniences at the Expense of Communication and Safety*. 12th ed. Warminster, Pa: Neil M. Davis Associates; 2005.
3. Should abbreviations from a foreign language be used? *ISMP Medication Safety Alert! Acute Care Edition*. May 6, 2004;9(9):3.
4. Joint Commission on Accreditation of Healthcare Organizations. Facts about the official "do not use" list. Available at: www.jointcommission.org/PatientSafety/DoNotUseList/facts_dnu.htm. Accessed June 23, 2006.

5. Joint Commission on Accreditation of Healthcare Organizations. The official "do not use" list. Available at: www.jointcommission.org/PatientSafety/DoNotUseList/. Accessed June 23, 2006.

6. Joint Commission on Accreditation of Healthcare Organizations. FAQs about the official "do not use" list. Available at: www.jointcommission.org/PatientSafety/DoNotUseList/. Accessed June 23, 2006.

7. Joint Commission on Accreditation of Healthcare Organizations. Implementation Tips for Eliminating Dangerous Abbreviations. Available at: www.jointcommission.org/PatientSafety/NationalPatientSafety Goals/abbr_tips.htm. Accessed June 23, 2006.

8. Institute for Safe Medication Practices. Hospital and medical staff leadership is key to compliance with JCAHO dangerous abbreviation list. *ISMP Medication Safety Alert! Acute Care Edition*. August 12, 2004;9(16):1.

9. Traynor K. Enforcement outdoes education at eliminating unsafe abbreviations. *Am J Health Syst Pharm.* 2004; 16:1314–5.

10. Joint Commission Resources. *A Guide to JCAHO's Medication Management Standards*. Oakbrook Terrace, Ill: Joint Commission on Accreditation of Healthcare Organizations; 2004: 142–6.

11. Institute for Safe Medication Practices. JCAHO NPSG survey change. *ISMP Medication Safety Alert! Acute Care Edition*. February 10, 2005;(10)3:2.

12. Abbreviations: a shortcut to medication errors. *PA-PSRS Patient Safety Advisory.* March 2005;2(1):19-21. Available at: www.psa.state.pa.us/psa/lib/psa/advisories/march_2005_advisory_v2_n1.pdf. Accessed May 31, 2005.

13. Schneider J. Pharmacy error leads to medicine overdose. *Lansing State Journal.* October 14, 2003.

14. Cohen MR. Medication error reports. *Hosp Pharm.* 1975;10:167.

15. Leape LL, Berwick DM, Bates DW. What practices will most increase safety? Evidence-based medicine meets patient safety. *JAMA.* 2002;288:501–7.

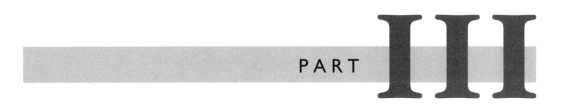

PART **III**

PREVENTING MEDICATION ERRORS: A SHARED RESPONSIBILITY

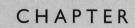

PREVENTING PRESCRIBING ERRORS

Michael R. Cohen

Although the root causes of medication errors reside in systems, each individual health care professional—beginning with the prescriber—must take every possible precaution to prevent errors. Many errors related to prescribing go undetected or unreported, but evidence suggests that the problem is substantial. Bates et al.[1] found 0.3 prescribing errors per patient day in hospitals. Lesar and colleagues[2] found an overall rate of 3.99 clinically significant prescribing errors per 1,000 orders written at a hospital. The most common errors during the 1-year study period were associated with failure to alter drug therapy in patients with impaired renal or hepatic function (13.9%); failure to recognize a patient's allergy to the prescribed medication class (12.1%); use of an incorrect drug name, dosage form, or abbreviation (11.4%); dosage miscalculation (11.1%); and use of an unusual or atypical but critical dosage frequency (10.8%). More recently, Bobb and colleagues[3] identified 62.4 prescribing errors per 1,000 medication orders; 30.8% of these were rated clinically significant. Most of the errors occurred upon admission and were most frequently related to the ordering of anti-infectives, the prescribing of incorrect doses, and deficiencies in medication knowledge.

In this chapter, the elements of a complete and safe medication order or prescription are discussed, as are specific prescribing practices and the pitfalls of various methods of communicating medication orders. Suggestions are offered for avoiding these pitfalls and reducing the risk of prescribing errors. This chapter also discusses the role of formulary systems in improving safety and describes methods for resolving disagreements about prescribed therapy. Pharmacists' clinical role in ensuring safe and appropriate prescribing is discussed in Chapter 10.

ELEMENTS OF THE MEDICATION ORDER OR PRESCRIPTION

It is the prescriber's responsibility to communicate complete information about the prescribed medication in a manner that is clear to the health care providers and patients who must carry out the order or take the medication. The following elements should always be included in the prescription or order:[4-6]

1. The patient's full name and location.
2. Applicable patient-specific data (e.g., allergies, age or date of birth, weight).
3. Generic and brand names of the drug. Ideally, both should be stated. If only one is used, the generic name is preferable, unless there is a possibility of confusion with another drug that has a similar name, or a specific brand or proprietary dosage form is desired. In these instances, the brand name should be added.

Research or chemical names, chemical symbols, abbreviations, and locally coined names should not be used.

4. The drug strength expressed in metric units by weight (e.g., milligrams [mg], grams [g], milliequivalents [mEq], or millimoles [mmol]). For liquid medications, the drug concentration should be expressed (e.g., 500 mg/10 mL). The outmoded and error-prone apothecary system should never be used.

5. The dosage form.

6. The amount to be dispensed, expressed in metric units. Package units (e.g., bottle, tube, ampul) should not be used.

7. Complete directions for use, including the route of administration and frequency of dosing. Ambiguous orders, such as "take as directed," should be avoided unless they are accompanied by further directions. Including specific directions reinforces proper medication use to the patient, helps differentiate the medication from others, and allows the dispenser to counsel the patient appropriately.

8. The purpose of the medication. Including the purpose provides the pharmacist, nurse, and patient with additional assurance that they have the correct medication. If patient confidentiality is of concern, the purpose may be omitted or generalized (e.g., heart disease, lung disease, neurologic disorder, skin disorder).

9. The number of authorized refills or the duration of therapy.

Patient Information

To choose the appropriate medication and dosage for the individual, the prescriber must consider the patient's age, weight, renal and hepatic function, concurrent disease states, laboratory test results, current medications (including nonprescription medications, vitamin and mineral supplements, and herbal or homeopathic remedies), allergies, and medical, surgical, and family history, including pregnancy or lactation status as appropriate.[2,5] The information should be reviewed for potential contraindications to the medication being considered and possible interactions with other medications the patient is receiving. Prescribers may wish to consult a pharmacist, particularly when a patient's drug regimen is complex. Prescribers should not rely solely on the checks and balances within the health care system, including technology, to ensure the appropriateness of the drug. The prescriber often has information about the patient that is not readily available to other health care professionals.

For instance, the primary prescriber may know about a patient's genetic predisposition to methemoglobinemia, a potentially life-threatening condition associated with the use of topical anesthetics.[7] The prescriber must communicate this information to the pulmonologist performing a bronchoscopy and other staff caring for the patient during and after a procedure in which a topical anesthetic is used, so that they are better prepared to assess the appropriateness of the order and care for the patient.[2,8]

Safe prescribing entails verifying the patient's identification. All staff involved in the medication-use process should use two identifiers (e.g., name, birth date, identification number), whether prescribing, dispensing, or administering medications. Making such identification available during prescribing presents a challenge. Computerized prescriber order entry (CPOE) systems can reduce prescribers' chance of entering orders on the wrong patient's record. For example, a CPOE system could be designed so that, once logged on, the physician would select the name from a list of his or her patients, rather than a list of all patients. In ambulatory care, a comparable list would be the schedule of patients seen that day. Enhancing the font of the patient's name on the screen can help ensure correct order entry by both prescribers and pharmacists. Some systems alert staff to similar names in the registry and require a second form of identification (e.g., birth date, identification number) before the practitioner can proceed.

Drug Information

Prescribing problems can involve doses beyond safe limits, confusion between formulations of similarly named products, off-label prescribing, inappropriate clinical use, unanticipated chemical reactions with products, and accidental prescribing of concomitant products that could have unintended effects, such as a toxic cumulative dose. Pharmacists can be a valuable source of information to prescribers. The 2005 edition of Lexi-Comp's *Drug Information Handbook* contains 4,900 entries for medications available in the United States and Canada. It is impossible for prescribers to remember everything about every product.

For example, many prescription analgesics contain acetaminophen. These combination products are often prescribed using brand names (e.g., Vicodin, Percocet), and nurses may overlook the fact that they contain acetaminophen. Since many of these products are kept as floor stock in hospitals, pharmacists may have difficulty tracking the amount of acetaminophen consumed by patients. Physicians may fail to recognize that various medications prescribed for use "as needed" or "prn" (in the hospital, often as standing orders) could cumulatively result in toxic amounts of acetaminophen. It is not uncommon for physicians to prescribe acetaminophen for fever or mild pain as well as a combination product containing acetaminophen for moderate pain. In 307 reports to the Food and Drug Administration of unintentional overdoses leading to hepatotoxicity between 1998 and 2001, 25% of the patients were taking more than one acetaminophen-containing product.[9]

One hospital confirmed this problem by printing usage reports from its automated dispensing cabinets each morning for all patients who exceeded 3 g of acetaminophen within the previous 24 hours.[9] A healthy patient with normal liver function can tolerate 6 g per day over a very short period without harm, but one patient had received 8 g of acetaminophen within a 24-hour period, and many others had received 6 g on several consecutive days. An average of one patient per day exceeded 4 g. Other hospitals have reported similar experiences, and several have identified combination products containing hydrocodone 5 mg plus acetaminophen 500 mg (e.g., Vicodin) as a contributing factor. Computerized prescribing systems with dose-checking capabilities can alert physicians if prescribed medications potentially exceed the 4 g daily limit of acetaminophen.

A lack of available or up-to-date prescribing information has resulted in overdoses of intravenous colchicine. A 72-year-old man with a history of gout successfully underwent surgery. Two days later he began to have symptoms consistent with acute gout. Previously, he had taken oral colchicine to relieve these symptoms, but since he could not yet take oral medications, the physician consulted a reference book and prescribed IV colchicine exactly as recommended: "2 mg IV bolus followed by 0.5 mg IV every 6 hours until pain resolved." Two days later, with the pain continuing, the dosage was increased to 1 mg every 6 hours. When the pain was still unrelieved, colchicine was discontinued and indomethacin was prescribed. Although the patient experienced some relief, he developed leukopenia, abdominal pain, renal failure, and metabolic acidosis. These symptoms, consistent with colchicine toxicity, led to respiratory distress. The patient had received a total of 11.5 mg of colchicine in a 3-day period. Intravenous colchicine is used in carefully selected patients when treatment with safer nonsteroidal anti-inflammatory drugs is unsuccessful. The dose must be reduced in geriatric patients with compromised renal or hepatic function. Any order for IV colchicine should indicate a specific stop time and reflect a limit of 4 mg/week. Although gastrointestinal (GI) symptoms often are used as a guide to oral colchicine dosing, they occur rarely with IV administration; therefore, GI status should not be used to gauge toxicity. The reference used by this prescriber had not clearly indicated the weekly dosing limits. Computerized alerts could have prevented this prescribing error.

System-based strategies should be used to help practitioners maintain familiarity with drug indications, interactions, and precautions. Most important, up-to-date, complete drug references must be made available at the point of prescribing. The Institute for Safe Medication Practices (ISMP) receives many reports of medication errors stemming from the use of information in outdated or inaccurate references. A section of the ISMP Web site (www.ismp.org) lists "Textbook Errata" discovered through error reports, and most publishers maintain a similar database.

Many practitioners use outdated hard copy references or the *Physicians' Desk Reference* (*PDR*). The *PDR* does not list every drug available; manufacturers choose the products they want to feature in the *PDR*, which consists of official product labeling. Unlike many other drug references, the *PDR* often lists products separately by dosage form; thus, certain information may be hard to find, which could lead to medication errors.

Prescribers can stay current through access to an electronic drug information database or hand-held devices that provide regular updates of the database. Ideally, information from these databases should interface with computerized prescribing systems to generate alerts and clinical decision support. Automated clinical decision support systems (see Chapter 15) help bring the most crucial information about the drug and the patient to the attention of clinicians, so that they can provide the best care. For example, a physician who uses an automated system with decision support to prescribe an antimicrobial may be alerted to the need for a dose adjustment based on the patient's most recent laboratory values.

Selecting the Correct Dosage Form or Formulation

Mix-ups among various formulations have occurred with many products. Hundreds of syphilis patients were inadvertently treated with Bicillin C-R (penicillin G benzathine and penicillin G procaine) instead of Bicillin L-A (penicillin G benzathine). Varivax (varicella vaccine) has been given to pregnant women instead of VZIG (varicella-zoster immune globulin). Mix-ups in dosing and routes of administration are bound to occur between the acetylcysteine products Mucomyst and Acetadote when prescribed for acetaminophen overdosage.

Many errors have involved drug name suffixes that are omitted from a prescription, ignored, or misinterpreted as an abbreviation, a dosage, or administration directions.[8,10] For example, when extended-release Procardia XL was first marketed, many people thought they heard "Procardia SL" (sublingual) when orders were spoken. Chapter 6 discusses the use of suffixes, and a list of problem suffixes has been published elsewhere.[11]

Drug Names That Look or Sound Alike

Look-alike and sound-alike drug names increase the risk for medication errors. Similar dosage ranges within a look-alike or sound-alike pair compound the problem. Errors may occur when prescribers interchange the two drug names, when someone misinterprets a poorly written order or prescription without consulting the prescriber, and when the person receiving a spoken order does not hear it correctly and fails to read it back to the prescriber.[8,12]

A common cause of name mix-ups is what human-factors experts call "confirmation bias." A practitioner confronted with a poorly written order may see the name with which he or she is most familiar and overlook any evidence to the contrary. Often the practitioner does not think of questioning the order.

Computer systems can reduce the risk of confirmation bias and drug name mix-ups (see Chapter 7). Many systems can be programmed to display on the monitor a clinical flag or a formulary note to alert the person entering the order when a look-alike or sound-alike danger is present. For example, when the drug name Norvasc is entered into the pharmacy computer at Erie County Medical Center in Buffalo, New York, a formulary note alerts the pharmacist that the handwritten word Norvasc (amlodipine) often looks like Navane (thiothixene). The pharmacist can then confirm the order if necessary. The medical center uses such notes for more than 100 name pairs.

When ordering medications for which there is a known look-alike or sound-alike danger, prescribers must take extra care to write or speak clearly and confirm that other health care providers understand what medication is intended. Errors may be avoided by expressing the purpose of the medication; few look-alike or sound-alike name pairs include two drugs with the same therapeutic indication.[4,5,13–15] Educating patients about their medications is another safety measure; including the medication's purpose on the prescription and the label facilitates this.[13]

Purpose of the Medication

Prescribers should indicate the purpose of all medications on outpatient prescriptions. This provides pharmacists with an additional way of confirming that they have interpreted the order correctly. The pharmacist should include the purpose of the medication on the label. This helps patients to confirm that they have the medication their physician prescribed and to distinguish among the medications they are taking.[14,15] A prescription form designed to remind prescribers to include the medication's purpose is shown in Figure 9-1.

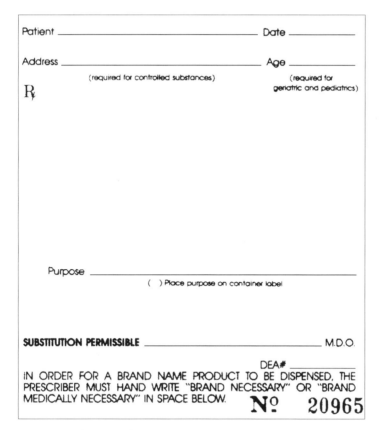

FIGURE 9-1 Prescription forms such as this one remind prescribers to specify the purpose of the medication.

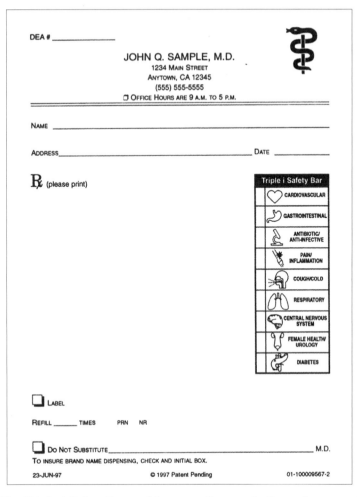

FIGURE 9-2 The Triple i Safety Bar enables prescribers to indicate the general purpose of a medication. More than 30 icons are available to meet the needs of prescribers in various specialties.

Prescribers may be concerned that specifying the purpose of a medication order will violate patient confidentiality. Some prescribers resist doing this because of the time it takes or because they think insurers will deny payment for medications prescribed for off-label indications.[5,14,15] Use of the "Triple i" Safety Bar (Figure 9-2) may allay some of these concerns. This vertical bar, which displays icons representing various therapeutic categories, appears on the right-hand side of some prescription blanks. The prescriber places a check in front of the appropriate icon.[15] Another way to avoid stating the clinical purpose would be to use the International Classification of Diseases (ICD) code. Precedent for this has been set for laboratory tests reimbursed through third parties; the ICD-9 code is required on prescriptions for laboratory tests.

An error that underscores the importance of including the purpose on prescriptions occurred in association with an outpatient prescription for Florinef. The physician did not write the strength on the prescription or include directions for use. The prescription was misread as Fiorinal. Had the dose and directions been included, this error could have been avoided, because the recommended dose and directions are different for the two drugs.

Including the purpose (the patient had Addison's disease and Florinef was prescribed to control electrolyte balance) would have helped prevent the mix-up, since Fiorinal is an analgesic.

In inpatient settings, the purpose of all prn medications should accompany the orders. Prescribers should use caution about listing the purpose of medications that are to be given on a regular schedule, since orders with an indication typically are reserved for prn medications and staff may interpret them as such. Some organizations have had success with a specially designed order form or electronic template that requires entering the purpose of all orders in a designated space.

Knowledge of Medication-Use Processes in Institutions

Prescribers should understand the medication ordering system of every institution at which they hold privileges.[4] They should make an effort to prescribe medications that are on the formulary, because those agents are familiar to other professionals working in the institution and thus less likely to be involved in errors than are nonformulary agents. If a nonformulary medication must be ordered, prescribers should know the process for this so that therapy can be initiated without delay. They should write the medication order clearly and reinforce it in conversations with the nurse or pharmacist.

In most hospitals, medication orders are taken from the patient's chart and sent to the pharmacy as a carbon or carbonless (no-carbon-required, or NCR) copy or a fax or are generated through a computer system. Prescribers should be familiar with standard medication administration times for institutional prescribing. Doses to be given at odd intervals (e.g., every 11 hours), or at regular intervals but nonstandard administration times, are more likely to be given at the wrong times or to be missed altogether. It is usually better to adjust the dosage of a medication and maintain a standard schedule than to adjust the dosing interval. For example, if a patient with renal failure needs a dosage adjustment for gentamicin, it is safer to order a smaller dose given on an even schedule (e.g., every 12 hours) than to order the medication in its normal dosage to be administered every 16 hours.

The procedure used for modifying an order that has been written is important in preventing errors. To correct or revise an order, the prescriber should write a new order and alert the nursing unit staff to this.[16] Once a prescriber has written an order, he or she should not alter the original order; if a copy of the original order has already been sent to the pharmacy, the change or correction will be missed, resulting in a medication error. If the prescriber makes a mistake while writing orders, the erroneous order should not be erased or otherwise obliterated. Instead, the prescriber should draw a single, thin line through all of the erroneous material, write the word error next to the lined-out area, date and initial this, and write the correct order as a new order.

ORDER-WRITING PRACTICES

Abbreviations

Prescribers may think the use of abbreviations saves time, but it can consume the time of other health care professionals and increase the potential for medication errors.[17] An abbreviation can be misunderstood for a variety of reasons. It may have more than one meaning, may be unfamiliar to the reader, or, if poorly written, may be mistaken for another abbreviation.[4,5,17–20] Chapter 8 discusses the need to minimize and standardize the use of abbreviations; it includes a list of abbreviations that have been associated with errors. Prescribers should avoid nonstandard abbreviations, including Latin directions for use. Certain abbreviations are consistently misunderstood and should never be used; these include the following:[5,18,20]

- Abbreviations for drug names,
- Any abbreviation for the word daily,
- The letter U for the word unit,
- "µg" for microgram (use "mcg"),
- "QOD" for every other day,
- "sc" or "sq" for subcutaneous (use "subcut"),
- "a/" or "&" for the word and,
- "cc" for cubic centimeter (use "mL" for milliliter instead), and
- "D/C" for discontinue or discharge.

Prescribers should also avoid "stemming," or creating shortened versions of drug names; these can be misinterpreted. For example, a physician who intended to prescribe Rheomacrodex (low molecular weight dextran) called the order in to a nurse as "Rheo 10 cc/hr." The nurse interpreted the order as ReoPro (abciximab) 10 cc/hr and immediately transcribed it onto an order form without verifying this interpretation by immediately reading it back to the physician. The pharmacy processed the order, and the patient received ReoPro for more than 24 hours before the error was noticed. The patient experienced no serious adverse effects.

Expressions of Weight, Volume, and Units

Prescribers should use the metric system to express all weights, volumes, and units. Use of the apothecary system can lead to errors because of unfamiliarity with the units and their abbreviations, confusion between apothecary and metric system units, and the need for conversion to metric units.[5,20-22] The antiquated apothecary system is rarely used today, but remnants can still be seen in prescription writing, and drug labeling and syringe scales that measure in minims can still be found in some countries. One milliliter contains 16.23 minims, but the symbol for minim (℥) has been confused with "mL," causing a 16-fold overdosage. For example, nurses have given 10 mL of opium tincture instead of 10 minims. Syringes marked with a minim scale have been confused with insulin syringes, resulting in massive insulin overdoses. The apothecary symbol for dram has also caused errors. An order for 1 dram (℥) was mistaken for 3 tablespoons (T), leading to a theophylline overdose in a child. The abbreviation for the apothecary unit grain (gr) has been confused with gram (g). Apothecary dosages expressed as fractions, such as "gr 1/200" have been misinterpreted; a nurse gave two nitroglycerin 1/100 grain tablets when a supply of 1/200 grain tablets ran out. If the metric system had been used, it would have been obvious that 1/100 (0.6 mg) plus 1/100 (0.6 mg) does not equal 1/200 (0.3 mg). The apothecary symbol "ss" for one-half led to the following error: A physician reduced the daily warfarin dosage for a patient in a long-term care facility from 3 mg to 2.5 mg. He wrote the order as "5 mg ss every day." The pharmacist dispensed the prescription with 5 mg tablets cut in half, and the nurse transcribed the order onto the patient's medication administration record (MAR) exactly as it had been written. A bottle of warfarin 5 mg remained in the patient's medication drawer, even though the patient had not taken 5 mg daily for some time. The other nurses overlooked the "ss" symbol on the MAR and administered 5 mg to the patient every day for 3 weeks. The patient died, and the death certificate stated that GI hemorrhage had been a significant contributing factor. (This example also shows the danger in keeping discontinued medications in a patient's medication drawer.)

The United States Pharmacopeia (USP) does not recognize the apothecary system as an official system for measurement of drug doses. USP states that all expressions of strength, including those on manufacturers' labels, medication orders and prescriptions, and dispensing labels, must be in metric units, with one exception: cases in which it is appropriate to express the medication's strength as a percentage of active ingredient.[21]

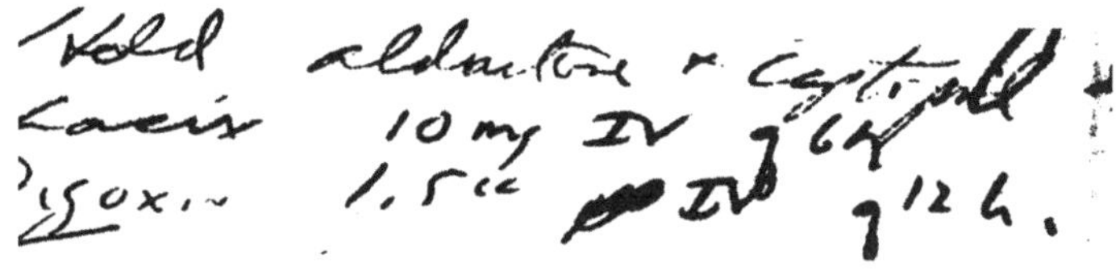

FIGURE 9-3 This order for IV digoxin includes only a volume and fails to include a strength.

In most cases, it is unacceptable to express doses or quantities in terms of dosage form or volume alone.[4,23,24] Volume may be used along with a strength or concentration; for example, it is acceptable (though unnecessary) to prescribe 5 mL of a solution of 100 mg/5 mL. It is acceptable to prescribe by volume when there is no strength because of a combination of many ingredients, or no active ingredient (e.g., cola syrup); when the active ingredient itself is available only as a liquid (e.g., paregoric); and for certain external-use items such as creams, lotions, and drops (e.g., "add 10 drops to vaporizer water"). Usually, however, prescribing by volume alone presents a hazard. For example, when Sudafed contained pseudoephedrine (available as Sudafed Children's Non-Drowsy), the liquid came only in a 15 mg/5 mL concentration, while many generic liquid pseudoephedrine products were available in a 30 mg/5 mL concentration. Some combination products also contained a 30 mg/5 mL concentration. If one of the more concentrated products was used but not recognized, patients, including children, could receive twice as much drug as intended. Health care providers should specify the dose in milligrams, as with all liquid medications, and alert parents if multiple concentrations are available. (Pharmacists should provide and demonstrate the use of metric-only measurement devices with all oral liquids dispensed.[11])

In another example, a pharmacy received a copy of a spoken order, transcribed by a nurse, for weekly methotrexate given subcutaneously at a dose of "0.7 mL (25 mg)." This was questioned and clarified as 0.7 mL of the 25 mg/mL strength. Ordering by volume rather than metric weight in milligrams caused the initial confusion.

An error involving IV digoxin prescribed for an infant illustrates the importance of including the strength in medication orders. Because the order (Figure 9-3) did not specify strength, the baby received 1.5 mL of the adult concentration, 0.25 mg/mL, instead of the pediatric concentration, 0.1 mg/mL. The child required digoxin immune Fab fragment (ovine) to bind and inactivate the digoxin in her blood.

Decimals and Spaces

Decimal points in dosages are a major source of errors. They can easily be missed, especially on lined (ruled) order sheets, carbon and NCR forms, and faxes. If a decimal point is missed, an overdose may occur. Decimals should be written with great care and should be avoided whenever a satisfactory alternative exists.[4,19,20] For example, the prescriber should write "500 mg" instead of "0.5 g," and "125 mcg" instead of "0.125 mg."

A decimal point should never be left "naked." Decimal expressions of less than 1 should always be preceded by a zero (0) to enhance the visibility of the decimal.[4,5,18–20] "Trailing" zeroes (e.g., "1.0"), however, should not be used; that is, a whole number should never be followed with a decimal point and a zero.[4,5,18–20]

A space should appear between the name of the medication and the dose, as well as between the dose and the units.[19] Otherwise, the last letter of the drug name can be mistaken as a number in the dose. For example, "Inderal40mg" could easily be misread as "Inderal 140 mg" instead of "Inderal 40 mg."

Dose Calculations

Patient-specific information (e.g., height, weight, age, and body system function) is often needed to calculate the correct dosage for an individual patient. For example, some drugs eliminated by the kidneys are adjusted for renal function as indicated by creatinine clearance. Chemotherapy doses are often calculated according to the patient's body surface area. Dosages may be adjusted to reduce the risk of toxicity, or to reduce expenses without sacrificing patient care. Dosage calculations are a well-recognized cause of errors. Perlstein et al.[25] reported that 1 of every 12 dosages calculated by 95 registered nurses in an intensive care unit (ICU) contained errors that would result in the administration of doses 10 times as large, or as small, as those prescribed. Eleven pediatricians, given the same examination, scored higher than the nurses but still made errors at the rate of 1 per every 26 computations attempted. Calculation errors can be prevented through (1) reducing the need for calculations and (2) requiring independent cross-checking of calculations. Standardizing drug concentrations and using commercially prepared dosage forms can reduce the need for calculations; however, prescribers must cooperate by prescribing standard concentrations. (The value of standardizing the concentrations of critical care drugs is discussed in Chapter 14.) Independent cross-checking is especially important when doses for pediatric, geriatric, oncology, and critical care patients are calculated. In orders involving a potentially dangerous drug, an unfamiliar calculation, or an especially sensitive patient population, prescribers should include both the dose they have calculated and the dosage in metric units per body weight (milligrams per kilogram) or body surface area (milligrams per square meter) that they used in their calculation.[26,27]

A 13-month study at Albany (New York) Medical Center[28] examined 200 consecutive prescribing errors arising from the use of dosage equations. Seventy percent of the errors involved pediatric patients. Errors were made in common calculations such as "mg/kg/day in four divided doses" and "mg/kg q6h." Although 60% of the errors involved decimal point placement, mathematical calculations, or expressions of dosage regimens, 30% involved misinterpretation of the dosage equation. Examples included prescribing the entire day's dosage as a single dose instead of properly dividing it, and using the entire day's dosage at each dosing interval throughout the day. Alternatives to using dosage equations include using preestablished dose ranges or tables, incorporating a calculator into a computer order entry system, and requiring both the calculated dosage and the dosage equation to appear on orders to facilitate independent checks.[28]

Dose Limits

Establishing and enforcing institutional, therapy-specific dose limits can reduce the chance of an improper dose reaching a patient. Such limits could include the maximum amount for a single dose, per 24-hour period, per cycle of therapy, or for a lifetime amount of a certain drug (e.g., anthracyclines). The established limits should be communicated to all personnel involved in ordering, dispensing, and administering medications. An easily retrievable list should be available for referral. When possible, maximum doses should be entered into pharmacy computer systems and "smart" infusion pumps (those with dosage-error-reduction software). Pharmacists and nurses should be aware that any dose exceeding a predetermined limit might not be dispensed without an independent review that includes input from clinicians other than the involved prescriber, nurse, and pharmacist.

"Bolus" Doses

The term "bolus" has been used inappropriately in ordering IV medications, sometimes with harmful consequences. *Stedman's Medical Dictionary* defines "bolus" as "a single, relatively large quantity of a substance, usually one intended for therapeutic use, such as a bolus dose of a drug," but medical dictionaries give practitioners no information about the rate of administration of a bolus. Practitioners may think "bolus" means the drug is to be injected "at once" or "immediately," but the term is sometimes used in orders for medications intended to be given slowly by direct administration into a vein or IV tubing.

Administering certain drugs over 2 or 3 seconds instead of over 5 to 30 minutes can produce an unintended response or tissue necrosis, as with colchicine, if extravasation goes unrecognized. In the past, confusion about orders for an "IV bolus" of potassium chloride resulted in direct, rapid IV administration that caused severe local pain and fatalities from cardiac arrhythmia. The term "IV bolus" should not be used because it does not indicate an appropriate rate of injection.

Incomplete Orders

Problems can arise from what is *not* included in orders. During a resuscitation, an emergency department (ED) physician ordered "10 of insulin." Distracted by the chaos, a new nurse drew up 10 mL of regular insulin instead of 10 units. Another nurse caught the error while double checking the syringe—a step that, understandably, may be bypassed during emergencies. Nurses may accept incomplete orders in the belief that they know what is intended. They may be accustomed to hearing "give an amp of magnesium sulfate" or seeing "Tylenol 2 tabs prn pain." But which size ampul? What strength of acetaminophen (Tylenol)? What route of administration? Clarification of an incomplete order is vital to patient safety, even during stressful situations.

Orders to "continue previous meds," "resume all pre-op medications," or "continue home medications" may result in serious misinterpretations and errors during the most vulnerable periods of a patient's care: admission, postoperative (or postprocedure) care, transfer to a different level of care, and discharge. Policies that prohibit orders to "resume" or "continue" therapy may not be successful and may simply transfer responsibility to nurses and pharmacists for clarifying incomplete orders. One pharmacist says that clarifying orders for "take home medications" constitutes the bulk of pharmacy interventions.

Prescribers may not know all the drugs a patient is taking at home, and they may not have easy access to a record of all therapy prescribed in the hospital. They may lack comprehensive knowledge about certain classes of drugs. Nevertheless, orders to "resume all previous medications" are not acceptable according to standards of the Joint Commission on Accreditation of Healthcare Organizations (JCAHO), because they can result in serious patient harm. For example, an order to "continue same meds" for a previously ventilated patient upon transfer from a critical care unit led to the fatal use of a neuromuscular blocking agent for a restless, but extubated, patient.

Unreconciled Medications

According to the Institute for Healthcare Improvement, experience from hundreds of organizations has shown that poor communication of medical information at transition points is responsible for as many as 50% of all medication errors and up to 20% of adverse drug events (ADEs) in hospitals.[29] The following examples resulted from failed communication about prescribed medications.

A patient who was transferred from one hospital to another received a duplicate dose of insulin because the receiving nurse did not know the medication had been given before transfer. The patient's medication history was not provided to the receiving facility until several hours after the patient arrived there.

Using a patient's handwritten list of medications taken at home, a physician misunderstood an entry for Desogen (ethinyl estradiol and desogestrel) and prescribed digoxin 0.25 mg daily. Later, a nurse discovered the error when she asked the patient why she was receiving digoxin.

A newly admitted patient with pulmonary hypertension had been receiving Flolan (epoprostenol) IV at home at 2.4 mL/hour. The physician prescribed Flolan at the same flow rate but did not specify the concentration. The hospital used a concentration of 0.5 mg/100 mL, whereas the patient had been using a 0.3 mg/100 mL concentration at home. The error was discovered after the patient experienced symptoms common with higher doses.

Enalapril 2.5 mg IV was administered to a patient after transfer from a critical care unit to a medical unit. The drug had been discontinued upon transfer, but the orders had not yet been transcribed.

A patient in an ED with chest pain received a 7,000 unit heparin bolus prior to the start of a heparin infusion. Upon the patient's admission to the critical care unit, the heparin bolus dose was repeated in error, delaying the patient's cardiac catheterization.

Examples like these led JCAHO to focus on medication reconciliation to reduce the risk of errors during transition points. A JCAHO National Patient Safety Goal (NPSG) requires hospitals to reconcile medications across the continuum of care. The sidebar below presents steps in the process. Medication reconciliation is also a NPSG for ambulatory care, assisted living, behavioral health, home care, and long-term care organizations. If reconciliation takes place in all these settings, it will be easier to obtain accurate medication histories and ensure continuity of appropriate therapy. The Institute for Healthcare Improvement Web site[29] provides further information on medication reconciliation.

MEDICATION RECONCILIATION PROCESS

Obtain a medication history. Obtain the most accurate list possible of the patient's current medications upon admission to the organization before administering the first dose of medications (except in emergency or urgent situations). The list should include prescription and nonprescription medications (including herbals and dietary supplements); the dose, route, frequency, and indication; and the time of the last dose. Most organizations use a specific form for this purpose, on which an assessment of patient compliance with drug therapy and the source of the medication history can also be documented. In addition to the interview with the patient and family, sources of information may include visual inspection of the medications brought into the facility, previous medical records, and the patient's pharmacy and physician office.

Prescribe medications. As soon as the list is reasonably complete, have the prescriber review and act upon each medication on the list while prescribing the patient's admission medications.

Reconcile and resolve discrepancies. Require another person to compare the prescribed admission medications with those on the medication history list and resolve any discrepancies.

Reconcile again upon transfer and discharge. Each time a patient moves from one setting to another, review previous medication orders alongside new orders and plans for care, and resolve any discrepancies. When the patient is discharged, the reconciled list of admission medications must be compared against the physician's discharge orders, along with the most recent medication administration record. Any differences must be fully reconciled before discharge.

Share the list. Communicate a complete list of the patient's medications to the next provider of service when transferring a patient to another setting, service, practitioner, or level of care within or outside the organization. This includes sending a list of medications prescribed upon discharge from the hospital to the patient's primary care physician, as well as encouraging patients to share the list with their pharmacy.

"Hold" Orders

Errors are likely to stem from orders to "hold" medications that lack explicit directions for restarting them. The medication may inadvertently not be resumed, or resumed too soon. For example, an elderly woman had been hospitalized for several days when the attending physician requested a gastroenterology consultation to determine if she was bleeding. He also wrote an order to "Hold Coumadin." According to protocol, the pharmacy interpreted this order as a discontinuation of Coumadin (warfarin). The gastroenterologist performed an endoscopy, with benign results; afterward, he rewrote the orders for all previous treatments and active medications, using the patient's current 24-hour computer-generated MAR as a reference. Since warfarin was no longer an active order, it was not listed on the MAR and thus was not prescribed after the procedure. Six days later, the patient suffered a stroke directly related to inadequate anticoagulation. Similar errors have been reported in outpatient settings when physicians have forgotten to restart warfarin after placing it on hold until a patient's international normalized ratio was within therapeutic range.

A physician wrote an order to hold a patient's Lovenox (enoxaparin) before implantation of a pacemaker and to resume the medication 48 hours after the procedure. However, the MAR did not instruct the nurse to wait 48 hours before restarting the drug, and she gave the patient a dose of Lovenox as soon as he returned to the ICU after the procedure.

Orders to hold a medication without specific instructions on when to resume it should not be allowed. Instead, prescribers should simply discontinue the medication. If a hold order is received, a nurse or pharmacist should ask the prescriber if specific conditions can be added for resuming administration. If not, the drug should be discontinued; the danger here, however, is that discontinued medications simply drop off the pharmacy and nursing profile, and resumption can easily be forgotten. Daily summaries from the pharmacy that list current and recently discontinued medications can help avoid this. Some pharmacy computer systems can generate a daily summary of prescribed therapy for each patient (prepared during the night) that is placed on the patient's chart for physician review. These summaries should include, in a discrete section, a list of medications discontinued within the past 3 to 5 days. Physicians should be required to review the summaries for accuracy of order interpretation. Thus, any inadvertent discontinuation or continuation of a drug can be quickly caught and adjusted. The summaries can also help physicians in reordering therapy after a procedure (or upon discharge). Electronic drug summaries can be used for this purpose if they include discontinued medications and physicians have easy access to them.

Orders to hold a medication until after a procedure should also be disallowed. All medications should be prescribed anew after such a transition in care, and the newly prescribed medications should be reconciled with the previously prescribed medications (as required by the JCAHO NPSG on medication reconciliation). If CPOE is available, it may be possible to place orders from before the procedure in a queue and represcribe them by releasing each individual drug as appropriate. Applicable postprocedure standardized order sets can also help if they contain prompts to remind prescribers to resume particular medications, such as anticoagulants.

In outpatient settings, physicians should establish a method of tracking medications placed on hold, with a tickler system for contacting patients with instructions for resuming the medication. Patients should be told when to expect a call and instructed to contact the physician's office before the end of the day if they are not called.

Medications Listed on Discharge Summaries

Hospital discharge summaries may not provide a reliable medication history. Transcription errors can occur on dictated discharge summaries or transfer forms, and physicians should not depend on these documents alone when prescribing medications for newly admitted patients. Summaries may include misplaced decimal points, misspelled or misheard drug names, misunderstood abbreviations, and wrongly transcribed doses and routes of administration. Summaries or transfer forms may not have been reviewed and corrected, and they may not include complete information about the patient's drug regimen.

In acute care settings, an admitting surgeon may reference the discharge summary from a previous admission and order maintenance medications exactly as listed there. An error occurred because a discharge summary listed Synthroid (levothyroxine) 0.5 mg as the patient's dose when the correct dose was 0.05 mg. The admitting physician prescribed the medication as written on the summary, but a pharmacist detected the error before the drug was dispensed.

The discharge summary may be dictated, transcribed, and sent with a patient to a long-term care or rehabilitation facility before the discharging physician has had an opportunity to review it for accuracy. The admitting physician at the new facility, who may be unfamiliar with the drugs used, may rely on the hospital discharge summary alone when prescribing medications. Furthermore, information in the discharge summary may differ from that in other forms transferred with the patient. Then, drug therapy may be delayed while correct dosages are determined, or prescribers may be unaware of all drugs previously administered to the patient.

Errors can also occur if prescribers misunderstand the way a drug order is communicated by the referring hospital. For example, an order for "methotrexate 10 mg p.o. b.i.d. weekly" appeared on a transferring hospital's pharmacy-generated medication list as "methotrexate 10 mg (4 tablets) p.o. b.i.d. weekly." In the receiving hospital, the admitting physician misunderstood the entry and ordered "methotrexate 40 mg p.o. b.i.d.," believing the reference to four tablets indicated a total dose of 40 mg, not the intended dose of 10 mg from four 2.5 mg tablets. "Weekly" was overlooked and omitted.

When completing institutional discharge summaries or transfer forms, physicians should use current MARs for reference and provide complete information, including doses and dosing schedules, about drug therapy. While dictating summaries, they should take time to spell each drug name and enunciate doses clearly. They should be sure to check the transcription as soon as possible. To promote timely and careful review and correction of discharge summaries, the potential for error should be discussed with the medical records department and at medical staff quality assurance committee meetings.

Physicians who are unfamiliar with a patient's medications should attempt to review as many documents as possible when the patient is admitted. MARs may be more accurate than dictated and transcribed discharge summaries or transfer forms. If necessary, the physician writing admission orders should contact the patient's family physician, internist, or community pharmacy for more information. Patients and family members knowledgeable about the current medications can also help detect errors.

METHODS OF COMMUNICATING ORDERS OR PRESCRIPTIONS

Written Orders and Prescriptions

Legibility

Illegible handwriting on medication orders and prescriptions is a widely recognized cause of errors.[8,30-33] Poorly written orders can delay the administration of medications. They can cause serious errors when the intended drug, dosage, route of administration, or frequency is misunderstood. When personnel must take time to clarify an order, their workflow is interrupted, further increasing the chance of errors.

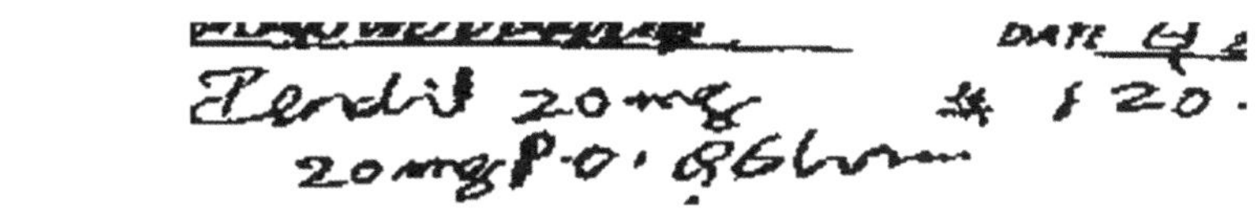

FIGURE 9-4 Prescription for Isordil misread as Plendil.

The prescriber's obligation to provide optimal patient care should in itself be adequate incentive to express all orders clearly. In addition, there are legal requirements that written orders be legible and that the prescriber's name be printed if the signature is not legible.[30] In 90,000 malpractice claims filed over a 7-year period, claims for medication errors related to misinterpreted prescriptions ranked second in prevalence and expense.[34]

A physician, pharmacist, and pharmacy were sued as a result of a death caused by an illegible order. The physician intended to order Isordil (isosorbide dinitrate) 20 mg every 6 hours. His handwriting was illegible, and the pharmacist misread the prescription (Figure 9-4) as Plendil (felodipine), a calcium-channel blocker. The patient suffered a myocardial infarction and died. The plaintiffs maintained that the physician, pharmacist, and pharmacy failed to provide reasonable standards of medical and pharmaceutical care. They noted that the physician wrote poorly and that the purpose of the medication was not indicated on the prescription. The pharmacist was involved because he did not question the illegible prescription or the high dose (the maximum dose of felodipine is 10 mg per day). The pharmacy was named because it failed to incorporate controls that could have prevented the error (for example, the pharmacy computer did not catch the excessive dose).

Prescribers with poor handwriting should fulfill their responsibility for clearly communicating orders and prescriptions by taking time to write or print more carefully.[31] They may need to dictate (and later review) or type their orders. Computers are playing a major role in solving the handwriting problem.[9,11] In addition, prescribers' handwriting may be improved if they are seated while writing.[31] Many institutions, clinics, and physicians' offices set aside areas for order writing and dictation where the prescriber can be seated and isolated from distractions.[8]

An additional step prescribers can take to ensure accurate interpretation of their handwritten orders or prescriptions is speaking to the nurse or pharmacist, as well as the patient, about the medication. Before they leave a patient care unit, prescribers should look over what has been written and be sure their orders have been understood. This is especially helpful if the medication is new to the market or unfamiliar to other health care providers.

Some hospitals are giving physicians courses in basic penmanship, but this may not yield lasting improvement. Handwriting is likely to remain a problem. Little has changed since 1979, when a study showed that it was difficult to interpret about half of all physicians' handwritten orders.[30] In a study at a large teaching hospital, published in 2005, one in three house physicians and medical students who believed their orders were always legible had been asked to clarify them because of poor legibility.[35] Another study[36] showed physicians' penmanship to be no worse than that of nonphysicians; the authors commented that problems with legibility are inherent in average human writing and that a systemic approach to this cause of error is needed. Computerized prescribing will do more to prevent errors than will efforts to improve penmanship.

Preprinted Orders and Standard Order Sets

The use of preprinted orders or order sets can help to standardize communication and reduce the risk of errors. However, if preprinted orders are not carefully designed and checked, they can contribute to errors. For example, a preprinted order form for managing acute pain listed six different analgesics (three injectable and three oral), all with dose ranges (e.g., "morphine 4–10 mg IM q 4 h," "Vicodin 1 tab PO q 4–5 h"). This meant the nurse had to choose the drug, dose, dosage form, route, and frequency of administration. On the form, this list of drugs was preceded by an instruction to "use minimum drug amounts initially in patients less than 120 pounds or over age 65." Errors can easily be made in transcribing such a list of drugs and dosages. Furthermore, drug orders with dose ranges are illegal in most states, and JCAHO prohibits their use.

The list of medications was followed by the statement, "May use any of the above medications unless the patient is allergic." Such statements are not acceptable. Transferring responsibility for allergy checking from the prescriber to others increases liability, including that of the hospital, if a patient receives a known allergen and has a reaction. Furthermore, eliminating redundant checking (i.e., allergy checking by both the prescriber and the nurse) increases the chance that allergies will be missed. In this example, placing the statement about allergies after rather than before the list of drugs made it more likely to be overlooked—and made it less likely that allergy screening would be properly performed.

Health care professionals may feel comfortable using preprinted orders or order sets, knowing that they have been approved by committees of the institution. But institutions need to establish procedures for evaluation and use of preprinted orders and order forms (sidebar, page 191). Safety recommendations for handwritten orders and prescriptions apply equally to preprinted orders and order sets.

Preprinted orders and order sets often include medications to cover every possible scenario. For example, a preprinted form might include orders for several analgesics, a laxative, an antacid, a bedtime sedative, an antidiarrheal, and an antiemetic. Each medication must be transcribed and entered on the MAR. A single analgesic order may require multiple MAR entries if it allows multiple administration routes and doses. The result can be MARs that are too many pages to be safe.

Printed forms providing a list of medications from which the prescriber may choose are not typically recommended; it is too easy to choose the wrong medication, especially when names look alike.[37,38] For example, vincristine has been confused with vinblastine, and carboplatin with cisplatin.

The goal of standardized orders and order sets is not simply to avoid illegible orders, but to reduce variation in how care is provided to patients. Individual physicians or groups should not have their own order sets. Instead, an institution or department's order sets should reflect consensus on the most effective way to manage patients with similar conditions, symptoms, or drug therapy requirements. The variety of medications, routes, and dosages should be minimized. Standard orders or order sets do not have to cover all possible contingencies; those that attempt to do so have been called "Don't bother me!" orders.

During the course of a hospital stay, a patient may have more than one set of standard orders. Unless medications such as bedtime sedatives, laxatives, and antidiarrheals are standardized across all preprinted order forms used in an institution, a patient could have orders for multiple drugs in each class.

Spoken Orders

Spoken ("verbal") orders should be avoided whenever possible. When orders are spoken and then transcribed by another person, errors are likely.[39] The prescriber assumes that the recipient of the order will understand and record it correctly. If a nurse receives and records a spoken order and then telephones it to the pharmacy, the pharmacist must assume that the nurse heard and transcribed the order correctly and is pronouncing it correctly. Thousands of pairs of drug names can easily be misheard. Some pairs of sound-alike drugs have overlapping strengths or dosage ranges, which increases the risk for error. Spoken orders for Celebrex 100 mg have often been misheard as Cerebyx 100 mg, for example.

RECOMMENDATIONS FOR SAFE DESIGN AND USE OF PREPRINTED ORDERS AND ORDER SETS

Involve professionals from all disciplines that may prescribe, dispense, or administer the orders or prescriptions (e.g., physicians, pharmacists, nurses) in the process for developing, reviewing, and approving preprinted order sets.[37,38]

Do not allow drug orders or conditions that are inconsistent with organizational policy. For example, "renew all previous orders" would not be acceptable, nor would a number of refills on a prescription that exceeds the organization's safe threshold.

Use generic drug names. Include the brand name for single-source items.

Avoid coined names and jargon such as "magic mouthwash" and "banana bag," since they can be misunderstood.

Do not include common allergenic medications, if possible. The prescriber can easily overlook the need to strike out an agent to which the patient is allergic. Statements such as "Unless allergic, give…" are not acceptable.

Do not use dangerous abbreviations or dose designations. Each health care provider should have a list of these, including the abbreviations and expressions specified by JCAHO and those identified as error-prone by ISMP (see Chapter 8).

Express doses in metric weight (e.g., 5 mg) rather than number of tablets, milliliters, and so forth, unless the drug is not measured by weight (e.g., milk of magnesia).

List the dosage per square meter or area under the curve for all chemotherapy orders when a calculated dose must be entered. Also include the daily dose and the number of days the drug should be taken for any multiple-day chemotherapy regimen.[37,38]

List the dosage per kilogram for all pediatric orders when a calculated dose must be entered.

Correctly spell drug names, and include proper spacing between drug names and dosages and between dosages and dosing units. For example, the U in 100Units can easily be misread as a zero (1,000 Units).

Specify the reason for each prescribed medication whenever possible.

Enhance readability by using professional quality fonts and print styles.

If multiple medications are listed as possible choices for prescribers, develop a uniform system by which they can indicate orders that should or should not be followed.

Omit lines on back copies of any carbonless order form. The lines can obscure decimal points or portions of a number or name.[37,38]

Include a tracking number and revision date on the form, to ease replacement.[37,38]

Avoid using preprinted order forms or prescriptions sponsored or prepared by pharmaceutical companies; such forms may promote a specific product or may list nonformulary items.

Ensure that blank order forms and prescriptions for use in preparing preprinted orders are accessible only through authorized personnel.

Review all preprinted orders or order sets every 2 to 3 years or when protocols change.[37,38]

A pharmacist received a telephone order from an oncologist to start a patient on what he heard as "thalidomide." He called the oncology pharmacist registered to dispense thalidomide under a restricted distribution program, who in turn called the oncologist to clarify. He learned that on rounds earlier that day, the team had suggested starting the patient on flutamide. Both products may be used to treat prostate cancer. Doses of thalidomide 250 mg may be prescribed daily, and flutamide dosing is typically 250 mg three times daily.

Spoken orders must be enunciated slowly and distinctly. Difficult drug names should be spelled out, and complete and nonambiguous information should be relayed. Only physicians, pharmacists, and nurses should be permitted to dictate and receive spoken prescriptions and orders.[4] The recipient should transcribe the order directly onto the patient's chart as it is being spoken, and then read it back to confirm that it was correctly understood, pronouncing the drug name and dose carefully. (Use of this read-back process is a JCAHO NPSG.) The prescriber should countersign the order as soon as possible, preferably within 24 hours, although a longer period may be necessary in long-term care facilities.[4]

In the mix-up between thalidomide and flutamide described above, read-back might not have been helpful unless the drug name had been spelled, since thalidomide and flutamide sound similar. In any case, spoken orders for cancer chemotherapy should never be accepted.

Not only drug names but dosages can be misunderstood in spoken orders. For example, an ED physician ordered morphine 2 mg IV, but the nurse heard morphine 10 mg IV. The patient suffered respiratory arrest after a 10 mg injection. Another physician called in an order for hydralazine 15 mg to be given IV every 2 hours. Thinking he had said 50 mg, the nurse gave the patient an overdose, leading to tachycardia and a significant drop in blood pressure.

A woman in premature labor had received various tocolytic agents. A perinatologist told the attending physician to order 100 mg of indomethacin, saying the words "two fifty milligrams" (meaning two 50 mg suppositories), if other agents were not effective in suppressing labor. The next day, the attending physician telephoned an order for 250 mg of indomethacin. The nurse hesitated to administer five suppositories. However, in communicating her concerns to the prescriber, she became intimidated and decided to give the medication. The patient was not harmed. Had the perinatologist used the words "one hundred milligrams" instead of "two fifty milligrams," the chance of error would have been less; had the dose been expressed in writing, the error would not have occurred.

An on-call pharmacist received a call during the night from a nurse working on the ventilator unit of a long-term care hospital. The nurse said she had a new order for 50 mEq of potassium phosphate for a "now" dose. The pharmacist questioned the dose, but the nurse said she was sure the physician had ordered that amount. The pharmacist insisted that the nurse verify the dose with the prescriber. The nurse called the prescriber and learned that he had said 15 mEq.

Practitioners reading back a spoken order should confirm the dose by expressing it in single digits (e.g., 5-2-0-0). Numbers in the teens can sound like multiples of 10; in two of the examples above, 15 was heard as 50. The following sidebar provides additional guidelines for reducing errors with spoken orders.

SAFETY RECOMMENDATIONS FOR SPOKEN ORDERS
Organizational Policies and Procedures

❑ Limit spoken orders to true emergencies or circumstances in which the prescriber is physically unable to write or electronically transmit orders (e.g., the prescriber is working in a sterile field).

❑ Limit spoken orders to formulary drugs. The names, uses, and dosages of drugs unfamiliar to staff are more likely to be misheard.

❑ Prohibit spoken orders for selected high-alert medications (e.g., chemotherapy, IV insulin for neonates) because of their complexity and potential for serious errors.

- ❑ To ensure familiarity with hospital guidelines and to enhance the ability to recognize callers and detect instances of fraud, limit the number of personnel who may receive telephone orders.
- ❑ Have a second person listen to the spoken order whenever possible. If the person taking the message is inexperienced, this should be required.
- ❑ Require prescribers to include the milligram per kilogram dosage along with the patient-specific dose for all neonatal and pediatric medication orders.
- ❑ Provide physician offices with appropriate order forms, and require that orders for newly admitted patients be transmitted by fax, pneumatic tube, or electronic means, rather than by telephone.
- ❑ To the extent possible, ensure that laboratory results are available when prescribers are on site, so that necessary dose adjustments need not be made later by telephone.
- ❑ Determine the time frame within which prescribers should validate (sign) spoken orders.

Prescribers and Receivers

- ❑ As an extra check, either the prescriber or receiver should spell unfamiliar drug names, using "T as in Tom," "C as in Charlie," and so forth.
- ❑ Pronounce each digit of a number separately, for example, saying "one six" instead of "sixteen" to avoid confusion with "sixty."

Prescribers

- ❑ Enunciate spoken orders clearly and ask the receiver to read back the order as transcribed directly onto the patient's medical record.
- ❑ To verify patient identification, ask the recipient of a spoken order to read back the patient's name on the order form that was used to transcribe the order.
- ❑ Provide the order recipient with a pager or telephone number for questions that arise.
- ❑ Verify, sign, and date transcriptions of spoken orders within a predetermined time frame.

Receivers

- ❑ Immediately transcribe spoken orders onto the patient's medical record as they are being transmitted. Transcription from a scrap of paper to the chart introduces another opportunity for error.
- ❑ Read the spoken order back to the prescriber for verification. This step is absolutely essential and should become habit even if the receiver is confident that he or she has initially heard the order correctly.
- ❑ Ensure that the spoken order makes sense in the context of the patient's condition.
- ❑ Obtain a telephone number in case it is needed for follow-up questions.
- ❑ Sign, date, record time, and note the spoken order according to procedure.
- ❑ When telephone communication results in the need to prescribe medications or change drug therapy, ask the prescriber to handwrite the orders and fax them to the facility when feasible, instead of communicating them by telephone.
- ❑ Do not accept spoken orders when the prescriber is present and the patient's chart is available.
- ❑ Whenever possible, have unit-based pharmacists receive spoken orders for medications in response to requested clarifications. Provide a mechanism for the unit-based pharmacist to transcribe the orders directly into the medical record.
- ❑ Do not request or dispense medications from the pharmacy unless the order has been transcribed and simultaneously faxed to or otherwise seen by a pharmacist.

Spoken orders may be necessary in emergencies. Despite the need for haste, safety measures such as read-back should be used. As with written and electronic orders, errors are more likely when the dose is expressed in number of tablets, ampuls, or vials, and when a volume but not a concentration is stated. When respiratory depression from meperidine occurred in an elderly patient, a physician ordered "naloxone one-half amp IV stat." The nurse took a 10 mL, 1 mg/mL vial of naloxone from an automated dispensing unit and administered half of the contents, a total dose of 5 mg. The physician had intended half of a 1 mL, 0.4 mg/mL vial, or 0.2 mg.

Another physician ordered "0.1 of flumazenil IV, repeat every 30–60 seconds," to reverse the effect of midazolam in an elderly patient. The nurse administered four doses of flumazenil 0.1 mL, and the patient's status remained unchanged. A second nurse noticed that the first nurse was giving 0.1 mL instead of 0.1 mg (1 mL). When the correct dose was administered, the patient became more alert.

Automated Voice Messages

Voice messaging systems and telephone answering devices are widely used to accept new and renewal orders, especially in community pharmacies. With these devices, interruptions of workflow are fewer, and presumably so are dispensing errors. When the pharmacy is called, the device asks for the patient's name, prescriber's name, and prescription information, but the information cannot be repeated to the prescriber for confirmation.

The safest way for prescribers to communicate telephone orders is to speak directly to pharmacy staff. If this is not possible, the prescription should be faxed to confirm the recorded telephone message, especially for high-alert drugs, or the patient should take the written prescription to the pharmacy when picking up the medication. Mentioning the drug's indication helps avoid misinterpretation. Patients should be told what has been prescribed and why. Patients taking the hard copy prescription to the pharmacy should be instructed to have the pharmacist check it against what was heard in the telephone order. When the medication order is complex or potentially dangerous, telephone orders should be avoided, or patients should be instructed to have the pharmacist call the prescriber. Many prescriptions are now being transferred to pharmacies electronically via the Internet, eliminating the risk of spoken orders.

When support personnel in physicians' offices phone in prescriptions, there is the additional risk that they may misread the prescriber's handwritten orders. Even when speaking directly with support staff, the pharmacist cannot ask clinical questions to learn more about the patient, the indication for use of the drug, and other information needed to detect an error.

Cellular Phones

The chance that telephone orders will be misunderstood is greater when cellular phones are used. Pharmacists surveyed on this topic by ISMP in 2002 reported that poor transmission clarity and failed connections requiring callbacks were common.[40] When follow-up calls were needed for clarification, the pharmacist often did not have the physician's cell phone number. Most respondents said they had had difficulty verifying a physician's identification in a cellular phone call. If prescribers must use cell phones, they should spell the patient's name and drug name and clearly state the dose. Before the call is terminated, the recipient should be given the opportunity to read back the order as it was understood.

Fraudulent Orders

A final concern about telephone orders is the possibility of fraud. In outpatient settings, a layperson may attempt to call in a prescription (often for a controlled substance).

Inpatient settings are also at risk for fraudulent orders. A teenage hospital employee who aspired to be a physician responded to pages intended for on-call surgical residents and ordered medications and procedures for six patients. The teen, a part-time unit secretary, had access to the hospital's computerized paging system and patient records, which enabled him to forward the physicians' pages to his own pager and respond to them. According to newspaper accounts, nurses followed the 16-year-old's orders, which included the administration of heparin, oxygen therapy, and laboratory tests, but no patients were harmed.

Pharmacists and nurses should be suspicious when an unfamiliar practitioner calls in an order for a patient. Minimizing the number of health care providers authorized to accept telephone orders helps ensure that callers are recognized. If the caller is not well known to the person taking the call, the caller's telephone number should be requested and verified in the medical staff directory, and the health care provider should then call the prescriber back for the order. As necessary and appropriate, cell phone numbers should be verified with the physician's office staff or answering service. For additional security, prescribers could be asked to provide an identification number (e.g., medical records dictation number) when issuing telephone orders; however, a list of identification numbers would need to be readily available to health care providers who accept telephone orders.

Electronic Order Transmission

Faxed Orders

To avoid telephone orders, many institutions now use electronic means of communicating orders, including fax (facsimile) transmission. However, faxed orders may not be clearly legible, as in the following example.

A physician ordered a test dose of bleomycin, followed by 8.2 units of bleomycin if no acute reaction was observed. Because the amount of the test dose was not specified, the pharmacist called the nursing unit. After the nurse received the order for the test dose, she faxed it to the pharmacy (Figure 9-5), noting that the original order would follow. The pharmacist prepared to fill the prescription, which would have totaled 13.2 units. Since he found only one vial, containing 15 units, in the refrigerator, he asked the pharmacy buyer to place a stat order. At this point, another pharmacist commented that it was odd that the test dose (believed to be 5 units) should be almost the same size as the therapeutic dose (8.2 units). Further preparation of the doses was halted until the original order was received. The original showed that the physician wanted a test dose of 0.5 units; an extraneous vertical line on the fax transmission had obscured the decimal point.

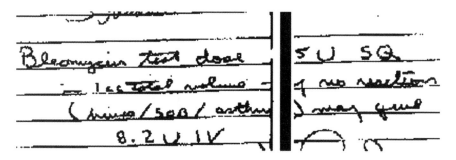

FIGURE 9-5 A vertical streak caused by transmission "noise" prevented accurate reading of this faxed order for bleomycin.

Fax transmission usually works well if order pages are free of printed lines, the handwritten order is written in the center of the writing space, and the pages are free of any debris that could cause distortions on the received image. However, transmission line "noise" can cause streaks and fadeouts on the faxed image. Debris such as dust, paper, correction fluid, hole punches, or stickers (e.g., "sign here") on the fax machine or scanner can cause black lines across every transmission. Information written on the edges of an order form will not be "read" and transmitted. Personnel sending and receiving orders by fax need to be aware of these potential problems. Regular equipment maintenance and platen (roller in a fax machine or glass surface of a scanner) cleaning can help prevent errors.

Ideally, no order faxed to a pharmacy should be filled until the original copy has been received, but this obviates the chief benefit of fax transmission: speed. The best compromise is to review each faxed order carefully. If the copy contains blackened or faded areas, or if there is significant phone line "noise" appearing as small, random black marks or streaks on the paper, the pharmacist should determine whether such marks appear on or near the order; if so, the pharmacy should verify the order before dispensing the drug or wait for the original order to arrive.

Electronic Prescribing

CPOE (see Chapter 15) could prevent many of the problems described in this chapter: poorly handwritten prescriptions, improper terminology, ambiguous orders, and omitted information. Prescribers could see vital information about the patient and drug, such as allergy alerts, overdose warnings, and drug interactions, at the moment of order entry, which would help avoid ADEs.

The vast majority of prescriptions issued in the United States are still handwritten. The use of computers would not only help prescribers clearly communicate medication orders and avoid dosing mistakes; it would also help in preventing serious drug interactions and monitoring and documenting adverse events and therapeutic outcomes.[41]

The authors of the 2006 Institute of Medicine (IOM) report *Preventing Medication Errors*[42] acknowledged that significant regulatory issues and problems with automated alerts still need to be worked out. Nevertheless, the report calls for all health care providers to have plans in place for CPOE by 2008. By 2010, IOM recommends that all prescribers be using electronic prescribing and that all pharmacies be capable of accepting electronic prescriptions.

CPOE has the potential to reduce medication errors by more than 50%,[43] but it can also introduce new sources of errors.[44-46] For example, after one hospital implemented CPOE, medications were prescribed for the wrong patient several times per month. In one case, the prescriber misspelled the patient's last name, thereby accessing the profile of another patient with a similar last name and the same first name. Also, physicians sometimes forgot to close one patient's records before prescribing medications intended for another patient. (Similar problems have occurred in pharmacy order entry.) Systems can be designed to avoid such errors, as described earlier in this chapter.

Errors in CPOE have also involved inadvertent ordering of laboratory tests instead of medications when options on the screen look like drug names. For example, "acetaminophen" may indicate a lab study for an acetaminophen level. Prescribers could see "acetaminophen," select it quickly, and fail to notice that they have not indicated a dose, route, and frequency for the intended medication. Systems would be safer if designed so that screens for drugs and those for laboratory tests cannot be accessed by the same route. Careful selection of nomenclature for pharmacy and lab studies could also reduce the chance of confusion.

Failure mode and effects analysis (Chapter 21) could be used to identify sources of errors introduced by CPOE systems. Chapter 15 discusses CPOE at length.

FORMULARY SYSTEMS

Many prescribers are under the impression that a drug formulary is a cost control mechanism and nothing more. In truth, it is first and foremost a means of ensuring medication safety. When drugs and administration methods are systematically included in (or deleted from) a controlled formulary, there are numerous benefits in addition to cost control. A carefully selected formulary guides clinicians in choosing medications determined to be the safest, most effective agents for treating particular conditions.

Each new drug added through a formulary system undergoes a peer review process that uncovers any safety concerns with the drug, enabling policies and protocols for use of that drug to be implemented prospectively. Examples include restricting the use of a chemotherapy agent to medical oncologists, and determining the maximum dose of a drug that can be safely dispensed. In addition, when drugs are systematically added to the formulary, there is adequate time to educate the staff before a drug is used.

A formulary also ensures that the number and variety of drugs is kept to a minimum so that the staff uses a limited number of drugs, with which they become familiar. When a nonformulary drug is ordered, pharmacists know to provide special instructions and appropriate hazard warnings to all practitioners involved in the medication-use process.

Misconceptions have prevented the full benefits of formularies from being realized. Rucker and Schiff[47] analyzed comments that were made by physicians during pharmacy and therapeutics (P&T) committee meetings and appeared in published sources; many of the comments illustrated misconceptions about the formulary system, rather than debate of the merits of a particular drug. An ISMP survey in 2004[48] indicated that physicians attending P&T committee meetings still had the same misconceptions, and that those "myths" affected formulary decisions. Most respondents had heard comments reflecting the following:

- **The specialist knows best.** Physicians' comments suggested that it was presumptuous for nonsubspecialists to play a role in formulary decisions for specialty drugs. Although specialists are particularly adept at interpreting and presenting data on drugs in their area of interest, a multidisciplinary group can best evaluate clinical efficacy and safety. Furthermore, a thorough formulary review can clearly separate drug prescribing for research purposes from patient therapy.
- **Causal empiricism.** Physicians used personal experiences to support the addition of a new drug to the formulary, at least for a trial period. Although physicians know the importance of scientific studies of a drug's safety and efficacy, they may be swayed by their own favorable experience.
- **Sicker patients need more drugs.** Arguments that more choices need to be available for sicker patients must be supported by evidence. Physicians may argue that strict formulary control can cause life-threatening delays when a nonformulary drug must be obtained, but poor outcomes in emergencies are more often due to failure to follow standard protocols than to the absence of a particular drug.
- **The formulary interferes with clinical freedom.** The tenets of an effective formulary include (1) acknowledgment that each clinician prescribes a very limited subset of available products, (2) recognition that a formulary prepared by a group of experts and peers with adequate resources is more likely than a clinician's personal formulary to provide optimal therapy, and (3) preservation of clinical freedom by providing broad therapeutic decision-making guidance, not interference with prescribing.

■ **Widespread use equals drug of choice.** Widespread use may be more a measure of marketing success than of the relative benefits of a product. Some drugs that have gained rapid acceptance have been prescribed inappropriately or proven to be potentially harmful.

The pharmaceutical industry has helped perpetuate such myths by asserting that formularies inhibit prescribers' knowledge of their products and freedom to use any approved medication. In addition, the role of formularies as a powerful patient safety and quality assurance tool, rather than a restrictive cost-containment strategy, is not emphasized in medical and pharmacy school training; this hinders progress and allows reinforcement of negative biases about formularies.

SAMPLE MEDICATIONS

Medication samples are widely used in hospital outpatient units, clinics, and physician offices. Physicians can provide samples to patients who might have difficulty paying for their medications or getting to an open pharmacy. Samples also enable physicians to see whether a new medication for a patient is effective and well tolerated.

The use of samples can be dangerous, however, for the following reasons:

■ Samples are usually dispensed before computerized safety checking such as screening for drug interactions, duplicate therapy, allergies, contraindications, and dose appropriateness.

■ Samples are often dispensed by physicians without an independent double check by another health care professional.

■ In hospitals, pharmaceutical representatives distribute samples of both formulary drugs and nonformulary agents that may be unfamiliar to staff.

■ Pharmacy oversight of sample procurement, storage, and dispensing is often lacking.

■ Patients may receive no written instructions on how to take a sample medication, or instructions may be on a separate form and not near the medication.

■ Special instructions such as "take on an empty stomach" are not provided as they would be with a prescription filled at a pharmacy.

■ The packaging of samples can be confusing. For example, each sample box of Protonix (pantoprazole) 40 mg is labeled as such, but inside the box is a card holding two tablets, which is also labeled as Protonix 40 mg. Patients instructed to take 40 mg daily have taken both tablets on the card, thinking the two tablets together equaled 40 mg, when each tablet contains 40 mg.

■ Samples may be overlooked in drug recalls, and expiration dates may not be checked.

■ Unsecured storage of samples allows unauthorized access to prescription and nonprescription drugs. According to a survey published in *JAMA*,[49] office staff frequently take samples for personal use.

Safe management of drug samples is difficult, especially in large teaching hospitals. Samples manage to find their way into facilities where they are prohibited. Pharmacists often have little control over their distribution and use; the entire process is influenced by the pharmaceutical industry and reimbursement concerns. Nevertheless, some practice sites have achieved safer use of samples when the following conditions are met:

1. Pharmacy maintains oversight of pharmaceutical representatives' visits by scheduling all appointments hospitalwide. Drug company representatives are instructed on the rules governing samples and required to sign an agreement to abide by them. If another department, such as materials management, schedules appointments, it must routinely send pharmacy a list of the areas representatives have visited.
2. Only samples of medications currently on the formulary are accepted.
3. The pharmacy stores samples and provides physicians with internal vouchers to prescribe from sample supplies, at no cost to the patient.
4. Samples that must remain in patient care areas or physician offices are stored in locked cabinets away from traffic.
5. As samples are received, staff enter each into a logbook, listing the drug name and expiration date. The patient's name and medical record number are entered in the logbook when samples are dispensed.
6. The physician writes an order in the medical record when samples are administered or sent home with a patient. A copy of the order is sent to the pharmacy for screening. Administration of samples is documented in the patient's medical record.
7. Pharmacy staff periodically visit patient care units and offices to ensure secure storage, check expiration dates, implement safety measures, and educate practitioners about the danger involved in using samples without pharmacy oversight and clinical order screening.
8. Physicians in office practices consult a local pharmacist about establishing safety measures such as keeping a logbook, monitoring drug storage and expiration dates, and providing staff with pertinent drug information.
9. When samples are dispensed, patients are educated about the drug and its potential adverse effects. Explicit written instructions are given on how much should be taken for each dose (since several doses may be packaged together and appear as a single dose). Patients are advised to keep the instructions with the sample. (Some offices and practice sites affix to the sample container stickers on which the directions are printed.) Patients are told how long they should take the sample medication and what to do when the samples run out. They are reminded to tell the pharmacy where they fill prescriptions about all sample use.
10. Patients are reminded to keep sample medications away from children. (Samples do not come in child-resistant packages.)

If it does not seem feasible to follow all these practices, they can be tried and fine tuned, a few at a time, before widespread implementation. In the end, it will be up to the pharmaceutical industry to recognize the risk that samples present to patients and take steps to improve safety.

RESOLVING CONFLICTS IN DRUG THERAPY

Communicating Conflicts

Poor communication can hinder the discovery of medication errors. A health care practitioner's persistence in communicating recognized problems, even when met with opposition from experts, can prevent errors from reaching patients.

This happened when one attending physician ordered pegaspargase (Oncospar) for a patient with acute lymphoblastic leukemia.[50] Pegaspargase is used solely for patients who have developed hypersensitivity to asparaginase (Elspar), as this patient had. The preferred administration route for pegaspargase is IM; the IV route increases the likelihood of cross-reactivity in asparaginase-sensitive patients and of liver toxicity, coagulopathy, and GI and renal disease.

Before pegaspargase was marketed, a protocol was used to desensitize patients to asparaginase by rapidly administering the drug IV, beginning with one unit and doubling the dose every 10 minutes until the total accumulated dose is equal to the planned daily dose. This physician ordered pegaspargase IV with a dosing schedule similar to that for the asparaginase desensitization regimen, rather than as the single IM dose indicated for pegaspargase. The pharmacist called the attending physician, who was reluctant to change the order; he had reviewed it with the director of the protocol under which pegaspargase was being used. Further questioning by the pharmacist revealed that the protocol director was unaware of the risks of administering pegaspargase IV and had never before prescribed it using a desensitization regimen. Eventually, all agreed that the drug should be administered as a single IM dose.

In this case, an experienced pharmacist was able to resolve the issue by being persistent and trusting his own expertise to augment the expertise of others. Many practitioners, particularly early in their careers, would not have challenged seemingly unimpeachable sources such as a protocol director or oncologist.

Another pharmacist received an order for topotecan 0.75 mg to be given subcutaneously. The topotecan (Hycamtin) labeling calls for the drug to be given as an IV infusion, and infiltration has caused local reactions such as erythema and bruising. The pharmacist checked with the prescriber, who said he had copied the order for topotecan from a protocol sent to him by an oncologist at a well-known university cancer center. Not satisfied, the pharmacist telephoned the university hospital oncologist who developed the protocol and asked him to fax the original. The protocol listed the dose per square meter ("topotecan 0.75 mg/sq m"), and the prescriber had misread "sq" to mean subcutaneously.

Pharmacists and nurses should not be afraid to question orders when they have reason to believe that a patient is at risk, or even when they just have a sense that something is wrong. Statements such as "the protocol says to do it this way" or "that's the way they do it at University Hospital" should never be taken as the final word when the safety of an order is being investigated. Timothy Lesar, of Albany (New York) Medical Center, has listed statements used as evidence that practitioners should carry out a questionable order, such as "A specialist prescribed it," "The patient has been 'titrated up to that dose,'" and "The drug [or dose] is 'from a published study.'"[50] These statements should be considered "red flags" that the order should be more fully investigated. When in doubt about their expertise in pursuing a questionable order, practitioners should ask themselves which would be worse: to be wrong, or to allow injury to a patient.

Conflict Resolution Guidelines

All health professionals involved in the medication-use system have an obligation to protect patients from harm. Conflicting opinions about patient care should be handled objectively and professionally. Guidelines for handling conflicts concerning drug therapy orders are discussed in the following paragraphs.[16]

If a nurse or pharmacist suspects that an order is potentially harmful, he or she should pursue the matter until satisfied that the therapy is safe for the patient or until the order is changed. The nurse may contact a pharmacist to help research the issue before contacting the ordering physician so that concerns and factual information can be clearly communicated. The pharmacist or nurse can review the medical record, talk with the patient, use reputable drug information resources, consult other pharmacists or physicians, or discuss the order directly with the prescriber. The pharmacist or nurse can ask the prescriber for documentation (e.g., protocols, journal articles) supporting the safety of the order and read the material carefully. Often the prescriber has misinterpreted published information or used references that contain misprints or ambiguous statements.

If the prescriber will not change the order and the pharmacist or nurse is not satisfied that the patient will not be harmed, the prescriber's chief resident, chief attending physician, department chair, or a specialist in the area of the ordered drug therapy should be contacted. If that person also believes the order may be unsafe, he or she should contact the ordering physician.

If concerns persist despite these efforts, the nurse or pharmacist should consider whether greater harm would result from administering the drug than from withholding it. Clinicians should refuse to administer or dispense a drug if they are reasonably sure that withholding it is the safest action. The issue should then be referred to an ad hoc group for peer review to determine the order's safety.

When concern about safety persists, the ordering physician should not be asked, nor allowed, to personally give the drug. Transferring responsibility to the physician for possible patient harm is not likely to legally or emotionally absolve the pharmacist or the nurse if the patient is injured. The pharmacist or nurse should be sure to document his or her actions objectively on a standard incident report.

Intimidation

Serious medication errors have often involved a drug order that at least one practitioner believed to be unsafe. Disruptive behavior or intimidation by the prescriber may have kept the practitioner from questioning the order. Of some 2,000 health care professionals, including more than 1,500 nurses and 350 pharmacists, responding to a November 2003 ISMP survey about intimidating behavior,[51,52] 7% said they had been involved in a medication error during the past year in which intimidation played a role. The intimidating behavior ranged from subtle questioning of judgment to more explicit threatening behavior. Nearly one-fourth of the respondents said they often encountered condescending language or tone of voice, and about 20% said they sensed impatience when questions were asked. Almost half of the respondents reported being the recipients of strong verbal abuse or threatening body language at least once during the past year.

Almost half of all respondents said such intimidation had altered the way they handle questions about or clarification of medication orders. Forty percent of the respondents said they had had concerns about the safety of an order in the past year but assumed that it was correct rather than interact with an intimidating prescriber. Almost half of the respondents said that when they did question the prescriber, they had felt pressured into dispensing or administering the medication despite their concerns.

Two-thirds of the respondents said a prescriber had, at least once in the past year, responded, "Just give what I ordered," when faced with a question. Although other health care providers exhibited intimidating behaviors, prescribers did so most often.

ISMP recommends that health care organizations create a code of conduct that encourages behaviors supportive of team cohesion, staff morale and sense of self-worth, and safety. Also recommended is a survey of staff attitudes about intimidation, to ascertain whether staff feel valued in the organization, how they handle stress and intimidation, how they treat others at work, and secret rules they share with new employees about how to interact with (or avoid) certain staff members. The resultant dialogue can lead to the development of more effective and respectful ways of interacting.

Health care providers should be assertive when conveying important information. For example, staff members can use the first names of colleagues, including physicians, when it is necessary to get their attention. This can help break down artificial barriers to effective communication. The problem, its rationale, and a potential solution should be clearly communicated, as described in Chapter 23. Furthermore, organizations should enforce a zero tolerance policy for intimidation, regardless of the offender's standing. Overcoming intimidation and reducing intimidating behavior will be a long process that requires the commitment of the entire staff and administration, as well as personal reflection on how each member of the health care team treats his or her colleagues.

CONCLUSION

Medication errors related to prescribing are common. Prescribers must take steps to prevent errors, but all practitioners involved in the medication-use process have a role in detecting and correcting errors in the prescribing phase.

REFERENCES

1. Bates DW, Boyle DL, Vander Vliet MB, et al. Relationship between medication errors and adverse drug events. *J Gen Intern Med.* 1995;10(4):199–205.
2. Lesar TS, Briceland L, Stein DS. Factors related to errors in medication prescribing. *JAMA.* 1997; 277: 312–17.
3. Bobb A, Gleason K, Husch M, et al. The epidemiology of prescribing errors: the potential impact of computerized prescriber order entry. *Arch Intern Med.* 2004;164:785–92.
4. American Society of Hospital Pharmacists. ASHP guidelines on preventing medication errors in hospitals. *Am J Hosp Pharm.* 1993;50:305–14.
5. National Coordinating Council for Medication Error Reporting and Prevention. Recommendations to Enhance Accuracy of Prescription Writing. Available at: www.nccmerp.org/council/council1996-09-04.html.
6. Rappaport HM. Consistency in prescription writing [letter]. *Ann Intern Med.* 1992;117:1059.
7. Moore TJ, Walsh WS, Cohen MR. Reported adverse event cases of methemoglobinemia associated with benzocaine products. *Arch Intern Med.* 2004;164:1192–6.
8. Vitillo JA, Lesar TS. Preventing medication prescribing errors. *Ann Pharmacother.* 1991;25:1388–94.
9. Institute for Safe Medication Practices. How are you preventing acetaminophen overdoses? *ISMP Medication Safety Alert!* August 8, 2003.
10. Cohen MR, Davis NM. Drug name suffixes can cause confusion. *Am Pharm.* 1992;NS32:301–2.
11. Cohen MR. Medication error reports. Naming drug products is serious business. *Hosp Pharm.* 1990;25: 747–8.
12. US Metric Association. Confusion over measurement units may be hazardous to America's health. *Metric Today.* 2005(May-June):2,4.
13. Davis NM, Cohen MR. More look-alike and sound-alike errors. *Am Pharm.* 1993;NS33(10):32.
14. Davis NM, Cohen MR. Purpose of medication will reduce errors. *Am Pharm.* 1992;NS32:878–9.
15. Institute for Safe Medication Practices. A novel way to prevent medication errors. *ISMP Medication Safety Alert!* Warminster, Pa: Institute for Safe Medication Practices; 1997.
16. Davis NM, Cohen, MR. *Medication Errors: Causes and Prevention.* Huntingdon Valley, Pa: Davis Associates; 1981.
17. Cohen MR, Davis NM. Avoid dangerous Rx abbreviations. *Am Pharm.* 1992;NS32:112–3.
18. Jones EH, Speerhas R. How physicians can prevent medication errors: practical strategies. *Cleve Clin J Med.* 1997;64:355–9.
19. Cohen MR, Davis NM. Expressing strengths, doses, and drug names properly. *Am Pharm.* 1992;NS32:216–7.
20. Cohen MR, Davis NM. The health sciences need a controlled vocabulary. *Am Pharm.* 1993;NS33(9):24.
21. United States Pharmacopeial Convention. Move to metric: apothecary system no longer recognized by USP. *Drug Product Quality Review No. 37.* 1993;1–2.
22. Cohen MR, Davis NM. Who needs the apothecary system? *Am Pharm.* 1992;NS32:482–4.
23. Hoffman RS, Smilkstein MJ, Rubenstein F. An "amp" by any other name: the hazards of intravenous magnesium dosing [letter]. *JAMA.* 1989;261:557.
24. Ward C. Medication errors: what's a dose? *Pharm-Fax of Fairfax Hospital.* 1989;5:19, 24.
25. Perlstein PH, Callison C, White M, et al. Errors in drug computations during newborn intensive care. *Am J Dis Child.* 1979;133:376–7.
26. Institute for Safe Medication Practices. Preventing death by decimal. *ISMP Medication Safety Alert!* July 31, 1996.

27. Rieder MJ, Goldstein D, Zinman H, et al. Tenfold errors in drug dosage [letter]. *Can Med Assoc J.* 1988;139:12–3.

28. Lesar TS. Errors in the use of medication dosage regimens. *Arch Pediatr Adolesc Med.* 1988;152:340–4.

29. Institute for Healthcare Improvement. Reconcile medications at all transition points. Available at: www.ihi. org/IHI/Topics/PatientSafety/MedicationSystems/Changes/Reconcile+Medications+at+All+Transition+ Points.htm.

30. A study of physicians' handwriting as a time waster. *JAMA.* 1979;242:2429–30.

31. Feldman H. Analyzing the cost of illegible handwriting. *Hospitals.* 1963;37:71, 74, 77, 80.

32. Brodell RT, Helms SE, KrishnaRao I, et al. Prescription errors: legibility and drug name confusion. *Arch Fam Med.* 1997;6:296–8.

33. Long KJ. The need for obligatory printing in medical records [letter]. *Hosp Pharm.* 1991;26:924.

34. Cabral JD. Poor physician penmanship. *JAMA.* 1997;278:1116–7.

35. Garbutt JM, Highstein G, Jeffe DB, et al. Safe medication prescribing: training and experience of medical students and housestaff at a large teaching hospital. *Acad Med.* 2005;80:594–9.

36. Berwick DM, Winickoff DE. The truth about doctor's handwriting: a prospective study. *BMJ.* 1996;313:1657–8.

37. Institute for Safe Medication Practices. Designing preprinted order forms that prevent medication errors. *ISMP Medication Safety Alert!* April 23, 1997.

38. Cohen MR, Davis NM. Developing safe and effective preprinted physicians' order forms. *Hosp Pharm.* 1992;27:508, 513, 528.

39. Fijn R, Van den Bemt PM, Chow M, et al. Hospital prescribing errors: epidemiological assessment of predictors. *Br J Clin Pharmacol.* 2002;53:326–31.

40. Institute for Safe Medication Practices. Don't have a bad "air" day. *ISMP Medication Safety Alert!* July 24, 2002;7(15):1.

41. Schiff GD, Rucker TD. Computerized prescribing: building the electronic infrastructure for better medication usage. *JAMA.* 1998;279:1024–9.

42. Committee on Identifying and Preventing Medication Errors; Aspden P, Wolcott J, Bootman JL, et al., eds. *Preventing Medication Errors.* Washington, DC: National Academies Press; 2006. Prepublication copy available at http://darwin.nap.edu/books/0309101476/html/R2.html. Accessed July 21, 2006.

43. Bates DW, Leape LL, Cullen DJ, et al. Effect of computerized physician order entry and a team intervention on prevention of serious medication errors. *JAMA.* 1998;280:1311–6.

44. Koppel R, Metlay JP, Cohen A, et al. Role of computerized physician order entry systems in facilitating medication errors. *JAMA.* 2005;293:1197–203.

45. Nebeker JR, Hoffman JM, Weir CR, et al. High rates of adverse drug events in a highly computerized hospital. *Arch Intern Med.* 2005;165:1111–6.

46. Han YY, Carcillo JA, Venkataraman ST, et al. Unexpected increased mortality after implementation of a commercially sold computerized physician order entry system. *Pediatrics.* 2005;116:1506–12.

47. Rucker TD, Schiff G. Drug formularies: myths-in-formation. *Med Care.* 1990;28:928–42.

48. Institute for Safe Medication Practices. The truth about hospital formularies. *ISMP Medication Safety Alert!* February 10, 2005. Available at: www.ismp.org/Newsletters/acutecare/articles/20050210.asp.

49. Westfall JM, McCabe J, Nicholas RA, et al. Personal use of drug samples by physicians and office staff. *JAMA.* 1997;278:141–3.

50. Institute for Safe Medication Practices. "Magic words" or "red flags"? *ISMP Medication Safety Alert!* February 24, 1999. Available at: www.ismp.org/Newsletters/acutecare/articles/19990224_2.asp.

51. Institute for Safe Medication Practices. Intimidation: practitioners speak up about this unresolved problem (part 1). *ISMP Medication Safety Alert!* March 11, 2004;9(5):1–3.

52. Institute for Safe Medication Practices. Intimidation: mapping a plan for cultural change in healthcare (part 2). *ISMP Medication Safety Alert!* March 24, 2004;9(6):1–3.

CHAPTER 10

PREVENTING DISPENSING ERRORS

Michael R. Cohen and Judy L. Smetzer

Pharmacies are responsible for dispensing medications accurately. Flynn and colleagues[1] have observed 98.3% accuracy in dispensing. However, if 1.7% of medications are dispensed inaccurately, that translates to four errors per day per 250 prescriptions, or 51.5 million errors in the 3 billion medications dispensed each year in the United States. Pharmacists must follow policies and procedures that prevent dispensing errors and ensure that drugs are distributed safely to patients. To improve accuracy, they must change their thinking about the causes of errors,[2] from finding fault with individuals to identifying system failures and updating practices to reflect new knowledge about the sources of error.

In this chapter, the term dispensing errors refers to medication errors linked to the pharmacy or to whichever health care professional dispenses the medication. Most dispensing errors are errors of commission (e.g., miscalculating a dose, or dispensing the incorrect medication, dosage strength, or dosage form), but some are errors of omission (e.g., failure to dispense a drug appropriately, counsel the patient, or screen for interactions and contraindications). Errors of omission may be less evident; failure to counsel the patient about a new prescription, for example, may not draw attention unless a serious error occurs. This chapter discusses causes and prevention of both types of dispensing errors. It also describes the role of pharmacists' clinical services in error prevention.

Pharmacy employers and supervisors can help ensure accurate dispensing by hiring well-trained staff, screening new employees for knowledge of error prevention methods, and providing continuing-education opportunities and access to professional publications. But they must take additional steps, such as those listed on page 206[3] and discussed in this chapter. Factors in the work environment can promote or detract from safe dispensing, as described in the first section of the chapter. Appropriate dispensing depends on clear and accurate information about the patient and the drug, as discussed in the next major section. The importance of patient counseling as part of the dispensing process is also discussed.

ERRORS RELATED TO THE WORK ENVIRONMENT

Many characteristics of the workplace can affect dispensing accuracy, including hours and workload, distractions, and product storage and labeling.

Need for 24-Hour Service in Hospitals

In hospitals, 24-hour pharmacy service is highly desirable. Patients are at risk when non-pharmacists have complete access to a pharmacy after hours. With current technology, planning, and cooperation from medical and nursing staff, night access to the pharmacy

STEPS FOR ENSURING ACCURATE DISPENSING[3]

1. Lock up or sequester drugs that could cause disastrous errors.
2. Develop and implement meticulous procedures for drug storage.
3. Reduce distractions, design a safe dispensing environment, and maintain optimum workflow.
4. Use reminders such as labels and computer notes to prevent mix-ups involving look-alike and sound-alike drug names.
5. Keep the original prescription order, label, and medication container together throughout the dispensing process.
6. Compare the contents of the medication container with the information on the prescription.
7. Enter the drug's identification code (e.g. National Drug Code [NDC] number) into the computer and on the prescription label.
8. Perform a final check on the prescription, the prescription label, and the manufacturer's container. When possible, use automation, such as bar coding.
9. Perform a final check on the contents of prescription containers.
10. Provide patient counseling.

can be eliminated, even in rural hospitals. Health systems may centralize night pharmacy operations at one location. Some companies provide order review via computer and video link or telephone; an example is Cardinal Health's Rx e-source service. Such a service can be used during periods of peak demand as well as when the hospital pharmacy is closed.

In the absence of 24-hour pharmacy service, a limited supply of medications should be accessible in a location outside the pharmacy for authorized nonpharmacists to use in initiating urgent orders. A pharmacist should be on call around the clock for questions and emergencies. The list of medications available after hours and policies and procedures governing their use, including a provision for outsourcing subsequent pharmacist review, should be developed by the pharmacy and therapeutics committee. The available items should be selected with safety in mind; the number, types, quantities, dosage forms, and container sizes should be limited.

Pharmacy departments that do provide 24-hour service must select and schedule the evening and night shift pharmacists and support staff carefully to ensure quality care during off-peak, potentially error-prone hours. Too often, staffing is thin during evening and night hours, and redundant checking systems are not fully operational. When possible, critical tasks such as the preparation of total parenteral nutrition (TPN) and cancer chemotherapy should be saved for daytime hours when staffing is typically greater.

Workload

Pharmacists in community, institutional, and mail-service practice regard work overload as the main cause of dispensing errors. The increasing prescription volume and continuing shortage of pharmacists make it difficult for departments and companies to maintain adequate staffing to ensure safe practice.[4] Factors straining the pharmacist workforce include the profession's move to the Doctor of Pharmacy (PharmD) as the entry-level degree, expansion of pharmacists' role to include disease management and in-depth patient counseling, changing workforce demographics, and increased opportunities for pharmacists to work in nontraditional, nondispensing roles. Researchers have noted that the transition to all-PharmD education has decreased not only the number of graduating pharmacists but also the pool of new entrants into the dispensing pharmacist workforce, because of PharmD programs' focus on preparing students for further education, residencies, and research.[4]

Easing the dispensing overload will require not only sufficient personnel but the elimination of quotas or time limits on dispensing. Explicit or tacit quotas for dispensing put pharmacists under stress and increase the risk of error. Demands to dispense a certain number of prescriptions per shift are put in place by misguided supervisors or companies that value productivity over accuracy. Although productivity must be maintained, pharmacies need to acknowledge that the speed at which pharmacists can safely work varies among individuals.

One state pharmacy association has served notice that pharmacists shall not dispense, and permit holders shall not allow a pharmacist to dispense, prescription drugs at such a rate per hour or per day as to pose a danger to the public health or safety; the statement mentions a threshold of 150 prescriptions per pharmacist per day.[5] This threshold may not take into account the increased level of safety that effective technician support can provide. Although limits on pharmacist work hours or prescription quotas have not been accepted professionwide, state boards of pharmacy and courts of law have disciplined employers for errors linked to unreasonable workloads.[6]

Regular rest breaks and meal breaks of at least one half-hour every day improve performance and the ability to organize workflow efficiently and safely. Pharmacists who perceive that break times are available and adequate have been shown to make fewer errors and detect more errors during self-monitoring than those who perceive that breaks are not an option.[6]

Clearly, pushing people past their limits for safe practice can lead to errors, but periods of low workload can also have a detrimental effect on accuracy. In a study of 36 community pharmacists, errors were more likely when the dispensing workload was low.[7] To measure their "task tension," the pharmacists were asked about the mental, physical, and temporal demands of the task; concerns about performing well; and the amount of effort and frustration on the job. Task tension was higher when prescription volume increased, but errors were more likely when prescription volume and task tension were low. Workload did not affect the pharmacists' concern about performance or their motivation to do well.

Boredom and disruptions in personal work rhythms (e.g., during a switch from high to low prescription volume) make it hard to focus on tasks. A brief warm-up period before restarting a task may help; pharmacists may need time to refocus on work, mentally rehearse what needs to be done, or work initially on noncritical task components. Pharmacies should prioritize and organize workflow to minimize fluctuations.

The use of pharmacy computer systems, bar code scanning of product labels for inventory replacement, robotic dispensing, and other forms of automation can enhance both workflow and the safety of dispensing. For example, a mail-service pharmacy claims that the use of sophisticated technology enables it to achieve a "six sigma" level of dispensing accuracy (a 99.9997% error-free rate), despite a prescription volume far exceeding that in hospital and community pharmacies.[8] This reflects the accuracy of dispensing *after* prescriptions have been transcribed correctly, verified, and approved, however.

Work Area and Workflow

A poorly designed work area can contribute to dispensing errors. A well-designed work area has proper lighting, adequate counter space, and comfortable temperature and humidity. It facilitates a smooth flow from one task to the next throughout the dispensing process. It is removed from areas of heavy traffic. The work area should be kept free of clutter; for example, containers no longer in use should be returned to the proper storage area or discarded. Telephones should be located where they are close enough for convenience without being a source of distraction or inefficiency. Working on one order or prescription at a time can prevent errors; pharmacists should fill one container at a time to avoid switching containers and ensure that the correct label is affixed.[9]

Distractions

For safe dispensing, pharmacy personnel need to focus on the task without interruption. Distractions are a major cause of error, and pharmacies could take a cue from the airline industry in preventing them. Federal regulations prohibit potentially distracting activities during the flight crew's performance of duties critical to the safe operation of an aircraft.[10] Activities specifically prohibited during a critical phase of flight (defined as taxi, takeoff and landing, and all other phases except cruise flight) include making calls to order supplies or confirm passenger connections, eating meals, and engaging in nonessential conversations.

It is unfortunate that no such prohibitions are in place to prevent distraction of health care practitioners during critical duties such as taking a patient's history, reviewing and assessing a prescription, consulting the prescriber for clarification, entering data in the computer, reviewing the patient profile, assessing computer alerts, selecting the proper medication (both in the computer and from the shelf), verifying the product expiration date, counting or measuring the medication, affixing the label, double-checking the prescription, returning the stock container to its proper location, and counseling the patient. Often, technicians are interrupted while returning medications to stock, and pharmacists are distracted by phone calls or questions while entering orders into the computer—or even while preparing or checking chemotherapy.

Critical work processes must be designed to reduce interruptions and distractions. For example, a community pharmacy could receive orders by fax. A telephone answering machine could be equipped with software that automates routine refill requests. Support personnel can answer the telephone if they are trained to know which calls to refer to the pharmacist.[3]

Cognitive and Social Factors

Although it is widely recognized that well-designed systems and technology offer the best chance of preventing errors, steps can also be taken to enhance staff members' performance. Grasha[6] suggested interventions that enhance memory and sensory input. Among his findings:

- Errors were reduced by 16% when pharmacists used a high-intensity task light and magnification lens to read prescriptions.
- Errors were reduced by 24% after a device was installed to hold prescriptions on the computer monitor, closer to eye level, during order entry.
- Posting alerts in strategic locations reduced errors with 30 error-prone products by 71% and potentially significant occurrences with these products by 45%. Heightened awareness as a result of these alerts also reduced errors with non-targeted drugs by 56%.
- Errors were reduced by 35% when sleeves with exaggerated, unconventional type fonts were affixed to products to enhance reading of sections of drug names and doses.

In Grasha's research, 12% of pharmacists had difficulty with details and focus, and they accounted for 33% of all the mistakes observed. These pharmacists in particular benefited from the use of high-intensity lights, copyholders, and exaggerated product labels.

Grasha also studied the roles that organizational dynamics (e.g., supervisory practices) and personal qualities (e.g., demeanor, patience, ability to manage stress, interpersonal relationships) play in performance. Pharmacists who had adequate coping skills and training in stress management made fewer errors. Pharmacists who made fewer errors had supervisors who fostered appropriate autonomy and were perceived as being democratic, facilitative, and helpful in goal setting. Pharmacists who made more errors had supervisors who were perceived as overly autocratic and punitive. Supportive supervisors who interacted well with their staff lowered stress levels and allowed staff to better focus on tasks at hand.

Pharmacists who received constructive feedback about errors from the research team and who established goals to enhance error detection were able to improve their ability to prevent errors by 103%. The pharmacists had been asked to set a goal of either improving their ability to detect mistakes or maintaining their current performance; even those who chose the latter goal increased their error detection by 22% compared with a control group that received no feedback. The pharmacists in this study benefited from receiving constructive feedback about errors and establishing personal improvement goals rather than comparing their performance with that of others.

Interventions such as Grasha's are applicable beyond pharmacy, although differences among facilities, processes, and individuals affect their success. Grasha believed that understanding how people react to systems and integrate them into their mental structures would reveal new ways of enhancing workflow, physical work spaces, sensory input, and memory; identify new applications for technology; and improve training for supervision, conflict resolution, and stress management. The long-term outcomes could be increased professional satisfaction and workforce retention, enhanced efficiency and productivity, and improved patient care and safety.

Storage

When medication storage areas are crowded, products are more likely to be interchanged or returned to an incorrect location. Adequate space should be allotted for each medication and each strength. All prescription bottles should be stored with the label facing forward. A separate area should be assigned for medications administered by each route, and some pharmacies prefer to separate oral liquids from other oral medications. Agents meant for external use, including chemicals and other nondrug substances, should never be stored with medications meant for internal use; look-alike containers have led to mix-ups of such products and resultant toxicity.

Auxiliary labels indicating the route of administration should be available in the individual storage areas for further differentiating products when a prescription is dispensed. For example, parents have instilled amoxicillin oral suspension prescribed for an ear infection into a child's ear rather than giving it by mouth; an auxiliary label reading "For Oral Use Only" would help prevent this error.

In most pharmacies, medications are stored on shelves or in bins, cabinets, or drawers that have external storage labels identifying the specific medications. These labels helps pharmacy staff locate medications for dispensing, but they may contribute to errors if a staff member reads the label and assumes that it accurately reflects the contents of the bin, cabinet, drawer, or shelf. If medications in similar packaging have been placed in the wrong storage area, staff who rely on the storage bin label for identification can select the wrong drug. Even if the storage bin label is used only to initially locate the product, confirmation bias can cause a person reading the actual product label to fail to recognize selection of the wrong drug. The use of bar code readers reduces the risk of selecting the wrong product.

In inpatient settings where a small number of medications are stored on patient care units, the drugs may be organized in bins with separators. The bins should be labeled with just the first letter of the drug name (or a range of letters, such as a through f); this forces staff to read the product label. Single compartments should never contain more than one product.

Container size and shape may not reliably differentiate medications that look alike or have similar names.[11] Rotating the placement of fast-moving medications can help staff avoid the habit of "reaching and grabbing" for products according to their usual position on the shelf. In another approach, called "prescription mapping," products are stored according to prescription volume, with the most frequently used products stored close to the center of fill stations to minimize staff travel time.[12] This storage arrangement is likely to separate different doses of the same product, and it can reduce the potential for errors involving look-alike products or names. Pharmacy computer software often has prescription-mapping features. Even without such software capability, organizations can use prescription mapping to separate look-alike and sound-alike products. It may be beneficial to separate frequently confused pairs (such as thiamine 100 mg and thioridazine 100 mg tablets) or strengths of drugs, especially medications available in strengths that vary by a factor of 10, such as 2.5 mg and 25 mg Compazine suppositories.[13]

High-alert medications, which include oral warfarin, oral methotrexate for nononcologic indications, heparin, insulin, and narcotics and opioids (Chapter 14), should be specially marked and placed in an isolated or locked storage area. If this is not possible, auxiliary labels can be used to warn the dispenser to take extra precautions.

Drug inventories should be inspected at least quarterly, and outdated products should be removed from storage areas. Keeping track of outdated items in the pharmacy can be a challenge. Even more difficult is tracking the expiration dates on manufacturers' samples used in ambulatory care areas; often, the expiration dates are not clearly marked, items are short dated when received from suppliers, and no specific individual is responsible for inspecting the products. To improve tracking and removal of outdated drugs, a list of dates for inspecting each area where medications (including samples) are stored and the individuals responsible for each area should be posted.

Dangerous chemicals, such as glacial acetic acid[14] (page 211), should not be stored anywhere in the pharmacy, including the compounding area. Unneeded chemicals should be discarded immediately, particularly those that have not been used in the past 6 to 12 months. If bulk chemicals must remain in stock, they should be stored in a locked, sequestered section of the pharmacy. If such substances are required for compounding, they can be obtained at the time they are needed.

Standard containers used for oral medications should never be used to store substances not meant for systemic use. Departments and individuals should not be allowed to requisition empty prescription containers or blank pharmacy labels; the pharmacy would not be able to control what was stored in those containers or written on the labels. A substance not intended or safe for ingestion could be taken accidentally.

Nomenclature and Packaging

As described in Chapter 6, medications with similar names can easily be mistaken for one another. For example, the Institute for Safe Medication Practices (ISMP) has warned practitioners about confusing Avandia (used in diabetes) and Coumadin (an anticoagulant) on handwritten orders. Both products are available as 4 mg oral tablets. One technician misread an order for Avandia 4 mg (Figure 10-1) and entered Coumadin 4 mg into the computer. A nurse, and a pharmacist who had just dispensed Coumadin for three other patients, reviewed the order and saw it as Coumadin. The pharmacist knew of Avandia, but it had not been considered for the formulary; neither the nurse nor the technician had heard of this drug. The patient received one dose before the physician detected the error while reviewing the medication administration record (MAR).

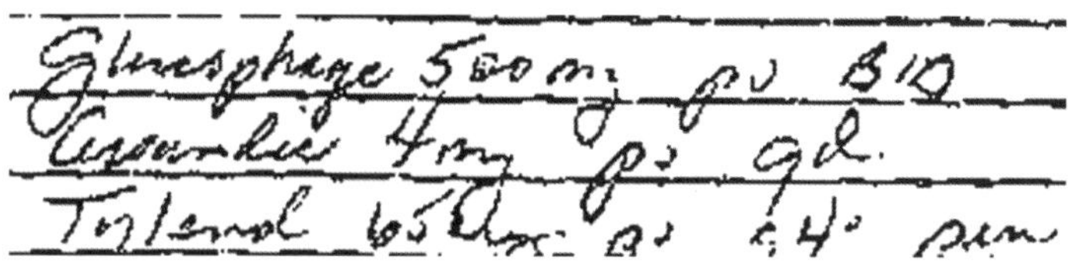

FIGURE 10-1   Avandia 4 mg (middle line) was misread as Coumadin 4 mg.

IS GLACIAL ACETIC ACID REALLY NEEDED?

The label of glacial acetic acid (pure acetic acid) bears a red skull and crossbones and strong warning statements: "POISON! DANGER! CORROSIVE. Liquid and mist cause severe burns to all body tissue. May be fatal if swallowed. Harmful if inhaled. Inhalation may cause lung and tooth damage." Nevertheless, this substance has been dispensed instead of diluted forms of acetic acid that are used for treating external ear infections, irrigating bladders and wounds, and identifying abnormal cells.[14] Patients have suffered severe pain, first and second degree burns, and even more serious consequences.

In one case, a nurse called the pharmacy for "acetic acid for irrigation" for a 31-year-old patient with paraplegia, osteomyelitis, and bilateral greater trochanter wounds. A pharmacist, who was experienced but new to that institution, placed glacial acetic acid at the window for pickup, and it was used for 2 days, resulting in severe burns that necessitated disarticulation at the hips because the wounds would not heal.

In another hospital where the pharmacy routinely restocks automated dispensing cabinets for patient care areas, the ambulatory surgery center sent a refill request for 30 mL of a 5% acetic acid solution. A technician poured 30 mL of glacial acetic acid directly into a 1 ounce bottle, unaware that it required dilution. Although the technician labeled the bottle "acetic acid—glacial," the pharmacist assumed that the technician had performed the required dilution. The nurses and physician in the ambulatory surgery department also assumed that the product had been diluted. The physician used the glacial acetic acid during a colposcopy. The patient experienced immediate vaginal bleeding and blistering and was in severe pain when she awoke from sedation, but she suffered no permanent harm.

In yet another case, a bottle of what should have been 3% acetic acid was sent to the operating room. A patient's skin was bathed with glacial acetic acid, causing first- and second-degree burns.

Despite the warning on the bottle, some practitioners do not recognize that this is the most concentrated form of acetic acid. If it must be kept in the pharmacy, more prominent warnings are needed; one hospital has designed a brightly colored label. Furthermore, when dangerous chemicals are handled, independent double checks before dispensing are crucial. In the second case above, the pharmacist assumed the technician had diluted the solution but did not observe what materials, calculations, and measurements were used. These cases also highlight the point that nothing should be dispensed without an order. Prescribers should specify the exact strength desired. Commercial products should be used whenever possible. Unusual requests such as these involving the dilution of acetic acid should be made at least a day before the product is needed.

The availability of both drugs in 4 mg tablet strength increased the likelihood of a mix-up. Had these health professionals known the medication's purpose, they could easily have prevented the error. This incident also highlights the need for a formal process for ordering nonformulary drugs; confusion of the two products would have been unlikely if a nonformulary request form accompanied the order, since Coumadin was on the formulary.

Pharmacists are more likely than nurses to be aware of newly marketed drugs that may be confused with familiar ones. The use of computerized prescriber order entry (CPOE) or scanning equipment (e.g., Pyxis Connect, McKesson MedDirect) to send orders to the pharmacy facilitates order review by the pharmacist. Pharmacists can view magnified images of scanned orders when parts are unclear. Electronic systems enable pharmacists to keep track of individualized messages and to process orders remotely.

Drug orders that are spoken rather than written can easily be misunderstood, especially when product names sound similar, such as Foradil (the bronchodilator formoterol) and Toradol (ketorolac), or Cerebyx and Celebrex. Such mix-ups have caused serious injuries. Doses can also be misheard. When morphine 2 mg IV was misheard as morphine 10 mg IV, the result was respiratory arrest. Tachycardia and hypotension occurred after 15 mg of hydralazine IV every 2 hours was misheard as 50 mg every 2 hours. Pharmacists must contact prescribers when clarification is needed. Spoken orders should be transcribed immediately and verified by reading back the order.[15] Chapter 11 gives additional recommendations regarding spoken orders.

Pharmacy staff should be aware of pairs of medications that are frequently confused. Some pharmacies post lists of such pairs to alert practitioners to the potential for error and the need for extra caution. A list of the most problem-prone name pairs is available at www.ismp.org. Many computer systems have a "clinical flag" or "formulary note" screen or field that prominently displays information on potential name mix-ups to the person entering an order. For example, when Norvasc is entered into the computer, the pharmacist sees a note that this name can look like Navane when handwritten. Orders can then be confirmed, if necessary. The Safety Briefs feature in the *ISMP Medication Safety Alert!* newsletters covers new reports of name pairs involved in errors.

Selecting brands and generic supplies carefully can help reduce the risk of mix-ups caused by look-alike labels (see Chapter 7). Pharmaceutical manufacturers design their labels to be recognized across their product line, so labels may look alike. Many manufacturers of generic medications have introduced label changes, particularly for injectables, that make it easier to distinguish one product from another, and pharmacies can choose these companies over others. Changing manufacturers for one product to reduce similarity to another is also an option. Pharmacists and pharmacy purchasers must watch for look-alike packaging within a manufacturer's product line or between products from different manufacturers; staff should be warned to send look-alike products back, separate them, or mark them with auxiliary labels.

Another way to avoid selecting the wrong medication among look-alike pairs, or the incorrect dosage strength or form, is to create vastly different computer mnemonics for potentially problematic drug pairs.[6] Mnemonics are not recommended, however, for high-alert medications such as cancer chemotherapy agents, neuromuscular blocking agents, and controlled substances. An error that illustrates the problem with mnemonics occurred in a children's hospital when a physician ordered buspirone 10 mg for a child with a seizure disorder. A pharmacist typed the mnemonic "BUS10" to bring buspirone 10 mg onto the computer screen, but that mnemonic had been assigned to the antineoplastic agent busulfan 10 mg, which the pharmacist dispensed in error. Another example involves the mnemonic "AZT100," which has been used for both azathioprine 100 mg and zidovudine (formerly named azidothymidine) 100 mg. If a patient with acquired immunodeficiency syndrome (AIDS) were to receive an immunosuppressant instead of an antiretroviral, the error could be fatal.

ERRORS RELATED TO INFORMATION ABOUT THE DRUG OR PATIENT

Misleading or Erroneous References

Some medication errors can be traced to mistakes in textbooks or use of outdated texts. For example, on the basis of information from the eighth edition of the *Handbook on Injectable*

Drugs, published in 1994,[16] sterile water was used to prepare 3,000 mL of 5% albumin from 25% albumin during a national shortage of 5% albumin. Albumin can be diluted with sterile water, 0.9% sodium chloride injection, or 5% dextrose injection, but large volumes of sterile water or dextrose injection cause a substantial reduction in tonicity. When such a solution is infused into a patient, hemolysis occurs. Preparation of large volumes of 5% albumin diluted with sterile water for use in plasma exchange resulted in several deaths. In subsequent editions of the *Handbook,*[17,18] the monograph for albumin was changed to note that if sterile water for injection is the diluent, the tonicity of the diluted solution must be considered because hypotonicity can cause hemolysis. Reports of hemolysis have since decreased, but errors could occur if old editions of the text were used. Another example, of a vincristine dosage error based on incorrect information in a journal, is described in Chapter 16.

Mistakes in books, journals, and reference charts are not uncommon. Any suspect information should be fully investigated, regardless of the source. New editions of references should be purchased as soon as they become available; it is well worth the cost. Computerized and online resources, such as Facts and Comparisons on monthly CD-ROM and Micromedex, are ideal for pharmacies and patient care areas because they are constantly being updated. Practitioners can augment their drug information resources with programs such as Epocrates and Lexi-Comp that are continually updated and designed for use with personal digital assistants.

Ambiguity in Handwritten and Typed Documents

Pharmacists must never second-guess prescribers. Illegible handwriting, nonstandard abbreviations, and incomplete information must be clarified with the prescriber before the prescription is processed. The clarification should be documented in writing.

Chapter 9 describes many prescriptions and orders that were misread because of poor handwriting and look-alike drug names, but letters and numbers can be misinterpreted even when handwriting is clear or the characters are typed on paper or a computer screen. For example, several overdoses were reported because a lowercase L, the final letter in the drug name, was misread as the number 1.

In the first case, an order for Tegretol 300 mg b.i.d. was misinterpreted as 1300 mg b.i.d. The patient had just been transferred from another facility, and the nurse transcribing this order onto a hospital form misread it. The lowercase L in Tegretol had been written very close to the number 300 on the patient's transfer order form (Tegretol300 mg). The pharmacist processing the order was unfamiliar with the medication, and the computer system did not alert him that the dose exceeded safe limits. The patient received only one dose in error before a clinical pharmacist caught the mistake. The overdose caused lethargy but no serious toxicity.

In the other case, a nurse misread an order for Amaryl 2 mg as 12 mg. Again, there was insufficient space between the last letter in the drug name and the numerical dose (Figure 10-2). In this case the pharmacist processed the order correctly; the error never reached the patient because the profile on the automated dispensing cabinet stated the dose correctly. Adequate spacing between the drug name and the dose also is crucial on medication history forms, preprinted order forms, and electronic formats such as the pharmacy computer, computer-generated MARs, and computerized order entry systems.

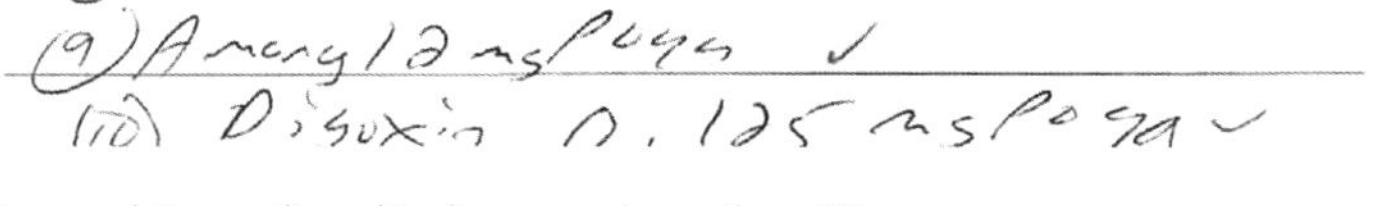

FIGURE 10-2 Amaryl 2 mg (top line) was misread as 12 mg.

Handwritten lists of patients' allergies have also been misread. While reviewing a handwritten, faxed order, a pharmacist read the word "Iodine" in the space for allergy alerts. A second pharmacist read "Lodine." When the prescriber was contacted, she identified Lodine as the drug to which the patient was allergic. In another case, a patient listed Lodine 400 mg b.i.d. as a medication she was taking before admission. The admitting resident misread this and ordered saturated solution of potassium iodide 400 mg b.i.d. The patient received two doses before the error was discovered.

Computerized Prescribing

CPOE can eliminate problems associated with handwritten orders. It also allow computerized drug-use review (DUR) by prescribers and a second DUR by pharmacists to further enhance safety. Through online prompting, CPOE can provide information about the drug and the patient at the time the order is entered, which further reduces the potential for error. Computer order entry also eliminates the need for transcription, thus preventing errors caused by incorrect interpretation of orders by the person transcribing them.

However, typed or computerized orders will not prevent all errors. Anyone who uses e-mail knows that it is easy to mistake a computer-generated lowercase L in an e-mail address for the numeral 1, or the letter O for zero. Similarly, computer software can translate drug names incorrectly. For example, if Lodine is typed with a lowercase L, the software will likely recognize it as Iodine. And even a clearly typed order for Levoxyl 25 mcg could be misread as 125 mcg if it appears without proper spacing (Levoxyl25 mcg), especially since both strengths are available. Research at Bell Laboratories has confirmed that some symbols are more likely than others to be misidentified.[19] The character pairs I and 1, O and 0, Z and 2, and 1 and 7 accounted for more than half of the errors in identification. In reading medication orders, the context does not always help with identification of characters. Although Zetar would not likely be read as "2TAR," "HCTZ50mg" could easily be read as either hydrocortisone 250 mg or hydrochlorothiazide 50 mg.

In the middle of the first decade of the 21st century, CPOE is not in widespread use; handwritten orders are still the norm. Until computerized ordering becomes the standard, outpatient prescription forms could be formatted so that prescribers must print the name and strength in designated blocks for each letter.[20] The rules outlining each block could be printed at a 30% screen so they appear light gray. These light rules would help prevent confusion among T, 7, and I, or E, F, and L. If used on inpatient order forms, such rules would be visible to prescribers but would not interfere with the legibility of alphanumeric characters. (The back copies of multiple-sheet [no-carbon-required, or NCR] order forms should never have rules.)

As commonly done in Europe, marks can be added to differentiate characters: a slash through a zero to differentiate it from the letter O, a bar through a 7 to prevent confusion with the number 1, a bar through a Z to distinguish it from the number 2.[1] The use of such symbolic differentiation would help reduce character misidentification.

Errors in Dosage

Dosing errors may occur when prescribers misplace a decimal point (e.g., ordering levothyroxine 0.25 mg instead of the intended dose of 0.025 mg). One pharmacist received an order for levothyroxine 0.75 mg p.o. daily but noticed in the patient's record from a prior admission that she had been taking 0.075 mg. While an experienced pharmacist may recognize 0.75 mg as an excessive amount, an order for 0.25 mg could slip by more easily, particularly since levothyroxine is available in a 0.3 mg tablet strength. Imagine the consequences if an elderly patient with a cardiac condition accidentally received 10 times the intended dose of levothyroxine.

Mathematical errors and decimal point misplacement are common in conversions between micrograms and milligrams. Errors of this type may not be easily detected with drugs such as levothyroxine and warfarin, which are available in a wide range of dosages to accommodate a variety of patient-specific orders. Since errors with levothyroxine are so frequent, pharmacies should consider using computer alerts triggered by the entry of a 0.25 mg dose; nearly always, the correct dose is 0.025 mg. In addition, prescribers should be encouraged to order the medication the same way manufacturers express the dosage—in micrograms, not milligrams—so no conversion is needed.

Many errors involving misplaced decimal points could be prevented if researchers, the pharmaceutical industry, and the Food and Drug Administration (FDA) agreed not to allow exact 10-fold differences in tablet strengths. For example, if Compazine were available as 3 mg and 25 mg, rather than 2.5 mg and 25 mg, 10-fold overdoses would be much less likely. Occasionally, using fractions instead of a metric designation could help prevent errors. For example, the dosage embossed on 2.5 mg Coumadin tablets is expressed as "2½ mg" to prevent confusion with 25 mg.

Stocking a single strength of a medication can help prevent errors, but often multiple strengths are needed. One hospital moved to a single strength after 10-fold dosing errors due to confusion between two patient-controlled analgesia hydromorphone concentrations (a low-dose concentration of 0.1 mg/mL and a high-dose concentration of 1 mg/mL). The pain management clinicians, nurses, and pharmacists subsequently realized that this did not meet patient needs. They decided to change the low-dose concentration from 0.1 mg/mL to 0.2 mg/mL, making confusion between the high- and low-dose strengths less likely.

Many dosage errors occur with oral liquid medications. This dosage form may seem to have less potential for harm than injectable medications, but oral liquids are the least likely form to be dispensed in unit doses, and they are prescribed most often for pediatric and geriatric patients. Improper dosing, incorrect or misunderstood directions for use, improper compounding, and inaccurate measurements of oral liquids have led to many errors. The cases described on page 216 and in Chapter 17 show the need for special care in dispensing oral liquid medications.

When writing prescriptions in inpatient and outpatient settings, prescribers should include both the calculated dosage (by metric weight) and its milligram per kilogram basis. This enables pharmacists and nurses to recalculate the dosage and recognize errors. Whenever possible, the pharmacy should calculate the volume to be administered and provide clear instructions to those responsible for administering the medication. Setting weight-based dose limits in the pharmacy computer system for oral liquid medications can alert staff when the volume selected exceeds a safe dose for the patient.

In community pharmacies, all new prescriptions for oral liquid medications (and other new prescriptions that suggest education is warranted) should be placed in a separate area away from other prescriptions. This helps remind the pharmacist to review directions with the patient or caregiver and to provide an appropriate measuring device and demonstrate its use. In reviewing the label directions, the pharmacist can detect any inaccuracies that may have been overlooked during the dispensing process.

In inpatient settings, oral liquid medications should be dispensed in unit doses in oral syringes whenever possible. Before discharge, health care providers should educate patients or caregivers about proper measurement. When feasible, they should provide an oral syringe and recommend going to a community pharmacy for a measurement demonstration.

The risk of errors is high when patients receive samples of oral liquid medications from physicians' offices, because the containers often lack directions and the products may require reconstitution before use. If such samples are provided, patient education in

ERRORS IN ORAL LIQUID DOSAGES

❑ A 12-month-old infant with a gastrointestinal virus was incorrectly prescribed a $2\frac{1}{2}$-fold overdosage of Donnatal (belladonna alkaloids w/phenobarbital) elixir (2.5 mL instead of 1 mL) in an emergency department (ED) and received two doses. (The infant also received two doses of 12.5 mg Phenergan [promethazine] suppositories, which are contraindicated in children under 2 years of age). The child was discharged but readmitted later that day, unconscious. The infant suffered permanent anoxic brain injury that resulted in delayed speech, seizures, and palsy of the lower extremities.

❑ A pharmacist received an order from an office nurse for Ventolin (albuterol) syrup 2 mg/mL, $1\frac{1}{2}$ teaspoonfuls (not $\frac{1}{2}$ teaspoonful as intended) t.i.d. for a 5-month-old infant. The pharmacist counseled the mother that the drug could cause hyperactivity or insomnia, but did not review the dosing directions or detect the error. After two doses, the infant, shaking uncontrollably, was admitted to the ED with a pulse of 140–200, but no permanent harm resulted.

❑ In five similar cases, the prescriber correctly ordered the weight and volume of an oral liquid medication, but the pharmacy dispensed the solutions with incorrect directions, most often confusing the prescribed volume in milliliters with teaspoonfuls. For example, Augmentin (amoxicillin and potassium clavulanate) was dispensed with directions to take $2\frac{1}{2}$ teaspoonfuls instead of $2\frac{1}{2}$ mL. In all of these cases, the directions for use were not reviewed with the caregivers when the medication was dispensed.

❑ A pharmacist dispensed metoclopramide syrup for an infant, labeled correctly with directions to give 0.7 mL (0.7 mg) every 6 to 8 hours. After misreading the directions, the infant's mother asked a pharmacy clerk how to measure 7 mL of the drug. The clerk, unaware that she was providing information about an incorrect dose, gave the mother an oral syringe and showed her the 7 mL marking. The child was admitted to the hospital for 2 days after receiving several 7 mL doses.

their use is imperative. Physicians could promote safe use of samples by making arrangements to send patients to a hospital or community pharmacy that will properly label the samples with instructions.

Wrong Patient Errors

"Wrong patient" errors may originate during any phase of the medication use process—including dispensing. In processing medication orders, pharmacists enter the patient's name or identification number to retrieve the patient's profile in the pharmacy computer system. Occasionally, orders are entered in the wrong patient's profile because of a poorly legible name or number on the paper prescription or order copy (often imprinted by an addressing machine), or because of look-alike last names.

In one case, a pharmacist tried using the identification number to access the profile and enter a new order for "Franklin Hope" (fictitious name used to illustrate this actual error). Because of difficulty reading the number, he could not locate the profile. He then entered the patient's name, and a profile appeared. But the pharmacist noticed that the profile was for a female patient, and he realized that he had been entering the order into Hope Franklin's profile, not Franklin Hope's.

An error that occurred during electronic prescribing could also occur during pharmacy order entry: The prescriber misspelled the patient's last name, inadvertently accessing the profile of another patient with the same first name as the intended patient and adding the orders to the wrong profile.

Since 2003, the Joint Commission on Accreditation of Healthcare Organizations (JCAHO) has required the use of at least two patient identifiers (neither can be the patient's room number) by personnel taking blood samples and administering medications or blood products. Initiated first as a JCAHO National Patient Safety Goal, this requirement is now a standard (PC.5.10, EP #4). However, the use of two identifiers is not required when physicians prescribe medications, when pharmacists and pharmacy technicians enter orders and dispense medications, when unit secretaries and nurses transcribe medication orders, or during other such critical processes. Perhaps all personnel should be required to use two patient identifiers. Hospitals would have to ensure that two identifiers (e.g., name, birth date, identification number) were readily available and clearly legible. During order entry, pharmacists and pharmacy technicians could compare the patient's name and identification number on the computer profile and the order. Using an enhanced type font for the patient's name on the screen could also improve accuracy. Some computer systems provide alerts and require a second form of identification (e.g., birth date, identification number) when the system contains similar names.

Pharmacists can help ensure that nurses administer medications to the correct patient. Pharmacy staff should place all doses delivered to patient care units between normal cart fills directly into patient bins and notify nurses that the drugs have been delivered. When a drug is discontinued, the remaining doses should be removed from the patient care unit, patient identification labels should be removed, and the doses should be returned to stock according to proper procedure.

Computerized Alerts

In addition to ensuring correct identification of the patient, the pharmacist must verify the safety and appropriateness of the prescribed medication and its dosage. The use of computerized alerts in order entry systems could prevent many serious adverse drug events (ADEs). For example, a fatal overdosage of colchicine could have been prevented if the pharmacist had been alerted to the maximum cumulative dose. The physician had prescribed 2 mg to be given intravenously every hour "until diarrhea develops or symptoms are relieved." Fatalities have occurred after a cumulative IV dose of as little as 5 mg, but the dispensing pharmacist did not notice the problem. The drug was stopped when the patient developed diarrhea after receiving 12 mg, but death ensued. A well-designed computer system could have alerted the pharmacist that the cumulative IV dose should not exceed 4 mg in 24 hours, and that no more colchicine should be given by any route for at least 7 days afterward.

Few hospitals or pharmacies can rely on their order entry systems to detect serious errors. In 2005, readers of the *ISMP Medication Safety Alert!* were asked to test whether safety warnings appeared in their pharmacy order entry systems when a series of orders was entered for a fictitious patient.[21] The test elements were associated with previously reported errors or hazards. Of 182 computer systems tested, only 4 were able to detect all the unsafe orders. Fewer than half of the systems were able to detect orders for medications exceeding a maximum safe dose. When unsafe orders were detected, most of the systems (9 out of 10) allowed users to override the warning, usually by simply pressing a function key. Most systems were capable of providing reports of drug warning overrides and enabling staff to build alerts for error-prone situations. Only one-fifth of the systems were able to intercept an order for a medication contraindicated by the patient's diagnosis or condition (pregnancy), and only one-fourth were able to detect a clinically significant drug–herbal interaction.

In some ways, the systems tested in 2005 performed less reliably than those similarly tested in 1999. For example, in 2005 fewer systems offered dose alerts based on the patient's age or weight and body surface area. Most systems tested in 1999 were able to intercept orders for drugs to which patients were allergic, but in 2005 fewer than half alerted staff when Fluzone (influenza virus vaccine) was ordered for a patient allergic to eggs. Some improvement since 1999 was observed in detecting drugs or doses contraindicated on the basis of lab results. More pharmacy computer systems today are directly interfaced with the laboratory system and able to automatically alert staff on the basis of current lab values. In 2005 the systems were also better able to detect duplicate therapy, and three-fourths of the systems were able to detect a significant drug–drug interaction.

More than half (56%) of the 2005 survey participants were using a pharmacy system that was at least 5 years old and not recently upgraded; 38% had been using the same system for 8 years or more without upgrades. Another reason for the poor results may be that drug information software was not updated. If a software vendor deems certain types of warnings unimportant, they may be omitted. If drug information is not current, important alerts may not appear.

The survey was not designed to test computerized *physician* order entry systems, but if independent screening by pharmacists is inadequate, unsafe orders may not be caught. Improving pharmacy technology to reduce the risk of serious patient harm should be a national priority. Pharmacy computer systems should be chosen for their ability to maintain patient profiles and alert the dispenser to medication overdoses, underdoses, duplicate therapy, overuse, contraindications, potential allergic reactions, and interactions with concurrently prescribed medications (page 219). Systems should be configured so the alert functions cannot be disabled and serious warnings cannot be easily or mistakenly overridden. A quality assurance system should be an integral part of any system that allows an override; the system should generate lists of overrides for retrospective review by management. Other desirable features of pharmacy computer systems include the neatness, clarity, organization, and understandability of the labels and reports generated and the display screens showing patient profiles and order entries.

Labeling

Pharmacy Computer-Generated Labeling, MARs, and Reports

The way information appears on pharmacy-applied labels and pharmacy computer-generated MARs has contributed to medication errors. The labeling process begins during order entry into the pharmacy computer system, with the selection and entry of the correct medication, dosage strength, dosage form, quantity, complete directions for use, number of refills, and prescriber name. The profiles of many pharmacy computer systems present first the dosage strength available in stock, followed by the number of tablets or volume of oral or injectable liquid that will be needed for the prescribed dose. This sequence may be transferred to a computer-generated MAR and pharmacy-applied product labels, so the drug name and available dosage strength, often in bold print, appear on the top lines and the patient's actual dose appears in lighter print below. This presentation also guides the selection of doses for daily cart distribution.

However, nurses who administer drugs tend to think first about the dose they must give, and then about the number of tablets or volume of liquid needed for the dose. Their eyes naturally go to the bold type in the topmost line to find the patient's dose on the MAR or label. As described in Chapter 11, errors may occur when the patient's dose differs from the available dosage strength listed on the top line.

To prevent such errors, the patient's dose should be accentuated, not the available dosage strength. Ideally, the drug name would be followed by the patient-specific dose in bold type, then the route and frequency (and indication, if applicable) on the next line, and any special instructions (e.g., 50 mg = 2 × 25 mg tabs) on the last line. Some hospitals print "Dose" in front of the patient-specific dose to avoid confusion with an available strength. To avoid dispensing dosage strengths that do not match the patient-specific dose, hospital pharmacies can carry multiple strengths of oral and injectable drugs and dispense in unit doses to the extent possible. If multiple tablets are needed for a single dose, they

OPTIMAL CAPABILITIES OF PHARMACY COMPUTER SOFTWARE

Dose limits. Computer screening for the predetermined dose limit of a medication can help prevent pharmacists from entering a prescription order that could result in overdosage. This function may require computer records of the patient's weight and height; in some cases, alerts rely on calculations of body surface area. Three types of dose checks are needed: (1) cutoff for a single dose, (2) cutoff for total amount of drug allowed in a 24-hour period, and (3) cutoff for an entire course of therapy. Products with multiple ingredients can contribute to excessive dosages, for example, when plain acetaminophen is given to a patient receiving Darvocet-N. Computer screening for dose limits should not overlook combination products.

Allergic reactions. Information on allergies is essential. Many pharmacists do not screen for allergies if allergy information has not been entered or has been inconsistently entered into the patient database. Orders should not be processed before this information is entered into the pharmacy computer system and coded so that the allergy alert system is functional. Some software packages do not flag ingredients to which the patient has reported an allergy.

Cross-allergies. Screening for cross-allergies to drugs such as codeine and oxycodone, codeine and morphine, and penicillin and cephalosporins is a minimum standard.

Duplication of drug ingredients. Screening for similar ingredients in different products is necessary to prevent drug duplication.

Duplication of therapeutic classes. Screening is needed to prevent duplications within therapeutic drug classes (e.g., giving omeprazole and a histamine H_2-receptor antagonist to the same patient).

Drug interactions. Fast and effective screening to detect drug interactions requires a significance level that catches major interactions but does not flag minor interactions. Even when the proper significance level is set, there is a risk that pharmacists may override the interaction and miss a dangerous situation. A system that flags important interactions but merely prints out less urgent messages without interrupting workflow might be effective. Having to justify an override would make the pharmacist think critically about interactions. Regular review by a clinical supervisor of all overridden interactions is recommended as a quality control measure.

Contraindicated drugs or drugs that need dosage modifications. The pharmacy computer system should be interfaced with the lab system to alert pharmacists when lab values suggest drug therapy changes. In addition, a database organized by patient diagnosis should be available from software vendors. This system could incorporate International Classification of Diseases (ICD) codes or, at a minimum, track a few important diagnoses. Such a system could, for example, prevent a patient with renal failure from receiving nephrotoxic drugs or alert the pharmacist when a dosage of a highly metabolized drug is too great for a patient with liver disease.

should be attached in some fashion. When liquids must be dispensed in bulk, the container's total volume should not be listed on the MAR.

The appearance of nonessential information (e.g., pharmacy mnemonics, pharmacy codes) can clutter labels and MARs, making it difficult for nurses to view the most important information. Adding the patient's name and location to a commercial unit dose product label may also foster errors. For example, a hospital pharmacist dispensing an order for oral ampicillin 500 mg wrote the patient's name and room number on the unit dose package. The order was discontinued before any of the labeled doses were administered, and the capsules were returned to pharmacy stock. A pharmacist dispensing an ampicillin 500 mg order for a different patient on the same unit selected three doses to last until the next 24-hour cart fill, placed them in a labeled zip-lock bag, and sent it to the nursing unit. He did not notice that the first patient's name was written on the unit dose packages. A nurse on the patient care unit saw ampicillin capsules in the bag, removed a dose, and wrongly assumed that the name and bed number written on the package identified the patient for whom the drug was intended. She remembered that ampicillin had been ordered for that patient but did not know it had been discontinued. She administered one dose to the wrong patient. Later, she noticed the correct patient's name and room number written on the zip-lock bag and discovered the error. This nurse may have read the label on the bag but been confused by a different patient's name on the unit dose package. If pharmacists believe it is necessary to label the unit dose package as well as the bag when sending oral solid medications to nursing units, a safer alternative is to affix a supplemental label that does not obscure the drug name, dose, or other important information and that can easily be torn off if the drug is returned to pharmacy. For example, the edge of a blank sticky label could be affixed to the edge of the unit dose packaging, the remainder of the label folded over on itself, and the patient's name and location printed on the label.

Syringe and Admixture Labels

Standardizing the way labels are placed on syringes can reduce errors. For medications used in hospital inpatient areas, the practice site's name and location should not appear anywhere on the label; it clutters the label. If state law requires this information to be on the label, it should be placed at the bottom. ISMP recommends this placement for all conventional pharmacy labels.

The patient's name and location should appear on line 1 at the top of the label, followed by drug name, dose (and strength if appropriate), and route of administration on line 2. This information (e.g., drug name, amount) should appear parallel to the long axis of the syringe and from the needle end of the syringe to the plunger (Figure 10-3). That way, the printing will be right side up for the 80% of practitioners who are right handed and usually hold a syringe by its plunger, in the right hand. Since the person administering the drug often will need to observe the syringe's volume scale, the top of the label should be placed flush against the scale but not covering it. Applying labels in this way improves safety by allowing practitioners to see the patient and drug names without turning the syringe.

Oral syringes, although they have tips that will not accommodate a needle, should always carry an auxiliary label stating "For Oral Use Only." Practitioners have mistaken oral syringes for improperly manufactured parenteral syringes and manipulated them to fit a needle or connect to an IV line. One nurse who was unfamiliar with oral syringes found a different way to inject the contents. The order was written for "Tussionex suspension," but the oral route of administration was not specified. Pharmacy dispensed the cough medicine in unit dose oral syringes. The nurse assumed that since the liquid was in a syringe and the patient had IV access, the drug should be given IV. A pharmacy label covered the words "For Oral Use Only" that the manufacturer prints on each oral syringe. Noting that the drug was rather thick, the nurse transferred it into a regular syringe,

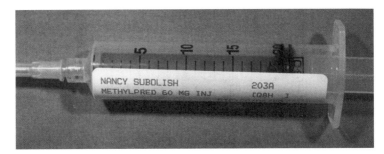

FIGURE 10-3 Properly labeled syringe.

diluted it with saline, and injected it. Afterwards, she commented to another nurse that the drug was quite sticky. Further queries revealed that the drug had been given by an incorrect route. The IV site was immediately removed, the patient was monitored, and no harm occurred.

During their orientation, all new staff members should be made aware of oral syringes and how they protect against inadvertent IV administration. Pharmacy labels should never cover the words "For Oral Use Only" printed on the syringe. For added protection, auxiliary labels are available with this warning printed in large red letters; they can be affixed to the syringe plunger whenever an oral liquid is dispensed in an oral syringe. When orders do not specify a route of administration, they should be clarified before initial transcription.

The manufacturers of IV solutions have been asked to label the bags on both sides but in most cases have not done so. That being the case, pharmacists have been divided on whether it is safer to place admixture labels on the front side bearing the name of the base solution as listed by the manufacturer. Such placement enables practitioners to easily check that all labeling agrees. Some practitioners believe, however, that placing the additive label on the reverse side reduces the chances of administration mix-ups because the content is identifiable in any position. In the absence of research indicating which method of labeling is safer, it is probably better to place the additive label on the front of the bag, without covering the product identity.

In both inpatient and outpatient settings, auxiliary labels should be used for vinca alkaloids. On syringes containing extemporaneously prepared vincristine and vinblastine, the U.S. Pharmacopeia requires a label stating, "Fatal if Given Intrathecally. For IV Use Only." The syringes must be placed in an overwrap (which accompanies the manufacturer's container) that also carries this labeling. Such labels and overwraps are available in the packaging of vincristine and vinblastine products. The package insert for vinorelbine, the other vinca alkaloid available in the United States, requires only a warning label that states, "For IV Use Only." However, to ensure safety, the same warning statements should appear on the syringe of any vinca alkaloid product.

Auxiliary Labels

The way auxiliary labels are stored in the pharmacy can be a factor in dispensing errors. A pharmacy student reported an incident in which a hospital nurse about to administer a TPN solution noticed a sticker on the bag stating, "For Irrigation Use Only." A call to the pharmacy revealed that the wrong sticker had been used; the roll of "For Irrigation Use Only" stickers was kept next to the roll of stickers stating "For Intravenous Use Only." Such stickers should be separated to prevent mix-ups. Similar incidents have been reported in which otic drops were dispensed with labels stating "For Use in the Eye Only."

Labeling Guidelines

To facilitate the adoption of standard formats for pharmacy computer-generated labels, MARs, and reports, a team was established in 2005 to begin drafting guidelines. Represented on the team are ISMP, pharmacy practitioners, vendors (McKesson, Siemens, and Cerner), and JCAHO. Team members are guided by human-factors concepts and computer-system-related reports submitted to the USP-ISMP Medication Errors Reporting Program. The team has completed guidelines for labeling oral solid and oral liquid medications dispensed and administered in the inpatient setting (appendix). Figure 10-4 shows an example of the proposed label format. Many concepts in these guidelines can be applied to pharmacy labels for other products and computer-generated MARs.

```
Patient Name***************************** Patient Location
Second patient identifier
generic drug name*****( BRAND name) Patient dose Route
(Dose= 2 X 75 mg tablets)
Bar code
                 expiration date if appropriate      space for RPh initials
```

1. **Patient name – 48 character field – bolded 12 point font**
2. Location – 12 character field – 12 point font
3. Second identifier – 10 character field (date of birth, financial #, encounter #, medical record #) – 10 point font
4. **Generic name – 40 character field – bolded 12 point font**
5. **BRAND name – 18 character field – 12 point font**
6. **Patient dose – 20 character field – bolded 12 point font**
7. **Route – 6 character field – 12 point font**
8. Dose composition
    For oral solids, number of tablets (e.g., "Dose = 2 × 75 mg tablets") – 30 character field – 10 point font
    For oral liquids, patient-specific dose with corresponding volume in milliliters – 30 character field – 10 point font *and, on next line,*
    Solution concentration per milliliter: 30 character field – 10 point font
9. Bar code
10. Pharmacist initials if needed – these may be handwritten or, if computer generated, 10 point font
11. Expiration date as needed in a MM/DD/YYYY format – 10 point font
12. Other information as required by state or federal law
13. Pharmacy information if required should be at the bottom of the label
14. Comments – 10 point font

FIGURE 10-4 Format for pharmacy-generated label for dispensing oral solid medications to inpatient care units (minimum content).

New Outpatient Prescription Label and Vial

In 2005, Target Corporation introduced a pharmacy prescription container and label called the ClearRx system. Its features for improving safety include added white space to reduce label clutter; a larger type font and colored background to enhance visibility of the drug name; placement of the most important information on the top of the label and the pharmacy information (name, address, phone number) at the bottom, below a horizontal line; and placement of the medication name in large print on the peak of the bottle to be easily read when viewed from above the container.

As shown in Figure 10-5, the unusually shaped bottle has wider front and back panels to allow for better presentation of information. The panels are flat to eliminate the need for rotating the bottle to read all pertinent information. The uncluttered format makes the information easier to locate and read.

The ClearRx system includes an abbreviated medication information card that tucks between the back label and the bottle. The card includes the patient's name, drug name, description of the medication's expected appearance, instructions for use, common uses, and common adverse effects. A traditional medication information leaflet is also provided to the patient.

The new containers use color to distinguish each family member's medication. Individuals select one of the six available colors for their prescriptions; it is used in a ring

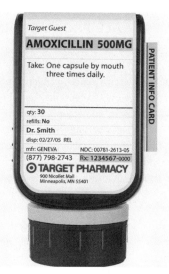

FIGURE 10-5 Example of Target's ClearRx prescription vial and label. Used with permission of Target Corporation.

around the neck of each bottle, or a colored sticker added to the front label if the medication is not packaged in a bottle.

With Target committed to making any necessary changes to improve safety, this new packaging and labeling initiative holds promise as a model for the community pharmacy industry.

ERRORS RELATED TO DISPENSING METHODS

Unit Dose Dispensing

The value of unit dose dispensing in preventing errors should not be underestimated. JCAHO standards require "medications to be dispensed in the most ready-to-administer form possible to minimize opportunities for error."[22] Most hospital pharmacists would say their facilities use unit dose dispensing, but often the system does not extend to all products (see sidebar on page 224). Pharmacies still receive many products in bulk packages; pediatric dosage forms, controlled substances, oral liquids, and injectable drugs often require repackaging for unit dose distribution. Some hospitals, ambulatory care centers, and long-term care facilities have moved away from robust unit dose dispensing systems, usually to cut costs.

Furthermore, in many hospitals, nurses are responsible for reconstituting or preparing some IV doses from floor stock drugs. This practice is especially prevalent with medications dispensed for neonates or pediatric patients, and often facilities have no policy for independent checking of doses to ensure that the order has been properly interpreted, the correct medication has been used, and dosage calculations, preparation, and labeling are accurate. Errors occur that a fully implemented unit dose system could have prevented.

For example, in a neonatal intensive care unit, a 7.4 mg loading dose of aminophylline was ordered for a premature infant who had episodes of apnea. Instead of 7.4 mg (0.3 mL of a 250 mg/10 mL solution), 7.4 mL (185 mg) was administered. Tachycardia and other signs of theophylline toxicity developed, and despite intubation, ventilator support, and other measures, the infant died within 36 hours of the incident. The nurse who administered the aminophylline dose had prepared it from floor stock, without an independent check by a second individual, which hospital policy did not require.

DOES PHARMACY SUPPLY ALL PRODUCTS IN UNIT DOSES?

Hospital pharmacies that purportedly use unit dose dispensing should consider the following questions:

- ❑ Are all drugs stocked in patient care units (including automated dispensing cabinets) in ready-to-use unit doses? Are the only exceptions topical products, nasal or throat sprays, ophthalmic solutions and ointments, otic solutions and ointments, and vaginal creams?
- ❑ Are manufacturers' prefilled syringes or single-dose vials or ampuls (rather than multidose vials) used for at least 90% of the injectable products commonly stored in patient care units, including narcotics and saline and heparin flushes?
- ❑ Are at least 90% of oral liquid medications dispensed from the pharmacy in oral syringes or cups containing the patient-specific dose (including medications sent to neonatal and pediatric units)?
- ❑ Are commercial premixed IV solutions used whenever they are available?
- ❑ Are all IV solutions that are not available commercially prepared in the pharmacy, except those needed in emergencies?
- ❑ Are at least 90% of all IV push medications used in the inpatient units (including neonatal and pediatric units) dispensed in unit dose form?
- ❑ For oral solid medications that are available in different strengths, is the inventory sufficient to avoid splitting tablets or using multiple tablets or capsules for patient-specific doses?

Such events underscore the need for the hospital pharmacy to prepare and dispense all nonemergency injectable doses when commercial unit dose products are not available. Mechanisms for quality assurance in the pharmacy and pharmacist–nurse checking systems reduce the chance that an error will reach the patient. These safety measures are particularly important when high-alert drugs such as aminophylline are used in the treatment of neonates; even minor dose miscalculations can prove disastrous. Nursing and pharmacy should work together toward the goal of patient-specific unit dose dispensing.

Dispensing Multiple Tablets

Many drugs such as warfarin and levothyroxine are available in a range of dosages to accommodate varied patient needs. Yet, to save shelf space or costs considered unnecessary, inpatient pharmacies may stock only some of the available strengths. As a result, the pharmacy may need to dispense multiple tablets, with potentially confusing directions for administering combinations of whole and half tablets. Quite often, partial doses are returned to the pharmacy because the full dose never reached the patient. Pharmacists and technicians should take note of drugs that often require dispensing of multiple tablets in different strengths to achieve the prescribed dose. Stocking additional strengths of these drugs will minimize the chance of error.

AUTOMATED AND MANUAL REDUNDANCIES

Independent Double Checks before Dispensing

To facilitate checking of the prescription label and the medication being dispensed, the original prescription order, label, and medication container should be kept together throughout the dispensing process, including patient counseling. This increases the likelihood that errors in computer order entry will be detected.[3]

In checking prescriptions prepared by a technician, the pharmacist should compare the label with the original prescription order, the original prescription order with the label on the stock container, and the medication in the stock container with that being dispensed. The pharmacist should also ensure that appropriate auxiliary labels are used. A final check should be performed to verify that the patient's name; the drug name, strength, and dosage form; and the directions on the label match those on the original order. All prescriptions prepared by a technician should be independently double-checked by a pharmacist. This is especially important for medications that could seriously harm the patient if given erroneously. Some pharmacists use a yellow felt-tipped marker and a checklist when dispensing medications prepared by technicians, looking at the original prescription, the typed label, and the prepared dose and marking through each item on the prescription (or hospital order) as they check it (e.g., patient's name, location, drug name, dose, route of administration, directions). This helps ensure that nothing is overlooked if the pharmacist is distracted during the checking process. In ambulatory care settings, the National Drug Code (NDC) number on the stock container should also be compared with the NDC number in the computer or on the dispensing label.

Self-Checking

Health care providers often cannot detect errors in their own work. Several methods have been suggested to improve safety when independent double-checks are not possible.[23] The first suggestion is to read the drug name on the label and then reread it backwards. Taking the name out of context in this way puts the focus on physical details (i.e., the actual letters). Proofreaders often use this technique, reading one word at a time, backwards. One retired pharmacist claimed that it had kept him from making many mistakes during his career.

ISMP senior advisor John Senders suggests reading the label while holding the container in one hand, then reading it again with the container in the other hand. By using different parts of the brain, this technique enhances re-examination of the label. Senders also suggests reading the medication order aloud and then immediately reading the container label aloud so that any difference can be heard. These methods help ensure that the checking process is more than a mechanical routine.

Grasha[6] offered yet another suggestion: Delay self-checking for a short time. He conducted a study in which community pharmacists randomly checked completed prescriptions awaiting pickup. Errors were reduced by 21% when the pharmacists periodically monitored their work to detect errors. Each subsequent check identified 95% of errors missed during a prior check. However, mistakes were detected less frequently as the amount of continuous time spent on the specific activity increased. Thus, taking a short break or changing to a different task before self-checking makes it more effective.

Reducing Calculation Errors

Errors in calculating or measuring doses are minimized if a second practitioner independently calculates the dose. Such checking might be required for all calculations or measurements, or only in certain cases. For example, checks could be mandatory when the patient is less than 12 years of age, when complex calculations are required (e.g., when a drug infusion in a critical care setting requires a dose in micrograms per kilogram per minute), and for insulin infusions, chemotherapy, and compounding of patient-controlled analgesia. Calculators and computer programs may improve accuracy, but they do not eliminate the need for independent practitioner review of calculations and solution concentrations.

The need to calculate doses can be avoided by using the unit dose system exclusively, using commercially available unit-of-use items (e.g., premixed injectable solutions for use in critical care), and standardizing doses and concentrations, especially for drugs used in critical care. When standard concentrations are used, dosage charts on patient care units and standard formulations in the pharmacy minimize the possibility of error. For example, in critical care settings, physicians need order only the amount of drug they want infused and the titration parameters; dosage charts show the appropriate flow rate for the patient's weight and the dose ordered. New "smart" infusion pumps offer an additional safeguard against calculation errors; the pumps incorporate drug libraries with established dosing parameters and provide alerts (with soft or hard stops) to prevent erroneous dosing.[24]

Verifying Compounded Products

Errors can occur during extemporaneous compounding of IV solutions and admixtures. Administering hypotonic or superconcentrated solutions of dextrose, for example, has resulted in brain injury and death. Compounding errors are most often attributable to poor training of staff, inadequate supervision, arithmetic errors, misuse or malfunction of automated compounders, look-alike labeling on manufacturer-supplied containers, or inadequate processes for checking before admixtures are dispensed.

Standard concentrations for frequently used formulations should be recorded and made accessible for reference in the sterile products area of the pharmacy. A second staff person should independently double-check all calculations; this check should be documented. Diluents as well as active drugs must be checked. To facilitate checking, the stock container of each additive and its syringe should be lined up in the order in which they appear on the container label. The plunger piston should be aligned with the calibration marks on the syringe barrel indicating the amount to be used. Even when these steps are followed, compounding errors can occur (sidebar, page 227).[25]

Many hospitals use automated compounders in preparing large- and small-volume injectable solutions, but errors can still happen. Errors have occurred because solutions were placed on the wrong additive channel or the wrong solutions were identified. The use of product bar codes and scanning can help prevent such problems. The software that drives automated compounders is complicated, and users can enter incorrect information without realizing it. Pharmacies must have an ongoing program for quality assurance in the use of this equipment; the program should include double checks and documentation of solution placement within the compounder.

Pharmacists always calculate the expected weight of the final product on the basis of the specific gravity of the ingredients and the final volume. Each bag should be within 5% of the calculated weight. Another technique is to mark the beginning volume of each container before mixing and at the end of the filling cycle and check each container to determine whether final volumes are appropriate. These checks require an investment of less than 5 minutes per patient.[2] Another way to perform a final check is to place a drop of solution in a refractometer to determine the approximate dextrose concentration. Pharmacies that prepare admixtures such as TPN base solutions or cardioplegic solutions in batches should use additional quality control checks, including sterility testing and quarantine until confirmation.

New technologies will facilitate quantitative and qualitative analysis of medications used in IV admixture preparation. For example, the ValiMed instrument from CDEX, Inc. uses light energy and a library of spectral fingerprints to determine whether the correct drug and dose have been added to a solution.

FATAL ERROR IN NEONATAL TPN COMPOUNDING[25]

In a 25-week gestational age neonate, arterial line fluid containing sodium acetate 80 mEq/L and heparin 0.5 unit per mL was being used with an inline bedside blood gas and chemistry monitoring device. On day 3 of life, when the neonate's sodium level was increasing, the arterial fluid was changed to sodium chloride 40 mEq/L with heparin 1 unit/mL. The nurses replaced the inline chemistry monitor twice, believing it was faulty, but 18 hours after the change in arterial fluid, the monitor displayed a sodium concentration above 190 mmol/L (normal range, 136–146 mmol/L). A serum sample sent to the laboratory had a sodium concentration of 266 mmol/L. All fluids were removed for analysis, and new fluids were hung. Despite treatment including dopamine, dobutamine, epinephrine, and exchange transfusions, the sodium level did not drop and the baby died.

Analysis of the original arterial line fluid and follow-up investigation revealed that instead of a 250 mL bag of sterile water, a 250 mL glass bottle of concentrated sodium chloride (23.4%) had been used as the base solution. The pharmacy had switched from glass bottles to bags of sterile water several months earlier but had not clearly communicated this change to all staff. The bottles of concentrated sodium chloride were kept on the same shelving as other IV solutions (along with other concentrated solutions for TPN compounding). The pharmacy shelving was set up as a pass-through cabinet between the central pharmacy and the IV cleanroom. When items were stocked, they were placed with the labels facing the central pharmacy. When the labels are not visible, bottles of concentrated sodium chloride and sterile water look exactly alike. The pharmacy technician, accustomed to preparing the arterial fluid in glass bottles, selected what he thought was a 250 mL bottle of sterile water. He drew up appropriate amounts of heparin and sodium chloride to make the ordered solution and left the syringes for the pharmacist to check. The pharmacist checked each additive but failed to catch the error. The additives were injected into the glass bottle, and a patient label was placed completely over the manufacturer's label, hiding the identity of the base solution (23.4% sodium chloride).

When a pharmacy purchases products whose appearance has changed, all staff must be alerted to the change. Furthermore, storing concentrated electrolytes in the same vicinity as other solutions creates an opportunity for serious error. Pharmacies should consider purchasing single-use vials of concentrated electrolytes for IV admixture so that bulk bottles are not introduced into the production line. Shelves must be stocked so that labels face the person who will be selecting products for use.

COUNSELING PATIENTS

Counseling patients is an important component of the dispensing process. Medication error databases are replete with events, including fatalities, that could have been prevented had the pharmacist counseled the patient before dispensing a medication. Some of these errors are directly related to dispensing the wrong drug, dose, or dosage form or providing the wrong directions for use.

Studies have shown that up to 83% of dispensing errors can be discovered during patient counseling and corrected before the patient leaves the pharmacy.[3] By reviewing the prescribed product's indication, dose, and directions for use with the patient, the pharmacist can discover anything that does not match what the physician told the patient. Opening the prescription bottle gives the patient an opportunity to see the medication and speak up if it looks different than expected.

Counseling can also avert patients' mistakes in medication use. For example, a patient died after he misunderstood the directions for use and took methotrexate 2.5 mg every

12 hours for 6 consecutive days instead of 2.5 mg every 12 hours for three doses each week. Another patient died after he misread the directions on a prescription bottle and took 10 mg every morning instead of every Monday. One patient took extra doses of methotrexate as needed to relieve arthritic symptoms, but survived the overdosage.

Another common patient mistake that counseling could prevent is concomitant use of Wellbutrin and Zyban or either of these products and the generic bupropion, or, similarly, of Coumadin and warfarin. Warfarin tablets may look different from the branded Coumadin, and seeing different names on the prescription labels may lead patients to think they should take both. One patient who was taking Coumadin obtained a new prescription for warfarin and took both for 6 weeks before experiencing a subarachnoid hemorrhage.

All patients should receive counseling when picking up prescriptions. Counseling is especially important with new prescriptions for high-alert medications or medications for high-risk patients (e.g., the elderly, patients obtaining several medications at once, pediatric patients); some pharmacies flag these medications to ensure counseling. One pharmacy stamps a red "C" (counsel) on the bag of all such prescriptions, indicating that the clerk should call a pharmacist when the patient picks up the medication. Simply asking the patient, "Do you have any questions?" is insufficient. Another pharmacy places new prescriptions for high-alert medications (and others as appropriate) in a separate area; only a pharmacist can give these medications to patients or their caregivers. At first, patients may dislike having to wait another few minutes to see the pharmacist, but in the long run they will appreciate the benefit, realizing that an educated patient (or caregiver) is the final safety check in preventing medication errors.[20]

CLINICAL PHARMACY ACTIVITIES

Although dispensing traditionally has been pharmacists' primary role in the medication-use process, pharmacists today are recognized as integral members of an interdisciplinary team with shared responsibility for safe and optimal patient care. Particularly in inpatient settings, pharmacists working alongside prescribers and nurses have helped prevent medication errors. The direct involvement of pharmacists throughout the medication-use process can minimize the risk of preventable ADEs, reduce morbidity and mortality rates, decrease costs associated with patient care, and improve patient outcomes associated with drug use.[26–36]

It is well established that pharmacists' retrospective review of medication orders helps prevent errors;[37–39] when pharmacists provide input earlier, at the time of prescribing, their effect is greater.[27,30,31,33,34] The presence of a pharmacist on rounds as a full member of the patient care team in a medical intensive care unit was associated with a 66% decrease in preventable ADEs; nearly all (99%) of the pharmacists' interventions were readily accepted by physicians.[27] Pharmacist participation in physicians' rounds on general medical units, where patients often have many comorbid conditions, has been shown to reduce preventable ADEs by 78%.[35]

The mounting costs of drug therapy make a compelling argument for the use of pharmacists' clinical services. Numerous studies have demonstrated an economic gain for health care facilities in which pharmacists are integral members of the clinical care team.[27,28,31,32,34,40] In one study, 4,959 interventions by clinical pharmacists during a 12-month period resulted in direct cost savings of $92,076 and estimated cost avoidance (because interventions prevented a potential ADE) of $488,436.[26] The net economic gain to the facility was $393,660 after deduction of the cost of providing clinical pharmacy services. Table 10-1 shows examples of pharmacist interventions studied for their effects on clinical and economic outcomes.

Pharmacists working in patient care areas help guide medication prescribing and administration through activities such as those listed on pages 229–230. A busy internal

TABLE 10-1   Pharmacist Interventions Studied for Their Effects on Adverse Drug Events

Type of Intervention	Intervention Type as Percent of All Interventions in the Study[a]		
	Leape et al.[27]	Nesbit et al.[26]	Kucukarslan et al.[35]
Clarification or correction of an order	45	8	4
Provision of drug information	25	13	NS
Recommendation of alternative therapy			
–General	12		
–Dose adjustment/frequency		20[b]	35
–Alternative route		12	5
–Addition of drug to therapy			21
–Deletion of drug from therapy			7
–Therapeutic alternative/preferred agent			6
Identification of drug interaction	4	2	NS
Identification of "system error"	3	NS	NS
Therapeutic consultation	NS	21	NS
Pharmacokinetic consultation	NS	14	NS
Identification of potential problem with continuing therapy after discharge	NS	NS	8
Laboratory monitoring	NS	NS	6
Therapeutic duplication	NS	2	1

[a] NS =not specified.
[b] Renal.

ACTIVITIES OF PHARMACISTS IN PATIENT CARE AREAS

❑ Support the collection of essential patient information, including a complete drug history on new admissions.

❑ Assess the patient's ability to access medications and overall financial ability to obtain prescribed medications upon discharge.

❑ Participate in the verification of medications taken at home by patients and reconciliation of these medications with those prescribed during inpatient admissions.

❑ Review patient records for necessary information related to drug therapy.

❑ Provide direct input into drug selection (per formulary guidelines) and dosing, and communicate directly with physicians about problem orders.

❑ Assess the need for intravenous medications and recommend a change to oral administration when appropriate.

❑ Participate in patient care rounds and discharge planning rounds. (If necessary, limit rounds with specific physicians so that pharmacists are available to consult with physicians and nurses about all patients on the unit.)

❑ Initiate and carry out selected pharmacokinetic dosing, dose adjustments for renal or hepatic impairment, or other related dosing protocols (e.g., dose adjustments for hypoglycemic agents, aminoglycosides, epoetin, anticoagulants).

❑ Observe and guide drug administration practices (e.g., compatibility, drug administration precautions, use of drug delivery devices).

❑ Monitor the effects of particular classes of high-alert medications on patients (therapeutic tracking of patients on anticoagulants, antibiotics, and other selected drugs).

❑ Perform drug-use evaluations on high-risk or problem-prone medications identified by risk assessment activities.

❑ Support limitations and restrictions established for the prescribing, dispensing, and administration of particular medications.

- ❑ Communicate with the pharmacy to prioritize order processing, speed turnaround time, intervene regarding stat or missing medications, and provide timely notification of discontinued or changed drug therapy (e.g., IV to oral).
- ❑ Enter orders (especially orders for new admissions or high-alert, stat, and urgent medications) so medications can be screened for safety before they are removed from floor stock. (The order entry function should not simply be transferred to the patient care units. Order entry in patient care areas should be limited to priority orders. If the pharmacist on the patient care unit is responsible for entering most orders, his or her workload should allow considerable time for clinical activities. For entering orders, clinical pharmacists need a sufficient number of dedicated computer terminals located away from traffic, or wireless laptop computers.)
- ❑ Review prescribed therapy for inpatients before drugs are removed from floor stock and administered, when applicable.
- ❑ Enter important patient information into the pharmacy computer system (e.g., allergies, height, weight, age, comorbid conditions) so data are available for computer screening.
- ❑ Serve as a source of drug information when questions arise during the prescribing or administration of medications.
- ❑ Participate in patient education, particularly when high-alert medications have been prescribed or for patients being discharged on multiple medications.
- ❑ Oversee the safety of drug storage on patient care units.
- ❑ Educate physicians and nurses about new drugs added to the formulary and priority drug safety issues.
- ❑ Actively participate in professional staff (e.g., medical, nursing, respiratory therapy staff) orientation programs.
- ❑ Assist in the application of medication-use technology in patient care units (e.g., computerized prescriber order entry, point-of-care bar coding systems, automated dispensing cabinets, electronic medication administration records).
- ❑ Report adverse drug events in the method determined by the organization.

---

medicine unit may derive as much benefit from pharmacists' clinical services as would a critical care unit. Health care organizations should identify the patient care units in which pharmacists' presence will have the greatest impact on patient safety. Determining factors might include staffing patterns, staff expertise, the availability of drugs on the units, the types of patients served, the types of medications frequently prescribed and administered, the volume of new admissions and patient turnover, the typical volume of medication orders, and the type of drug distribution system used. Pharmacists should be present during peak hours when physicians make rounds and write orders. The greatest benefit from pharmacist review of orders can be achieved by focusing on the most critical and error-prone times in a patient's care: admission, postoperative care, changes in the level of care, and discharge.

In some facilities, pharmacists process physician orders on computer terminals located in patient care areas or satellite pharmacies; this has resulted in decreased error rates. In a disguised observational study, the medication error rate was 6.9% at a hospital in the United States, compared with 3% at a hospital in the United Kingdom, where pharmacists visited the wards several times daily to review each patient's chart.[41] Transcription was obviated by use of the same physical chart on which the physician ordered medications.

Interpersonal relationships are key to the success of pharmacists' clinical services and influence on patient care. The personality and cooperative spirit of both pharmacists and medical staff are critical factors, especially during the establishment of a clinical pharmacy program.[27] The results may be less than optimal if an interdisciplinary care model is not in place, or if nurses and medical staff do not perceive the important role pharmacists play in safe and effective medication use.

Effective communication between clinical pharmacists and the pharmacy staff providing distributive services is also essential. In some organizations, staff pharmacists rotate between clinical and distributive services. Where the clinical and distributive staffs are separate, they should meet regularly to collaborate on improvement strategies, understand their respective roles in the medication-use process, maintain strong working relationships, and promote the perception of a single, united pharmacy service. A daily, face-to-face report between clinical and distributive pharmacists to discuss anticipated admissions, pending orders, and any unresolved issues or problem areas may be useful.

Barriers to pharmacists' clinical interventions were identified by 600 respondents to a 2002 ISMP survey.[42] Lack of technology support, inadequate staffing, and an inefficient documentation process were cited most frequently. Most respondents reported that they had easy access to drug information (70%) and patient information (55%). Only 30% of all respondents believed pharmacists had sufficient clinical intervention skills, and 31% believed pharmacists were highly motivated to perform interventions.

These pharmacists, from hospitals of all types, indicated that the interventions most commonly performed were ensuring that orders were complete, checking allergies, and verifying doses. Fewer than one-third reported performing interventions on patient care units.

Overall, however, the respondents said prescribers responded well to pharmacists' interventions and accepted most of their recommendations. Two-thirds of the respondents said their hospitals had used pharmacy interventions to improve the prescribing process in the past year.

REFERENCES

1. Flynn E, Barker KN, Carnahan BJ. National observational study of prescription dispensing accuracy and safety in 50 pharmacies. *J Am Pharm Assoc*. 2003;43:191–200.
2. Davis NM, Cohen MR. Changing how pharmacists think about errors. *Am Pharm*. 1995; NS35(2):11, 46.
3. Ukens C. Deadly dispensing: an exclusive survey of Rx errors by pharmacists. *Drug Top*. March 13, 1997:100–11.
4. Fraher EP, Smith LM, Dyson S, et al. The Pharmacist Workforce in North Carolina. Report by the Cecil G. Sheps Center for Health Services Research, University of North Carolina at Chapel Hill, August 2002.
5. North Carolina Board of Pharmacy. Board Statement on Pharmacist Workload. March 26, 1997. Available at: www.ncbop.org/workload.htm. Accessed January 3, 2006.
6. Grasha A. A cognitive systems perspective on human performance in the pharmacy: implications for accuracy, effectiveness and job satisfaction. Executive Summary Report. Alexandria, Va: National Association of Chain Drug Stores; October 2000. Report No. 062100.
7. Grasha A. Misconceptions about pharmacy workload. *Can Pharm J*. 2001;134(3):26–35.
8. Medco Health. www.medco.com/medco/corporate/home.jsp?ltSess=y&articleID=CorpMedcoByMail. Accessed January 3, 2006.
9. Cohen MR, Davis NM. Pharmacy label mix-ups. *Am Pharm*. 1992;NS32(1):26–7.
10. Code of Federal Regulations. 14 CFR 121.542. Title 14: Aeronautics and Space, Chapter I: Federal Aviation Administration, Department of Transportation, Part 121: Operating requirements: Domestic, flag, and supplemental operations, Subpart T: Flight Operations, Section 121.542: Flight crewmember duties. Doc. No. 20661, 46 FR 5502, Jan. 19, 1981, Revised as of January 1, 2003. U.S. Government Printing Office. Available at: http://a257.g.akamaitech.net/7/257/2422/14mar20010800/edocket.access.gpo.gov/cfr_2003/14cfr121.542.htm. Accessed January 3, 2006.
11. Tranum D, Grasha AF. Susceptibility to illusions and cognitive style: implications for pharmacy dispensing. *Percept Mot Skills*. 2002;95(3 Pt 2):1063–86.
12. Caverly WM. Improving efficiencies and preventing dispensing errors [monograph]. Quebec, Canada: Efficient Pharmacy Institute; 2001. Available at: www.rxconference.org/rxconference/2002/Improving_Efficiences_and_Reducing.pdf. Accessed January 3, 2006.
13. Davis NM, Cohen MR. Learning lessons from dispensing errors. *Am Pharm*. 1994;NS34(5):27–8.

14. Institute for Safe Medication Practices. End the ice age; is glacial acetic acid really needed? *ISMP Medication Safety Alert! Acute Care Edition.* May 5, 2005.

15. Davis NM, Cohen MR. More look-alike and sound-alike errors. *Am Pharm.* 1993;NS33(10):32.

16. Trissel LA. *Handbook on Injectable Drugs.* 8th ed. Bethesda, Md: American Society of Hospital Pharmacists; 1994.

17. Trissel LA. *Handbook on Injectable Drugs.* 9th ed. Bethesda, Md: American Society of Health-System Pharmacists; 1996.

18. Trissel LA. *Handbook on Injectable Drugs.* 10th ed. Bethesda, Md: American Society of Health-System Pharmacists; 1998.

19. Nierenberg GI. *Do It Right the First Time.* New York: John Wiley and Sons; 1996.

20. Davis NM. Drug names that look and sound alike. *Hosp Pharm.* 1999;34:1160–78.

21. Institute for Safe Medication Practices. Safety still compromised by computer weaknesses. Comparing 1999 and 2005 pharmacy computer field test results. *ISMP Medication Safety Alert!* August 25, 2005.

22. Joint Commission on Accreditation of Healthcare Organizations. *Comprehensive Accreditation Manual for Hospitals—The Official Handbook.* Oak Brook Terrace, Ill: 1998:TX.3.5–TX.3.5.2.

23. Institute for Safe Medication Practices. Safety briefs. *ISMP Medication Safety Alert!* May 6, 1998.

24. Rothschild JM, Keohane CA, Cook EF, et al. A controlled trial of smart infusion pumps to improve medication safety in critically ill patients. *Crit Care Med.* 2005;33:533–40.

25. Institute for Safe Medication Practices. Unfortunately, this time it wasn't the equipment. *ISMP Medication Safety Alert! Acute Care Edition.* October 6, 2005.

26. Nesbit TW, Shermock KM, Bobek MB, et al. Implementation and pharmacoeconomic analysis of a clinical staff pharmacist practice model. *Am J Health Syst Pharm;* 2001;58:784–90.

27. Leape LL, Cullen DJ, Clapp MD, et al. Pharmacist participation on physician rounds and adverse drug events in the intensive care unit. *JAMA.* 1999;282:267–70.

28. Schumock GT, Meek PD, Ploetz PA, et al. Economic evaluations of clinical pharmacy services—1988–1995. *Pharmacotherapy.* 1996;16:1188–208.

29. Bond CA, Raehl CL, Franke T. Clinical pharmacy services and hospital mortality rates. *Pharmacotherapy.* 1999;19:556–64.

30. Bond CA, Raehl CL, Pitterle ME, et al. Health care professional staffing, hospital characteristics, and hospital mortality rates. *Pharmacotherapy.* 1999;19:130–8.

31. Bond CA, Raehl CL, Franke T. Clinical pharmacy services, clinical staffing, and drug costs in United States hospitals. *Pharmacotherapy.* 1999;19:1354–62.

32. Bond CA, Raehl CL, Franke T. Clinical pharmacy services, pharmacy staffing, and the total cost of care in United States hospitals. *Pharmacotherapy.* 2000;20:609–21.

33. Bjornson DC, Hiner WO, Potyk RP, et al. Effect of pharmacists on health care outcomes in hospitalized patients. *Am J Hosp Pharm.* 1993;50:1875–84.

34. Boyko WL Jr, Yurkowski PJ, Ivey MF, et al. Pharmacist influence on economic and morbidity outcomes in a tertiary care teaching hospital. *Am J Health Syst Pharm.* 1997;54:1591–5.

35. Kucukarslan SN, Peters M, Mlynarek M, et al. Pharmacists on rounding teams reduce preventable adverse drug events in hospital general medicine units. *Arch Intern Med.* 2003;163:2014–8.

36. Kaboli PJ, Hoth AB, McClimon BJ, et al. Clinical pharmacists and inpatient medical care: a systematic review. *Arch Intern Med.* 2006;166:955–64.

37. Folli HL, Poole RL, Benitz WE, et al. Medication error prevention by clinical pharmacists in two children's hospitals. *Pediatrics.* 1987;79:718–22.

38. Broyles JE, Brown RO, Vehe KL, et al. Pharmacist interventions improve fluid balance in fluid-restricted patients requiring parenteral nutrition. *Ann Pharmacother.* 1991;25:119–22.

39. Kilroy RA, Iafrate RP. Provision of pharmaceutical care in the intensive care unit. *Crit Care Nurs Clin North Am.* 1993;5:221–5.

40. Mutnick AH, Sterba KJ, Peroutka JA, et al. Cost savings and avoidance from clinical interventions. *Am J Health Syst Pharm.* 1997;54:392–6.

41. Dean BS, Allan EL, Barber ND, et al. Comparison of medication errors in an American and a British hospital. *Am J Health Syst Pharm.* 1995;52:2543–9.

42. Institute for Safe Medication Practices. Pharmacy interventions can reduce clinical errors. *ISMP Medication Safety Alert!* June 26, 2002. Available at: www.ismp.org/Newsletters/acutecare/articles/20020626.asp.

APPENDIX

PRINCIPLES OF DESIGNING MEDICATION LABELS FOR PATIENT-SPECIFIC INPATIENT USE

Poorly designed labels can increase the risk of medication error. To prevent errors related to misinterpretation of labels, ISMP offers the following recommendations, which are based on analysis of actual medication errors reported, a survey, and a review of pharmacy-generated labels produced by a number of systems. *Except where noted, the recommendations presented here pertain to both oral solids and oral liquids.*

1. Use bold type for the **patient name, generic drug name,** and **patient-specific dose** on all labels.

2. For all products, use the generic name, in lowercase letters, as the primary drug nomenclature (unless tall-man letters are used as a safety strategy), ensuring that each name matches FDA-approved nomenclature. As appropriate, list associated brand names in a requisite field, in all uppercase letters (e.g., LASIX) to differentiate them from generic names, ensuring that all product labels match the way the drug name appears on the original order and medication administration record. Trademark symbols (e.g., ™ or ®) should not be used. For medications that contain multiple ingredients, use the brand name to provide clarification and reduce the risk of error.

3. Use tall-man letters (e.g., hydrOXYzine and hydrALAZINE) to help distinguish look-alike products on screens and reports in order to minimize the risk of selecting the wrong product when medication names appear alphabetically in look-up lists. Establish and disseminate a list of products for which tall-man letters are used, specifying which letters are affected, to ensure standard application for all uses (see Table 6-1).

4. Do not include the salt of the chemical when expressing a generic name, unless there are multiple salts available (e.g., hydroxyzine hydrochloride and hydroxyzine pamoate). If the salt is listed as part of the name (e.g., USP-approved abbreviations such as K, Na, HBr, and HCl), it should follow the drug name, not precede it (e.g., hydroxyzine HCl, not HCl hydroxyzine).

5. *Pertains only to oral solids:* Express suffixes that are part of the brand name (e.g., SR, SA, CR) within both the generic name field and the brand name field (e.g., diltiazem XT and DILTIA XT).

6. If state law prohibits printing the brand name when the specific brand is not dispensed, then the words "used for" may be inserted before the brand name.

7. The frequency of administration may be displayed, if available and desirable; if used, it should appear in 10-point, light-face (not bold) type.

8. Use Arial, Verdana, or an equivalent typeface for all text and numbers.

9. Minimum type size for the patient name, generic drug name, and patient-specific dose should be 12 point or equivalent.

10. Allow for text wrap and continuation on an additional label (expandable label stock) to accommodate large numbers of characters for drug names, patient names, or doses. Set parameters so that breaks in patient or medication names are intelligible.

11. Set the comments field with a minimum capacity for 250 characters. The printing of order comments must support carriage returns within the note to allow formatting of tabular data such as dosing nomograms. The minimum type size should be 10 point or equivalent.

12. Use a white background color for labels for better visualization of the text and bar codes (when applicable). Use black for all bar codes. If a different-colored label is needed to highlight certain classes of high-alert drugs (e.g., chemotherapeutic agents), use yellow label stock.

13. When the drug name, strength, dosage form, and dosage units appear together, avoid confusion by providing a space between them (e.g., propranolol20 mg has been misread as 120 mg and 10Units has been misread as 100 Units).

14. Provide adequate space in the data fields for drug name, dosing units, route of administration, and frequency. Using two- or three-character fields forces the use of potentially dangerous abbreviations (q.d. for daily, often misread as q.i.d.; q.o.d. for every other day, often misread as q.i.d.; U for units, often misread as a zero or four). Seeing dangerous abbreviations in electronic formats may encourage practitioners to use them. The fields for route of administration and for frequency should have space for a sufficient number of characters to clearly communicate the intended route and frequency.

15. Ensure that the application and the printer support both uppercase and lowercase fonts, characters that drop below the lower line (such as lowercase y and g), and mixed cases within a line or format to allow tall-man lettering when indicated, or doses per square meter (such as 100 mg/m^2).

16. Avoid the use of all potentially dangerous abbreviations and dose expressions (see Table 8-3).

17. Consideration must be given to the role that symbols and certain letters may play in creating errors during electronic communication. For example, slash marks and hyphens have been misread as the number one, and symbols for more than and less than (> and <) are frequently misinterpreted as the opposite of what was intended. Also, the letter O can be misread as a zero (0), the letter z as the number 2, and a lowercase L (l) as the number 1 or the letter i (I).

18. To avoid confusion, do not abbreviate drug names (e.g., MTX for methotrexate has been misunderstood as mitoxantrone; MSO$_4$ for morphine sulfate has been misinterpreted as magnesium sulfate). The field for drug names should be large enough for a sufficient number of characters to prevent truncating drug names, whether single entity or multi-ingredient.

19. All *combination products* should include the brand name on the label. If a product contains two ingredients, they should both appear in the generic name field. If the product contains more than two generic ingredients, the two primary ingredients should be placed in the generic field, followed by the words "and others."

20. When the drug name, patient dose, dosage form, and dosage units appear together, the generic name should be listed first, followed by the brand name, patient dose, dosage units, and dosage form (e.g., propranolol [INDERAL] 5 mg oral solution):

propranolol (INDERAL) **5 mg Oral Solution**

Dose = 5 mg/1.25 mL
Conc. = 4 mg/mL

When the patient dose of an oral solid and the tablet strength differ, also list the amount needed for the dose; fractions should be displayed in fraction format, not as 1 slash 2 (1/2). For example,

propranolol (INDERAL) **5 mg Oral**

Dose = ½ × 10 mg tablet

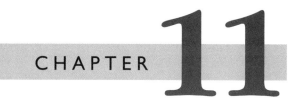

PREVENTING DRUG ADMINISTRATION ERRORS

Judy L. Smetzer and Michael R. Cohen

In addition to their highly visible role of administering patients' medications, nurses in health care organizations perform other important functions that support safe medication use:[1]

- Obtaining and documenting the patient's medication history;
- Reconciling the medications prescribed upon admission, transfer, and discharge;
- Transmitting orders to pharmacy;
- Transcribing orders and verifying orders on the medication administration record (MAR);
- Documenting medication administration;
- Assessing patients' response to medications and notifying prescribers; and
- Educating patients and families about medication use.

Also, information provided by nurses helps other members of the health care team to choose patients' drug therapy, evaluate orders, and prepare medications. These complex interactions among nurses, other clinicians, and patients suggest that an interdisciplinary approach to medication use is needed. The team of nurses, physicians, pharmacists, unit secretaries, pharmacy technicians, respiratory therapists, and others must ensure that systems are in place within the organization to support safe medication use.

This chapter discusses system-based causes of drug administration errors and nurses' role, as part of an interdisciplinary team, in reducing medication errors.

OBTAINING PATIENT INFORMATION

To safely administer medication to a patient, the nurse must know the patient's identification, age, weight, height, current medications, allergies, diagnoses, laboratory and diagnostic test results, pregnancy and lactation status, and vital signs. Health care providers should also know the patient's cultural influences and ability to read instructions and labels and to purchase medications. Lack of access to any of this information can contribute to errors.

Age, Weight, and Height

Dosages of many medications, including antithrombotic and chemotherapeutic agents, are based on the patient's weight, height, or age. For example, pediatric drug dosages often are based on weight. Doses of cancer chemotherapy may be based on body surface area. Dosage adjustment may be needed for elderly patients.

Dosages based on weight can be optimal only when accurate weights are obtained. Estimates by the patient or family are often unreliable. One patient with deep vein thrombosis purposely understated her weight as 160 pounds in the emergency department (ED) so that her husband would not know her actual weight of 180 pounds. Although this 20-pound difference may not have caused a problem with her antithrombotic dosage, discrepancies of up to 100 pounds between a patient's stated weight and measured weight have been reported.

All patients should be weighed upon initial assessment, and height should be measured. Weights should be documented in one standard measurement unit, preferably kilograms. In the ED, all walk-in patients should be weighed during triage. Bedridden patients can be weighed on stretchers with built-in scales. For patients whose weight can be expected to change (e.g., children, the elderly, oncology patients), a standard routine for reweighing should be established.

Diagnoses

Knowing a patient's diagnoses can prevent errors, particularly with drugs whose names look or sound alike. Nurses are less likely to make an error if they match patients' medications to their diagnoses and ensure that each drug's intended purpose makes sense for the patient. Each time nurses administer a medication, they should mention the drug's purpose so that the patient can question anything unusual.

Pregnancy and Lactation Status

A number of drugs that can cross the placental membrane are considered teratogenic, or capable of causing developmental abnormalities in utero. Examples include Accutane (isotretinoin), for the treatment of acne, and sulfonamides. The particular developmental abnormality depends on the type of teratogen and when it interacts with the fetus.[2] Most organ development occurs during the first 3 months of gestation, so the first trimester is the time of greatest risk. Nurses should ask whether the patient is attempting to conceive or might be pregnant.

Almost all drugs transfer into breast milk. The risk to the infant depends on a particular drug's effects and the dose received.[3] Many medications are considered safe for use by breastfeeding mothers, but nurses should always ask mothers with young children whether they are lactating.

Allergies

Some 550,000 serious allergic reactions to medications occur annually in hospitals.[4] The greatest number of allergy-associated deaths in the United States each year are caused by medications; reactions to penicillin account for 75% of the deaths attributable to drug allergies.[5,6] Other drugs known to cause severe allergic responses include opioids, sulfonamide anti-infectives, medications for seizures and arrhythmias, nonsteroidal anti-inflammatory drugs (NSAIDs), vaccines, antihypertensives, insulin, and radiocontrast media.

Even if patients have been asked about allergies, nurses may not think of possible cross-allergies, such as between aspirin and NSAIDs (e.g., ketorolac). There are numerous reports of nurses administering NSAIDs to patients with a known aspirin allergy, sometimes with fatal results.

Allergies may also escape detection when products contain two or more medications. For example, it may not be readily apparent that Vicodin contains hydrocodone and acetaminophen or that Percodan contains oxycodone and aspirin. Some of the medications most often involved in serious allergic reactions—most notably NSAIDs and combination products that contain NSAIDs—are sold without prescription in community pharmacies and may be kept as floor stock in inpatient settings. These medications may not be included in pharmacists' screen for a patient's allergies. In inpatient settings, an opioid could be administered from floor stock before a pharmacist has screened the order.

During drug administration, nurses must also consider latex allergy. Some drug delivery catheters are coated with latex, and the rubber stopper on some vials may contain latex.

Nurses should ask patients to describe the type of allergic reaction they have experienced. Patients often refer to adverse drug effects such as nausea or fatigue as allergies; such effects (intolerance to a medication or food) should be documented but should not be grouped with allergies. All allergy information should be prominently documented on the patient's MAR and in a standard location in the patient's medical record. For inpatients, a colored armband can be used to alert nurses to an allergy. The armband should not contain information about the specific allergy; rather, it reminds the nurse to check the patient's chart before administering medications. Also helpful are charts of common cross-allergies and the ingredients of combination products; these can be placed in areas where medications are prepared and administered.

Current Medications

Obtaining a list of all medications used by a newly admitted patient, including herbals, vitamins, and nonprescription products, can be a challenge. Patients and their families often cannot accurately report all of their medications and dosages. They may be reluctant to report the use of herbals or other home remedies. Previous medical records may not be up-to-date. The nurse or pharmacist may need to call physicians' offices or outpatient pharmacies to correctly identify the patient's medications.

Poor communication about medications at transition points—admission, transfer, and discharge—is responsible for up to 50% of all medication errors and 20% of adverse drug events in hospitals.[7] For this reason, a National Patient Safety Goal (NPSG) of the Joint Commission on Accreditation of Healthcare Organizations (JCAHO) asks hospitals to compare a list of the patient's home medications with medications ordered upon admission and reconcile any discrepancies. Each time a patient moves from one setting to another, the new medication orders and plan of care must be compared with the previous medication orders, and any discrepancies must be resolved. The patient's discharge orders must be compared and reconciled with the most recent inpatient medication orders and the original list of medications taken at home. Nurses often have a major role in this reconciliation process.

A list of medications taken at home can be obtained during the preadmission process from patients undergoing an elective surgical or other invasive procedure. Thus, the patient can be questioned about any medications or herbals that might interact with medications administered during the procedure or cause an adverse outcome. For example, aspirin, warfarin, and other anticoagulants must be discontinued before most surgical procedures. Some herbs can accelerate heart rate (e.g., ephedra), inhibit blood clotting (e.g., ginkgo, garlic), alter the immune system (e.g., echinacea), and change the effects and duration of anesthesia (e.g., kava).[8]

IDENTIFYING THE PATIENT

Errors that result in administration of medications to the wrong patient can originate in any phase of the medication-use process. Physicians may order a medication for the wrong patient, unit secretaries or nurses may transcribe the order onto the wrong patient's MAR, and pharmacists may enter a medication into the wrong patient profile. However, the most common image of a "wrong patient" error is the nurse giving one patient's medication to another patient. Errors of this type tend to occur when more than one patient's medications are prepared for administration at the same time and when a nurse is caring for two patients in the same room.

Medications have also been prescribed for or administered to the wrong patient after mix-ups in patients' test results. In one case, a physician prescribed Cardizem (diltiazem) 20 mg IV followed by 30 mg orally for a patient in bed A after a telemetry unit nurse reported that the patient's cardiac monitor showed atrial fibrillation and flutter with a heart rate of 140. The patient's heart rate and rhythm did not change after receiving the medication, so the nurse called the physician again and received an order to administer 150 mg of amiodarone IV push followed by a 60 mg per hour infusion. A short time later, the nurse realized that the rhythm she was viewing on the monitor at the nurses' station was for the patient in bed B. The names of the patients in bed A and bed B had been mixed up and posted on the wrong channel of the central monitoring unit at the nurses' station.

A spoken affirmation of the patient's name does not replace the need for reading the patient's armband. One patient received her roommate's medications after she misheard the nurse's pronunciation of her roommate's name and verified that she was, indeed, her roommate.

In outpatient settings, where identification bracelets may not be used, nurses typically rely on patients to verify their identification. However, one oncology clinic patient, tired of waiting for his turn, responded when the name of another patient was called. He assumed that all patients in the clinic received the same therapy. The patient's wife clarified his identification, and he did not receive the wrong chemotherapy.

Since 2003, JCAHO has required health care organizations to use at least two unique patient identifiers (name, birth date, identification number, but not the patient's room number) whenever taking blood samples or administering medications or blood products. This requirement, initiated as an NPSG, has been a standard since 2004 and applies to both inpatient and outpatient settings.

The patient's MAR should be taken to the bedside for the required verification of patient identifiers. Even when this process is used, an error can occur. Two infants' MARs were mixed up, resulting in administration of Synagis (palivizumab), used to prevent respiratory syncytial virus, to the wrong child. The infants were in adjacent isolettes, and both infants' MARs were on the counter between the two isolettes. The infants had the same first name, similar last names, and nearly identical hospital identification numbers. The nurse administered a dose of Synagis to the wrong infant after failing to notice that she was referring to the wrong MAR.

System changes can make patient identification easier. Patients can help prevent errors if they are educated about the need to identify themselves—even if staff is well known to them—by holding out their name bracelets, spelling their names, and giving their birth dates (especially if their last name is common).

Unit dose medications should be kept in manufacturer or pharmacy packaging up to the point of administration. Nurses can show patients the packages and open them at the bedside while stating the drug's name, dose, and purpose. Patients who are educated about their drug therapy can then alert staff to potential errors. Point-of-care bar-code systems can also help confirm accurate drug administration to the correct patient; the drug dose and the patient's identification band are scanned for verification.

Outpatient settings can use name bracelets or provide registration cards listing name, record number, and birth date for routine clinic patients, such as oncology patients. Photographs of long-term patients can be used on their registration cards. Before administering medications, nurses can use the cards to find two patient identifiers, rather than relying solely on a spoken response to a patient's name.

MONITORING THE PATIENT

Nurses and other caregivers must continually evaluate the effects of medications to ensure both efficacy and safety. For example, vital signs and level of consciousness can be monitored to evaluate the effectiveness of cardiac medications, antihypertensives, and analgesics. Pain scales are frequently used to evaluate the effectiveness of analgesics, but the patient's level of sedation and risk of oversedation cannot be evaluated with a pain scale alone.

Many health systems, spurred by 2001 JCAHO pain management standards, have made patient comfort a high priority, but the need for safety is equally compelling. Although patients are still undertreated for pain,[9] error reports suggest occasional over-aggressive attempts to ensure that patients experience no discomfort.

For example, a 24-year-old woman died from fentanyl toxicity less than 24 hours after giving birth by cesarean section. She had been given several doses of fentanyl IV before and after the birth. That evening, she fed and cared for her daughter. In the early morning, she again complained of pain and the dose of fentanyl was increased. She asked for a blanket 30 minutes later; in another 30 minutes she was found in cardiac arrest.

Oversedation can be linked to insufficient patient monitoring. Too often pain scores are elicited but not reevaluated after each dose of analgesic. Respiratory rates are counted, but depth and quality may not be considered. Treatment and monitoring may not be altered for patients with a history of sleep apnea. The cumulative effects of narcotics given at the end of a surgical procedure and then again in the postanesthesia care unit (PACU) may not be considered, especially after the patient is transferred out of the PACU.

A serious problem is orders for multiple pain management options with routes and dosages based on the patient's assessment of pain. A patient may be prescribed acetaminophen 650 mg by mouth every 4 hours for pain scale 1 to 3; codeine 30 mg by mouth every 4 hours for pain scale 4 to 6; morphine 2 mg IV every 3 hours for pain scale 7 or 8; and morphine 4 mg IV every 4 hours for pain scale 9 or 10. If a patient with a low threshold for pain reports discomfort on the high end of the scale, the nurse may administer morphine at the higher dose without careful consideration of the patient's clinical status and the cumulative effects of drug therapy. If a patient with a high threshold for pain rates his discomfort on the low end of the pain scale, the nurse may simply administer acetaminophen.

Although clinicians' judgment should not be substituted for patient self-reports of pain, a nurse's objective evaluation of patient response to medication and safety considerations must be integrated with the patient's assessment of pain.

Diagnostic data such as lab results can indicate the effects of medications or signal that a medication is contraindicated. If determination of the serum concentration of a drug is ordered, the result should be reviewed before the next dose is given. Platelet counts must be evaluated to quickly detect and treat heparin-induced thrombocytopenia. Complete blood counts must be monitored for patients receiving cancer chemotherapy so that doses can be postponed if necessary.

Nurses need to know the patient's most recent international normalized ratio (INR) for anticoagulant monitoring before administering a dose of warfarin, and the patient's blood glucose level before administering insulin or another antidiabetic medication. A flow sheet for recording each dose of medication and corresponding lab values allows nurses to review previously administered doses and track the patient's overall response to therapy.

Accurate communication of diagnostic results is necessary to avoid erroneous decisions about drug therapy. A JCAHO NPSG addresses this issue: When critical test results are spoken aloud in person or by telephone, the receiving clinician must verify the results by reading back the transcribed information. Each organization must define critical test results. Although organizations may not think of blood glucose determinations at the patient's bedside by a hand-held glucometer as critical test results, they should define high and low readings that would be considered critical and should be communicated.

The following example illustrates how errors in communicating results can lead to patient harm. After performing bedside glucose testing, a nursing assistant told a nurse that the patient's blood sugar was 217 mg/dL. Thinking the aide was talking about a different patient, the nurse administered a sliding-scale dose of insulin to a patient whose blood sugar was just 116 mg/dL. The error was soon recognized, and the patient was fed and monitored. Another nurse saw a list of several patients, with a number next to each name. All of the numbers were above 200, and the nurse thought they were blood glucose levels. She gave each patient a dose of insulin according to a sliding-scale protocol. She later realized that the numbers were patient room numbers.

Each health care provider must determine the safest way to receive, document, communicate, and verify glucose meter readings. In some hospitals, nursing assistants record the readings onto flow sheets or MARs. In others, the nurse responsible for administering insulin performs the glucose monitoring.

COMMUNICATING PATIENT INFORMATION TO PHARMACY

In inpatient settings, nurses can supply crucial patient information to pharmacists so they can properly screen all medication orders before dispensing products. Pharmacists should know a patient's diagnoses, weight, height, allergies, and other information such as the patient's nothing-by-mouth (NPO) status or inability to swallow tablets. Knowing a patient's chronic conditions can help a pharmacist avoid mistaking a prescribed medication for a look-alike medication that has a different indication.

The pharmacy can initially receive information by computer, in the admission orders, or in a faxed admission assessment form or other such patient information document. Pharmacists will also need follow-up information (e.g., daily weights).

Nurses who telephone prescriptions to community pharmacies can provide the same types of information. Often this is the only way for pharmacists to obtain crucial information about the patient.

DRUG AND DOSING INFORMATION

To safely administer medications, nurses need access to reliable drug information. During morning medication administration to several patients, a nurse might need to know

- The typical dose and route of administration for a new medication recently added to the formulary,
- The compatibility of a piggyback medication with the primary IV solution,
- The typical dose in milligrams per kilogram of a common analgesic prescribed for a pediatric patient,
- The correct dose of an IV opioid, on the basis of the oral dose the patient was taking before admission,
- How fast an IV push medication can be administered safely,
- Whether a medication can be crushed for administration, and
- The rate of infusion for heparin.[1]

Improving access to drug information is a key principle of safe medication use.

Drug and Herbal References

Nurses must have an up-to-date drug reference book or electronic database and a textbook or reliable Internet source for information on herbal products. References that are not up-to-date may lack new information on incompatibilities, adverse events, and changes in drug administration practices, as well as information on new products. Budgets should allow nurse managers to provide a sufficient number of standardized medication and herbal references annually. Outdated texts should be discarded. As a rule, nurses should not bring personal references, which may be outdated, to work. Electronic references that are updated frequently, either online (e.g., Micromedex, Lexi-Comp) or on a personal digital assistant (PDA) (e.g., ePocrates, Davis's Drug Guide), should also be available to nurses.

Dosing Guidelines

In addition to a basic drug information book or electronic database, several tools and principles can help nurses avoid harmful dosing errors.

Dosing Charts

Dose determination charts can eliminate the need for error-prone mathematical calculations. When standard concentrations of medications and solutions are used, as recommended for safety, charts can be used to determine a dose or infusion rate. Pharmacists should provide nurses with approved and updated dosing charts and should affix labels to IV solution containers that clearly list the total amount of drug in the container, volume of diluent, and concentration. The pharmacy can also apply computer-generated or commercially printed labels that include dosing tables.

No More Than Two

It is unusual for a single dose to be composed of more than two or three dosage units (e.g., tablets, capsules, vials), and nurses should question all orders that exceed that number. If a dose does require several tablets or capsules, pharmacists can often formulate it into a single dosage unit to make it easier for the patient to swallow. The same principle applies to the preparation of IV solutions. If more than two or three dosage units are needed to prepare the solution, this may signal an error, as in the following example:

While the pharmacy was closed at night, an intensive care unit (ICU) nurse prepared what she believed to be a 25 mg per 250 mL infusion of phenylephrine. The vials of phenylephrine stated, in bold print, "1%." The drug name and "10 mg/mL" appeared in smaller print that was partially obscured by a colored band. The nurse thought each vial contained 1 mg and prepared the infusion by using 25 vials (250 mg). A nurse on the next shift hung the infusion. Shortly thereafter, the patient's systolic blood pressure rose to 208 mm Hg. The nurse suspected that something was wrong with the infusion; after she remade and hung the infusion, the patient's systolic blood pressure decreased to 100 mm Hg. Upon investigation, the 25 empty vials were found in the trash.

Change in Dose with Change in Route

A change in route may require a change in dose. When a patient who has been NPO becomes able to ingest oral medications, or when a patient previously taking oral medication is placed on NPO status, medication doses may change because the bioavailability of most medications is higher when they are given intravenously.

For example, levothyroxine is only 50% bioavailable when given orally; a patient who is switched from the oral to the IV route with no change in the dosage will, in effect, receive twice the necessary dose. Opioid analgesics are another example. Prescribing errors have been reported when physicians were not aware that the oral dose and the IV dose of most opioid analgesics are quite different. In one case, a physician covering for an oncologist admitted a patient with Hodgkin's lymphoma to a medical unit. At home, the patient had been taking hydromorphone (Dilaudid) 2 to 4 mg orally for pain. The covering physician prescribed the same medication but also wrote an order for hydromorphone 2 to 4 mg IV every 3 hours for pain if the patient was unable to tolerate oral fluids. The generally accepted oral to IV conversion of hydromorphone is 3 to 5 mg of oral product for every 1 mg IV. A nurse administered 4 mg IV; the patient developed respiratory depression and became unresponsive. Two IV doses of naloxone reversed the effects of the medication. To help prevent errors, pharmacy could create an oral-to-IV conversion chart for opioids and other narcotics and post it on patient care units where physicians prescribe and nurses prepare these medications.

Doses Expressed as a Ratio or Percentage

The concentration of most injectable medications is expressed in milligrams per milliliter or micrograms per milliliter, but concentrations of a few drugs are expressed as a dilution ratio (e.g., epinephrine 1:1,000) or percentage (e.g., lidocaine 1%). Physicians and other practitioners may not know how to accurately calculate dosages expressed as ratios or percentages.[10–12] There may be little risk in expressing concentrations of topical products and local anesthetics in this way, but harmful errors have occurred with IV medications. Practitioners have administered undiluted epinephrine 1:1,000 (1 mg/mL) IV to patients instead of using the 1:10,000 (0.1 mg/mL) concentration. A nurse in radiology who infrequently administered medications made such a mistake. When her patient had an adverse reaction to the contrast medium, with visible hives and respiratory distress, the physician prescribed 3 mL of epinephrine 1:10,000 IV. The nurse administered the 1:1,000 concentration, not understanding the difference. The two concentrations are hard to distinguish; on the small label, 1:1,000 could look like 1:10,000.

Many drugs used for resuscitation (e.g., calcium, epinephrine, lidocaine, magnesium sulfate, neostigmine, sodium bicarbonate) have these unusual expressions of concentration. To avoid an inappropriate dose or a life-threatening delay in treatment, the pharmacy could create a dose conversion chart for all concentrations of epinephrine, lidocaine, calcium, magnesium sulfate, sodium bicarbonate, and other emergency drugs whose concentrations are expressed as a dilution ratio or percentage. The charts could be posted on code carts and in other areas where emergency medications are prepared and administered. The charts should be reviewed as part of training in cardiopulmonary resuscitation. If possible, facilities should store a single concentration of these drugs (e.g., a code cart might contain epinephrine in 1:10,000 prefilled 10 mL syringes only). If more than one concentration must be available, warning labels should be used to alert staff to the different concentrations. Bold labels should be affixed to epinephrine 1:1,000 ampuls to warn nurses to dilute the drug before IV use.

Liposomal Products

Some medications, such as the antifungal amphotericin B and the antineoplastics doxorubicin and daunorubicin, are available in both conventional and liposomal formulations. Dosages are not interchangeable between the two types of formulations. Liposomal drugs have enhanced activity because the medication, entrapped in synthetic fat globules, can circulate in the bloodstream for several hours after injection and selectively accumulate at the targeted disease site. As a result, healthy cells are shielded from the drug's toxic effects, less medication is concentrated in vulnerable tissues such as the kidneys and liver, and adverse effects (e.g., nausea, fatigue, hair loss) of cancer drugs are often lessened.

Confusion between liposomal and conventional forms of the same drug has resulted in serious patient harm, including death. Doses of conventional amphotericin B desoxycholate (Amphocin, Fungizone) should not exceed 1.5 mg/kg/day, while doses of the liposomal form (Abelcet, Amphotec, Ambisome) are higher but vary from product to product. In one case, while the pharmacy was closed, a nurse retrieved seven 50 mg vials of conventional amphotericin B instead of what was actually ordered: 350 mg of the liposomal form, Abelcet. The result was a fatal overdosage.

Conventional doxorubicin hydrochloride (Adriamycin) and liposomal doxorubicin (Doxil) are dosed differently and administered differently, although both are given at 3- or 4-week intervals. Giving the liposomal form by IV push, without further dilution, can lead to serious harm. In one case, conventional doxorubicin 35 mg was prescribed, but the dose was prepared using the liposomal form, Doxil. The nurse noticed that the red medication in the syringe appeared cloudy (both forms are red, but the conventional product is clear). However, since the pharmacist and another nurse had already checked the drug, the nurse decided to administer it IV push, as prescribed. When the patient became cyanotic, the nurse quickly realized the mistake and stopped administering the medication, averting further harm.

To help prevent errors, the pharmacy should provide patient care areas with a list of drugs for which there are both liposomal and conventional forms, with notations about dosing differences. All antineoplastics and other products available in both liposomal and conventional forms should be stored in and dispensed by the pharmacy to preserve a system of double-checking by pharmacists and nurses. Physicians should be encouraged to include the brand name when prescribing liposomal products; this is necessary for liposomal amphotericin B because various brands are dosed differently. Both the brand and generic names should be listed on MARs, as should "liposomal form." The pharmacy should add bold cautionary labels to liposomal products (e.g., "Doxil, **liposomal** doxorubicin"). An independent double check before administering all chemotherapy, amphotericin B, and liposomal forms of other medications is highly advisable. If staff, patients, or family members notice a change in the medication's appearance from previous doses, nurses should stop and verify that the correct drug is being used.

Adverse Drug Reactions

The Food and Drug Administration (FDA) defines a suspected adverse drug reaction (ADR) as "a noxious and unintended response to any dose of a drug for which there is a reasonable possibility that the product caused the response."[13] ADRs result in more than 100,000 deaths annually.[4] Approximately 7% of hospitalized patients are affected by ADRs, about 50% of which occur before hospital admission.[4] These statistics do not include ADRs that occur in long-term care facilities or outside organized health care settings.

The drugs most commonly implicated in ADRs include antimicrobials, NSAIDs (including aspirin), diuretics, warfarin, and cytoxics, and the most common reaction is an allergy or gastrointestinal bleeding.[14] Fatal ADRs in children have most often involved anticonvulsants, cytotoxics, and antibiotics, and the most common reaction has been hepatic failure.[4,15] Patients sometimes report symptoms they have experienced since taking a new medicine, but it is typically nurses, pharmacists, and physicians who identify ADRs.

One ADR that nurses should be attuned to is methemoglobinemia induced by benzocaine topical sprays such Cetacaine (benzocaine 14%, tetracaine 2%) and Hurricaine (benzocaine 20%). This life-threatening condition is characterized by abnormal levels of oxidized hemoglobin.[16] The oxidized hemoglobin binds so firmly with oxygen that little oxygen is available to tissues. Normally, methemoglobin accounts for 1% of circulating hemoglobin. Cyanosis occurs as the level rises above 10%. Anxiety, fatigue, and tachycardia appear at levels between 20% and 50%. With levels ranging from 50% to 70%, coma and death may result.

About 100 life-threatening cases of methemoglobinemia related to benzocaine have been reported to FDA.[16] With millions of doses of topical anesthetics used annually for intubation, endoscopy, and other procedures, this ADR probably occurs far more often than reported. In most reported cases, clinicians have used multiple sprays of benzocaine-containing products, or sprays of longer duration than recommended, forgetting that the benzocaine is absorbed systemically.

Prompt recognition and treatment can be a challenge. Pulse oximetry readings can be normal when methemoglobin levels are significantly elevated, and arterial blood gas readings may not be helpful in diagnosing the condition. An arterial blood sample for co-oximetry, which directly measures methemoglobin levels, is needed for evaluation. Methemoglobinemia should always be considered if cyanosis develops after application of topical anesthetics, even if pulse oximetry readings are normal. The brown appearance of arterial blood also provides a clue.

Some patients may be predisposed to methemoglobinemia: infants under 6 months of age, elderly patients with cardiac problems, and patients with altered hemoglobin, such as those with glucose-6-phosphate dehydrogenase (G6PD) deficiency or methemoglobin reductase enzyme deficiency.[16]

Any nurse who administers topical benzocaine should become familiar with the treatment of methemoglobinemia. Supplemental oxygen should be readily available, as should methylene blue, which is administered (1 to 2 mg/kg IV) to enhance the oxygen-carrying capacity of hemoglobin. Patients with G6PD deficiency should be treated with transfusion or dialysis, since methylene blue can cause hemolytic anemia in these patients.

COMMUNICATING DRUG INFORMATION ACCURATELY

Nurses obtain information about the medications they administer from two main sources: the prescriber's order or prescription and the MAR. Errors can originate in either of these sources. Failure to control and standardize prescribing vocabulary, order transcription, and MAR formats can lead to misinterpretations that result in patient harm. Errors are also possible when nurses' communication of orders to the pharmacy is incomplete, untimely, or illegible (e.g., in faxed orders).

The Order or Prescription

Written Orders

The Institute for Safe Medication Practices (ISMP) 2004 Medication Safety Self Assessment indicated that only about 15% of U.S. hospitals use computerized prescriber order entry (CPOE) systems or other means of electronically communicating medication prescriptions, and such technology is used even less in outpatient settings. Most medication orders are handwritten, usually on NCR (no-carbon-required) order forms; the original written order is placed in the patient's chart and a copy is sent to the pharmacy. Lines printed on the first page of these forms make it easier to write neatly, but they can also obscure parts of a drug order. They may hide the top of a 7 and make it look like a 1; they may obscure decimal points and other marks.

For example, a physician who intended to order 0.5 mg of terbutaline failed to place a zero before the decimal point. The transcriber failed to see the decimal point because the line obscured it. As a result, the patient received 5 mg instead of 0.5 mg of the drug. In another instance, an unnecessary decimal point and a zero were added to an order for 1 mg of warfarin (i.e., the order was expressed as 1.0 mg), and a patient received 10 mg instead of the intended 1 mg.

Errors such as these can best be prevented by adding a zero before a decimal point and by eliminating trailing decimal points and zeroes. Also, the printed lines could be eliminated from the back copy of the NCR form. The person receiving it could then clearly see decimal points or other marks that might be obscured by lines on the top copy. (If orders written on NCR forms are scanned or faxed, as discussed below, only the original, top copy should be used for this purpose.)

Chapter 9 contains examples of poor handwriting that led to errors. When an order is completely illegible, the nurse must call the prescriber. Marginally legible orders are more likely to lead to errors because nurses may try to read them, using their experience with a particular physician's handwriting or enlisting the help of a colleague to decipher the order.

Error-Prone Abbreviations

Inappropriate use of error-prone dose expressions, abbreviations, acronyms, coined names, symbols, and other ambiguous means of communicating drug information can lead to errors. For example, "HCTZ 50 mg," used as an abbreviation for hydrochlorothiazide 50 mg, can easily be mistaken for hydrocortisone 250 mg if the Z looks like a 2. More than 1 in 10 medication errors are directly related to the use of incorrect drug names, confusing expressions of dosage forms, error-prone dose expressions, and misunderstood abbreviations.[17] As discussed in Chapter 8, JCAHO prohibits the use of certain abbreviations and expressions. Chapter 8 suggests ways in which nurses, pharmacists, and physicians can avoid errors related to abbreviations and other ambiguous expressions.

Incomplete Orders

Nurses must question any incomplete or unclear order before administering a medication. Even if the course of action seems obvious, the nurse must not make any assumptions about the prescriber's intent. For example, a physician ordered "Mycostatin (nystatin) suppository, one at bedtime" for a woman recovering from a cerebrovascular accident. The route of administration was not noted. A nurse prepared the tablet according to instructions in the package insert and placed it in the patient's vagina. The physician had intended that the tablet dissolve in the patient's mouth, an accepted means of treating oral yeast infections.

"Verbal" Orders

Orders that are spoken aloud in person or by telephone can easily be misheard. Various pronunciations, accents, and dialects contribute to misunderstanding, as do background noise, interruptions, sound-alike drug names, poor cell phone reception, and unfamiliar terminology. No one except the prescriber can verify that the recipient heard the message correctly.

Doses in particular are easily misunderstood; for example, when spoken, 15 can sound like 50. One physician phoned in an order for 15 mg of hydralazine to be given IV every 2 hours. The nurse, thinking he had said 50 mg, drew up the contents of two 20 mg vials and half of a third vial and administered this to the patient. Within a few minutes, the patient experienced tachycardia and a significant drop in blood pressure. The nurse called the physician, and a rapid infusion of fluids restored the patient's blood pressure to a safe level.

Errors can occur when spoken orders are incomplete and a nurse assumes the prescriber's intention. A nurse took a spoken order to "increase Lasix to 40 an hour" for a patient who was receiving a furosemide infusion (10 mg/mL). The prescriber had wanted the solution to infuse at 40 mg an hour, but the nurse thought he wanted to run the infusion at 40 mL an hour. The patient received 400 mg of furosemide per hour, a 10-fold overdose, for nearly 15 hours before the error was discovered. The patient's serum potassium level remained within normal limits, and he did not suffer hearing loss or other harm.

Since 2003, JCAHO has required nurses to first transcribe each spoken order onto the patient's record as received and then read back the complete order. Nurses should not hesitate to ask prescribers to speak slowly, spell drug names, and provide the indication for each drug. When repeating back dosages, nurses should pronounce each digit separately (e.g., "five-zero" rather than "fifty," which can sound like "fifteen"). Before reading an order back to the prescriber, it is helpful to pause to be sure it is complete and fully understood. Table 11-1 presents additional safety strategies for accepting and transcribing spoken orders.

Order Transcription

Medication errors can result from mistakes in order transcription—both transcription of spoken orders and transcription of written orders from the order sheet onto the MAR or other forms. The use of CPOE eliminates order transcription and thus, transcription errors.

When transcribing spoken orders—either writing them on an order form or entering them by computer—nurses and other health care providers should not number orders, even on preprinted order forms. If orders must be numbered, each digit should be circled; otherwise, an order number could be read as part of the dose or as the quantity of tablets. Furthermore, transcribed orders should always list the dose after the drug name, not before it. One nurse transcribed an order that the pharmacist read as "1.25 mg of Toradol × 1." Since the dose did not make sense, the pharmacist checked with the transcribing nurse, who said she had numbered the order for 25 mg of Toradol (ketorolac) IV, using the number 1 followed by a period.

In transcribed orders, stray marks as well as marks intended as initials, letters, check marks, and so forth can also obscure or change the appearance of a medication order, as illustrated in the following error reports. A unit secretary conscientiously checked off on the order sheet each order that she transcribed. But when a pharmacist read a handwritten order for Levbid (hyoscyamine extended release), he saw Enbrel (etanercept), because the "L" in Levbid had been obscured by the check mark. He realized his mistake because Enbrel is given subcutaneously and the order specified the oral route. In another case, "40 mg Tylenol Infants' Drops" looked like 140 mg because a check mark preceding the dose looked like the number 1. In other cases, the transcriber's initials have been placed at the beginning of each order, or the letter P, M, K, or O has been used to indicate that the order was *p*ulled or entered on the *M*AR or *K*ardex or that the medication has been *o*rdered. In one case, Monopril (fosinopril) was dispensed instead of Accupril (quinapril) because an M had been placed in front of the drug name.

The order sheet should be sent to the pharmacy before the orders are transcribed onto other forms. "Clean" orders help the pharmacist interpret the order correctly and thus speed the dispensing process. If notations are needed to signal completed transcription or verification of the order, such notations should be made at the bottom of the page of the written order form so they are less likely to obscure the drug name or dose. If check marks or notations must be used to track completed transcription within large order sets, order forms should be designed with a separate column or box for these marks.

Medication Administration Records

MARs can be created by hand, generated on paper by the pharmacy computer system, or created electronically as a screen in a computerized system. Handwritten MARs can contribute to errors if they are crowded or illegible or present drug information in an inconsistent manner. Typically, orders are transcribed onto the MAR exactly as written; the presentation of information may not be consistent, and error-prone abbreviations and dose expressions may be carried forth from the order. If a product is prescribed (and thus

TABLE 11-1   Safety Strategies for Accepting and Transcribing Spoken Orders

Problem	Causative Factors	Strategy	Examples
Overuse of spoken orders	Convenience, habit, poor access to patient record, insufficient environment and space	Limit use	■ Reserve spoken orders for true emergencies or for when prescriber is physically unable to write or electronically transmit orders (e.g., working in a sterile field) ■ Prohibit all spoken orders for selected high-alert medications (e.g., chemotherapy, IV insulin for neonates) ■ In hospitals, limit spoken orders to formulary medications
		Simplify	■ Establish standing orders with corresponding preprinted order forms for areas where spoken orders tend to be prevalent (e.g., emergency department, critical care units) ■ Provide physician offices with appropriate order forms and request transmission of orders for new admissions via fax, pneumatic tube, or electronically, rather than by telephone
		Improve access	■ Locate and hand the patient's medical record to any prescriber who is physically present and attempting to issue spoken orders (and capable of writing or entering the orders) ■ Stock blank order forms in patient records for easy access ■ Provide adequate space (and computer terminals, as appropriate) for prescribers to write orders, in a low-traffic area if possible
Mistranscribed spoken orders	Delayed transcription, chart unavailability, mental slip, transcription onto wrong patient's chart	Simplify	■ Document a spoken order directly onto the patient's medical record immediately as it is being received, before reading back the order for verification
		Redundancies	■ To verify patient identity, read back the patient's name on the order form that was used to transcribe the spoken order ■ When taking a telephone order, obtain prescriber's phone number for questions that arise
Misheard, misinterpreted, or fraudulent spoken orders	Sound-alike drug names, sound-alike numbers, momentary inattention, distractions, noise, phone interference, hearing impairment, unfamiliarity with prescriber and prescriber's voice	Limit use	■ Maximize ability to recognize caller's voice by limiting the number of nurses who may receive telephone orders (reduces the risk of fraudulent orders)

		Redundancies	■ After writing the order on the patient record (immediately as received), read entire order as documented back to prescriber for confirmation
			  – Spell all drug names
			  – Confirm numbers using single digits ("one-four" for 14, "one-zero" for 10)
			  – Ask for the drug's indication, or communicate an understanding of its intended purpose
			  – Ensure that the medication makes sense in context of the patient's condition
			■ If medication prescribed requires emergency administration (or nurse is working within a sterile field), repeat back order as above, and, if prescriber is at patient's bedside, announce medication again just before administration ("I am now giving heparin 2,000 units IV")

```
DAPSONE 25 MG TAB
12.5 MG (0.5 TAB)
PO DAILY


DIGOXIN ELIXIR 0.05 MG/ML 60 ML
0.125 MG (0.25 mL)
PO DAILY
```

FIGURE 11-1   Error-prone MAR entries.

transcribed onto the MAR) only by brand name and the pharmacy dispenses a generic form, confusion can result. Patient allergies and other important information may not be present on a handwritten MAR.

Pharmacy-generated MARs, usually produced every 24 hours from orders entered into the computer, can help prevent errors. With electronic MARs, new, changed, or discontinued orders appear on the MAR in "real time," awaiting verification by the pharmacist and nurse. Both electronic and pharmacy computer-generated MARs often contain the generic name of a product as well as the brand name if prescribed by brand. Pharmacy-generated and electronic MARs provide consistency (e.g., in spelling and dose documentation) and enable nurses to compare their transcriptions with those of the pharmacist. Also, pharmacy-generated and electronic MARs can provide consistent drug messages, warnings, and information on patient allergies, current diagnoses, and chronic conditions.

Despite the benefits of computer-generated MARs, the appearance of orders can be confusing to nurses. In pharmacy-generated MARs, an entry typically begins with the medication name and the strength available in the pharmacy; the next line of the entry is the number of tablets or volume of oral or injectable liquid needed to equal the patient's prescribed dose (Figure 11-1). This presentation mirrors the pharmacy inventory, but nurses tend to think first about the dose they must give and second about the number of tablets or volume of liquid needed for the dose. Their eyes are naturally drawn to the top line of the entry to locate the patient's dose. When the patient's dose differs from the available dosage strength listed on the top line, errors can occur.

For example, a hospital patient received cyclosporine 50 mg IV after a nurse misinterpreted the 50 mg/mL dosage strength listed in bold on the top line as the patient's actual dose, which was listed as 30 mg on a subsequent line. In another case, a patient received 2 mg of digoxin after a nurse misinterpreted the total volume dispensed in the bottle (listed on the first line as "Digoxin Elixir 0.05 mg/mL 60 mL") as the patient's dose, which was listed below (0.125 mg). The error was detected after the nurse gave the patient the amount left in the bottle (40 mL) and called the pharmacy for the remaining 20 mL.

In another case, a single tablet that matched the available tablet strength listed on the first line was administered when the patient's dose required two tablets. Similar errors often go unrecognized and likely account for some of the doses returned to the pharmacy and calls to the pharmacy for missing doses.

The ideal presentation for nurses would list the drug name (generic first with brand name in parentheses, if applicable) on the first line; the patient-specific dose, route, and frequency (and indication, if applicable) in bold print on the second line; and the product strength or special instructions (e.g., 50 mg = 2 × 25 mg tabs) or warnings (e.g., IM only) on the third line. If oral liquids must be dispensed in multidose bottles, the container's total volume should not be listed on the MAR.

Computer-generated MARs guide drug administration far more safely than handwritten MARs. However, it is essential to ensure that the presentation of orders is clear to nurses.

Interdisciplinary meetings are needed to identify and prioritize MAR format problems that could contribute to errors. Information system staff should attend so that they understand the problems and can work with the pharmacy software vendor to make changes.

Regardless of the format, MARs that are too long can lead to inadvertent omissions. Lengthy MARs result in part from the use of preprinted order sheets that include medications to cover every possible patient need. An order set might include several analgesics, a laxative, an antacid, a bedtime sedative, an antidiarrheal, an antiemetic, and an antipyretic. Each medication requires transcription and a separate entry on the MAR, even if electronic prescribing is used. A single analgesic order may require multiple MAR entries if the order allows different doses and routes of administration. Patients may have multiple preprinted order sets that overlap; these patients may have orders for several different bedtime sedatives, laxatives, antidiarrheals, and so on unless medications are standardized among the various preprinted order forms.

Preprinted orders do not have to cover all contingencies. (Those that do have been called "Nurse, don't bother me!" orders.) If MARs have too many pages, the problem should be brought to the attention of nurses who serve on the pharmacy and therapeutics committee so that they can work with the pharmacists and medical staff to minimize the variety of prescribed medications, routes of administration, and dosages on preprinted orders.

Documenting Administration

Once a medication dose has been administered, it must be immediately recorded on the MAR. If a nurse records administration before it actually takes place and then is called away from the patient care unit before all doses are administered, other nurses may assume that the medication has been administered. This may lead to a dose omission. On the other hand, if a nurse elects to chart doses for all of her patients later, rather than immediately after administration, and is called away before completing the task, another nurse may administer a duplicate dose.

Dose administration should be documented in a part of the patient record designated for only that purpose. Administration should not be documented within narrative notes, even in settings such as the ED, clinics, and outpatient surgery units. Special administration records for drugs such as anticoagulants, cardiac medications, and insulin provide extra space for recording monitoring variables. However, if these records are kept separately in the patient's chart, the MAR will not give a complete picture of drug therapy. This has led to errors.

For example, a nurse administering aspirin was surprised when the patient said he had been told not to take aspirin while he was taking warfarin. The nurse had not seen an order for warfarin on the patient's MAR because the record of anticoagulants was kept separately in the patient's chart. Had the patient not intervened, the nurse would not have known to question the order for aspirin.

When patients refuse doses, the prescriber must be informed and an explanatory note left in the patient's bin or sent electronically to alert the pharmacist to the situation. When unadministered doses are returned to the pharmacy without adequate explanation, follow-up should take place to learn the reason for the returned dose. This helps detect errors of omission and ensure that drugs are not accidentally discontinued prematurely.

Communicating Orders to the Pharmacy

Modes of Communication

Except where CPOE systems are fully implemented, nurses are responsible for communicating orders to the pharmacy. Often, unit secretaries send orders to the pharmacy as a fax or a scanned image (e.g., Pyxis Connect from Cardinal Health, MedDirect from

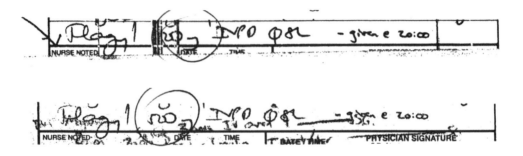

FIGURE 11-2   Faxed copy (top) and original order (bottom) for Flagyl.

McKesson Automation). In some institutions, the pharmacy staff makes regular rounds to the nursing units to pick up copies of the orders.

When a fax machine or scanner is being used to send prescriptions or medical orders, the equipment must be maintained and the roller (of a fax machine) or glass surface (of a scanner) cleaned regularly. Figure 11-2 shows an order that originally was read incorrectly as 250 mg of Flagyl (metronidazole) but was correctly interpreted as 500 mg when the original order was checked. Dirt, dust, stuck paper, correction fluid, and hole punches can cause streaks or fadeouts on fax or scanned image transmissions. Because fax machines are connected to telephone lines, line "noise" can obliterate important information such as part of a drug name or dose.

Orders may be obscured when unit secretaries or coordinators affix small stickers (e.g., a "sign here" arrow for prescribers) and forget to remove them before scanning or faxing the order. Stickers can obscure information on scanned documents or become caught in a fax machine and cause a black line across every order.

Another potential problem with these modes of transmission is that prescribers sometimes write to the very edge of the order form and the fax machine or scanner cannot "read" the entire order. An order for "Lomotil QID PRN" could appear as "Lomotil QID" if "PRN" were in the extreme right margin.

Send All Orders

All orders should be sent to pharmacy, including orders for floor stock medications and orders that do not mention medications. Pharmacists should be aware of all tests and procedures that patients will be undergoing, as well as the patient's dietary status, additional therapies, and planned discharge. Having all of the patient's orders helps pharmacists critically assess each medication order for appropriateness, safety, and efficacy. Without this context, pharmacists could contribute to a medication error by dispensing the wrong drug, dose, or dosage form, as in the following example.

Lovenox (enoxaparin) and warfarin were prescribed upon admission for an elderly woman with a history of atrial fibrillation, hypertension, and constipation. Because a colonoscopy was scheduled, warfarin was discontinued and a heparin infusion was ordered. Lovenox was not discontinued, however. The order for the heparin infusion was never sent to the pharmacy because the solution was stocked on the unit. If this order had been entered in the pharmacy computer system, an alert would have appeared to warn the pharmacist that the patient had two active orders for heparin products, Lovenox and heparin. Several hours after the patient received both of these drugs, her activated partial thromboplastin time was above 90 seconds. The heparin infusion was decreased, but the patient suffered internal bleeding. Despite immediate discontinuation of both heparin products, she died.

   In settings such as long-term care facilities, clinics, and physician offices, nurses often telephone the pharmacy to communicate a prescription. The error-reduction strategies in Table 11-1 should be followed. Voice mail or other message systems should not be used to communicate prescriptions, because the receiving pharmacist has no opportunity to read back the prescription for verification. Faxing a copy of the actual prescription may be a safer alternative.

Admissions from ED

Pharmacists may not be dispensing all medications administered to patients in hospital EDs. ED nurses may not send orders to the pharmacy for medications that are available as floor stock. However, if a patient is admitted to the hospital, the ED nurse must communicate all of the drug therapy that has been prescribed and administered. These medications must be on the pharmacy profile so that medications prescribed upon admission can be screened against those administered in the ED for drug interactions and duplicate therapy.

   Duplicate therapy with heparin products could be particularly harmful. In one case, a patient with unstable angina died from internal bleeding after he received Fragmin (dalteparin) in the ED and then received a thrombolytic and IV heparin immediately upon admission to a cardiac care unit and confirmation of an acute myocardial infarction. The heparin infusion was started too soon after Fragmin administration because of failure to communicate the drugs given in the ED.

   As a further precaution against unintentional concomitant use of heparin products, patients' current and recent MARs should be reviewed before any heparin product is administered. Reminders on heparin protocols and order forms to discontinue low molecular weight (LMW) heparin are helpful, as is listing the time interval (8 to 24 hours, depending on the dose) before heparin therapy can be initiated when a patient has received a dose of LMW heparin. When transferring a patient to an inpatient setting, the ED nurse should mention all doses of LMW heparin administered, as well as clearly documenting those doses.

Communication Barriers

Rigid, hierarchical structures in health care can make it difficult or uncomfortable for nurses and others—regardless of their of rank, education, and experience—to voice their opinions or concerns about the safety of an order. The difficulty is compounded when there is no effective policy for handling disagreement between practitioners. The effect is workplace intimidation and faulty interaction between health care professionals, which contributes to at least 10% of medication errors that occur in the administration phase.[18] Chapter 23 provides strategies that nurses at all levels of an organization's structure can use to overcome workplace intimidation and promote effective communication.

DRUG LABELING, PACKAGING, AND NOMENCLATURE

All of us have, on occasion, picked up the wrong product from a shelf because it looks so similar to the item we intended to select. Accidentally picking a can of Pepsi rather than Diet Pepsi is a perfect example—the containers are similar in color, print, size, and shape, and both have Pepsi as part of the product name. Similar mix-ups occur with medications that have look-alike or sound-alike names or look-alike packages, but here the consequences can be more serious; choosing the wrong medication may cause a life-threatening or fatal event. Table 11-2 lists strategies for preventing errors with these products, and Chapter 6 discusses this topic in more detail.

TABLE 11-2 Safety Strategies for Look-Alike and Sound-Alike Drug Names and Look-Alike Packages

Problem	Strategy	Examples
Look-alike brand or generic names	Differentiate items	■ For name pairs known to be problematic, include both generic and brand names on orders, storage shelf and product labels, computer screens, and medication administration records (MARs) ■ Change the appearance of look-alike names on storage shelf and product labels, computer screens, and MARs by using color, bold type, or tall-man lettering (hydrOXYzine, hydrALAzine) ■ When feasible, use magnifying lenses and good lighting during transcription to improve the likelihood of proper interpretation of look-alike product names ■ Do not list medications with look-alike names sequentially on computer screens, preprinted order forms, or MARs
	Improve access to information	■ Include the drug's indication on all prn orders ■ Match purpose of the medication to patient's diagnosis before administering it (many products with look-alike names are used for different purposes)
	Use reminders	■ Affix "name alert" stickers to areas where look-alike products are stored
	Redundancies	■ Require pharmacy to review all medication orders before drug administration whenever possible ■ Double-check with the patient: ensure that the medication's purpose makes sense and that the medication looks similar to what the patient took at home ■ Investigate further if patient says the medication does not look similar to prior doses
Sound-alike brand or generic names	Simplify Standardize	■ Accept spoken orders only when truly necessary ■ Prohibit all spoken orders for high-alert medications such as chemotherapy ■ Require staff who accept spoken orders to write them immediately as received onto the patient's chart
	Redundancies	■ Read back all transcribed spoken orders, spelling drug names, stating numerical doses in single digits ("one-five," not "fifteen"), and stating the drug's intended purpose to verify understanding
	Use reminders	■ Affix "name alert" stickers to areas where sound-alike products are stored
Look-alike packaging	Differentiate items	■ Purchase products with look-alike packaging from different manufacturers ■ Circle important information on the package to draw attention to differences
	Limit access or use	■ Segregate medications with look-alike packages by storing in separate areas ■ Return medications to their segregated storage area after use (e.g., multiple-use vials of insulin, heparin)
	Use reminders	■ Add shelf stickers to draw attention to the medication's name ■ Add "look-alike alert" stickers to medications in look-alike packaging ■ Create alerts to appear on the screen of automated dispensing cabinets for medications in look-alike packages
	Redundancies	■ Require pharmacy to review all medication orders before drug administration whenever possible ■ Double-check with the patient: ensure that the medication's purpose makes sense and that the medication looks similar to what the patient took at home ■ Investigate further if patient says the medication does not look similar to prior doses

TABLE 11-2 Safety Strategies for Look-Alike and Sound-Alike Drug Names
and Look-Alike Packages (continued)

Problem	Strategy	Examples
New medications	Failure mode and effects analysis (FMEA; see Chapter 21)	■ Anticipate errors with new medications when a name looks or sounds like another product already in use or the packages look similar ■ Perform FMEA for new high-alert medications before use

Look-Alike and Sound-Alike Drug Names

With so many medications on the market, similarities in names and packaging are common. Not a week goes by without reports of practitioners' confusing products with similar names, such as the following:

- A nurse misheard a spoken order for Neurontin (gabapentin, an antiepileptic) 400 mg b.i.d. as Noroxin (norfloxacin, an antimicrobial) 400 mg b.i.d. and administered several doses in error.
- A patient told a nurse he was allergic to Lodine (etodolac, an anti-inflammatory). This was written on the admission assessment, but another nurse misread it and added an allergy to iodine to the patient's record.
- A pharmacy technician accidentally stocked an automated dispensing cabinet (ADC) with 100 mg tablets of chlorpromazine (an antipsychotic) instead of chlorpropamide (an antidiabetic). Four patients received the wrong drug, some with fatal results.

If the intended medication is new to the practitioner, the likelihood of misreading or mishearing the name as a familiar drug name is greater.

Manufacturer Labeling and Packaging

Even when product names are not similar, errors can result when medication packages or labels look alike (Figure 11-3). Nurses are taught to read labels three times: when selecting the medication, when opening and preparing the medication, and before discarding the empty package or returning the remainder to stock. Although this is a good practice, it is not always enough to prevent errors. Particularly under suboptimal conditions (e.g., poor lighting, distractions, emergencies), mix-ups can still occur.

Humans tend to perceive confirming evidence more readily than disconfirming evidence. This confirmation bias causes us to see what is familiar, rather than what is actually

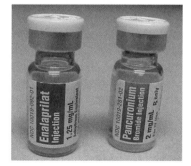

FIGURE 11-3 (also in color section following page 120) Enalaprilat and pancuronium. The vial size and labels of these two drugs look similar.

there. A health care provider who selects an incorrect medication with a label or package similar to that of the correct medication may have "read" the label but not "seen" it correctly. Our minds create pictures of how familiar medications look. When we use these mental pictures to locate or recognize medications, we may be blind to disconfirming evidence if the wrong product is selected.

Labeling Challenges

All medications must be labeled, and two categories present particular challenges: syringes of medications or flush solutions prepared by the nurse, and medications and solutions used within a sterile field.

Syringes

Any syringe of medication or solution that leaves the hand of the person filling it and will not be administered immediately must be labeled. Thus, syringes prepared anywhere but at the patient's bedside for immediate use must be labeled. Many errors have occurred despite nurses' good intentions to go directly to the patient's bedside and administer the medication in an unlabeled syringe; the nurse may be interrupted and forced to put down the syringe.

For example, just before a Persantine (dipyridamole) stress test, a hospital nurse prepared a syringe of aminophylline 75 mg from a multidose vial. She did not label the syringe. The aminophylline (used for emergency reversal of the effects of dipyridamole) was not needed, and the unlabeled syringe was left in the room with the patient. The nurse stepped out of the room as a nuclear medicine technician entered to administer an IV dose of thallium. Since the unlabeled syringe of aminophylline had been placed where saline flushes were usually kept, the technician assumed that it was saline and injected the patient. The nurse returned just as the technician finished giving the aminophylline. The patient experienced no serious adverse effects.

Tape should not be used to label syringes. If the roll of tape has disappeared from the medication preparation area, the nurse has to either walk around with an unlabeled syringe or leave it behind while searching for tape. Commercially available labels for syringes should be provided and regularly restocked in all medication preparation areas.

Medications on a Sterile Field

Failure to label all medications and solutions used on a sterile field in operating rooms and other settings has caused many errors, some with tragic outcomes, as in the following examples.

A 15-year-old boy with a history of malignant hyperthermia was undergoing repair of a torn tendon. A nurse initially drew half of the contents of a 30 mL vial of epinephrine 1:1,000 into a syringe to begin compounding bags of epinephrine and normal saline for use during the procedure. She was called away unexpectedly and left the unlabeled syringe on the table. When the surgeon asked for Marcaine (bupivacaine) with epinephrine, he saw the unlabeled syringe lying next to him and thought it contained the anesthetic. He injected the syringe contents into the surgical site, and the patient's blood pressure increased. The staff at first thought the patient was experiencing malignant hyperthermia, but they recognized the error when he developed ventricular tachycardia and pulmonary edema. The boy was sent to the ICU and recovered without permanent harm.

During coil placement under cerebral angiography to repair a brain aneurysm, a patient was accidentally injected with a skin preparation antiseptic, chlorhexidine, instead of contrast medium. Chlorhexidine is highly toxic when injected intravascularly. Both solutions were clear and available on the sterile field in unlabeled basins. Within 2 hours, the patient suspected that something was very wrong. Acute chemical injury to the blood vessels of her leg restricted circulation to the muscles, causing profound injury and swelling. The patient's leg was amputated, and she subsequently suffered a stroke and multiple organ failure leading to death. The hospital's recent decision to switch antiseptics, from a brown povidone–iodine solution to a clear chlorhexidine solution, had resulted in a latent failure: two look-alike, clear solutions on the sterile field that previously had been distinguishable by color.

Of some 1,600 hospitals participating in the 2004 ISMP Medication Safety Self Assessment, only 41% said they always label containers (including syringes, basins, and other vessels) used on a sterile field, even when just one product or solution is present. Eighteen percent said they do not label medications and solutions on the sterile field at all, and another 42% apply labels inconsistently. It is surprising that this basic safety measure is not widely implemented, although the 2004 findings showed improvement from a similar self-assessment in 2000 (25% reported full labeling; 24% reported no labeling).[19] This breach in safe practice is particularly disturbing because patients undergoing a surgical procedure are highly vulnerable to errors. Since they usually are sedated or anesthetized, they cannot intervene on their own behalf.

Policies and procedures must be implemented for safe labeling of medications and solutions used on a sterile field in any setting, including the ED, traditional operating rooms (ORs), ambulatory surgery units, labor and delivery rooms, physicians' offices, cardiac catheterization suites, endoscopy suites, and radiology departments. A 2006 JCAHO NPSG requires such labeling in both inpatient and outpatient settings. The sidebar on page 256 provides a starting point for the development of policies and procedures.

Labeling to the Point of Administration

Medications should not be removed from unit dose packages until the point of administration. Opening the packages before they reach the patient's bedside defeats the purpose of the unit dose system. Once medications have been removed from their packaging, it is difficult to identify them. An unlabeled dose is at increased risk of being mixed up with another drug. The loss of identity of each dose also means that a drug cannot be returned if it is unused. The following example illustrates the importance of keeping medications in their packaging until at the bedside.

A night-shift nurse was preparing medications for three patients when a patient with Parkinson's disease requested aspirin. After confirming the order, the nurse placed two aspirin tablets in a cup. She then picked up that cup plus the other three into which she had opened the three patients' medications. Heading for the patients' rooms, she remembered that the patient who requested the aspirin often complained about getting her medications late. The nurse administered that patient's medication first, but she soon realized that she had switched the cups and given the woman who requested aspirin the morphine sulfate tablets intended for another patient with cancer. Had the medications remained in their packages, the nurse could have confirmed that they were correct.

DRUG STORAGE AND STANDARDIZATION

Many medication orders can be prevented by simply safeguarding or restricting high-alert drugs and dangerous chemicals that are available on patient care units. Products stored on patient care units bypass the safety checks present in the pharmacy dispensing system. When a pharmacist does not screen patient-specific doses before drug administration, problems such as drug interactions, excessive doses, duplicate therapy, and drug allergies

STRATEGIES TO ENSURE LABELING OF MEDICATIONS AND SOLUTIONS USED IN A STERILE FIELD[a]

Provide labels. Make labeling easy by purchasing sterile markers, blank labels, and preprinted labels prepared by the facility or commercially available (e.g., from Healthcare Logistics) that can be opened onto the sterile field during all procedures. To minimize staff time, prepare surgical packs ahead of time with sterile markers, blank labels, and preprinted labels for all anticipated medications and solutions that will be needed for the case. Labels that can be viewed more clearly on basins, or basins that can display labels more effectively, will soon be available.

Require labels. Require labels on all medications, medication containers (e.g., syringes, medicine cups, basins), or other solutions on and off the sterile field, even if there is only one medication or solution involved. Also require labels on all solutions, chemicals, and reagents (e.g., formalin, saline, Lugol's solution, radiocontrast media) that are used in perioperative units.

Differentiate look-alike products. If drug or solution names are similar, use tall-man lettering on the labels to differentiate them, or highlight or circle the distinguishing information on the label. When possible, purchase skin antiseptic products in prepackaged swabs or sponges to clearly differentiate them from medications or other solutions and eliminate the risk of accidental injection.

Label one at a time. Individually verify each medication and complete its preparation for administration, delivery to the sterile field, and labeling on the field before another medication is prepared. Verify any medication listed on the physician's preference list with the physician before delivery to the sterile field, labeling, or administration.

Confirm medications and labels. Require the scrub person and the circulating nurse to concurrently verify all medications and solutions visually and verbally by reading the product name, strength, and dosage from the labels. (If there is no scrub person, the circulating nurse should verify the medication or solution with the licensed professional performing the procedure.) When passing a medication to the licensed professional performing the procedure, visually and verbally verify the medication, strength, and dose by reading the label aloud. Keep all original medication and solution containers in the room for reference until the procedure is concluded.

Verify again with relief staff. At shift change or relief for breaks, require the entering and exiting personnel to concurrently note and verify all medications and their labels on the sterile field.

Discard unlabeled medications. Do not assume that you know what is contained in an unlabeled syringe, cup, or basin. Discard any unlabeled solution or medication found in the perioperative area (including the sterile field), and report the event as a hazardous condition. Nothing should leave the hand unless it is labeled.

Conduct walk-arounds. Perform regular safety rounds in perioperative areas to observe labeling procedures, promote consistency, and inquire about barriers to implementing this important safety practice.

Establish pharmacy presence in the OR. Although an OR is sometimes considered foreign ground for a pharmacist, establishing close ties between pharmacists and the OR staff (via satellites or regular onsite presence) can help spur improved labeling on the sterile field.

Enhance awareness. Tell memorable stories to perioperative staff about tragic mix-ups that have occurred in other facilities when medications and solutions on a sterile field were not labeled. Forming a multidisciplinary perioperative safety team comprising nurses, technicians, pharmacists, and physicians from various sites where invasive procedures are performed might also help improve labeling.

[a] Many of these recommendations also appear in guidelines published by the professional organization of perioperative registered nurses (www.aorn.org/About/positions/pdf/7f-safemeds-2004.pdf).

may not be detected. In addition, nursing staff may be required to calculate drug doses and mix or draw up medications from bulk supplies sent from pharmacy or floor stock medications. Each of these operations provides opportunity for error.

Unit Dose Distribution

A comprehensive unit dose drug distribution system reduces the need for floor stock in patient care areas. JCAHO and other credentialing organizations recognize unit dose distribution as the standard of practice for inpatient settings. However, pharmacies receive a substantial number of drugs in bulk packages and need to repackage them for dispensing in patient-specific unit doses. Pediatric dosage forms, controlled substances, oral liquids, and injectable drugs available from the manufacturer only in multidose vials are especially problematic in this regard. Innovative methods for hospital pharmacy repackaging of bulk medications into unit doses can be used to reduce the risk of error.

Hazardous Drugs and Solutions in Floor Stock

Chemicals

Nurses routinely use chemicals (e.g., testing reagents) that could be mistaken for medications. Hemoccult Sensa (hydrogen peroxide, denatured ethyl alcohol) and Seracult (hydrogen peroxide, ethanol) solutions (Figure 11-4) are examples. Patients, family members, and nurses have mistaken these products for eye drops. Such chemicals should never be left in bedside stands, medicine carts, patient bathrooms, or other areas where they could be confused with medications. Furthermore, chemicals used for cleaning, equipment maintenance, or other purposes should never be poured into empty saline, water, or medication containers, even if the containers are relabeled, nor kept in areas where medications are stored or prepared.

Concentrated Electrolytes

To prevent medication errors that have great potential for patient harm, access to concentrated electrolytes must be restricted or eliminated. JCAHO requires that concentrated electrolytes (e.g., potassium chloride, potassium phosphate, sodium chloride solutions more concentrated than 0.9%) be removed from patient care units. Such products have caused countless deaths when mistakenly administered too rapidly without proper dilution. Many patients have died as a result of receiving concentrated potassium chloride

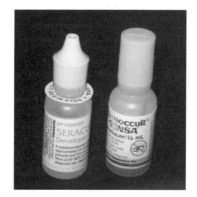

FIGURE 11-4 (also in color section following page 120)   Hemoccult and Seracult solutions. The containers are similar to those used for eye drops.

(KCl) as a bolus instead of in a diluted infusion. Aggravating the situation is the fact that some physicians have prescribed it as "KCl 40 mEq IV bolus." To some people, "bolus" means "at once."

Most potassium-containing IV solutions used today are premixed in the pharmacy or by commercial vendors. JCAHO reports that sentinel events involving potassium chloride have decreased. However, other concentrated electrolyte solutions pose a similar danger.

For example, a nurse mistakenly removed a vial of concentrated (23.4%) sodium chloride from floor stock and administered the solution IV, instead of a normal saline (0.9% sodium chloride) flush, to a neonate. The infant died of acute hypernatremia. In many similar cases, death or permanent central nervous system impairment has resulted.

There is no reason to risk serious errors by using concentrated electrolytes. Treatment for severe hyponatremia can be initiated with typical concentrations of sodium chloride until the pharmacy can prepare a patient-specific infusion or dispense a more concentrated premixed solution (e.g., 3% sodium chloride). Precautions with electrolytes and other high-alert medications are discussed in Chapter 14.

Other Concentrated Medications

Two additional concentrated medications warrant mention as hazardous floor stock.

Concentrated Morphine Oral Solution

Several manufacturers distribute concentrated morphine oral solution in different formulations, primarily labeled (and listed in drug references) in milligrams per milliliter (e.g., 20 mg/mL) or milligrams per 5 mL (e.g., 100 mg/5 mL, 20 mg/5 mL). When concentrated oral morphine is stocked on patient care units, it can easily be confused with conventional concentrations (e.g., 10 mg/5mL, 20 mg/5 mL). Some physicians have prescribed the medication in milliliters instead of milligrams, which has led to errors when multiple concentrations were available. In other cases, patients have been given the prescribed milligram dose in milliliters, often of the more concentrated solution when it was available as floor stock.

For example, one elderly man being treated for a mild heart attack was mistakenly given a 100 mg dose of Roxanol, likely contributing to his death. Instead of the prescribed 5 mg, he was given 5 mL of Roxanol 20 mg/mL.

Patient care units, including the ED, should avoid stocking concentrated oral morphine solutions. The drug is used primarily to treat chronic pain. If it is prescribed for a specific patient, pharmacy should dispense the concentrated solution in unit dose oral syringes for inpatients. Orders without a specified dose in milligrams (not just milliliters) should not be accepted. Unused supplies should be returned to the pharmacy immediately after the patient is discharged. If possible, the pharmacy should dispense concentrated solutions in dropper bottles (available from at least two manufacturers) to help prevent dose measurement errors and differentiate the concentrated product from conventional products. If a larger supply of the drug must be stored on a patient care unit, an auxiliary label should be affixed to the bottle, and the concentrated solution should be segregated from the other concentrations. ADCs alone will not prevent errors; the wrong strength could be stocked or removed by mistake.

Concentrated Insulin

Concentrated insulin (500 units/mL, referred to as U-500) can be used for patients with insulin resistance who would otherwise need large volumes of U-100 insulin. A red label on U-500 Humulin R (regular insulin, from Eli Lilly and Company) warns "high potency" and "not for ordinary use," but the type size is small and easily overlooked, as noted in the following error report.

A nurse removed what she thought was a dose of Humulin R from the refrigerator, but she failed to notice that it was the U-500 concentration. The vial of U-500 insulin had been dispensed for another patient, who had been discharged. The nurse withdrew the prescribed dose using a U-100 syringe, which resulted in a fivefold overdose. The error was recognized when the nurse was documenting administration, so the patient was monitored and treated accordingly.

U-500 insulin should not be routinely stocked in patient care units. Ideally, pharmacy should dispense each dose in a syringe when it is prescribed for a patient. If a full vial must be dispensed for an individual patient, it should be segregated from other supplies and returned to the pharmacy when it is no longer needed for that patient. Also, U-500 insulin should never be given IV because of the harm that could result from an inadvertent overdose.

Sterile Water

Numerous cases of accidental IV administration of sterile water for injection have resulted in serious patient harm, including death, from hemolysis (destruction of red blood cells). Some of the errors reflect a lack of knowledge about the hazards of IV administration of this solution, as in the following example.

A physician prescribed "free water" IV at 100 mL/hour for an elderly patient with severe hypernatremia, hyperglycemia, and congestive heart failure, because he was reluctant to give the patient IV solutions containing sodium or dextrose. "Free water" refers to water not associated with organic or inorganic ions (plain water). Hypernatremia usually results from a deficit of free water, and the physician most likely intended to replace that. Free water can be replaced orally, but it should never be given IV as plain sterile water for injection without additives to increase osmolarity; if it is, hemolysis will occur. Before writing the order, the physician had called a pharmacist to ask if "large bags of sterile water for injection" were available. Without giving it much thought, the pharmacist had confirmed their availability; the bags were typically used in the pharmacy for preparing total parenteral nutrition.

When the pharmacy received the order, a technician retrieved a 2 L bag of sterile water and sent it to the ICU. The nurse began the infusion without question because she was aware of the patient's severe hypernatremia and had overheard the physician asking the pharmacist if bags of sterile water were available. She failed to see a red statement on the bag, "Pharmacy Bulk Package, Not For Direct Infusion," because the label that the technician had applied was on the opposite side of the bag. The label imprinted on the bag also stated that the product was not suitable for IV injection without first being made approximately isotonic through the addition of a suitable solute, but this warning blended in with the other text and was not seen. Another nurse noticed the problem and stopped the IV, but not before 550 mL had infused. The patient had a hemolytic reaction, resulting in acute renal failure and death.

To avoid errors like this, protocols for the treatment of hypernatremia should be established. Severe hypernatremia is generally treated with infusions that contain low concentrations of sodium to reduce serum levels slowly; too rapid correction may lead to cerebral edema, seizures, or death. Excess fluid volume and elevated blood glucose can be managed with diuretics and insulin. Pharmacists should use 2 L containers (or larger) of sterile water in the pharmacy for preparing solutions; nurses would notice the large size if a bag was mistakenly dispensed.

Bags of sterile water have been inadvertently stocked on patient care units and mistaken for look-alike bags of IV solution. Hospital purchasing departments have provided patient care units with 1 L bags of sterile water, most often when the supplier accidentally

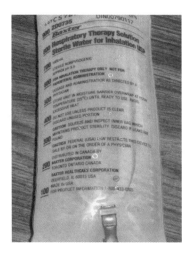

FIGURE 11-5 This bag of sterile water for use in respiratory therapy could be inadvertently attached to IV tubing.

sent sterile water for injection instead of 5% dextrose injection. Although the sterile water bags (from Baxter) are labeled in red with the warning "For Drug Diluent Use Only," they look quite similar to IV solution bags. Purchasing departments have also provided patient care units with 1 L bags of sterile water for injection because the pour bottles of sterile water were on backorder.

Emergency malignant hyperthermia boxes found in ORs and PACUs are another source of sterile water bags. In response to a recommendation by the Malignant Hyperthermia Association, these boxes are often stocked with 1 L bags of sterile water for use in diluting Dantrium (dantrolene). Hospitals have reported concern that unused or partially used bags of the solution may find their way into IV stock or be hung as an IV solution during emergencies. Replacing the 1 L sterile water bags with 50 mL vials would help prevent errors.

Respiratory therapy staff may store bags of sterile water in patient care units or take them to patient rooms for humidification devices used with ventilators or continuous positive airway pressure devices. These bags are labeled in blue print as "Respiratory Therapy Solution, Sterile Water for Inhalation" (Figure 11-5). However, the bags easily attach to IV tubing and may look similar to IV bags labeled in blue print, especially if they are left in a patient's room or hung for convenience on an IV pole. Some humidification units for ventilated gases use plastic bottles rather than sterile water bags; to avoid errors, these units should be used when possible.

Neuromuscular Blocking Agents

Many health care providers have reported deaths when neuromuscular blocking agents (e.g., vecuronium, pancuronium, succinylcholine, rocuronium) have been mistakenly administered to patients who were not mechanically ventilated. This has most often occurred when a neuromuscular blocking agent is inadvertently removed from the refrigerator instead of the intended drug with a similar vial label, or when an inexperienced nurse medicates an agitated patient with a neuromuscular blocking agent that a physician has inadvertently failed to discontinue after extubation. Outside the OR, these drugs should be stocked only in critical care units and the ED. In these areas, they should be stored in zip-lock bags with "WARNING: Paralyzing agent" labels (available from label vendors) affixed. They should be sequestered in some manner (e.g., placed in a closed box in the refrigerator).

Multidose Vials

One cost-saving measure that warrants further scrutiny is the use of multidose vials (MDVs). Any potential savings is quickly consumed if MDV contamination results in an outbreak of infections. Faulty aseptic technique is the primary cause of vial contamination, especially with products (e.g., saline, heparin, local anesthetics such as lidocaine) that may require more than one entry into the vial for a single patient.[20,21] Contamination occurs when, for example, a practitioner needs "just a little more" lidocaine, or another saline flush, and forgets to use a new needle and syringe for reentering the vial.

MDVs have also been linked to harmful medication errors. In one case, vecuronium was administered to a 3-year-old child who was not on a ventilator. Prefilled saline syringes were not available, so nurses had drawn up a daily supply of saline flushes from MDVs, labeled the syringes by hand, and placed them in a container. Earlier, syringes containing vecuronium had been prepared for another patient. An unused vecuronium syringe, hand-labeled similarly to the saline syringes, found its way into the saline flush supplies and was used to flush the child's IV line. The child became flaccid, and all respiratory effort ceased. She was quickly intubated and ventilated.

Whenever possible, prefilled syringes, either purchased commercially or prepared by the pharmacy, should be used instead of vials for heparin flushes, saline, and bacteriostatic water. Single-dose vials of local anesthetics such as lidocaine should be provided, and they should not be reused after initial entry. These vials contain no preservatives to prevent microbial growth.

If MDVs must be used for heparin, saline, bacteriostatic water, or local anesthetics, pharmacy should dispense labeled vials for each individual patient with a blood-borne pathogen. The vials should be kept with the patient's medications and discarded upon discharge. Before each entry of an MDV, nurses should check the expiration date, visually inspect the solution for signs of contamination (i.e., cloudiness), decontaminate the vial membrane, use a new sterile syringe and needle, and properly label the syringe. MDVs contain preservatives to inactivate bacteria (not viruses), but bacteria may remain viable for up to 2 hours.[21] The frequency of entering the vial and the environmental air injected into the vial can be risk factors for contamination. MDVs should be stored and discarded according to manufacturers' recommendations. Any used but undated MDVs should be discarded.

Flammable Products

About 100 surgical fires occur each year, of which 10 to 20 are serious.[22] Given the 50 million inpatient and outpatient surgeries per year, the number of fires is small; however, the outcome can be devastating or disfiguring.[23,24] A number of fires have involved flammable medications in the form of skin preparation agents (alcohol and alcohol-containing iodophors), eye lubricants, ointments, and wound dressings (tincture of benzoin and collodion).

For example, a fire occurred in an ambulatory care surgery unit. An assistant surgeon had prepared an operative incision for bandaging by spraying it with tincture of benzoin (which protects the skin and acts as an antiseptic). The primary surgeon had nearly finished suturing the patient's incision, but he noticed a small area of bleeding along the incision line and decided to cauterize it. The flammable benzoin ignited briefly, but the patient was not harmed.

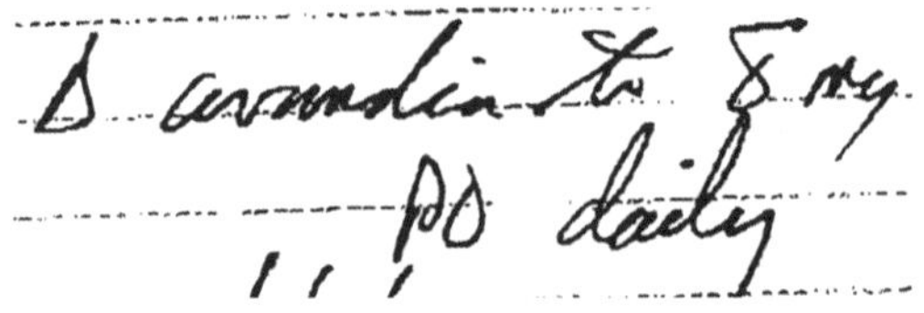

FIGURE 11-6   Order for Avandia interpreted as Coumadin.

Staff working in surgical areas should be aware of the potential for fire and burns when flammable products are used in conjunction with a heat source. Even a static discharge is enough to ignite highly flammable products such as ethyl chloride. The need for flammable products should be evaluated; often, there are safer alternatives, especially for topical anesthetics.

Missing Medications

What appears to be a missing dose is often a sign of a potential error. Finding a dose "missing" could mean any of the following:

- The medication was already given but not documented,
- The medication was already given on another unit or in a procedure area,
- The medication was prescribed using a brand name and dispensed as a generic or therapeutic substitution,
- The medication time or frequency was scheduled incorrectly,
- The prescriber's order was incorrectly interpreted or mistranscribed at some point in the medication-use process,
- The medication was not dispensed by pharmacy because of a safety problem (e.g., allergy, unsafe dose, interaction),
- The order was not sent to pharmacy, or
- A discontinued drug remains active on the MAR.

For example, a patient received unintended warfarin doses (8 mg) when a nurse misinterpreted a poorly handwritten order for Avandia (rosiglitazone) as Coumadin (warfarin) (Figure 11-6). The pharmacy dispensed Avandia, but for 2 days nurses called for the missing warfarin. On the third evening, when a nurse called again, the pharmacist added warfarin to the patient's profile as a daily dose, but this was done improperly, without an actual order for verification. After 5 days, a physician discovered the error while reviewing a computer-generated list of the patient's medications. The patient required fresh frozen plasma and vitamin K. After this and appropriate antidiabetic therapy, the patient recovered.

Missing doses are an inconvenience and could certainly be related to system problems with pharmacy dispensing or delivery. However, even if it means a delay in therapy, missing doses should never be borrowed from other patients' supplies. The original order should be verified before a "missing" medication is requested and administered.

Nurse Preparation of IV Solutions

When preparing a drug infusion on a patient care unit, the nurse must assemble the right drug and the correct volume and solution of diluent, calculate the amount of drug to add to the solution, obtain a syringe and properly measure the drug additive, mix the solution, and prepare an accurate label with the right patient's name. This is often accomplished on a cramped, crowded counter area of the nursing unit, with many other medications nearby and no independent double-check system or documentation for prepared doses. Distractions and interruptions during the process are likely. The situation is not conducive to safe drug preparation.

A far simpler and safer approach is the use of commercially available or pharmacy-prepared admixtures. When 24-hour pharmacy services are available, the pharmacy should prepare and dispense all injectable solutions that are not available commercially, except in rare cases when a nurse must mix and hang a solution immediately.

Preparation of admixtures on the nursing unit eliminates the opportunity for one practitioner's mistake to be caught by another before an error can reach the patient. If a nurse must prepare an IV admixture in the absence of a pharmacist, all calculations should be independently verified by another nurse, and preparation of the admixture should undergo another independent check before administration to the patient.

In EDs, critical care units, and other areas where nurses may need to mix IV solutions in emergencies, mixing protocols should be readily available and should be followed. If emergency boxes are used for particular medications such as thrombolytics, the mixing protocols should be inside the box for immediate reference.

Chapter 17 discusses admixture preparation for pediatric patients and the importance of minimizing preparation by nurses, using standardized concentrations, and avoiding reliance on the "rule of 6."

Nurse Access to Pharmacy

In hospitals that do not have 24-hour pharmacy services, open access to the pharmacy by nurses after hours is not safe and does not ensure medication quality. JCAHO standards do not allow pharmacy access by nurses, and some state regulations prohibit nurses from entering the pharmacy after hours.

Many harmful or potentially harmful errors have been reported when nonpharmacists have retrieved the wrong medication, dose, or dosage form from a closed pharmacy. Most errors are linked to nurses' lack of familiarity with the wide variety of tablet strengths; vial sizes, concentrations, and strengths; and dosage forms stocked in the pharmacy.

For example, nursing access to the pharmacy after hours led to an error in which an IV solution containing potassium 132 mEq/L and phosphate 90 mmol/L was prepared and partially administered to a patient. An order had been written during the night for 30 mEq of potassium phosphate in 1,000 mL IV to run over 6 hours. A nursing supervisor entered the pharmacy and attempted to determine the contents of 15 mL vials of potassium phosphate injection. On the side of the vial, the label stated, "Each mL contains monobasic potassium phosphate (anhydrous) 224 mg; dibasic potassium phosphate (anhydrous) 236 mg; water for injection q.s. 7.4 mOsmol/mL. Each mL provides: potassium 170 mg (4.4 mEq); phosphate ($H_2PO_4^-$ + HPO_4^{2-}) 285 mg (equivalent to 3 mM phosphorus)." The front of the label prominently listed "Potassium Phosphate," followed by "Phosphorus 3 mM/mL" and "Potassium 4.4 mEq/mL" in much smaller print. Below this, "15 mL" was listed in large bold print. The label information overwhelmed the supervisor, and she misread "15 mL" as 15 mM. Believing that 15 mM and 15 mEq were equivalent, she dispensed two vials.

The patient's nurse, equally confused, added both vials to the IV fluid and started the infusion. The pharmacy reopened about an hour later and the error was immediately detected. The supervisor documented removal of 2 vials of potassium phosphate 15 mM, but she left a sample of the 15 mL vial on the counter for inspection. The patient received just 150 mL of the solution (about 20 mEq of potassium and 14 mM of phosphorus), and serious harm was avoided.

When pharmacy services are not available, the use of an outside pharmacy, nighttime floor stock in automated or nonautomated dispensing cabinets, and access to a location containing selected medications should be considered, as allowed by state law and regulation. A limited supply of specific medications on a "night formulary" could be stocked in a centralized dispensing cabinet. Where such a cabinet is used, it should be stocked with premixed IV solutions and unit dose medications. Nonformulary drugs should not be available. The number of doses or vials stocked should be minimized. Dosing errors have been averted simply by allowing access to only a small quantity of a drug. If the quantity seems insufficient for an order, the nurse is likely to recalculate the dose, clarify the dose with the prescriber, or call a pharmacist, resulting in recognition and correction of the error.

Alerts and special instructions can be posted on night drug containers. A pharmacist should be on call for questions, and an independent double-check system should be established to verify all calculations and drugs removed from the night cabinet. Each morning, pharmacy staff should immediately compare all drugs removed from the night cabinet with the physicians' orders.

Centralized order processing systems have also been used to prevent errors related to a lack of 24-hour pharmacy services.[25] Order entry can be performed by pharmacists at a remote location that has access to each hospital's pharmacy computer system and other electronic data (e.g., lab, radiology). Orders are sent to the remote pharmacy by digital scanning or fax. Although the remote pharmacy is isolated from other pharmacy functions, each pharmacist on duty has the ability to contact staff at the referring hospital when necessary. After order entry, the drug is accessible in automated dispensing equipment. The potential benefits of such a system include minimal distractions, improved staffing patterns, high satisfaction levels, and reduced medication errors.

ENVIRONMENT, WORKFLOW, AND STAFFING PATTERNS

Noise, lighting, interruptions, distractions, flawed workflow, and other characteristics of the environment can make it difficult for nurses to remain focused on the critical tasks involved in drug administration. Mental slips due to inattention are responsible for 11% of prescribing errors, 12% of administration errors, and 73% of transcription errors.[18]

Distractions are common during the transcription and entry of orders, because unit secretaries and nurses often have to answer telephones and requests for information during this process. Staffing deficiencies and excessive workload contribute to errors. Because of fluctuations in census and in patients' severity of illness, the availability of qualified staff may be inadequate.[18]

Poorly designed work processes are especially vulnerable to environmental stresses. When processes are inefficient, rework, interruptions, inadequate information and supervision, poor prioritization, and unproductive time management are likely—and the chance for errors is increased.

Distractions

Medication error reports to the United States Pharmacopeia (USP) indicate that distractions are a greater problem for nurses than for pharmacists, pharmacy technicians, and physicians.[26] Over a 5-year period (1998–2002), nearly 35,000 errors related to distractions were submitted to USP's MEDMARX database. Nurses were the most frequent category of personnel involved in these errors, which occurred most often during drug administration.

The proportion of errors categorized as wrong patient errors doubled when distractions played a role.[26] Interruptions can cause nurses to confuse one patient's medications with those of another patient. After receiving a call to send a patient to physical therapy, a nurse interrupted her sequence of administering medications to prepare that patient's medications. She found the patient's MAR, selected the correct medications, and opened the medications and placed them in a cup. But she took the cup into the room of the next patient in her sequence of administration and gave the medications to the wrong patient. The nurse detected her error while documenting the medication administration. The patient was transferred to ICU because antihypertensive drugs were among the medications given in error.

Minimizing distractions during drug administration is difficult, but the following measures have been moderately effective:[27]

- Establishing "do not disturb" times (during drug administration) and places (in the medication room),
- Educating staff on the importance of working as a team, staying focused during drug administration, and avoiding unnecessary distractions while others are administering medications, and
- Providing phone and call-bell support for nurses who are administering medications.

Staffing Level

A November 2003 report by the Institute of Medicine (IOM), *Keeping Patients Safe: Transforming the Work Environment of Nurses,*[28] concluded that the environment in which nurses work cultivates error, not safety. According to that report, research confirms that how well patients are cared for by nurses affects their health and safety. For example, nearly half of all prescribing errors and one-third of transcription and dispensing errors are intercepted, largely by nurses, before they reach the patient.[18] The number of patient deaths is greater when there are fewer nurses to provide care.[29] Nurses' ongoing monitoring of patients' health status is directly related to better outcomes.[30]

Despite compelling evidence that higher nurse staffing levels result in safer patient care, staffing levels vary widely in hospitals and nursing homes. Data from 135 hospitals showed that a medical–surgical day nurse was typically responsible for about 6 patients; in 23% of the hospitals, however, such a nurse was responsible for as many as 12 patients.[31]

Federal regulations governing nursing home staffing are outdated and do not reflect recent information on safe staffing levels. For example, for each facility only one registered nurse (RN), for 8 consecutive hours every day, is required, regardless of patient capacity. Furthermore, the regulations do not specify minimum staffing levels for nursing assistants, who provide most of the care in nursing homes.

The 2003 IOM report concluded that, to improve patient safety, nurse staffing patterns should

- Incorporate estimates of patient volume that count admissions, discharges, and "less than full-day" patients in addition to a census of patients at a point in time,
- Involve direct-care nursing staff in selecting and evaluating the approaches used to determine appropriate unit staffing levels for each shift,
- Provide for staffing "elasticity" or "slack" within each shift's scheduling to accommodate unpredicted variations in patient volume and acuity and resulting workload (e.g., scheduling excess staff, creating cross-trained float pools), and
- Empower nursing unit staff to regulate unit workflow and set criteria for unit closures to new admissions and transfers as nursing workload and staffing necessitate.

The report also recommended ongoing evaluation of the effectiveness of nurse staffing practices if staffing levels fall below the following for a 24-hour day:

TABLE 11-3   Effects of Fatigue[32-36]

Slowed reaction time
Reduced accuracy
Diminished ability to recognize significant but subtle changes in a patient's health
Inability to deal with the unexpected
Lapses of attention and inability to stay focused
Omissions and neglect of nonessential activities
Compromised problem solving and decision-making
Impaired communication skills
Inability to recall
Short-term memory lapses
Reduced motivation
Irritability or hostility
Indifference and loss of empathy
Intrusion of sleep into wakefulness
Decreased energy for successful completion of required tasks
Decreased learning of new activities
Reduced hand–eye coordination

- In hospital ICUs—one licensed nurse for every two patients (12 hours of licensed nursing staff per patient day);
- In nursing homes, for long-stay residents—one RN for every 32 patients (0.75 hour per resident day), one licensed nurse for every 18 patients (1.3 hours per resident day), and one nursing assistant for every 8.5 patients (2.8 hours per resident day).

Long Hours and Overtime

Health care providers' long work hours and the resulting fatigue pose a serious threat to patient safety. As shown in Table 11-3, the detrimental effects of fatigue on performance are well documented.[32-36] Prolonged wakefulness can degrade performance, leaving a health care provider with the equivalent of a blood alcohol concentration of 0.1%, which is above the legal limit for driving in most states.[37]

Although other industries have taken actions to defend against the effects of fatigue, health care has largely disregarded the problem, partly because of the ongoing shortages of licensed practitioners. The *Keeping Patients Safe* report[28] recommends that nurses work no more than 12 hours a day and 60 hours a week, in any combination of scheduled shifts, mandatory overtime, or voluntary overtime. The Anesthesia Patient Safety Foundation offers additional suggestions for reducing worker fatigue (page 267).[38]

Workflow and Workload

Timing of Medication Administration

Health care institutions define the specific time frame in which medications are to be administered—usually within 60 minutes of the scheduled time. Use of a unit dose system has improved the timeliness of medication administration because it reduces medication preparation time.

The potential for medication errors is greatest in the morning, because more medications are given in the morning than at any other time. For this reason, many hospitals have adopted standard alternative times for medications that require laboratory monitoring or specific patient assessment before administration. For example, warfarin is often given late in the afternoon or at bedtime so that the INR can be checked earlier in the day and the daily dose adjusted if necessary. Digoxin is frequently given at noon or in the

---

REDUCING FATIGUE IN THE WORKPLACE[38]

Education. Using multiple educational forums, provide practitioners and managers with information about the science of sleep, risks associated with fatigue, mechanisms that underlie sleep disorders and fatigue, circadian rhythm disturbances, and approaches to optimize performance. An assessment of staff perceptions about the impact of fatigue on safety may offer a helpful starting point for ongoing education in this area.

Scheduling. Conduct a fatigue analysis on current staffing patterns, looking at the minimum off-duty time, consecutive work periods, and rest/recovery opportunities. Establish work schedules with off-duty requirements (intended for rest), limitations on hours worked each day and week, and time limitations for specific, potentially fatiguing physical and mental tasks within each workday. Disruptions in circadian rhythms, or our biological clock, can also result in fatigue. Whenever possible, recognize the circadian rhythm principles when designing work schedules. Also establish contingency plans to manage staff who have suffered a particularly fatiguing work schedule and consider themselves unfit to continue work.

Planned naps. Establish policies that sanction planned naps in the workplace for staff prone to fatiguing schedules, and procedures that address the timing of naps and required coverage. Even short naps of 45 minutes have been shown to be beneficial in improving alertness, without undue grogginess upon awakening. Create quality accommodations and space for these planned rest periods.

Routine rest and meal breaks. Provide for periodic rest breaks; a 15–30 minute break away from the work area decreases the effects of sleep deprivation. If unable to take breaks, report the inadequacy to supervisors. Good-quality meals and nutritious refreshments should be available at all times for health care workers, including at night.

Light therapy. Application of higher levels of ambient light has helped reduce the effects of disrupted circadian rhythm for night-shift workers. Special facilities may be needed to allow workers to obtain light therapy at designated times, though, since timing is crucial to its success.

Use of evidence-based safety practices. While not a replacement for well-rested staff, the use of proven safety practices and technologies such as CPOE, bar coding, and "smart" infusion pumps may help overcome some of the errors caused by any impairment from fatigue.

---

early evening, when few medications are given, so that the nurse will have time to check the patient's apical and radial pulses as indicators of digoxin level.

Nurses must consider the timing of each medication in relation to others the patient is receiving. For example, oral antacids should not be administered with quinolone antimicrobials, because the antacid will bind to the quinolone. Incompatibilities among IV medications must be checked before medications are added to the same infusion container or administered via a Y site. At the time medications are ordered and added to the MAR, drug interactions or incompatibilities should be noted, and nursing and pharmacy should cooperate in determining an appropriate administration schedule.

Standard Administration Schedules

Standardized drug administration times should be established throughout the facility. Nonstandard times can result in delayed, omitted, or duplicate doses. If the administration times determined by nurses differ from those anticipated by pharmacy, "missing" medications will delay therapy; furthermore, when the missing dose, now off schedule, is received, the nurse may not remember to administer it. Omissions can also occur because nurses are not accustomed to administering medications at nonstandard times. Duplicate doses may be given if a nurse administers the drug at the conventional time as well as the nonstandard time.

Dosing Windows

When a first dose is administered at a nonstandard time, nurses need an agreed-upon method of converting subsequent doses to the standardized schedule. Many hospitals have guidelines for this purpose. These "dosing windows" or "staggered dosing times" provide a matrix for determining the safest time to administer the second dose according to when the first dose was administered. Patients usually are back on a standard dosing schedule by the third dose. Dosing windows help ensure that nurses and pharmacists consistently follow the same schedule. Exceptions must be made for drugs such as aminoglycosides that require individualized scheduling by pharmacy after the nurse communicates the time of the first dose.

Schedules must sometimes be changed to accommodate patient procedures or to prevent the administration of incompatible medications at the same time. A clear method of communication between nursing and pharmacy is needed so that dosing times can be safely returned to the standard schedule. The dosing window matrix is useful for this purpose.

STAFF COMPETENCY AND EDUCATION

Many newly licensed nurses are not prepared to provide safe, effective care, according to surveys of new graduates and nursing leaders.[39,40] In particular, they lack skills in critical thinking, working as part of an interdisciplinary team, and recognizing subtle but important changes in patients' health. Like newly licensed physicians, new nurses need additional training and education once they enter the workforce. Similarly, experienced nurses need ongoing education to keep up with advances in medical knowledge and technology.

It is unrealistic to assume that nurses can know all they need to know about all medications on the market. Most nurses (72%) responding to a 2005 survey on patient safety said medication errors are more likely to occur when nurses are unfamiliar with the medication being administered.[41]

Education alone cannot effectively close the gap in nurses' knowledge and insure against medication errors. A more effective strategy is providing nurses with immediate access to the right quantity and quality of information about medications, exactly when needed, through the use of information technology. In the 2005 patient safety survey, nurses indicated that automatic notification of important information would improve their jobs and help protect their patients.

Practices that result in a culture of safety are another area of staff competency and education that should be addressed and periodically assessed. Many of the actions recommended for nurses in the 2006 IOM report *Preventing Medication Errors*[42] are directly related to safety practices; examples include the following:

- Establish safe work environments for medication preparation, administration, and documentation.
- Maintain a culture of rigorous commitment to principles of safety in medication administration.
- Enhance communication skills and team training so as to be prepared and confident in questioning medication orders and evaluating patient responses to drugs.
- Work to improve systems that address most common near misses in the work environment.

TABLE 11-4 Priorities for Nurse Education

Medication Errors
Risk assessment methods for identifying, reporting, and analyzing errors and hazards in care
Medication errors that have occurred in the facility and related error prevention strategies
Medication errors that have occurred in other organizations and error prevention strategies (including
    information in the *ISMP Medication Safety Alert!*)
System-based causes of medication errors

Safety Design Principles
Human error (cognitive and psychosocial basis for human error)
Principles and strategies for error reduction (e.g., standardization, simplification, reducing handoffs, restricting
    access, minimizing reliance on memory, redundancy for critical functions, forcing functions, fail-safes)
Measurement of medication safety in terms of structure, process, and outcomes

Medications
Safe use of high-alert medications or drugs with unusual or critical dosing considerations
New medications added to the formulary (or inventory) and associated policies, procedures, and guidelines
Existing and new black box warnings or life-threatening adverse drug reactions reported in the literature

Processes
Institutional efforts to deal with current and projected drug shortages
Institutional efforts to deal with current and projected staff shortages
Guidelines for using the override feature on automated dispensing cabinets
High-risk processes such as patient-controlled analgesia

Interdisciplinary Teams
Interdisciplinary team training
Team communication and decision-making
Managing intimidation in the workplace

Patient-Centered Care
Patient health literacy
Patient diversity
Pain management
Patient education about medication error prevention

Informatics
Knowledge of information technology capabilities and clinical applications
Specific technology (e.g., computerized prescriber order entry, bar-coded drug dispensing and administration,
    electronic medical records) to enhance medication safety
Automated drug information resources available for staff or patients
Automated forms of interdisciplinary and team communication
Use of informatics for decision support
Use of informatics to search for evidence-based practices

Evidence-Based Practices
Integration of clinical expertise, patient values, and evidence-based practice
Ongoing quest for improved safety and patient outcomes
Commitment to lifelong learning

- Play a role in evaluating the efficacy of new safety systems and technology.
- Contribute to the development and implementation of error reporting systems,
  and support a culture that values accurate reporting of medication errors.

To help reduce the risk of serious medication errors, the orientation and ongoing education
of nurses and other health care practitioners should focus on these priorities and the core
competencies listed in Table 11-4.

PATIENT EDUCATION

Patients should be encouraged to ask questions about their medications and seek satisfactory answers. Many errors have been prevented by observant and informed patients and their families.

For example, when a patient with diabetes insisted that a dose of 85 units of NPH insulin was too much, the nurse checked the order and the MAR. Although both indicated that the dose was correct, the nurse took the patient's concern seriously and called the attending physician. She learned that the dose had been ordered in error because another physician had relied on medical records from the patient's prior admission.

A tragic example in which patient concerns were not immediately addressed is the highly publicized death of a well-informed patient at the Dana-Farber Cancer Institute. She told her health care providers that she felt something was wrong after 2 days of treatment. Both the patient and her husband repeatedly asked the staff to check her chemotherapy orders. Without investigating thoroughly, the providers reassured the patient that her orders were correct. Each day for 4 days, she received a dose equivalent to the entire course of therapy (i.e., she received a fourfold overdose). It is impossible to know whether the patient would have survived if the error had been caught after 2 days, but there is no doubt that 4 days of course-dose therapy was the cause of death.

Patient education can present some challenges for nurses. More than 250 nurses participated in a 2003 ISMP survey on teaching patients about their medications.[43] The respondents indicated that discussion at discharge (94%) or during drug administration (84%) was the method most often used to teach patients about their medications. Written information about medications was provided to patients much less frequently; one in four nurses said they never provide it. One-third of nurses said the available written materials did not cover the most important information clearly for their patients. Half of the nurses said they did not use videos, television, or an intranet site to teach patients about medications or medication safety.

More than two-thirds (68%) of the nurses said they required all patients to repeat back information or demonstrate drug administration techniques that they had been taught. Nurses who worked in teaching hospitals (75%) were even more likely to require this validation. Most nurses (80%) said patients were given a way to contact them with questions after discharge; the response for patients who visited outpatient settings was 92%.

Fifty-six percent of nurses in teaching hospitals and 41% in nonteaching hospitals had little or no written information to give patients about preventing medication errors. One in four nurses cited lack of written materials about medications as a frequent problem; one in three said they often lacked written materials in the patient's native language; and one in four said written materials might not be suitable for their patients' level of reading or health literacy. Most respondents believed they had sufficient knowledge about medications to educate patients, readily available drug references, and access to pharmacy resources. However, nearly half (43%) of all responding nurses said they lacked time for teaching (47% of nurses in inpatient settings, compared with 29% in outpatient settings).

Table 11-5 provides tips for teaching patients about medications and error prevention. Also see Chapter 13.

QUALITY PROCESSES AND RISK MANAGEMENT

About one in five medications (19%) reach patients in error.[44] More than one-third (38%) of these errors originate during drug administration.[18] About the same proportion of errors (39%) occur when physicians prescribe medications, but nurses and pharmacists detect about half (48%) of those errors before they reach the patient. In contrast, just 2% of errors

TABLE 11-5 Patient Teaching Tips

Install a computerized drug information system (e.g., Micromedex, Lexi-Pals) that offers patient leaflets in different languages and appropriate reading levels.

Provide patients with written drug information if they are taking error-prone medications (e.g., metered-dose inhalants) or high-alert medications (e.g., warfarin, heparin, insulin, opioids, chemotherapy).

Include the family or caregivers, when appropriate, during patient education. Do not wait until discharge to begin education about complex drug regimens.

Clearly explain the directions for using each medication, including obvious information. (For example, patients have eaten the oranges that they used to practice insulin injections, believing that is how they should take their insulin; drunk a capful of medication while sitting in the bathtub instead of putting a capful in the bathtub; spread contraceptive jelly on their toast each morning for birth control; taken warfarin prn because they were told the medication was "for leg pain and swelling.")

Always require repeat demonstrations or explanations about medications that will be taken at home.

Use the time you already spend with patients (e.g., during assessments and daily care) to evaluate their level of understanding about their medications.

Develop standing orders for pharmacy consultations to educate patients who are being discharged on five or more prescription medications.

Identify patients at risk for nonadherence with medication regimens. Consider a referral to home care services, and alert a pharmacist to design a drug administration schedule that minimizes the number of times per day that medications must be taken or administered.

---

that originate during drug administration are intercepted and corrected. Thus, errors made when administering medications are much more likely to reach the patient. Furthermore, it has been reported that more than half of the medication errors that cause harm originate during drug administration.[18] These findings make a powerful case for enhancing double-check systems during drug administration so that potentially harmful errors are detected and corrected before they reach patients.

Interdisciplinary Double-Check Systems

Because there are many opportunities for error, the ideal medication administration system is one in which there is more than one practitioner between the drug and the patient. Persons who prescribe, dispense, and administer drugs must rely on one another to detect and prevent errors. For example, while screening orders, a pharmacist may detect a prescribing error such as an inappropriate dose, duplicate therapy, or a drug interaction. While checking medications before administration, a nurse may detect a pharmacy dispensing error. While reviewing a daily computer printout of a patient's current medication regimen, a physician may detect the inadvertent discontinuation of a drug by nursing or pharmacy staff.

Most pharmacies have a system of double-checking medications. Multiple staff members are involved in entering the order, using software to screen it for appropriateness and safety (allergies, contraindications, safe dosage range, interactions), preparing the medications, and checking the drugs against the order before they are dispensed. However, this safety system is bypassed when doses are prepared from floor stock on the nursing unit, borrowed from other patients, or obtained from an ADC before a pharmacist has screened the order. The following example shows what can go wrong without such independent double checks.

A nursing staff development director was asked to fill in as a staff nurse on the ICU. One of her patients was supposed to receive pentobarbital. She misread the MAR and thought the patient was to receive phenobarbital IV. When she could not find phenobarbital in the patient's medication bin, she assumed that the pharmacist had forgotten to put it there. She retrieved a supply from floor stock and administered the drug. Had the nurse called the pharmacist about the "missing dose," this error could have been detected.

Interdisciplinary double checks are also vital at the time of order transcription. The unit secretaries or coordinators who often transcribe orders are less familiar with medications and dosage forms than a nurse or pharmacist would be. It is less likely that the wrong drug, dose, or dosage form will reach a patient when both pharmacy and nursing staff have reviewed the orders.

For example, a physician wrote an order for "Rocephin 1 gm IVPB q12." Because of the poor handwriting, the unit secretary and nurse interpreted the "q12" as "qid." The nurse was unaware that Rocephin is usually given only once or twice daily. Following procedure, a copy of the order was sent to the pharmacy. The pharmacist recognized the error and immediately called the nursing unit. Without this intervention, the patient might have received twice the prescribed amount. Dose omissions are also less likely under a system that requires double-checking, because an order that is missed on the nursing unit has a chance of being recognized in the pharmacy, and vice versa.

Most hospitals have adopted the unit dose drug distribution system. Medications arrive in ready-to-use, single-dose form. The nurse can check each dose to make sure it matches the order transcribed onto the MAR. The greatest safety advantage of the unit dose system is that the pharmacist and the nurse can independently interpret, transcribe, and verify each dose before dispensing or administering it. When a pharmacist dispenses a dose of medication that does not correspond to the MAR, it is a signal that something may be incorrect. A pharmacist or nurse may have misinterpreted the order, a mistranscription or an error in computer order entry may have occurred, or the wrong drug may have been selected. The process is halted until the situation is investigated and corrected if necessary. In contrast, when a single nurse interprets, transcribes, prepares, and administers the dose, it is unlikely that the system will provide adequate checks to capture errors.

Independent Double Checks

The examples above involve interdisciplinary double checks by nurses, physicians, pharmacists, pharmacy technicians, and unit secretaries. Effective double-checking can also be accomplished by two nurses who work separately and verify each component of the other's work. For example, one nurse calculates and prepares a dose, and another independently checks the order, makes the same calculation, and compares the results.

Two people are unlikely to make the same mistake if they work independently. But if they work together or influence the checking process by offering hints, both nurses could follow the same path to an error. Therefore, holding up a syringe and a vial and saying, "This is 5 units of regular insulin; can you check it?" is not effective. Each person should independently start with the order and end up with the same result. The person asking for the double check must not influence the checker in any way.

Asking one nurse to double-check the work of another can be an important safety strategy, but it is a practice that may not be readily accepted. Some nurses may think the time required for the checking process is not justified by what they believe to be a small number of problems that would be detected. Others may think double checks could lead to more mistakes if staff members come to rely on the checker to catch problems. As staff shortages continue, the value of double checks is under increased scrutiny, especially because errors have reached patients despite double checks. Although research on double checks by nurses is lacking, studies involving other clinicians suggest that independent double checks are worth the time they require.[45,46]

Double checks identify a higher rate of errors than most people realize. Pharmacists who independently checked 5,700 prescriptions awaiting pickup uncovered 240 (4.2%) that were filled in error.[45] Of these, 2.1% were considered potentially harmful to the patients. In another study, errors were artificially introduced into the medication-use process; 93–97% of the errors were identified during an independent double check.[45,46] Over time, a significant number of mistakes can be identified through an independent double check.

In simulations, participants are much better at finding mistakes made by others than at finding their own mistakes.[45] Confirmation bias may keep the nurse calculating a dose from recognizing his or her own mistake; independent calculation by another nurse is likely to be more accurate. However, certain environmental conditions can lead both nurses, working independently, to make the same mistake; both may misread a poorly legible order or a confusing drug label.

Independent double-checking should never be the only safety strategy. It should be limited to situations that involve high-alert drugs, complex processes, and high-risk patients. Overall, processes that prevent errors are more effective than processes for detecting them.

Automated Double-Check Systems

Technology can enable an automated double check during drug administration. Bar code scanning at the point of care can be used to verify the five rights of drug administration. "Smart" infusion pumps can help ensure safe dosage ranges and accurate programming. However, nurses should carefully consider whether technology can replace all manual checkpoints. Bar coding cannot verify that an infusion pump is programmed correctly. Smart pumps cannot verify that a line is attached to the correct access port or that it is connected to the correct channel of a multichannel pump. In designing appropriate double-check systems, each component of the checking process should be evaluated against the capabilities of the technology, and manual checks should remain in place for critical components not addressed by the technology.

REFERENCES

1. Institute for Safe Medication Practices. *Mosby's Nursing PDQ for Medication Safety.* St Louis: Mosby; 2005.
2. Huskey RJ. Teratogens. Biology 121: human biology web site. Available at: www.people.virginia.edu/~rjh9u/terato.html. Accessed May 29, 2005.
3. Gardiner S, Begg E. Drug safety in lactation. Prescriber update No. 21:10–23. Available at: www.medsafe.govt.nz/Profs/PUarticles/lactation.htm#Safety. Accessed May 29, 2005.
4. Lazarou J, Pomeranz BM, Corey PN. Incidence of adverse drug reactions in hospitalized patients: a meta-analysis of prospective studies. *JAMA.* 1998;279:1200–5.
5. Bochner BS, Lichtenstein LM. Anaphylaxis. *N Engl J Med.* 1991;324:1785.
6. Hunt KJ, Valentine MD, Kagey-Sobotka A, et al. Anaphylaxis. *J Allergy Clin Immunol.* 1998;101:S465–S528.
7. Institute for Healthcare Improvement. Medication reconciliation. Available at: www.ihi.org/IHI/Topics/PatientSafety/MedicationSystems/Measures/Errors+Related+to+Unreconciled+Medications+per+100+Admissions.htm. Accessed May 10, 2005.
8. University of Chicago Hospitals. New recommendations proposed for safe use of herbal medications by patients having surgery. July 10, 2001. Available at: www.uchospitals.edu/news/2001/20010710-herbs.html. Accessed May 5, 2005.
9. Promoting pain relief and preventing abuse of pain medications: a critical balancing act. A joint statement from 21 health organizations and the Drug Enforcement Administration. Available at: www.ampainsoc.org/advocacy/pdf/consensus_1.pdf. Accessed June 15, 2005.
10. Rolfe S, Harper NJ. Ability of hospital doctors to calculate drug doses. *BMJ.* 1995;310:1173–4.
11. Jones SJ, Cohen AM. Confusing drug concentrations. *Anaesthesia.* 2001;56:195–6.
12. Nelson LS, Gordon PE, Simmons MD, et al. The benefit of houseofficer education on proper medication dose calculation and ordering. *Acad Emerg Med.* 2000;7:1311–6.
13. Raczkowski VF. Safety reporting requirements: proposed rules. June 19, 2003. Available at: www.fda.gov/cder/Offices/ODS/SADRDIA061903/sld024.htm.
14. Pirmohamed M, James S, Meakin S, et al. Adverse drug reactions as cause of admission to hospital: prospective analysis of 18,820 patients. *BMJ.* 2004;329:15-9.

15. Moore TJ, Weiss SR, Kaplan S, et al. Reported adverse drug events in infants and children under 2 years of age. *Pediatrics*. 2002;110:e53.
16. Moore TJ, Walsh CS, Cohen MR. Reported adverse event cases of methemoglobinemia associated with benzocaine products. *Arch Intern Med*. 2004;164(11):1192–6.
17. Lesar TS, Briceland L, Stein DS. Factors related to errors in medication prescribing. *JAMA*. 1997;277:312–7.
18. Leape LL, Bates DW, Cullen DJ, et al. Systems analysis of adverse drug events. *JAMA*. 1995; 274:35–43.
19. Smetzer JL, Vaida AJ, Cohen MR, et al. Findings from the ISMP Medication Safety Self-Assessment for Hospitals. *Jt Comm J Qual Patient Saf*. 2003;29(11)586–97.
20. Multidose vial linked to nosocomial HCV outbreak. *Hosp Infect Control*. May 2000:68–9.
21. Kirschke DL, Jones TF, Stratton CW, et al. Outbreak of joint and soft-tissue infections associated with injections from a multiple-dose medication vial. *Clin Infect Dis*. 2003;36:1369–73.
22. ECRI. A clinician's guide to surgical fires: how they occur, how to prevent them, how to put them out [guidance article]. *Health Devices*. 2003;32(1):5–24.
23. Hall MJ, Lawrence L. *Ambulatory Surgery in the United States, 1996*. Advance data from vital and health statistics; No. 300. Hyattsville, Md: National Center for Health Statistics; 1998.
24. Hall MJ, Owings MF. *2000 National Hospital Discharge Survey*. Advance data from vital and health statistics; No 329. Hyattsville, Md: National Center for Health Statistics; 2002.
25. Cronk J. Digital scanning and consolidated entry of medication orders in a multihospital health system. *Am J Health Syst Pharm*. 2002;59:731–3.
26. United States Pharmacopoeia. Distractions contribute to medication errors. *USP Patient Safety CAPSLink*. September 2003:2–4.
27. Pape TM. *The Effect of Nurses' Use of a Focused Protocol to Decrease Distractions during Medication Administration* [doctoral dissertation]. Denton, Tex: Texas Woman's University, College of Nursing; 2002.
28. Institute of Medicine. Keeping patients safe: transforming the work environment of nurses. In: Page A, ed. *Committee on the Work Environment for Nurses and Patient Safety*. Washington, DC: National Academies Press; 2004. Available at: www.iom.edu/report.asp?id=16173. Accessed May 23, 2005.
29. Aiken L, Clarke S, Sloane D, et al. Hospital nurse staffing and patient mortality, nurse burnout, and job satisfaction. *JAMA*. 2002;288:1987–93.
30. Kahn K, Rogers W, Rubenstein L, et al. Measuring quality of care with explicit process criteria before and after implementation of the DRG-based prospective payment system. *JAMA*. 1990;264(15):1969–73.
31. Cavouras C, Suby C. *Perspectives on Staffing and Scheduling. 2003 Survey of Hours Report: Direct and Total Hours per Patient Day (HPPD) by Patient Care Units*. Phoenix, Ariz: Labor Management Institute; 2003.
32. Gillberg M, Kecklund G, Akerstedt T. Relations between performance and subjective ratings of sleepiness during a night awake. *Sleep*. 1994;17(3):236–41.
33. Linde L, Bergstrom M. The effect of one night without sleep on problem-solving and immediate recall. *Psychol Res*. 1992;54(2):127–36.
34. Howard SK. Fatigue and the practice of medicine. *Anesth Patient Saf Found Newsletter*. 2005;20(1):1–4.
35. Rosekind MR, Gander PH, Connell LJ, et al. Crew factors in flight operations X: alertness management in flight operations. NASA Technical Memorandum # 1999-208780. Moffett Field, Calif: NASA; 1999.
36. Howard SK, Gaba DM, Smith BE, et al. Simulation study of rested versus sleep deprived anesthesiologists. *Anesthesiology*. 2003;98:1345–55; discussion 5A.
37. Dawson D, Reid K. Fatigue, alcohol and performance impairment. *Nature*. 1997;388:235.
38. *Anesth Patient Saf Found Newsletter*. 2005;20(1):1-24.
39. Smith J, Crawford L. *Report of Findings from the 2001 Employers Survey*. NCSBN Research Brief. 3. Chicago: National Council of State Boards of Nursing, Inc; 2002.
40. Smith J, Crawford L. *Report of Findings from the Practice and Professional Issues Survey—Spring 2001*. NCSBN Research Brief. 2. Chicago: National Council of State Boards of Nursing, Inc; 2002.
41. Harris Interactive. McKesson Survey of Frontline Nurses' Perceptions of the State of Patient Safety, 2005. Available at: http://mpt.mckesson.com/harris/splash.asp?&nlv=0&bct=Harris%20Survey. Accessed June 17, 2005.
42. Committee on Identifying and Preventing Medication Errors; Aspden P, Wolcott J, Bootman JL, et al., eds. *Preventing Medication Errors*. Washington, DC: National Academies Press; 2006. Prepublication copy available at http://darwin.nap.edu/books/0309101476/html/R2.html. Accessed July 21, 2006.
43. Institute for Safe Medication Practices. As you see it: patient education survey results. *ISMP Nurse Advise-ERR*. 2003;1(5):2.
44. Barker KN, Flynn EA, Pepper GA, et al. Medication errors observed in 36 health care facilities. *Arch Intern Med*. 2002;162(16):1897–903.
45. Grasha AF, Reilley S, Schell KL, et al. Process and delayed verification errors in community pharmacy: implications for improving accuracy and patient safety. Tech Report No. 112101. Cincinnati: Cognitive Systems Performance Lab; 2001.
46. Campbell GM, Facchinetti N. Using process control charts to monitor dispensing and checking errors. *Am J Health Syst Pharm*. 2000;55:946–52.

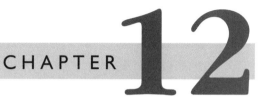

CHAPTER 12

PREVENTING MEDICATION ERRORS RELATED TO DRUG DELIVERY DEVICES

Judy L. Smetzer and Michael R. Cohen

Health care professionals use a wide variety of devices—from sophisticated infusion pumps to oral syringes—in medication administration. Research indicates that misuse of infusion pumps and other parenteral device systems is the second most frequent cause of medication errors during drug administration.[1] This suggests that safety features and intuitive use should be as important as price and service when pumps and other medication delivery devices are being evaluated for purchase or continued use.[2] Failure mode and effects analysis (FMEA) can be applied in the evaluation of these devices.[3,4] FMEA, as initially used in industries outside health care, closely examines the human–machine interface that is necessary for successful operation of equipment.

INFUSION PUMPS

Purchase

Using FMEA before purchasing new pumps can help health care providers predict how and when errors and other failures may occur. In this process, an interdisciplinary team (e.g., nurses, physicians, pharmacists, engineering staff, risk and quality staff) tries to identify all possible errors and other failures that could occur during pump use and predict how harmful those failures could be. Action can then be taken to eliminate or at least reduce the risk of pump failures that could harm patients. Chapter 21 further describes the use of FMEA to assess high-risk processes in health care.

The questions on page 276 offer a starting point for discussion of potential sources of infusion pump failure.[5] These questions can be applied to pumps being considered for purchase, or they can be used to evaluate the safety of an organization's current pumps.

Preventing Programming Errors

Harm is more likely to result from errors in administering medications by the IV route than by other routes.[1] Nurses like infusion pumps because they deliver IV medications at a much more accurate rate of infusion than can be maintained with gravity-flow drip. Pumps are a great improvement in terms of both therapeutic outcomes and patient safety. However, a tragic outcome can be just a keypunch away.

To limit pump size, manufacturers may design programming keys to be used for several functions, and small display screens may be cluttered with information. Some pump menus are so complex that they confuse even experienced nurses. A 2006 report from the Institute of Medicine (IOM) calls on the Agency for Healthcare Research and

USING FAILURE MODE AND EFFECTS ANALYSIS TO PREDICT INFUSION PUMP FAILURES

1. Basic functionality (How well does the pump perform the required task?)
   a. Is this the correct pump for the desired task(s)?
   b. Can the pump deliver the volume and increments needed under the correct pressure?
   c. Are any features (e.g., size, weight, number of channels) incompatible with the environment where the pump will be used?
   d. Will the pump deliver medications in the concentrations most typically used?
   e. What tubing and other supplies does the pump require to perform effectively and safely? Are these items usable with other pumps? Could other tubing be used for this pump, rendering it unsafe?
   f. Are users alerted to pump-setting errors? Wrong patient errors? Wrong channel errors? Wrong medication or solution errors? Mechanical failures?
   g. Does the pump have memory functions for settings and alarms with an easily retrievable log? If the pump is turned off, does it retain settings for a period of time?
2. User–machine interface (How easy and intuitive is it for people to use the pump?)
   a. What functionalities do users expect the pump to have?
   b. Is the number of steps for programming minimal?
   c. Are the touch buttons used in programming clearly labeled, logically positioned, and of an appropriate size?
   d. Are the screens readable, with appropriate font size, lighting, and contrast?
   e. Do the pump's units of medication delivery (e.g., micrograms per kilogram, micrograms per kilogram per minute) match current practices?
   f. Do the medications, units of delivery, and strengths appear in a logical sequence for selection?
   g. Is there any information that defaults to a predetermined value? If so, is it safe?
   h. Is it easy to install and prime administration sets and to remove air in the line?
   i. Are special features such as drug dose calculations and dose alerts helpful and easy to use?
   j. Are the screens free of abbreviations, trailing zeros (e.g., 1.0 mg), and naked decimal points (e.g., .1 mg)?
   k. Do the alarms clearly guide staff to the problems? Is it possible to permanently disable audible alarms or set them too low to be heard?
   l. If the infusion rate is changed, but not confirmed, does the device continuously alert the user that the solution is infusing at the old rate?
   m. Could the administration sets be mispositioned during installation or accidentally dislodged, separated, or removed by patients?
   n. Does the administration set prevent gravity free-flow of the solution when it is removed from the pump?
   o. Is the device tamper resistant?
   p. Does the pump fit into the typical workflow?
   q. How does the pump compare with the pumps now in use?

Quality and the medical device industry to develop and consistently apply user interface designs based on cognitive and human factors principles and appropriate for the clinical environment.[6] Until this occurs, programming errors when a pump's information is presented in a disorderly or illogical way, or when keys do not function as expected, are likely to continue.

For example, an error occurred when a nurse accidentally set an infusion pump to deliver an infant's total parenteral nutrition (TPN) solution at 130 mL/hour. She had intended to program the pump at 13.0 mL/hour, but the decimal point key failed to engage when she pressed it. (Setting the pump at 13, not 13.0, would have been safer.) The error was noticed about an hour after the start of the infusion. The infant's blood glucose level had risen to 363 mg/dL. The TPN infusion rate was decreased for several hours, and the infant suffered no permanent harm.

Errors can occur with pumps that automatically calculate an infusion rate, although this feature is intended to reduce the potential for errors. The process of programming the pump to calculate the infusion rate is error-prone. Nurses must enter, in the correct sequence, the total amount of drug in the solution, the volume, and the ordered dose. The need to program three different numbers into the device increases the opportunity for error.

In many reported errors, nurses have accidentally deleted or added a zero to the diluent volume or the total amount of drug in the solution, or entered the prescribed dose incorrectly. The pumps have then calculated an infusion rate based on the erroneous entries and delivered an overdose or underdose of medication.

For example, one patient received heparin 12,000 units/hr instead of 1,200 units/hr after the diluent volume was entered as 5,000 mL, not 500 mL. The pump automatically set the infusion rate at 240 mL/hr. Two other patients received heparin 7,000 units/hr instead of 700 units/hr after the total drug in the solution was entered as 2,500 units, not 25,000 units, and the pump automatically set the infusion rate at 140 mL/hr. The nurses assumed that the device would calculate an accurate infusion rate. They did not notice that the calculated rate far exceeded typical dosing for IV heparin infusions.

To detect device programming errors, infusions of high-alert medications should undergo independent checking before administration. One individual should ready the solution and program the pump, and another should independently verify the drug, dose concentration, line connection, patient identification, and infusion pump settings. When using pumps that automatically calculate an infusion rate, both practitioners should also observe the device's final infusion rate; simply recognizing an atypical infusion rate for the solution being administered can avert an error. Whenever possible, a single standard concentration for each high-alert drug solution should be established and used consistently throughout the facility to promote accurate programming.

Pharmacists should affix auxiliary labels to the containers of high-alert drug solutions that clearly list the data (the total amount of drug in the container, the volume of diluent, and the ordered dose) that must be entered into the infusion pump for calculation of an accurate infusion rate. For commonly used drug infusions, pharmacists can apply labels with dose/infusion rate tables so nurses can verify that the final infusion rate calculated by the pump is accurate.

Smart Pumps

Since 2002, "smart" infusion pumps have been available to warn nurses about programming errors so the errors can be corrected before an infusion is started. With smart pumps, a traditional IV pump becomes a computer capable of intercepting and preventing wrong dose and wrong infusion rate errors that may be due to misprogramming, miscalculation, or an inaccurately prescribed dose or infusion rate.[7] For each IV solution with a standard concentration, dose limits can be set in the pump and individualized for each patient type (e.g., adult, pediatric, neonate) or treatment type (e.g., chemotherapy). Then, when the pump is being programmed, an alert will appear if the infusion rate does not fall within the dose limits. Some pumps also offer compatibility information, special infusion directions, and other reminders. Chapter 15 provides more information on smart pumps.

One problem with smart pumps is that they are often used as a standalone system, rather than an integrated component of a comprehensive clinical information system; thus, they are not used to their full advantage.[6] Furthermore, dose limits for the pumps are loaded by each individual hospital, using drug terminology from its particular pharmacy system.

The 2006 IOM report[6] recommends development and application of standard data terminology to promote communication among smart pumps and other clinical information systems, including point-of-care bar-coding systems.

Protection from Free-flow

The Joint Commission on Accreditation of Healthcare Organizations requires hospitals to ensure free-flow protection on all general-use infusion pumps and patient-controlled analgesia (PCA) pumps used in the organization. Free-flow is accidental, uncontrolled gravity flow of IV fluids and drugs after the removal of an IV administration set from a pump.[8–10] Free-flow is possible with IV sets that lack a mechanism to prevent flow if the operator fails to close a manual control clamp. Free-flow of infusions has caused patient death. Most infusion pumps today are designed with fail-safe mechanisms that eliminate the risk of solution free-flow, but older pumps may not offer this protection.

Preventing Line Mix-ups

Multiple-channel IV pumps may be used when several solutions are being infused into a patient. This allows more room around the patient for providing care and facilitates the transport of patients who have several solutions infusing. However, the likelihood of mixing up administration lines increases when more than one pump or a dual-channel pump with the capacity for multiple rate settings is used.

In one example, a nurse accidentally switched the lines when using a two-channel pump to infuse tirofiban through one channel and heparin through the other. While hanging a new bag of each solution, she inadvertently threaded the tirofiban tubing through the channel already programmed for heparin, and vice versa. Another nurse noticed the error before patient harm occurred.

When using multiple-channel pumps, nurses should handle just one IV solution at a time. Physically tracing the line from the solution, through the pump, and to the patient (insertion site) helps ensure that the correct channel has been used to program the infusion. For selected high-alert drug infusions, one nurse should hang the solution and ready it for infusion, and another nurse should independently validate the original order, the patient's identification, the dose and concentration, the insertion site (route), and the pump or channel setting.

Affixing the name of the drug being infused to each IV line (at the end closest to the patient) and above each channel on the pump can also help; however, nurses should not rely on the label alone to select the proper channel. The label must be removed when the drug is discontinued. Nurses should conduct patient rounds more than once each shift to double-check all IV solutions and should take time to trace each line from the solution to the patient to validate proper channel selection. A multiple-channel pump should never be used to infuse solutions into two different patients. (This unsafe practice has been observed in inpatient and outpatient settings.)

The risk of a line mix-up should be factored into the decision to purchase and use multiple-channel pumps, but the same type of error could happen if two single-channel pumps on the same pole were in use. For instance, a patient was ordered infliximab 5 mg/kg IV infused over 2 to 3 hours. Tubing from a bag of saline solution that was hanging on the patient's IV pole was accidentally threaded through the pump instead of the tubing attached to the intended admixture. Since its tubing was not inserted in the pump, the infliximab admixture infused at an uncontrolled rate. The error was discovered 20 minutes later after the solution infiltrated and caused a 4×2 inch inflamed, indurated area. Phlebitis developed at the IV site.

Current technology cannot prevent line mix-ups. Bar coding could verify the solution being hung, but if the tubing had been switched during pump setup, the incorrect rate of infusion would not be detected. Similarly, current smart pumps that alert nurses to pump setting errors would not detect a line mix-up, although future models may be able to do so. The best approach is to label each infusion line and have two nurses independently trace the line back to the insertion site.

Protecting Epidural Lines

To prevent epidural administration of drugs or solutions not intended for use by this route, tubing used for epidural infusion should contain no side ports. Special tubing is available for this purpose; it has a yellow line running along the lumen to distinguish it from other tubing. Some organizations use a distinctive infusion pump for all epidural solutions to help ensure that IV solutions are not given epidurally.

Removing Lines

To prevent line mix-up and drug administration by an incorrect route, tubes or catheters that are no longer needed should be removed as soon as possible, especially when the patient has some lines still in use. One patient was transferred from the intensive care unit to the medical unit with an unneeded intra-arterial line in place. When the patient requested pain medication, the nurse prepared an IV dose of meperidine 25 mg. Since the IV line had infiltrated, she administered the meperidine into the intra-arterial line, which she thought was another venous line. The stopcock ports on the intra-arterial line had a male adapter, allowing easy access for blood draws. The nurse assumed the male adapter was an access site, since this type of adapter is often present on central venous lines used to monitor pressure. The patient suffered extreme pain and flushing during administration, but no permanent harm resulted. Clearly labeled access lines and removal of the unnecessary line before the patient's transfer could have helped prevent this error.

PATIENT-CONTROLLED ANALGESIA DEVICES

In contrast to the administration of analgesics by nurses, PCA allows the patient to self-administer smaller, more frequent doses as needed to control pain. When used as intended, this administration method reduces the risk of oversedation. However, errors with PCA occur and are sometimes serious. Factors contributing to these errors are discussed in the following paragraphs, and strategies for reducing the risk of errors are presented in Table 12-1.[11]

PCA by Proxy

PCA devices are intended to be activated by the patient. A sedated patient will not press the button to deliver more opioid, but family members and health professionals have administered doses, hoping to keep the patient comfortable. Such "PCA by proxy" has resulted in respiratory depression leading to death.

One postoperative patient asked her husband to press the button on her meperidine PCA device if she moved or made any noise as she slept during the night. He complied, and by morning the patient had suffered respiratory arrest and could not be resuscitated. In another instance, a nurse consistently woke an elderly patient, assessed his pain, and pressed the button on his morphine PCA device, believing she was helping a stoic patient. Extreme oversedation contributed to the patient's death.

Improper Patient Selection

Patients selected for PCA should have the mental alertness and cognitive, physical, and psychological ability to manage their pain. However, the benefits and convenience of PCA

TABLE 12-1 Safety Strategies for Patient-Controlled Analgesia (PCA)

Problem	Strategy	Examples
PCA by proxy	Improve access to information	■ Educate patients about the proper use of PCA; begin during the preoperative testing visit, when patients are not too groggy to understand
	Limit access	■ Warn caregivers, family members, and visitors about the dangers of PCA by proxy ■ Identify rare instances in which critical care patients may be suitable for nurse-controlled analgesia (nurse delivers each dose via PCA device) and the level of enhanced monitoring necessary for these patients
	Use reminders	■ Place warning labels on activation buttons that state "For Patient Use Only" ■ Provide visual and auditory feedback to patients when the button is pressed
Improper patient selection	Limit use	■ Establish patient selection criteria; candidates should have appropriate level of consciousness and cognitive ability to manage their pain and physical ability to use PCA device; infants, young children, and confused or agitated patients may not be suitable candidates
Inadequate patient monitoring	Careful monitoring	■ At a minimum, evaluate pain, alertness, and vital signs (including rate, quality, and depth of respirations) every 4 hours ■ Monitor patients more frequently during the first 24 hours and at night (when hypoventilation and nocturnal hypoxia can occur) ■ For an accurate assessment of patients' level of sedation, use minimal verbal and tactile stimulation before evaluation ■ Identify risk factors that could increase respiratory depression (e.g., obesity, low body weight, concomitant medications that potentiate opioids, asthma, sleep apnea) and determine the necessary level of enhanced monitoring (e.g., capnography, apnea alarms at night) ■ When nurse-controlled analgesia with a PCA device is used, require special monitoring (e.g., more frequent observation, vital signs, capnography) ■ Do not rely on pulse oximetry readings alone to detect opioid toxicity (oxygen saturation is usually maintained even at low respiratory rates) ■ Keep PCA flow sheets at the bedside to document doses and patient monitoring ■ Have oxygen and naloxone readily available at the bedside for use in the event of oversedation or respiratory depression
Drug product mix-ups	Standardize	■ Establish one standard concentration for each opioid used for PCA ■ Use prefilled syringes/bags/cassettes whenever available commercially; have pharmacy mix all PCA products that are not commercially available (hydromorphone)
	Limit access	■ Stock only the standard concentrations for morphine and hydromorphone in patient care units (dispense any other drugs used for PCA from the pharmacy) ■ Separate the storage of morphine and hydromorphone to avoid mix-ups
	Use reminders	■ Ask pharmacy to affix prominent warnings if dispensing an opioid in a nonstandard concentration
	Differentiate items	■ Ask pharmacy to label hydromorphone using tall-man letters (HYDROmorphOne) to differentiate it from morphine
	Require redundancies	■ Require pharmacy to review all PCA orders before initiation ■ Require an independent double check for patient identification, drug and concentration, pump settings, and the line attachment before initiation of PCA and at each syringe/cassette change ■ Use bar coding to verify the drug and concentration

TABLE 12-1   Safety Strategies for Patient-Controlled Analgesia (PCA) (continued)

Problem	Strategy	Examples
Prescribing errors	Standardize and simplify	■ Accept PCA orders only from prescribers who possess requisite proficiency ■ Use standard order sets to guide drug selection, doses, and lockout periods; patient monitoring; and precautions such as avoiding concomitant analgesics (which should also appear on the medication administration record) ■ Accept spoken/telephone orders only for dose changes ■ Ensure that prescribers have a list of other medications the patient has received (e.g., at home, intraoperatively) for consideration in determining the loading dose ■ Use morphine as opioid of choice; use hydromorphone for patients needing very high doses
Device misprogramming	Improve access to information	■ Train nurses to program PCA pumps; offer practice sessions as needed to maintain proficiency ■ Provide laminated instructions for use that are attached to each pump
	Limit access (reduce options)	■ To promote ongoing user proficiency, limit PCA pumps to a single model
	Forcing functions and fail-safes	■ Establish default settings on the PCA pump of zero or the highest concentration available for opioids delivered by PCA
	Require redundancies	■ Require an independent double check for patient identification, drug and concentration, pump settings, and the line attachment before initiation of PCA and at each syringe/cassette change ■ Verify PCA settings each shift, immediately after receiving report ■ Use "smart" PCA pumps that immediately alert the nurse if a programming error has been made
	Failure mode and effects analysis	■ To help identify potential failure points, include frontline nurses in the evaluation of new PCA pumps under consideration for purchase

Source: Adapted with permission from reference 11.

have led providers to extend its use to less than ideal candidates such as infants, young children, and confused patients. This facilitates the dangerous practice of PCA by proxy and can result in oversedation and sometimes death. PCA use in unsuitable patients may also result in undertreatment because of their inability to clearly communicate pain.

PCA use has led to oversedation of patients at risk for respiratory depression because of conditions such as obesity, asthma, or sleep apnea and patients concurrently receiving drugs that potentiate the action of opioids (e.g., benzodiazepines, barbiturates).

Inadequate Monitoring

Even at therapeutic doses, opioids can suppress respiration and decrease heart rate and blood pressure. Thus, standard monitoring intervals may not be adequate to alert caregivers to opioid toxicity. Patients may not be checked often enough during the first 24 hours and at night when nocturnal hypoxia can occur. Opioid toxicity can be overlooked if the nurse arouses the patient for the purpose of assessment; patients with induced respiratory depression or oversedation can easily be stimulated to a higher level of consciousness and an increased respiratory rate. Once the stimulus is removed, the patient may fall back into an oversedated state.

Reliance on pulse oximetry readings can also offer a false sense of security. Oxygen saturation is usually maintained even at low respiratory rates, especially if supplemental oxygen is being administered. One elderly patient on morphine PCA was found with a respiratory rate of 4 and an oxygen saturation of 96%. The patient's daughter, who had been advised not to press the button, was afraid the medication would wear off during the night, so she woke her mother frequently and encouraged her to push the button. Despite frequent monitoring during the night, the respiratory depression was not noticed until the next morning, partly because of the high pulse oximetry readings. The patient was given naloxone and responded quickly.

Improper Patient Use

Failure to control pain with PCA is often related to inadequate patient education. Most patients who are suitable candidates for PCA can be taught to use the device successfully. However, those who are taught to use the device during the immediate postoperative period are often too groggy to understand its use and have reported poor pain control during the first 12 hours after surgery. But alert, appropriate patients can also misunderstand the directions for use, believing they must press the button every 6 minutes or so even when they are sleepy and comfortable.

Design flaws can prevent patients from using PCA properly. The device activation button may look like a call bell, and patients have inadvertently given themselves a dose of analgesic while attempting to call a nurse. Many pumps fail to provide visual or auditory feedback, so patients are unable to tell whether a press of the button has been successful. Frustration and inadequate pain control may result.

Misprogramming

Misprogramming of PCA pumps is much too frequent, even when nurses are properly educated in use of the device. Complex programming sequences and pump design flaws often contribute. Programming a PCA pump requires multiple steps, and the device design is often far from intuitive. Common pump design flaws include the following:

- Some pumps contain manufacturer-set defaults for drug concentrations; this may be unknown to the users and result in overdosage or underdosage.
- Some do not require users to review all settings before the infusion starts, which makes verification of the programming difficult.
- Some require users to program the dose in milliliters, not milligrams, making it easy to overlook the drug concentration and amount of drug the patient is actually receiving.
- Some have hidden programming defaults, which may be unknown by the user.

The following adverse event was related to hidden programming defaults: A patient died from an overdose of fentanyl delivered as a bolus dose by a clinician. The two nurses who initially programmed the pump likely set the concentration at 50 mcg/mL as prescribed. However, the Deltec CADD-Prizm PCS Pain Control System pump (model 6101) defaulted to a prior setting, 1 mcg/mL, when the Enter key was not pressed within a set time period, so the pump delivered 50 mL.

Programming errors have been linked to mental slips or mix-ups. For example, a pump was programmed to deliver 5 mL (50 mg) of meperidine at each demand dose instead of the prescribed 5 mg, resulting in oversedation, and a morphine PCA pump was set to deliver 10 mg every 2 minutes, not 2 mg every 10 minutes as prescribed, again resulting in oversedation.

Mechanical Problems

Mechanical problems, such as siphoning of air from broken syringes or cassettes, short circuits, and insufficient batteries, can lead to failures in drug delivery. Some devices also obstruct the view of labels on syringes or cassettes once they are in the pump, thus limiting ongoing verification of the drug.

Inadequate Staff Education

Nurses may not always receive adequate education on PCA device programming, potential adverse events with PCA and how to avoid them, and patient monitoring requirements. Even when their training is adequate, nurses may not retain proficiency if multiple types of PCA pumps are used or if PCA is encountered infrequently. The result may be programming errors or failure to detect the signs of opioid toxicity.

Prescribers may not undergo a process for verifying proficiency in this form of pain management. Physicians have made mistakes in converting oral hydromorphone dosages to IV dosages. The correct oral to IV conversion range is between 3:1 and 5:1; patients have received overdosages when physicians assumed a 1:1 ratio. Prescribers have also made mistakes in selecting and calculating an appropriate drug and dose for a morbidly obese, opioid-naïve, or elderly patient. Occasionally, one opioid has been prescribed but the accompanying dose has been appropriate for a different opioid. Concurrent orders for other opioids (oral or injectable) during PCA use have resulted in opioid toxicity. In addition, clinicians have misheard or misread spoken or written PCA orders, sometimes with serious consequences.

Drug Mix-ups

Name similarities among the drugs used for PCA have led to mix-ups. Morphine and hydromorphone are most often confused; some nurses have thought that hydromorphone is the generic name for morphine (1.5 mg of hydromorphone is equivalent to about 10 mg of morphine). Morphine is available in prefilled syringes in two concentrations (1 mg/mL and 5 mg/mL), but the packaging may not help distinguish them, which leads to errors. Since opioids are typically unit stock, such errors are rarely detected. These errors most often result in overdoses, but they can also result in allergic reactions or undertreatment of pain.

ORAL SYRINGES

Liquid medications meant to be given through gastric or nasogastric tubes have been accidentally given intravenously because of failure to identify the correct tubing before administration. If given in a large enough dose, a suspension not intended for IV use can lodge in the pulmonary capillaries and lead to embolism and death.

The patients at greatest risk are those who have both IV lines and small-bore polyurethane nasogastric feeding tubes or percutaneously inserted gastric tubes in place. The distal ends of these small-bore tubes can accommodate Luer connections like those on the end of an IV administration set. Thus, an oral or enteral solution intended for administration through one of these small-bore tubes could be connected to an IV line.

For example, the manufacturer of Nimotop (nimodipine) oral capsules, Bayer Pharmaceutical Division, states that the drug may be given via nasogastric tube by extracting the contents of the capsule into a syringe, administering it via the tube, and flushing the tube with 30 mL of saline. In several instances, because the drug was in a parenteral syringe, nurses have given it IV, resulting in cardiac arrest.

The same mistake has been made when liquid medications meant to be given orally are drawn into parenteral syringes. In one reported case, the mother of a hospitalized child gave an oral medication intravenously. The nurse had drawn a dose of amoxicillin and clavulanate oral suspension into a parenteral syringe, but she had to leave the room for an emergency before administering the dose. Since the mother had been helping nurses administer other oral medications to her child, the nurse handed the mother the syringe, saying, "Can you give this to her?" The mother had previously watched nurses give her child IV anti-microbials via an indwelling intermittent injection port—which was still in the child's arm. She uncapped the port, attached the syringe, and administered the oral suspension intravenously. The child stopped breathing but was resuscitated. The nurse, devastated by the error, resigned. This error would not have happened if the child's IV access port had been removed as soon as it was no longer needed. But the use of specially designed oral syringes without Luer connections would prevent all errors involving the administration of oral solutions via IV ports. Parenteral syringes should never be used for oral or enteral medication administration.

Oral syringes are labeled "oral only." Manufacturers may also provide labels printed with the word "ORAL" in large, red, upper-case letters for nurses to affix to the plunger so that the syringe contents cannot be expelled until the label is removed. Ideally, pharmacy should dispense each oral liquid dose in an oral syringe with the warning label attached to the plunger.

The best solution to this problem would be to make the connectors on nasogastric tubes and intravenous lines incompatible. A standard for enteral feeding set connectors and adapters implemented by the Association for the Advancement of Medical Instrumentation (ANSI/AAMI ID54-1996) is helping to accomplish this. However, until the use of oral syringes becomes a widely accepted standard of practice, many manufacturers of nasogastric tubes are continuing to provide both a Luer connection port and an oral syringe port.

ENTERAL FEEDINGS

Efforts to avoid harmful connections between enteral and parenteral delivery devices have focused on the distal ends of administration sets. However, enteral feeding containers can also be spiked at the proximal end with an IV administration set, making the container look similar to that of a three-in-one parenteral nutrition admixture. Many ready-to-hang, closed enteral nutrition containers (e.g., Mead Johnson Kangaroo, Nestle UltraPak, Ross Ready-to-Hang) will allow the formula to flow freely through a standard IV infusion set. An inline filter may not prevent IV administration. An administration set with a 0.22-micrometer filter will quickly become occluded, but larger filters (1 to 5 micrometers) may allow some of the enteral feeding suspension to enter the vascular system before the pump's occlusion alarm is triggered.

In one reported event, a patient who was to receive TPN was given 200 mL of enteral feeding by IV infusion over 1 to 2 hours. The enteral product had been discontinued 1 week before but had not been removed from the nursing unit refrigerator. An agency nurse who had never seen enteral products dispensed in anything but a can mistook the enteral product in the bag for TPN and administered it IV. The patient died several days later.

Enteral product containers have label warnings against IV administration, but this is not sufficient to eliminate the risk. The appropriate enteral administration set should be attached with a rubber band to the enteral product container before the product is stocked in or dispensed to patient care units. As with any medication dispensed for a specific patient, discontinued enteral products should be removed from patient care areas immediately and returned to their source.

Reports indicate that some nurses have purposely used an IV pump to administer an enteral feeding or other enteral solution. This is an accident waiting to happen. For example, when a nurse could not find an enteral feeding set, she improvised and spiked the bottle's cap with IV tubing. Since the enteral pump would not accept the IV tubing, she used an IV pump to deliver the feeding. The patient was being weaned from a three-in-one TPN admixture, and both pumps were on the same pole. Although the solutions looked similar (the TPN admixture was white with a yellow tint and the enteral product was tan) and the tubings were wound around one another and hard to distinguish, an error did not occur.

IV tubing and pumps have also been used with GoLytely (PEG-3350 and electrolytes), a bowel preparation product that may be administered via nasogastric tube to patients who are vomiting or cannot tolerate the large volume of solution necessary for effective preparation. A typical enteral pump may not be capable of delivering the solution at the desired rate (e.g., 600–1,000 mL in 1 hour). The following error occurred when IV tubing and an IV pump were used to administer GoLytely.[12,13]

A 4-year-old child was taken to an emergency department after ingesting a large number of tablets of the chemotherapeutic agent 6-mercaptopurine. After treatment with activated charcoal, the child was started on GoLytely, to be administered at 400 mL/hr via IV tubing attached to a nasogastric tube. After 1 hour, a nurse discovered that the solution was actually being administered through an IV access line; 391 mL had already infused. The child showed no evidence of acidosis or renal failure, and glycol levels were undetectable. She was discharged several days later without further complications.

The use of IV tubing and an IV pump may seem like a necessary "work around" for the administration of GoLytely, but there are safer methods. If an enteral solution like this must be administered quickly in a large volume, an adapter can be used to connect two enteral feeding pumps, each delivering half the desired volume simultaneously. Some nasogastric tubes have a dual port to facilitate such a connection. Also, a few enteral pumps are capable of delivering higher than usual volumes (e.g., 500 mL/hr with the Ross Embrace pump). Use of these alternatives and clear labeling of each access line can help prevent the inadvertent connection of an enteral solution to an IV tubing port.

OTHER TUBING MISCONNECTIONS

Tubing intended for uses other than medication delivery has been inadvertently connected to IV ports, with serious or fatal results. For example, tubing from a blood pressure (BP) monitoring device has been connected to a patient's IV line. Although this seems improbable, there have been several such reports.

One patient who was connected to a portable BP device was transported to the radiology department. A length of tubing that led from the monitor's BP cuff inflator had a male Luer connector. This fit into a female connector on a shorter length of white tubing that was attached to a Critikon disposable BP cuff (Figure 12-1). Because of the metal Luer connector on the monitor's tubing, the tubing and cuff were disconnected before the patient underwent magnetic resonance imaging. After the test, a radiology employee reconnected the tubing and transported the patient back to his room. A family member noticed that the tubing from the BP monitor was attached to a needleless Y injection port on the patient's IV line. He immediately contacted a nurse, who disconnected the tubing. More than 1,500 mL of air could have entered the patient's vascular system, but the machine had not yet cycled to take a BP reading.

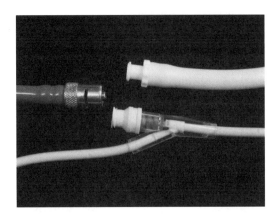

FIGURE 12-1   Tubing from a blood pressure (BP) cuff inflator (top left) was erroneously connected to the needleless Y injection port of an IV line (bottom) instead of to the BP cuff tubing (top right).

Other patients have not been as lucky. One nurse accidentally connected the BP monitor tubing to a needleless IV port. Propofol, which is white and opaque, had been infusing through the patient's IV line. Thus, the IV tubing and port looked very similar to the white length of tubing and connector on the BP cuff (shown in Figure 12-1). In another case, an agitated patient died after removing the tubing from his BP cuff and attaching it to his IV line. These inadvertent connections are most likely to occur at the Y sites of needleless IV tubing, but it is possible to connect BP monitor tubing to any other tubing with a Luer connector.

The following mistakes have also happened:

- A hospitalized patient was easily able to connect an air supply hose from an Albahealth sequential compression device, used to prevent deep vein thrombosis, to his needleless IV tubing. The device was turned off at the time, and the erroneous connection was found before harm occurred.

- A young child died when her oxygen tubing was mistakenly connected to her IV line. The child had been receiving asthma medication by nebulizer. While it was still attached to a wall outlet, the oxygen tubing (Airlife, from Allegiance Healthcare Corporation) became disconnected from the nebulizer fluid chamber (Figure 12-2). A staff member accidentally connected the oxygen tubing to the Y injection port on the patient's IV line (Baxter Clearlink needleless access system). Oxygen tubing does not have a Luer connector, but it can be connected to Baxter's Clearlink valve (Figure 12-3), albeit with excessive force. The oxygen tubing disconnected from the IV tubing in seconds, but not before the compressed oxygen supply forced the needleless valve open and allowed air into the tubing. The child died instantly.

- A hospital employee inadvertently attached oxygen tubing instead of suction tubing to a total joint drainage system, which resulted in the patient's death from a gas embolism.

- Medications intended for injection into catheters or other tubes have been inadvertently injected into the balloon inflation ports of endotracheal tubes, gastrostomy tubes, and Foley catheters. In each case, the balloon expanded when the medication was injected, causing harm to the patient.[14] Medications intended for IV use were inadvertently infused into the balloon of a tracheostomy tube, resulting in hyperinflation of the cuff, constriction of the tube's

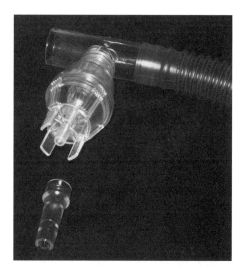

FIGURE 12-2 Oxygen tubing (bottom) connected to a wall outlet became disconnected from a nebulizer fluid chamber (top) and was mistakenly connected to an IV line.

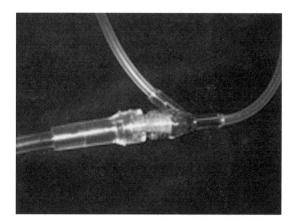

FIGURE 12-3 Oxygen tubing (left) can be forcibly connected to the Y site of the Baxter Clearlink needleless access system.

lumen, and airway obstruction that led to respiratory arrest. The port on the pilot line is compatible with slip tip and Luer lock syringes for easy inflation or deflation—and therefore with IV tubing. The risk of error was heightened in this case because the patient's triple-lumen catheter was not secured, so the IV tubing hung down at the same level as the tracheostomy cuff tubing, and the connection ports on the needleless tubing appeared very similar to the tracheostomy pilot line.

Health care organizations should review the medical equipment used in their facilities to identify the potential for misconnections to IV tubing. Before the implementation of new tubes, catheters, and connectors, an interdisciplinary team should identify the potential for connectivity with other medical equipment as part of FMEA. Before connecting or reconnecting a patient's tubing, staff should always trace the tubing from the patient to the point of origin. Appropriately labeled IV lines can help prevent inadvertent access to these lines.

The Association for the Advancement of Medical Instrumentation Human Factors Committee is engaged in a global initiative to address the dangers of compatibility of various health care device connections. To avoid unintended consequences, any change in the design of non-IV connectors would need to be made by all manufacturers. It may be years before new standards are implemented.

REFERENCES

1. Leape LL, Bates DW, Cullen DJ, et al. Systems analysis of adverse drug events. *JAMA*. 1995; 274:35–43.
2. ECRI. Evaluation of infusion pumps. *Health Devices*. 2002;31(10):352–84.
3. Cohen MR, Senders J, Davis NM. Failure mode and effects analysis: a novel approach to avoiding dangerous medication errors and accidents. *Hosp Pharm*. 1994;29:319–30.
4. Senders JW. FMEA and RCA: the mantras of modern risk management. *Qual Saf Health Care*. 2004;13:249–50.
5. Institute for Safe Medication Practices. Using FMEA to predict failures with infusion pumps. *ISMP Nurse Advise-ERR*. February 2004;2(2):3.
6. Committee on Identifying and Preventing Medication Errors; Aspden P, Wolcott J, Bootman JL, et al., eds. *Preventing Medication Errors*. Washington, DC: National Academies Press; 2006. Prepublication copy available at http://darwin.nap.edu/books/0309101476/html/R2.html. Accessed July 21, 2006.
7. Rothschild JM, Keohane CA, Cook EF, et al. A controlled trial of smart infusion pumps to improve medication safety in critically ill patients. *Crit Care Med*. 2005;33:533–40.
8. Cohen MR, Davis NM. Free flow associated with electronic infusion devices: an underestimated danger. *Hosp Pharm*. 1992;27:384–90.
9. ECRI responds to FDA public health advisory on IV free-flow. *Health Devices*. 1994;23(6):256–7.
10. Food and Drug Administration. Avoiding Injuries from Rapid Drug or I.V. Fluid Administration Associated with I.V. Pumps and Rate Controller Devices. Public Health Advisory. March 1, 1994. Available at: www.fda.gov/cdrh/ivfluid.pdf. Accessed June 16, 2005.
11. Institute for Safe Medication Practices. *Mosby's Nursing PDQ for Medication Safety*. St Louis: Mosby; 2005.
12. Guzman DD, Teoh D, Velez LI. Accidental intravenous infusion of Golytely(R) in a 4-year-old female [abstract]. *J Toxicol Clin Toxicol*. 2002;40:361–2.
13. Tucker V, Cramm K, Martinez J. Accidental large intravenous infusion of Golytely [abstract]. *J Toxicol Clin Toxicol*. 2002;40(5):687.
14. Institute for Safe Medication Practices Canada. Devices with inflation ports—risk for medication error-induced injuries. *ISMP Canada Safety Bulletin*. May 2004;4(5). Available at: www.ismp-canada.org/download/ISMPCSB2004-05.pdf. Accessed June 17, 2005.

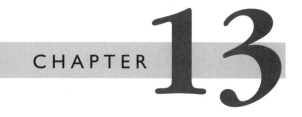

CHAPTER 13

THE PATIENT'S ROLE IN PREVENTING MEDICATION ERRORS

Stacy A. Aimette, Nancy R. Tuohy, and Michael R. Cohen

Patients can do a great deal to decrease their chances of experiencing a medication error. They do not need to spend hours researching their medications and diseases; rather, they need to know what questions to ask their health care providers, how to insist on answers, and how to recognize situations that could result in a medication error.

The public has been exposed to extensive coverage of medical error by the mass media. Most respondents to a 1997 survey by the National Patient Safety Foundation believed carelessness and negligence were the most frequent causes of medical error.[1] Three-fourths thought the most effective solution was to prevent "bad" professionals from providing care. Most of the respondents (92%) believed they themselves could have a positive effect on safety; they believed only a patient's personal physician has a greater role in safety than the patient. However, only 1 in 10 respondents said they had taken precautions to ensure their safety, perhaps because health care providers have not encouraged patients to participate and taught them practical ways of doing so.

Public interest in preventing medical errors was heightened by the Institute of Medicine's *To Err Is Human* in 2000 and *Crossing the Quality Chasm* in 2001, but substantial error rates continue to be reported. In 2002, more than one in five Americans surveyed by the Commonwealth Fund reported that they or a family member had experienced some type of medical error.[2] Of the 16% reporting a medication error, more than one-fifth said the error turned out to be very serious. In a 2004 survey by the Kaiser Family Foundation, Agency for Healthcare Research and Quality (AHRQ), and Harvard School of Public Health,[3] 55% of respondents said they were dissatisfied with the quality of health care in this country. More than one-third (34%) of respondents or their family members had been involved in a preventable medical error, and 21% said it had caused serious consequences such as severe pain; loss of time at work, school, or other important life activities; disability; or death. More than half of the respondents (52%) believed mistakes made by individual health professionals were the most important cause of medical errors, compared with 36% who cited mistakes made by institutions. Of 13 possible ways to reduce errors, the respondents ranked fines and license suspension for health professionals eighth. Requiring hospitals to develop better systems ranked second. The lowest-ranked solution was malpractice lawsuits. When asked what information is useful in comparing hospitals, 70% of the respondents said reports of medical errors would tell them a lot about the quality of a hospital.

HEALTH CARE PROVIDERS' CHALLENGES IN ENGAGING PATIENTS AS EQUAL PARTNERS

We will not be able to engage patients and families in their health care and safety unless this is a top priority, fully supported by senior leadership.

We will not connect with our patients on a personal level unless we are willing to take the time to listen to their stories—not just their medical stories, but how their medical stories interact with their personal stories.

We will not empower our patients until we include them and their families as equal members of our interdisciplinary clinical teams, actively participating in patient care and the decision-making process.

We will not improve our patients' adherence to a jointly developed plan of care unless we provide good instructions and make even the most complex of processes clear and easy to follow.

We will not earn our patients' respect unless we treat them with dignity and pay attention to the whole patient.

We will not earn our patients' trust unless we disclose our errors. We will not feel comfortable disclosing errors until we change our culture. Our patients will not listen to us unless we begin to tell them what we are doing about the problem of medical errors.

We will not demonstrate our moral responsibility and our just accountability for medical errors until disclosure is accompanied by a fair offer of compensation for injuries, not through the litigious avenues currently available to patients and families, but through thoughtfully considering the financial burden placed on the victims of an error and sharing in that burden up front.

We will not truly show compassion to patients and families until we can offer them emotional, physical, spiritual, and psychological support in the wake of a sentinel event.

We will not be able to motivate all patients to engage in their own health care and safety without providing them with the knowledge to do so and strong encouragement from programs like the Speak Up: Help Prevent Errors in Your Care campaign from the Joint Commission on Accreditation of Healthcare Organizations.

We will not have time to engage our patients until we improve the efficiency and safety of our systems and free our workforce to carry out tasks such as talking to patients and their families.

We will not be able to give patients what they really want unless we ask them what they want.

The Kaiser, AHRQ, and Harvard study found that patients are taking precautions to reduce the risk of error. Sixty-nine percent of respondents said they had checked the medication a pharmacist dispensed against the physician's prescription; 48% had taken a list of all medications, including nonprescription drugs, to a medical appointment; and 38% had told a health care practitioner about a drug allergy without being asked for this information.

As patients become better-informed consumers of health care, many are embracing the motto "Nothing about me without me." As providers, we need to engage patients and families not just as victims of disease or injury in need of our expertise and care, but as equal partners—an approach that presents some challenges (see above).

Clinicians should take advantage of patients' willingness to participate in their care by suggesting actions to reduce the risk of error. For example, after years of frustration over not being able to get physicians and nurses to wash their hands before they touch patients, researchers coordinated a study at four community hospitals to educate patients about the importance of hand washing by staff.[4] Patients were told to ask anyone who came in direct contact with them whether they had washed their hands. Patients who were hesitant to ask could wear stickers that said, "Did you wash your hands?" The researchers measured a 42% increase in liquid soap use at the end of the study.

The same principle—that patients can have an impact—could be applied to medication error prevention. The Institute for Safe Medication Practices (ISMP) has received reports about errors that occurred because nurses did not check patients' armbands. A hospital could make up buttons for patients to wear that say, "Did you read my armband?"

Some hospitals have included patients and consumers in internal quality improvement and safety initiatives. For example, the Dana-Farber Cancer Institute in Boston has established a patient and family advisory council. When the staff wanted to change from IV to oral antiemetics to reduce patients' time in the clinic, the advisory council said patients were not interested in reducing clinic time. Instead, they were concerned that changing to oral therapy would reduce the quality time that they now spend with staff, asking questions and talking about their fears while receiving their IV antiemetics. The advisory council receives aggregate information about medication errors and system-based remedies. Dana-Farber staff members initially were concerned about patients' reactions to aggregate error data. However, patients told the staff they were well aware that errors occurred and were relieved to know the hospital was aware of them and doing something about the problem.[5] Legal counsel should always be obtained before sharing any error data, but the benefits have been enormous for the few hospitals that have adopted this courageous practice. If we continue to hide our error reduction efforts, we cannot expect to regain the public trust.

This chapter discusses the questions all patients should ask when they receive a medication in the hospital or when they purchase a product at the pharmacy. It also addresses patients' adherence to their drug regimens as an important part of safe and effective medication use. It concludes with considerations for safe medication use in three specific populations: hospitalized patients, elderly patients, and children.

THE BASIC QUESTIONS

Most pharmacists, physicians, and consumer advocates believe that to ensure safe medication use, all patients must have the answers to the following questions:

1. What are the brand and generic names of the medication?
2. What is the purpose of the medication?
3. What is the strength and dosage?
4. What are the possible adverse effects? What should I do if they occur?
5. Is there any other medication I should avoid while using this product?
6. I am allergic to _____. Should I take this medicine?
7. How long should I take this medication? What outcome should I expect?
8. When is the best time to take the medication?
9. How should I store the medication?
10. What do I do if I miss a dose?
11. Should I avoid any foods while taking this medication?
12. I'm also taking _____ (which I got at another pharmacy). Can I take both safely?
13. Is this medication meant to replace any other drug that I am already taking?
14. May I have written information about this drug?

FIVE STEPS WHEN PICKING UP A PRESCRIPTION

1. Take the medication out of the bag and read the label.
   Are your name and your doctor's name correct? A misspelled name could mean you have someone else's prescription.

2. Read the directions on the label.
   Make sure that it is what your doctor told you, and that you understand how much medicine to take and how many times a day you should take it.

3. While you are still in the pharmacy, read the drug information sheet stapled to the bag to learn what the medicine is supposed to treat.
   Is that what you are being treated for? If not, it could signal an error, so check with your pharmacist.

4. Read about the possible side effects.
   If you are picking up a refill and realize you have been having these side effects, tell the pharmacist immediately. He or she may want to call your doctor.

5. If you are getting a refill, make sure the medicine looks the same as it did last time.
   If it looks different, ask the pharmacist about it. Most likely, the pharmacist has filled your prescription with a generic drug that looks different from what you are used to. But mistakes are possible, so check with the pharmacist to be sure.

The answers to these questions give patients the tools they need to take responsibility for safe drug use. To be most effective, the answers must be provided at the time the medication is prescribed, whether this is at the patient's bedside in a hospital or in the physician's office. After the initial encounter, patients should have an information resource available, such as a medication handbook or access to the Internet. Information must be presented in a form and at a rate that the patient can understand, and it must be periodically reinforced. Patients should be urged to question anything that they do not understand or that does not seem to be in keeping with their understanding.

In addition, patients should be taught to follow a five-step checking process (above) each time they pick up a medication at a pharmacy.[6] More questions for patients to ask and tips for preventing errors are provided in the Joint Commission on Accreditation of Healthcare Organizations (JCAHO) Speak Up Campaign.[7] A 2007 JCAHO National Patient Safety Goal is to "encourage patients' active involvement in their own care."[8]

PROVIDING INSTRUCTIONS TO PATIENTS

Clinicians should not take for granted that patients understand their instructions. Health care providers may think that what is obvious to them will be obvious to their patients; they may therefore omit discussion of routine parts of proper medication use.

ISMP heard about one asthmatic patient who was not responding to therapy.[9] During follow-up, the patient described how he was using his inhaler. He would get into his car, roll up the windows, release two puffs of medication into the air, and breathe deeply for 15 minutes. At first, he did this in his house, but later he thought it might be more effective to use the inhaler in a confined space. He said he had been instructed to do this by his physician, who had picked up an inhaler, held it in the air, and released two puffs to demonstrate its use. The physician had provided no additional instructions.

Label directions on a prescription bottle can be similarly confusing. Adding verbs to prescription directions can lead to errors (verbs such as "give" or "take" often are not part of the original prescription).[10] When the label on a coal tar bath preparation read "Take four capfuls in bath," the patient sat in the tub and swallowed concentrated coal tar solution meant for dilution in the bath water.

Clinicians need to be clear and complete in their instructions. It is important to assume nothing regarding the patient's knowledge base and to leave no room for patients to make erroneous assumptions. The American Medical Association recommends six steps for improving communication with patients:[11]

1. Slow down. Speak slowly and spend a small amount of extra time with each patient.
2. Use plain, nonmedical language.
3. Show or draw pictures.
4. Limit the amount of information provided, and repeat it.
5. Use the teach-back or show-me technique.
6. Create a shame-free environment.

PATIENT RECORD KEEPING

Patients should keep records of all their medications, including nonprescription products they are taking. Such records are especially important for patients who have chronic diseases, who see more than one physician, or who take many medications. The following information should be included:

- Name, strength, dose, and frequency of dosage of all prescription medications,
- Names of all nonprescription medicines, vitamins, and herbal products,
- Known medication or food allergies,
- Special diets, and
- Medications that the patient previously took and the reason why the medication was discontinued.

Patients need to know that they should include herbal products on their medication lists. Herbals can have pharmacologic effects in the body as well as interactions with other medications. In one reported case[12] a young woman developed temporary nerve damage 4 weeks after taking 500 mg of St. John's wort for mild depression. She began to feel stinging pain on the areas exposed to sun, and she sought medical attention when the pain worsened. Her symptoms gradually disappeared 2 months after she stopped taking the herb. The active ingredients in this herb, known as photoactive hypericins, produce substances that can damage myelin when exposed to light. In addition, St. John's wort interacts with many drugs; this must be considered before taking it with other prescription and nonprescription products. In another example,[13] a patient taking warfarin after a heart valve replacement had maintained an international normalized ratio (INR) of between 2.5 and 3.5 for many months. After he started taking ginseng, an herb said to improve well-being, his INR dropped to 1.8. After discontinuing the herb, his INR returned to therapeutic levels with no warfarin dosage adjustments. The patient denied medication or dietary changes that could have resulted in the same effect. Another patient, who had been taking the same dose of digoxin for years, experienced an elevated digoxin level. Common causes of an elevated serum digoxin were ruled out before the patient admitted he was taking ginseng. His digoxin level again became acceptable after he stopped taking ginseng.

Patients should update their medication lists whenever their medication regimen changes. Many health care providers give patients forms to simplify record keeping. The South Carolina Hospital Association offers a form in English and Spanish versions (www.scha.org/documents/English-UMF_904_1_1.doc and www.scha.org/documents/Spanish-UMF_904_1_1.doc). Another form is available from ISMP at www.ismp.org/Newsletters/consumer/consumerAlerts.asp.

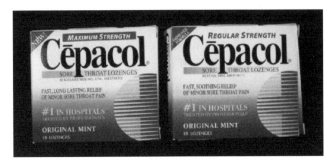

FIGURE 13-1   These packages look nearly identical, but only one of the products contains benzocaine.

SAFE DRUG USE BY PATIENTS: KEY POINTS

Medication Packaging

Poor packaging is a major reason for medication errors. Many manufacturers package their products in containers that are virtually identical, as illustrated by the two boxes of lozenges shown in Figure 13-1. Only on careful examination does the reader note that one box is labeled "Maximum Strength" and that it contains benzocaine. The other product does not contain benzocaine. Some patients are allergic to benzocaine or could become sensitized to it. Because of the similarity in packaging, patients and health care professionals could find it difficult to distinguish these two products.

Packaging and labeling can mislead users of a product about the correct dose to take. For example, as originally marketed, the packaging of Children's Tylenol Meltaways (acetaminophen), shown in Figure 13-2, could lead a practitioner or a parent to accidentally double a child's dose. The inner packaging looked like a typical unit dose package for institutional use, although it was intended as a convenience for parents with children who might require one, two, or three tablets per dose. The front of the carton stated "medicine per dose 80 mg," but the individual blister packs that contained either one or two 80 mg tablets all were labeled "Children's Tylenol 80 mg." With the two-tablet blister packs, a practitioner or parent might have concluded that both tablets should be given to provide an 80 mg dose, resulting in a 160 mg double dose (or a 320 mg dose if 160 mg is intended). This situation is especially troubling because the medication is a nonprescription product, and pediatricians often provide parents with dosing instructions in milligram amounts rather than a per tablet dose. The manufacturer and the Food and Drug Administration (FDA) were made aware of this problem. The manufacturer agreed to change the "medicine per dose 80 mg" message on the front label panel to "80 mg per tablet," and the blister packaging now clearly indicates the exact milligram amount enclosed.

Dissimilar products can have similar packaging. Mix-ups have been reported between products packaged in low-density polyethylene containers (Figure 13-3). In particular, respiratory medications can look like ophthalmic products. The similar shapes and the absence of a large printed label can make it difficult to distinguish between products at a quick glance. Often, the medication name is embossed into the clear plastic.

Mix-ups have also occurred with products whose containers resemble the containers often used for eye drops.[14] For example, a patient's wife accidentally administered Hemoccult Sensa (hydrogen peroxide, denatured ethyl alcohol) solution into the patient's eyes. A nurse had left the Hemoccult bottle at the bedside, and the patient's wife thought it was her husband's artificial tears. The patient experienced pain, which resolved when his eyes were flushed. Hemoccult developer and other generic developers are available in

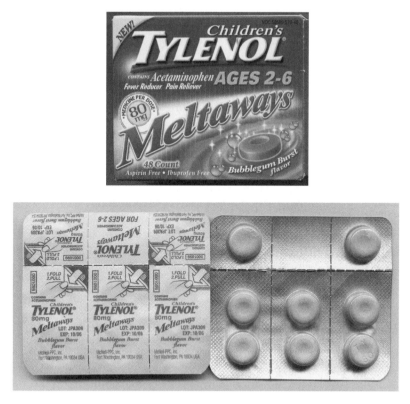

FIGURE 13-2 Outer and inner packaging of Children's Tylenol Meltaways; each tablet contains 80 mg. This packaging has been changed. The front label panel now states "80 mg per tablet," and the blister packages state, in milligrams, the amount enclosed.

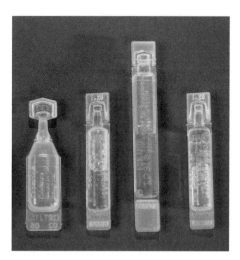

FIGURE 13-3 Various products in similar-looking low-density polyethylene containers.

what looks like a typical ophthalmic dropper bottle. About 10 years ago, after reports of accidental ophthalmic administration, the manufacturer began packaging Hemoccult with a "stovepipe" cap and added an icon (encircled eye with red line through it) to signal that it should not be used in the eye (Figure 11-4). Neither change has been fully effective in preventing errors. A similar product, Seracult (hydrogen peroxide, ethanol), is packaged with a cardboard ring around the bottle's neck stating, "Do not use in the eyes" (Figure 11-4). However, the ring is easily torn off, and a small warning to avoid contact with eyes and skin is poorly visible. These solutions should never be left in areas where they could be confused with eye drops (e.g., bedside tables, medicine carts, patient bathrooms). For safe storage, the bottle can be secured (with string around the neck) to a fixed object in the location where stool specimens are tested.

All information on packaging must be large enough for people to read. Because of difficulty seeing an indicator, patients have failed to receive medication from a device. A long-term care patient who had received no medication (salmeterol inhalation powder) from the Serevent Diskus for 5 weeks required hospitalization because of exacerbation of chronic obstructive pulmonary disease.[15] The delivery system, like other dry powder inhalation medications, incorporates a dosage indicator with numbers to indicate the number of doses remaining. The last five numbers are in red ink but are very small. In this case, the dosage indicator read zero but neither the patient nor the facility staff noticed. Furthermore, the Diskus continued to make a clicking sound, as if it were loading the medication for delivery, even after it was empty. Packaging features that alert patients to an empty device would be helpful.

Brand Names and Extensions

Many patients have received overdoses because of confusion about brand and generic names. A patient who did not know that warfarin is the generic name for Coumadin could take both simultaneously for the same condition. Pharmaceutical companies add to the confusion by using different brand names for the same drug when it is used to treat different conditions. For example, finasteride is named Propecia when used to treat alopecia and Proscar when used to treat benign prostatic hyperplasia. Fluoxetine is marketed as Prozac when used to treat depression, obsessive–compulsive disorder, and bulimia, and as Sarafem when used to treat premenstrual dysphoric disorder.

One middle-aged man accidentally took too much bupropion, which sent him to the emergency department (ED) with severe nausea, vomiting, and a reported seizure.[16] He had a long history of depression treated with Wellbutrin (bupropion). Six weeks previously, his physician had given him new prescriptions for all of his medications but had prescribed them by generic name. The patient had continued taking his original prescription for Wellbutrin, along with his new prescription for generic bupropion. About the same time, he had attended a smoking cessation program where another physician gave him a prescription for Zyban (bupropion). Even though the patient had given the ED staff a list of his current medications, which included Zyban, bupropion, and Wellbutrin, the nurses and physicians did not recognize the problem. A third-year medical student finally noticed the error after looking up the generic names of all the patient's medications. The patient was discharged from the hospital after 24 hours of intravenous hydration.

The suffixes used for line extensions of medications increase the potential for mix-ups. There are no standard definitions of suffixes such as XL, SR, and ER. Confusion has been reported between Wellbutrin (bupropion immediate release) and Wellbutrin SR (bupropion extended release), between Metadate ER and Metadate CD (methylphenidate hydrochloride extended-release formulations), between Ritalin LA (methylphenidate extended release) and Ritalin SR (methylphenidate hydrochloride sustained release), and between Depakote and Depakote ER (divalproex sodium extended release).[17] Some formulations are not substitutable. Some are available in identical strengths, making mix-ups even more likely.

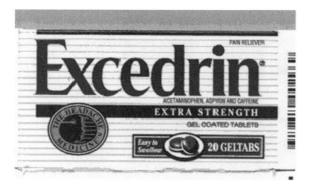

FIGURE 13-4 This product contains aspirin, but the active ingredients are printed in small type between the brand name and "Extra Strength."

Brand-name extensions may also cause problems. Popular brand names have become associated with certain ingredients; for example, Tylenol is associated with acetaminophen and Bayer with aspirin. Consumers and health care providers may not realize that whereas the chief ingredient of Anacin is aspirin, the chief ingredient of Anacin-3 is acetaminophen. A patient taking glipizide for type 2 diabetes who takes Anacin instead of Anacin-3 might experience adverse effects such as dizziness, because aspirin increases the hypoglycemic effect of glipizide.

Similarly, Excedrin caused an anaphylactic reaction in an 18-year-old woman.[18] She required intubation and treatment with epinephrine, methylprednisolone, and diphenhydramine. She was resuscitated and admitted to the respiratory intensive care unit, where she eventually recovered. The patient knew she was allergic to aspirin, but she was unaware that it was in the Excedrin Extra Strength tablets that she took for headache. Although the product lists aspirin as an ingredient on the carton label (Figure 13-4) and the bottle and warns allergic patients not to take it, the word "aspirin" appears below the brand name in very small print that may not be easily seen by people in a hurry or those with poor eyesight.

In another example, a patient needing a colonoscopy was handed printed instructions by his physician's office staff that called for a bottle of magnesium citrate and two tablets of "Dulcolax" each day for 2 days before the procedure.[19] Although bisacodyl is needed for bowel preparation, only the brand name Dulcolax appeared in the printed instructions. At the drugstore, the patient was directed to the laxative aisle, where he selected a product boldly labeled Dulcolax. He took two tablets on the first day, but on the second day his son, a pharmacist, recognized that his father was taking the stool softener (docusate sodium), not the laxative. The patient's son went to the drugstore to purchase bisacodyl and found the two Dulcolax products (Figure 13-5) side by side. Patients should be warned against confusion between these products; taking the wrong product could necessitate repeating the colonoscopy.

Clinicians must teach patients that all medications have one generic name and may have one or more brand names. Patients should know both the generic and the brand name (if applicable) of medications they are taking, and they should understand the risk of duplicate therapy if the medication prescribed is also marketed under other brand names. When possible, patients should obtain all medications from the same pharmacy. They should tell their pharmacist about any prescriptions dispensed elsewhere so that duplicate therapy and drug–drug interactions can be avoided. Patients should be provided

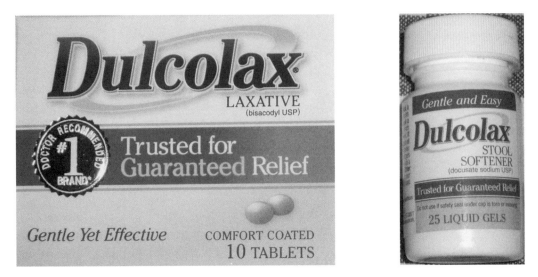

FIGURE 13-5 Two Dulcolax products that contain different medications: bisacodyl (left) and docusate (right).

with written instructions about which drug previously taken at home is being replaced by a newly prescribed drug, and they should be encouraged to properly dispose of discontinued medications.

Pharmacists should encourage patients to choose single-ingredient products when possible. They should explain that multi-ingredient products contain medications that are not needed or that may cause adverse effects. For example, a patient with nasal congestion that is not caused by allergy should take only a decongestant; a decongestant–antihistamine may cause unnecessary drowsiness.

Readability of Labels

Most medication packages have limited space for label information, but FDA requires that certain information appear on all labels. Before 1999, there was no standard format for the placement of product information on the label. In 2002, use of a new Drug Facts label format (Figure 13-6) was required for almost all nonprescription products. It uses simple language and a larger type size. The following information must appear, in this order:[20]

- The product's active ingredients, including the amount in each dosage unit;
- The purpose of the medication;
- The uses (indications) for the drug;
- Specific warnings, including when the product should not be used under any circumstances and when it is appropriate to consult a physician or pharmacist; the warnings section also describes adverse effects that could occur and substances or activities to avoid;
- Dosage instructions addressing when, how, and how often to take the medication; and
- The product's inactive ingredients; this is important information for those with specific allergies.

Problems can still arise, however, because of the limited space on a container. Some manufacturers have placed this information on a peel-away portion of the label, which can be missed or torn from the container.

Drug Facts

Active ingredient (in each tablet)	Purpose
Chlorpheniramine maleate 2 mg	.Antihistamine

Uses temporarily relieves these symptoms due to hay fever or other upper respiratory allergies:
■ sneezing ■ runny nose ■ itchy, watery eyes ■ itchy throat

Warnings
Ask a doctor before use if you have
■ glaucoma ■ a breathing problem such as emphysema or chronic bronchitis
■ trouble urinating due to an enlarged prostate gland

Ask a doctor or pharmacist before use if you are taking tranquilizers or sedatives

When using this product
■ You may get drowsy ■ avoid alcoholic drinks
■ alcohol, sedatives, and tranquilizers may increase drowsiness
■ be careful when driving a motor vehicle or operating machinery
■ excitability may occur, especially in children

If pregnant or breast-feeding, ask a health professional before use.
Keep out of reach of children. In case of overdose, get medical help or contact a Poison Control Center right away.

Directions

adults and children 12 years and over	take 2 tablets every 4 to 6 hours; not more than 12 tablets in 24 hours
children 6 years to under 12 years	take 1 tablet every 4 to 6 hours; not more than 6 tablets in 24 hours
children under 6 years	ask a doctor

Other information store at 20-25° C (68-77° F) ■ protect from excessive moisture

Inactive ingredients D&C yellow no. 10, lactose, magnesium stearate, microcrystalline cellulose, pregelatinized starch

FIGURE 13-6 Sample of the label information required by the Food and Drug Administration on nonprescription products.

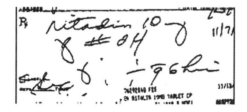

FIGURE 13-7 Ritodrine order misread as Ritalin.

Readability of Physicians' Handwriting

Patients should be able to clearly read all information on their prescriptions before leaving a physician's office or hospital. They should ask their physician to print drug names and indicate the purpose of the drug on the prescription. This will reduce the likelihood of pharmacist misinterpretation of "look-alike" drug names; of the confusing drug name pairs that have been identified, it is rare for both drugs in a pair to have the same purpose.

A woman who was 6 months pregnant received Ritalin (methylphenidate) 10 mg by mouth every 6 hours instead of ritodrine (Yutopar).[21] Reportedly, the error originated with an obstetrician's poorly written prescription (Figure 13-7). Then, a pharmacist misread the ritodrine prescription as Ritalin and failed to ask the patient or physician why the drug was being used. The pharmacist also did not ensure that the dosage was reasonable or question why Ritalin would be prescribed around the clock. The patient's pregnancy was also overlooked. According to the reporter, the child is now 6 years old and suffers from developmental delay. This outcome might have been avoided if questions had been asked as recommended above, and if the brand name and the reason for giving ritodrine had been on the prescription.

Spoken Orders

To Pharmacists

When prescriptions are phoned in to a pharmacy, mix-ups with sound-alike names can occur. For example, when a man complained of allergy symptoms, his physician called the pharmacy with a prescription for Allegra (fexofenadine).[22] After picking up the prescription, the man called the physician to ask why he had prescribed something so expensive ($450). When the physician then called the pharmacy, the pharmacist realized he had misheard the prescription as "60 Viagra" (sildenafil).

A prescriber giving a spoken order to a pharmacist or nurse should be asked to spell the name of the drug, and the pharmacist or nurse should be required to read back the name and spelling to the caller. Providing information such as the purpose of the medication is an additional safeguard. Patients should be made aware that spoken orders can be misinterpreted and should be advised to minimize their requests for telephoned prescriptions. It is preferable to fax prescriptions or use electronic order entry and processing.

To Patients

Patients are often instructed by telephone about changes in their medication regimens. One patient taking warfarin required numerous dose changes to maintain a therapeutic level. The patient was accustomed to taking 5 mg tablets. On one occasion, he was called and told to take 7.5 mg daily. He misunderstood the directions and took 7½ of the 5 mg tablets (37.5 mg total) for 2 days.

When a medication regimen is changed without a new prescription, the directions on the prescription bottle may differ from the actual administration directions. To reduce the risk of error, the patient's dose in metric units (e.g., milligrams) should be provided first, followed by instructions on the number of tablets needed for each dose.[23] When patients are given instructions by telephone, they should be asked to (1) retrieve a pen and paper to write any dosage changes, (2) write the information as received and the date, and (3) read back the dose and instructions to verify understanding. The patient should be advised to keep the dated instructions with the prescription bottle for quick reference.

Misidentification

Errors may occur because patients are misidentified. For example, a prescription may be entered into the profile of the wrong patient, often a family member or another person with the same name. The possibility for error can be reduced if the patient insists on counseling and, before leaving the pharmacy, checks to see that his or her name is on the label and that the name of the drug is the same as that provided by the physician. In other situations, the patient's address or Social Security number may be incorporated into the method of identification.

Storage

The medicine cabinet in the family bathroom is probably the worst possible place to store medications. The heat and humidity of bathrooms may affect the shelf life of the product. For this reason, medications should be kept on a kitchen shelf or in the linen closet, well out of the reach of children and pets. Similarly, medications should never be left in an automobile, where their potency can be reduced by extreme heat or cold.

Storing medications in the bathroom, often next to toiletries, poses a risk of dangerous mix-ups. In one instance, a woman reached for the toothpaste and inadvertently grabbed a tube of her husband's nitroglycerin paste.[24] Brushing her teeth with the nitroglycerin, a vasodilator, caused her blood pressure to drop suddenly. Her husband found her unconscious in the bathroom.

Tablet organizers have been suggested to help patients remember when to take their medications, but careful attention is needed to avoid mix-ups between look-alike tablets or capsules. A hospitalized patient in Australia was discharged with instructions to take two orange-and-white capsules each night to treat seizures (phenytoin 100 mg capsules).[25] However, the patient was also handed a prescription for calcitriol 0.25 mcg capsules; in Australia these are also orange and white. The patient was supposed to take four capsules of calcitriol each Tuesday and Friday. After discharge, he took two calcitriol each night and four phenytoin twice weekly. He was soon readmitted with seizures. During this admission, the patient insisted that he had followed his medication regimen. When he was asked to demonstrate, it became clear that he had mixed up the capsules.

Some patients may use containers such as old prescription bottles to store their medications. One patient went to the ED with an acute dystonic reaction and was treated successfully with diphenhydramine.[26] The patient said she had never before had this type of reaction. Inspection of her prescription vials at the hospital revealed that one of the vials, labeled Zocor (simvastatin), actually contained haloperidol 10 mg tablets. The patient had been taking this medication twice daily for several days, causing the dystonic reaction. A call to the community pharmacist who filled the patient's prescriptions established that the prescription vial taken to the hospital was from an older refill and that another family member was currently taking haloperidol. The patient admitted that she reused prescription vials occasionally to store small supplies of medications for herself and her spouse (e.g., when they were traveling). Patients should be advised to discard empty prescription vials and to never store multiple drugs in the same container.

ADHERENCE: THE OTHER SIDE OF SAFE DRUG USE

Patient nonadherence to drug therapy can be defined as any one of the following:

- Not filling a prescription initially,
- Not having a prescription refilled,
- Omitting doses,
- Knowingly taking the wrong dose,
- Stopping a medication without the physician's advice,
- Knowingly taking a medication incorrectly,
- Knowingly taking a medication at the wrong time, or
- Taking someone else's medication.

Nonadherence is a major problem. Although the median rate of nonadherence is around 50%,[27] some form of failure to comply with prescribed therapy is associated with up to 93% of the 1.8 billion prescriptions filled annually in the United States.[28,29]

Consequences of Nonadherence

The results of nonadherence (also called noncompliance) are substantial. Studies show that noncompliant patients are more likely to be hospitalized and to require more clinic visits than compliant patients. The National Council on Patient Information and Education estimates that nonadherence is a cause of 10% of all hospital admissions and 25% of admissions among the elderly. Estimates of the annual cost to the economy range from $100 billion to $300 billion.[30,31] (In comparison, the total amount spent purchasing prescription drugs in the United States in 2004 was $235.4 billion.[32])

Certain groups of patients are more likely to be noncompliant than others. These include persons who take more than one drug, who have a chronic condition, who take a drug more than once a day, or who have a condition that produces no overt symptoms or physical impairment.[29,33–35] Compliance decreases as the complexity of drug therapy increases. Patients with chronic diseases are often noncompliant because of the complexity of their drug therapy, adverse effects, and social factors. Compliance often hinges on how important or desirable the outcome of treatment appears to the patient. Effective treatment of diseases such as hypertension that have few or no symptoms is difficult, because the patient may think the adverse effects are worse than the disease itself. In one study, 76% of cardiology and internal medicine patients had discrepancies between their prescribed regimens and how they were taken.[36]

In the 2001 Commonwealth Fund Health Care Quality Survey, 24% of the respondents said there was a time during the previous 2 years that they did not follow their physician's advice.[2] A 2005 Harris poll indicated that 33% of U.S. adults are often or very often noncompliant with their medication regimens.[37] The reasons given for noncompliance were as follows: symptoms went away (36%), to save money (35%), medications were not effective (33%), there was no need to take them (31%), and unpleasant side effects (28%).

Health care providers must help patients understand the consequences of treatment and nontreatment. For example, a man with hypertension is more likely to be compliant if he is told that the medication will reduce his risk of heart attack or stroke than if he is told only that it will reduce his blood pressure. A woman with glaucoma will probably be more compliant if she is told that using the prescribed eye drops will save her eyesight than if she is told that it will reduce her intraocular pressure.

Nonadherence may be unintentional. One cause of unintentional nonadherence is visual impairment. Unintentional nonadherence also may occur if patients do not understand instructions for taking their medication. For example, a patient taking Sinemet CR (carbidopa 50 mg and levodopa 200 mg extended-release) told the pharmacist he had trouble swallowing the tablets.[38] The pharmacist jokingly suggested that the patient coat them with petroleum jelly. The patient followed the pharmacist's advice and, within a few days, suffered a marked decline in function, became fatigued, and lost coordination. The patient called his pharmacist to report that the new drug was not working. Upon questioning, the pharmacist discovered that the patient had taken literally his advice on coating the tablets. The coating was impairing the drug's absorption.

Reasons for Nonadherence

Reasons for nonadherence can be divided into three categories: knowledge deficits, practical barriers, and attitudinal barriers.

Knowledge Deficits

Unintentional nonadherence may occur when patients lack knowledge about their medications and conditions. In one study of emergency department visits related to medication misadventures, one-third of the patients had little or no understanding of proper medication use.[39] Knowledge deficits can be overcome by providing more information or providing the information in a more understandable form. Dispelling myths about treatment and disease may be part of this process. The way in which health care providers present information should be tailored to the patient's level of understanding and cultural and ethnic background.

Literacy problems, a key contributor to knowledge deficits, may not always be immediately discernible. The National Institute for Literacy estimates that 90 million Americans, nearly half of the U.S. population, are marginally or functionally illiterate.[40] The American

TABLE 13-1   Indicators of Limited Literacy

Behaviors
Incomplete or inaccurate patient registration forms
Frequently missed appointments
Nonadherence to medication regimens
Lack of follow-through with tests or referral appointments
Discrepancies between patient reports of medication compliance and lab or other test results

Responses to Questions about Medication Regimens
Unable to name medications
Unable to explain the purpose of a medication
Unable to explain timing or medication administration
Unable to identify medication names from a label on a bottle; able to do so only by looking at actual product
   inside container

Responses to Receiving Written Information
"I forgot my glasses. I'll read this when I get home" or "Can you read this to me?"
"Let me take this home so I can discuss it with my children."

Medical Association Foundation estimates that as many as half of American adults lack "sufficient general literacy to effectively undertake and execute the medical treatments and preventive health care" they need.[11] In 2001, low functional literacy resulted in $32 million to $58 million in additional health care costs.[41]

Those most likely to have limited literacy include persons who are elderly, have low incomes, are unemployed, did not finish high school, belong to minority ethnic groups, are recent immigrants to the United States who do not speak English, or were born in the United States but use English as their second language.[11] Table 13-1 lists behaviors and responses to questions that may indicate limited literacy.[11]

Many individuals with low literacy have jobs and function quite well. They may hide their inability to read, in some cases so well that members of their own families are unaware of their deficit. These individuals rely on memory, association, color, shape, and other cues. If such a patient must take several medications, errors are inevitable unless a system is designed that can compensate for illiteracy. This might entail, for example, color coding the bottles. Color coding has also been shown to improve determination and measurement of pediatric doses.[42]

Language barriers may contribute to knowledge deficits. Brochures about patients' medications should be professionally translated into the most commonly spoken foreign languages. Ad hoc translations can cause problems. One Spanish-speaking mother applied Oxistat (oxiconazole) 1% cream to her baby's inflamed rash up to 11 times each day instead of the prescribed once a day. The prescription label directions were half in English and half in Spanish: "*Aplicarse* once *cada dia* til rash is clear." *Once* is the Spanish word for 11. If this had been an oral medication, the harm to the patient could have been much more serious.

Practical Barriers

Practical barriers to adherence include poor eyesight, inability to pay or lack of insurance coverage, adverse drug reactions, confusing dosing schedules, containers that are difficult to open, and cognitive impairment.

Visual impairment has been shown to be a significant barrier. In one study of ophthalmic medications, the optimal type size was determined to be almost three times the size normally used on medication labels.[43] Tactile cues can be very effective for patients with poor eyesight. For instance, placing a rubber band around a vial of regular insulin helps to differentiate it from other insulin vials of the same size. In another example, when 20 prefilled syringes with 100 units of NPH insulin were dispensed instead of the prescribed 15 units, the patient, who was legally blind, realized by the feel of the plunger position that the dosage was not correct and waited until a family member could verify the dose.[44]

Inability to pay for medications (or health care in general) is one of the most frequently cited reasons for nonadherence.[2,45,46] In a February 2004 Associated Press poll, one in three respondents said paying for prescriptions was a problem for their families.[47] Of those, three out of four said they had put off filling their prescriptions or cut back on doses because of the cost. In a survey of older patients, 26% reported nonadherence because of cost; this included not filling a prescription at all, skipping doses, and taking smaller doses to make the medication last longer.[46] In every case, older patients without insurance coverage reported more cost-related nonadherence than those with insurance coverage.

When patients seek alternative sources of medications to save costs, such as purchasing medications from another country, potential problems include counterfeit medications and confusion among brand names. As discussed in Chapter 6, there are many instances in which brand names used for U.S. medications are used in other countries for products with completely different ingredients. Table 6-5 lists a few examples.

Adverse effects are another barrier to medication compliance. Some of these, such as urinary incontinence, are not only very disturbing to the patient but also difficult to admit to the health provider.

Attitudinal Barriers

These may be the most difficult barriers to overcome because they are rooted in the patient's health belief system, which is formed by his or her culture, ethnicity, family, personal values, and previous experience with the health care system. Patients may deny their condition or express frustration with treatment. Some may exhibit a lack of trust for the health care establishment and seek alternative treatments such as homeopathy or herbal remedies.

Compliance is based on the patient's understanding of the disease and medication and the belief that treatment is necessary and beneficial.[48–50] Some patients of various ethnic backgrounds, such as African Americans, Native Americans, and Hispanic Americans, may stop using their medications when symptoms ease. They may discontinue antidiabetic medications or not complete a course of antimicrobial therapy. In some developing countries, medications are customarily prescribed for just a few days; people from these countries may not understand the value of drugs with a delayed onset of action, such as antidepressants. Because diabetes mellitus is uncommon in Asia, Asian Americans may find it difficult to grasp the relationship between blood glucose and diet.

SPECIFIC PATIENT POPULATIONS

Hospitalized patients, the elderly, and children require special considerations for safe medication use.

Hospitalized Patients

During a hospital stay, a patient is placed in a dependent role. All responsibilities that he or she normally bears, including that of safe drug use, are transferred to professionals. It is understandable that patients are reluctant to ask questions. They do not want to be labeled "troublesome." As a result, they hesitate to question anything, even if they believe something is wrong. Such a climate increases the likelihood of medication errors.

Hospitalized patients need to play an active role in their treatment. They should take their medicine record and medications with them to the hospital. Medications should be in their original containers. After the physician, nurse, or pharmacist has seen the medications, a family member should take them home. Most hospitals do not allow patients to take their own medications while they are hospitalized. One reason for this is to prevent the patient from receiving a double dose—one from the nurse and one that is self-administered. Another reason is that the patient's drug regimen often changes during a hospital stay.

To guard against receiving another patient's medication, patients should make sure the nurse has read their armband before administering each dose. Some hospitals use bar code technology to reduce errors in drug administration. As described in Chapter 15, the nurse uses a bar code scanner to scan the patient's armband and the medication package to ensure that the medication matches the patient's orders.

Hospitalized patients should ask the name and purpose of their medications. Because the patient may not be well enough to do this, a family member or friend should be fully aware of the patient's medication regimen and be prepared to ask questions on the patient's behalf. The literature contains many examples in which a family member has intervened to prevent a medication error. The mother of a child with leukemia who was to receive a daily injection of interferon noticed that the solution in the syringe the nurse was about to use was brown instead of its usual color.[51] The mother questioned this and learned that the syringe actually contained Imferon (iron dextran).

Before discharge from the hospital, the patient should have the opportunity to talk with a health care provider about any new prescriptions and any changes in the medications the patient was taking before hospitalization. If the patient brought a medication list to the hospital, it should be updated. If not, a list should be created. This medication reconciliation process is now a JCAHO requirement.[52] A complete list of patient medications is to be obtained upon admission, with the involvement of the patient. The list is then compared with medications subsequently prescribed. Upon each transfer of care, including discharge, the list is communicated to the next provider of service, including providers outside the institution.

The importance of patient education at the time of discharge is underscored by the following example.[53] A child with leukemia was discharged from the hospital with a nasogastric tube in place for intermittent enteral feeding. He was readmitted for chemotherapy. During this admission, he developed an infection, and a peripherally inserted central catheter (PICC) was placed for administration of IV antimicrobials. The patient improved and was discharged to home care with the PICC still in place. When the PICC line clotted, the child's mother called the home care nurse. The nurse arrived to find that the mother had drawn up ginger ale into a syringe and was about to inject it into the PICC line. Having been taught to clear the child's nasogastric tube with ginger ale, the mother assumed that it could be used to clear all tubes. Had the home care nurse not intervened, the child would have been at risk for infection and carbon dioxide-induced air embolism. Predischarge counseling would have greatly reduced the potential for this error.

Older Patients

Ninety percent of older patients take prescription medications.[46] Of those who use at least one prescription drug, almost half use five or more medications. Furthermore, a majority of older patients use medications prescribed by more than one practitioner, and about one-third fill their prescriptions at more than one pharmacy.

The physiological response to a medication may be different in an older patient. An estimated 25% to 30% of hospital admissions of elderly patients are linked to medication-related problems.[30,54] Because of the lack of controlled studies on medication use in the

Time	Medication	Date		
		10/11	10/12	10/13
8:00 am	Diltiazem 60 mg capsule			
	Aspirin 81 mg tablet			
12 noon	Diltiazem 60 mg capsule			
6:00 pm	Diltiazem 60 mg capsule			
10:00 pm	Warfarin 2 mg tablet			
	Diltiazem 60 mg capsule			

FIGURE 13-8   Example of a medication schedule kept by a patient.

elderly, a list of medications that should generally be avoided in patients age 65 and older has been created.[55] Called the Beers criteria, this list, based on evidence and consensus of experts, identifies medications that lack effectiveness or pose an unnecessarily high risk, as well as medications that should not be used in older patients with specific medical conditions. Practitioners should be aware of such risky medications so that they can educate their older patients about potential adverse effects and drug–drug interactions of both prescription and nonprescription medications. An educated patient who experiences such effects is more likely to call the prescriber, rather than deciding to take a lower (and possibly subtherapeutic) dose or stop the medication altogether.

Because they often take several medications, older patients are at risk for drug–drug and drug–disease interactions. In one study of patients age 65 and older, 0.74% of outpatient visits to a health care provider in which the patient received two or more prescriptions involved at least one inappropriate drug–drug combination.[56] When patients had a prescription for warfarin, 6.6% were prescribed another medication with a potentially harmful interaction. The risk of inappropriate and potentially dangerous combinations of drugs increases with every additional prescription.

Older patients may have some degree of mental impairment, and practitioners should be sensitive to this during counseling. If possible, a family member or friend should be engaged in the counseling process.

A medication schedule can be especially helpful for these patients. It can be hand drawn or produced on a computer. Figure 13-8 shows a sample chart for an elderly patient taking diltiazem, warfarin, and aspirin. The medications should be listed by time of day so the patient can mark the schedule each time he or she takes a dose. Patients who use charts are less likely to inadvertently repeat a dose. The chart must be updated when the drug regimen is changed.

Older patients may want to use medication organizers that allow them to prepackage up to a week's worth of medicine. The organizers are divided by time of day and provide space for multiple daily doses. Patients using these organizers must be able to identify their medications by sight (or by touch—organizers marked in Braille are available), in case the contents spill or the dosage is changed while the organizer is full. Unless a medication organizer is used, patients should be instructed to keep all medications in their original containers. Medications should never be mixed in a single bottle.

Older patients may have trouble swallowing medications. Cutting or crushing a tablet or capsule may not be safe[57] and may impair the action of some products. In one case, an 83-year-old woman died after chewing Cardizem CD (diltiazem).[58] The first time the medication was dispensed, a pharmacist suggested to the patient's son that he ask the prescriber about using immediate-release diltiazem, which comes in tablets that are easier to swallow. The patient was changed to immediate-release tablets and did well for several months until she returned to her physician for a checkup. The physician was not reminded about the previous problem with the CD product and neglected to review patient records. A pharmacist who was unaware of the problem dispensed Cardizem CD according to the new prescription. The patient either forgot about the past problem or was never warned about the consequences of chewing Cardizem CD, so she began chewing the capsules. She became weak and died 3 weeks later. According to her family, the patient was alert and intelligent but had such faith in her health professionals that she would not question their advice.

Patients should ask questions about their medications at the time of prescribing. They should check with a pharmacist before manipulating (splitting or crushing) a dosage form.

Pediatric Patients

Rates of compliance with drug therapy are virtually the same for children and adults, but children may have some unique reasons for noncompliance.[59] If they do not understand the difference between drugs that help people and those that hurt people, children may be reluctant to take any medication. Children with chronic illnesses may be noncompliant because they feel hopeless about their disease. Children lack control over many aspects of their lives, and compliance with drug therapy is one thing they can control. In addition, children may have erroneous beliefs, such as thinking that a higher dose will lead to a faster cure.

Accidental poisonings are a separate but related concern with respect to children and safe medication use (error prevention in pediatric patients is discussed in Chapter 17). If a medicine tastes too good, children may consume the entire bottle; this is quite common with cough syrups, chewable analgesics, vitamins, and antibiotics. Children may also consume cleaning substances and personal care products such as toothpaste and shampoo that are left in accessible locations.[60]

Child-resistant packaging has decreased the number of childhood poisonings, but it has not eliminated the risk. The American Association of Poison Control Centers reported that among children under the age of 6 years, there were 568,939 exposures to potentially harmful pharmaceutical products and 721,556 exposures to potentially harmful nonpharmaceutical products in 2003.[61] Approximately one ED visit every 7 minutes by a child under 5 years old is due to unintentional poisoning.[62] Many of these poisonings occur because containers are not properly closed, products sold in non-child-resistant packaging are not secured, or medications are repackaged and stored in containers that are not child resistant.[62-64]

According to the Poison Prevention Act of 1970, packaging is considered child resistant if 85% of children between 3½ and 4 years of age would be unable to open the package within 10 minutes and 80% would be unable to open it even after being shown how to do so and given 5 minutes to try.[65,66] However, one study performed in an ED showed that properly closed child-resistant packaging failed to deter children under the age of 5 in 20% of cases.[67]

Adults can promote children's safety by storing medications with caps securely fastened, on a high shelf or in a locked box. Adults should never take medications in the presence of children, because a positive or negative reaction on the part of the adult may influence the child's perception of medications. When taking their children to visit in another home, parents should ask their hosts whether their medications are stored in a place that is not accessible to children.

Parents should post the universal number for poison control (1-800-222-1222) near a telephone so it is available to family members, babysitters, and visitors. The American Academy of Pediatrics no longer recommends keeping syrup of ipecac in the home, nor does it recommend home use of activated charcoal.[68] Parents should be instructed to safely dispose of syrup of ipecac and to contact a poison control center before any home treatment, including having the child drink water or milk or inducing vomiting. Parents can help determine how much a child has ingested if they mark bottles of liquid medication after each appropriate use.

Unit dose packaging of oral solids, especially blister packaging, makes it more difficult for children to accidentally ingest drugs. Many new nonprescription drugs, as well as some prescription products, are packaged this way.

CONCLUSION

Patients can play an important role in their medication therapy by asking questions of health care providers and by providing information to their physicians, nurses, and pharmacists. Patients should maintain accurate, up-to-date medication records.

Informed patients have prevented many medication errors, and health care providers should encourage patient involvement in medication safety. Health care facilities should not only make patients aware of errors and what is being done at a system level to prevent them, but they should ask patients to participate in safe practices.

One way to prompt patients to adopt the safety strategies in this chapter is to make them more aware of the prevalence of errors and provide examples. Resources for patients include ISMP's brochure "How To Take Your Medications Safely," which is included at the end of this chapter and available at www.ismp.org/Newsletters/consumer/alerts/Brochure.asp, and the ISMP consumer newsletter *Safe Medicine,* which includes error stories and safety strategies. Medication safety strategies are also available from consumer groups such as PULSE (Persons United Limiting Sub-standards and Errors in Healthcare) and CAPS (Consumers Advancing Patient Safety), which were formed in response to personal experiences with medical errors. PULSE (www.pulseamerica.org) is a nonprofit support group for consumers involved in medical errors; it uses actual error stories to educate the community and advocate for a safer health care system. CAPS (www.patientsafety.org/index.htm) is another nonprofit group promoting a safer health care system.

REFERENCES

1. Louis Harris & Associates. Public Opinion of Patient Safety Issues: Research Findings. Prepared for National Patient Safety Foundation at AMA. September 1997. Available at: www.npsf.org/download/1997survey.pdf. Accessed June 16, 2006.
2. Davis K, Schoenbaum SC, Collins KS, et al. Room for improvement: patients report on the quality of their health care. New York: The Commonwealth Fund; 2002. Available at: www.cmwf.org/publications/publications_show.htm?doc_id=221270. Accessed May 19, 2005.
3. Kaiser Family Foundation, Agency for Healthcare Research and Quality, Harvard School of Public Health. National survey on consumers' experiences with patient safety and quality information. November 2004. Available at: www.kff.org/kaiserpolls/pomr111704pkg.cfm. Accessed May 19, 2005.
4. McGuckin M, et al. Handwashing Compliance: the Effect of a Patient Education Program. Paper presented at: Society for Healthcare Epidemiology in America annual meeting, April 1997, St Louis, Mo.
5. Want a savvy participant in your error-prevention program? Put a consumer on your team! *ISMP Medication Safety Alert!* May 17, 2000;5(10):2.
6. Do you know…how to check your prescriptions? *ISMP Safe Medicine.* November/December 2003;1(5):2.
7. Joint Commission on Accreditation of Healthcare Organizations. Speak Up Campaign. Available at: www.jointcommission.org/GeneralPublic/Speak+Up/about_speakup.htm. Accessed June 23, 2006.
8. Joint Commission on Accreditation of Healthcare Organizations. 2007 National Patient Safety Goals—Hospital & Critical Access Hospital Programs. Available at: www.jointcommission.org/PatientSafety/NationalPatientSafetyGoals/07_hap_cah_npsgs.htm. Accessed June 23, 2006.
9. Safety brief. *ISMP Medication Safety Alert!* August 12, 1998;3(16):2.

10. Safety brief. *ISMP Medication Safety Alert!* May 5, 1999;4(9):2.

11. Weiss, BD. *Health Literacy: A Manual for Clinicians.* American Medical Association Foundation and American Medical Association. 2003. Available at: www.ama-assn.org/ama1/pub/upload/mm/367/healthlitclinicians. pdf. Accessed May 4, 2005.

12. Naturally speaking. *ISMP Nurse Advise-ERR.* July 2003;1(4):1.

13. Warfarin and digoxin interactions with ginseng. *ISMP Nurse Advise-ERR.* August 2003;1(5):2.

14. This will bring tears to your eyes. *ISMP Nurse Advise-ERR.* June 2004;2(6):1.

15. Running on empty. *ISMP Medication Safety Alert!* September 23, 2004;9(19):3.

16. A medication error trifecta! *ISMP Nurse Advise-ERR.* August 2004;2(8):1.

17. Inappropriate designation of dosage form is a common source of error. *ISMP Medication Safety Alert!* November 28, 2001;6(24):2.

18. Excedrin: headache for aspirin-sensitive patients? *ISMP Medication Safety Alert!* July 30, 1997;2(15):2.

19. Caution: Dulcolax brand name extensions. *ISMP Medication Safety Alert!* April 8, 2004;9(7):1.

20. US Food and Drug Administration. New OTC drug facts label. *FDA Consum.* July–August 2002. Available at: www.fda.gov/fdac/features/2002/402_otc.html. Accessed May 19, 2005.

21. "Rit" or wrong? Is it Ritalin or ritodrine? *ISMP Medication Safety Alert!* May 21, 1997;2(10):1.

22. Safety brief. *ISMP Medication Safety Alert!* June 17, 1998;3(12):1.

23. What's my dose of Coumadin today? *ISMP Safe Medicine.* September/October 2004; 2(5):1.

24. O'Keefe JH, Kwong EM, Tancredi RG. Transgingival nitrate syncope. *N Engl J Med.* 1986;315:1030.

25. Appearances are deceiving. *ISMP Medication Safety Alert!* June 1, 2004;9(12):2.

26. Safety brief. *ISMP Medication Safety Alert!* April 5, 2000;5(7):1.

27. Kyngas H, Duffy ME, Krol T. Conceptual analysis of compliance. *J Clin Nurs.* 2000;9(1):5-12.

28. Berg JS, Dischler J, Wagner DJ, et al. Medication compliance: a health care problem. *Ann Pharmacother.* 1993;27: S5–S19.

29. Greenberg RN. Overview of patient compliance with medication dosing: a literature review. *Clin Ther.* 1984;6:592–8.

30. Task Force for Compliance. *Noncompliance with Medications: An Economic Tragedy with Important Implications for Health Care Reform.* Washington, DC: National Pharmaceutical Council; 1992:1–16.

31. McGhan WF, Peterson AM. Pharmacoeconomic impact of noncompliance. *US Pharm.* 2001; ImPact suppl:1–13.

32. IMS reports 8.3 percent dollar growth in 2004 U.S. prescription sales [press release]. February 14, 2004. Fairfield, CT: IMS. Available at: www.imshealth.com/ims/portal/front/articleC/0,2777,6599_3665_70069264,00. html. Accessed May 19, 2005.

33. Hulka BS, Kupper LL, Cassel JC, et al. Medication use and misuse: physician–patient discrepancies. *J Chron Dis.* 1975;28:7–21.

34. Eraker SA, Kirscht JP, Becker MH. Understanding and improving patient compliance. *Ann Intern Med.* 1984;100:258–68.

35. Col N, Fanale JE, Kronholm P. The role of medication noncompliance and adverse drug reactions in hospitalizations of the elderly. *Arch Intern Med.* 1990;150:841–5.

36. Harris L & Associates. Prescription drug compliance a significant challenge for many patients, according to a new national survey [press release]. March 29, 2005. Rochester, NY: Harris Interactive. Available at: www.harrisinteractive.com/news/printerfriend/index.asp?NewsID=904. Accessed May 19, 2005.

37. Bedell SE, Jabbour S, Goldberg R, et al. Discrepancies in the use of medications. *Arch Intern Med.* 2000; 160(14):2129–34.

38. Cohen MR. Caution: what patients hear may be taken literally. *Hosp Pharm.* 1996;31:603–4.

39. Schneitman-McIntire O, Farnen TA, Gordon N, et al. Medication misadventures resulting in emergency department visits at an HMO medical center. *Am J Health Syst Pharm.* 1996;53(12):1416–22.

40. Kirsch IS, Jungeblut A, Jenkins L, et al. Executive summary of adult literacy in America: a first look at the results of the national adult literacy survey. National Center for Education Statistics, US Department of Education, 1993. Available at: http://nces.ed.gov/naal/resources/execsumm.asp. Accessed May 19, 2005.

41. Potter L, Martin C. Impact of low health literacy skills on annual health care expenditures [fact sheet]. September 2003; Center for Health Care Strategies, Inc, Lawrenceville, NJ. Available at: www.chcs.org/publications3960/publications_show.htm?doc_id=213128. Accessed May 19, 2005.

42. Frush KS, Luo X, Hutchinson P, et al. Evaluation of a method to reduce over-the-counter medication dosing error. *Arch Pediatr Adolesc Med.* 2004;158:620–4.

43. Drummond SR, Drummond RS, Dutton GN. Visual acuity and the ability of the visually impaired to read medication instructions. *Br J Ophthalmol.* 2004;88:1541–2.

44. Safety brief. *ISMP Medication Safety Alert!* March 24, 1999;4(6):1.

45. Malhotra S, Karan RS, Pandhi P, et al. Drug related medical emergencies in the elderly: role of adverse drug reactions and non-compliance. *Postgrad Med J.* 2001;77:703–7.

46. Safran DG, Neuman P, Schoen C, et al. Prescription drug coverage and seniors: findings from a 2003 national survey. *Health Aff* [serial online]. 2005. Available at: http://content.healthaffairs.org/cgi/content/abstract/hlthaff.w5.152. Accessed May 19, 2005.

47. Associated Press/Ipsos. Almost a third of Americans say paying for drugs is a problem in their families. February 25, 2004. Available at: www.ipsos-na.com/news/pressrelease.cfm?id=2064. Accessed May 19, 2005.

48. Levy R, Hawks J. *Cultural Diversity and Pharmaceutical Care* [monograph]. Reston, Va: National Pharmaceutical Council; May 1999.

49. Burroughs VJ, Maxey RW, Levy RA. Racial and ethnic differences in response to medicines: towards individualized pharmaceutical treatment. *J Natl Med Assoc.* 2002;94:1–26.

50. Pavlovich-Danis S. Ethnicity and culture vary medicinal effects. *Nurs Spectrum* (Phila/TriState). 1999;Oct 4:18–9.

51. Cohen MR. Do not confuse interferon with imferon. *Hosp Pharm.* 1992;27:784–5.

52. Joint Commission on Accreditation of Healthcare Organizations. 2005 National Patient Safety Goals. Available at: www.jointcommission.org/PatientSafety/NationalPatientSafetyGoals/05_hap_npsgs.htm. Accessed June 23, 2006.

53. Patient teaching needed before home care patients leave the hospital. *ISMP Medication Safety Alert!* March 26, 1997;2(6):2.

54. Hanlon JT, Schmader KE, Kornkowski MJ, et al. Adverse drug events in high risk older outpatients. *J Am Geriatr Soc.* 1997;45:945–8

55. Fick DM, Cooper JW, Wade WE, et al. Updating the Beers criteria for potentially inappropriate medication use in older adults. *Arch Intern Med.* 2003;163:2716–24.

56. Zhan C, Correa-de-Araujo R, Bierman AS, et al. Suboptimal prescribing in elderly outpatients: potentially harmful drug–drug and drug–disease combinations. *J Am Geriatr Soc.* 2005;53(2):262–7.

57. Mitchell JF, Leady MA. Oral solid dosage forms that should not be crushed: 2004 revision [wall chart]. *Hosp Pharm* 2004;33(7): suppl.

58. Patient dies after chewing Cardizem CD. *ISMP Medication Safety Alert!* April 10, 1996;1(7):2.

59. Thompson CA. Children's drug-information needs are explored at USP conference. *Am J Health Syst Pharm.* 1996;53:2782–3.

60. Litovitz TL, Felberg L, White S, et al. 1995 Annual Report of the American Association of Poison Control Centers Toxic Exposure Surveillance System. *Am J Emerg Med.* 1996;14:487–94.

61. Watson WA, Litovitz TL, Klein-Schwartz W, et al. 2003 annual report of the American Association of Poison Control Centers Toxic Exposure Surveillance System. *Am J Emerg Med.* 2004;22(5):335–404. Available at: www.aapcc.org/Annual%20Reports/03report/Annual%20Report%202003.pdf. Accessed May 19, 2005.

62. National Poison Prevention Week warns: most child poisonings result from common household products [press release]. March 15, 2005. Washington, DC: US Consumer Product Safety Commission.

63. McIntire MS, Angle CR, Grush ML. How effective is safety packaging? *Clin Toxicol.* 1976;9:419–25.

64. Jacobson BJ, Rock AR, Cohn MS, et al. Accidental ingestions of oral prescription drugs: a multicenter survey. *Am J Public Health.* 1989;79:853–6.

65. Poison Prevention Packaging Act of 1970. Pub Law 91-601; December 30, 1970.

66. Code of Federal Regulations, Title 16 Commercial Practices, Chapter II–Consumer Product Safety Commission, Part 1700–Poison Prevention Packaging. Available at: www.access.gpo.gov/nara/cfr/waisidx_98/16cfr1700_98.html. Accessed May 19, 2005.

67. Lembersky RB, Nichols MH, King WD. Effectiveness of child-resistant packaging on toxin procurement in young poisoning victims. *Vet Hum Toxicol.* 1996;38:380–3.

68. Committee on Injury, Violence, and Poison Prevention, American Academy of Pediatrics. Poison treatment in the home. *Pediatrics.* 2003;112(5):1182–5.

APPENDIX

CONSUMER BROCHURE FROM THE INSTITUTE FOR SAFE MEDICATION PRACTICES

Be an Informed Consumer

Unfortunately, medication errors happen. They happen in hospitals, in pharmacies, or even at home. And sometimes people get hurt because of these errors.

The more information you have, the better able you are to prevent errors and to take care of yourself. You have to ask your pharmacists, doctors, and nurses about your medications, and you have to expect answers.

Also, if you have any chronic illnesses, pick up one of the consumer guides about medications at a bookstore or from the library. Find out all that you can about your illnesses and the medications you are taking. What you learn will help protect you later.

Your doctors, nurses, and pharmacists work hard to keep you healthy, but you are also responsible. Learn what questions to ask. Expect answers—it's your life and your health!

Key Questions

Your pharmacist can be your partner to prevent medication errors. Find one who offers services like monitoring your therapy and keeping a complete list in the pharmacy computer of all your medications and chronic medical conditions. Include over-the-counter medications, vitamins, nutritional supplements and herbal products even if you bought them somewhere else. It's worth the cost. With this information in one place, your pharmacist can help to protect you against harmful drug interactions, duplicate medications, and other potential problems.

Before you leave the pharmacy, your pharmacist should give you printed information about the medication and make sure that you understand the answers to these questions:

1. What are the brand and generic names of the medication?
2. What does it look like?
3. Why am I taking it?
4. How much should I take, and how often?
5. When is the best time to take it?
6. How long will I need to take it?
7. What side effects should I expect, and what should I do if they happen?
8. What should I do if I miss a dose?
9. Does this interact with my other medications or any foods?
10. Does this replace anything else I was taking?
11. Where and how do I store it?

When you buy over-the-counter medications, read the labels carefully because they might contain ingredients you do not want or should not take. Maybe they will interact with your other medications, cause an allergic reaction, or not be correct for your symptoms. Ask your pharmacist for help if you have trouble selecting the right product.

What You Can Do at Home

Make a list of medications you are taking now. Include the dose, how often you take them, the imprint on each tablet or capsule, and the name of the pharmacy. The imprint can help you identify a drug when you get refills.

Any time that your medications change, change your list, too. Double-check the imprints on the tablets and capsules.

Also list your medication and food allergies and any over-the-counter medications, vitamins, nutritional supplements, or herbal products that you take regularly.

Keep medications in their original containers. Many pills look alike, so by keeping them in their original containers, you will know which is which and how to take them.

Never take someone else's medication. You don't know if it will interact with your medications. The dose may be wrong for you, or you may be allergic to it.

Read the label every time you take a dose to make sure that you have the right drug and that you are following the instructions.

Turn on the lights to take your medications. If you can't see what you're taking, you may take the wrong thing.

Don't store medications in the bathroom medicine cabinet or in direct sunlight. Humidity, heat, and light can affect medications' potency and safety.

Store medications where children can't see or reach them, for example, in a locked box or cabinet.

Keep medications for people separate from pets' medications or household chemicals. Mix-ups are common and can be dangerous.

Don't keep tubes of ointments or creams next to your tube of toothpaste. They feel a lot alike when you grab quickly, but a mistake could be serious.

Don't chew, crush, or break any capsules or tablets unless instructed. Some long-acting medications are absorbed too quickly when chewed, which could be unsafe. Other medications either won't be effective or could make you sick.

What You Can Do in the Hospital

Take your medications and the list of your medications with you when you go to the hospital. Your doctors and nurses will need to know what you are taking.

After your doctor has seen them, send your medications home with your family. While you are in the hospital you may not need the same medications.

Tell your doctor you want to know the names of each medication and the reasons you are taking them. That way, if anyone tells you anything different, you'll know to ask questions, which might prevent errors.

Look at all medicines before you take them. If it doesn't look like what you usually take, ask why. It might be a generic drug, or it might be the wrong drug. Ask the same questions you would ask if you were in the pharmacy.

Do not let anyone give you medications without checking your hospital ID bracelet every time. This helps prevent you from getting someone else's medications.

Before any test or procedure, ask if it will require any dyes or medicines. Remind your nurse and doctor if you have allergies.

When you're ready to go home, have the doctor, nurse, or pharmacist go over each medication with you and a family member. Update your medication list from home if any prescriptions change or if new medications are added.

What You Can Do at the Doctor's Office

Take your medication list every time you go to your doctor's office, especially if you see more than one doctor. They might not know about the medications other doctors prescribed for you.

Ask your doctor to explain what is written on any prescription, including the drug name and how often you should take it. Then when you take the prescription to the pharmacy, you can double-check the information on the label.

Tell your doctor you want the purpose for the medication written on the prescription. Many drug names look alike when written poorly; knowing the purpose helps you and the pharmacist double-check the prescription.

If your doctor gives you samples, make sure that he or she checks to be sure that there are no interactions with your other medications. Pharmacies have computers to check for drug interactions and allergies, but when your doctor gives you samples, this important check may be missed.

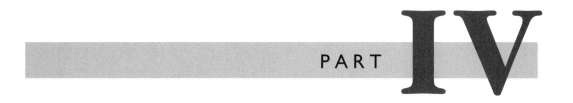

PART **IV**

PREVENTING MEDICATION ERRORS: SPECIFIC MEDICATIONS, PATIENTS, AND CONDITIONS

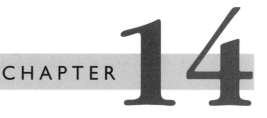

CHAPTER **14**

HIGH-ALERT MEDICATIONS: SAFEGUARDING AGAINST ERRORS

Michael R. Cohen, Judy L. Smetzer, Nancy R. Tuohy, and Charles M. Kilo

Although most medications have a wide margin of safety, a few drugs have a high risk of causing patient injury or death if they are misused. Special precautions are needed to reduce the risk of error with these "high-alert" medications. Errors with these drugs may not be more common than with other medications, but their consequences can be more devastating.

High-alert medications can be targeted for specific error-reduction interventions. For example, they can be packaged, stored, prescribed, and administered differently than other medications. Forcing functions (i.e., methods that make it difficult for the drug to be given in a potentially lethal manner) can be developed and instituted. The use of these products can be standardized and simplified, or restricted.

This chapter consists of two major parts. The first part presents a framework for safeguarding the use of high-alert drugs and discusses changes to make the use of these products safer. The second part of the chapter provides detailed discussion of some of the most commonly used high-alert drugs (Table 14-1). The high-alert designation is based on review of voluntarily submitted reports of errors that have caused significant patient harm and on the results of a survey of more than 350 practitioners by the Institute for Safe Medication Practices (ISMP), described on page 319.[1] The potential list of high-alert medications was also reviewed by the clinical staff at ISMP, members of a clinical advisory board, and safety experts throughout the United States. The discussion of individual high-alert drugs summarizes the problems that have occurred and outlines error-reduction strategies based on practitioners' experience, the professional literature, and human-factors concepts.

Some of the recommendations presented here have not been proven effective by scientific clinical trials.[2] However, we agree with the following assessment by other patient safety experts: "Evidence from randomized trials is important information, but it is neither sufficient nor necessary for acceptance of a practice. For policymakers to wait for incontrovertible proof of effectiveness before recommending a practice would be a prescription for inaction and an abdication of responsibility."[3] The more obvious safety interventions have been likened to the use of parachutes[4]: The effectiveness of parachutes has never been subjected to rigorous evaluation in randomized controlled trials. Rather, it is based on anecdotal evidence and obvious benefit. So, too, are some of the recommendations in this chapter for reducing the risk of errors with high-alert drugs.

TABLE 14-1   ISMP List of High-Alert Medications

Class/Category

Adrenergic agonists, IV (e.g., dopamine, dobutamine, ephedrine, epinephrine, isoproterenol, norepinephrine)

Adrenergic antagonists, IV (e.g., amiodarone, beta-blockers such as propranolol, esmolol, labetalol)

Anesthetic agents, general, inhaled and IV (e.g., propofol, thiopental, methohexital, etomidate)

Cardioplegic solutions

Cancer chemotherapy agents, injectable and oral (e.g., carboplatin, cisplatin, cyclophosphamide, doxorubicin, daunorubicin, methotrexate, vinblastine, vincristine)

Dextrose, hypertonic, 20% concentration or greater

Dialysis solutions, peritoneal and hemodialysis

Epidural and intrathecal medications (e.g., bupivicaine, opioids, baclofen, fentanyl, intrathecal antineoplastics)

Glycoprotein IIb/IIIa inhibitors (e.g., abciximab, eptifibatide, tirofiban)

Hypoglycemics, oral

Inotropic medications, IV (e.g., digoxin, milrinone)

Liposomal forms of drugs (e.g., liposomal amphotericin B [Abelcet, Ambisome, Amphotec], daunorubicin [DaunoXome], doxorubicin [Doxil])

Moderate sedation agents, IV (e.g., midazolam)

Moderate sedation agents, oral, for children (e.g., chloral hydrate, midazolam syrup)

Neuromuscular blocking agents (e.g., atracurium, doxacurium, pancuronium, pipecuronium, succinylcholine, vecuronium)

Opioids, IV, epidural, transdermal, and oral, including liquid concentrates and immediate-release and extended-release forms (e.g., morphine, fentanyl, hydromorphone [Dilaudid], meperidine [Demerol])

Radiocontrast agents, IV (iohexol [Omnipaque], diatrizoate meglumine [Hypaque])

Thrombolytics/fibrinolytics, IV (e.g., alteplase [Activase], tenecteplase [TNKase], reteplase [Retevase])

Total parenteral nutrition solutions

Medication

IV amiodarone

Colchicine injection

Heparin, low molecular weight, injection (e.g., dalteparin [Fragmin], enoxaparin [Lovenox], ardeparin [Normiflo], danaparoid [Orgaran], fondaparinux [Arixtra])

Heparin, unfractionated, IV

Insulin, subcutaneous and IV

Lidocaine, IV

Magnesium sulfate injection

Methotrexate, oral, nononcologic use

Nesiritide (Natrecor)

Nitroprusside sodium for injection (Nitropress)

Potassium chloride for injection concentrate

Potassium phosphates injection

Sodium chloride injection, hypertonic, greater than 0.9% concentration

Warfarin (Coumadin)

A FRAMEWORK FOR IMPROVEMENT

Three principles can be applied for the safe use of high-alert medications: (1) reducing or eliminating the possibility of errors, (2) making errors visible, and (3) minimizing the consequences of errors. These principles provide a framework for developing specific error-reduction strategies.

Principle 1: Reduce or Eliminate the Possibility of Error

The occurrence of errors can be reduced by limiting the number and variety of medications on the formulary, limiting the available number of concentrations and volumes

PRACTITIONER SURVEY ON HIGH-ALERT MEDICATIONS

ISMP surveyed practitioners in 2003 about which drugs or drug categories they considered to be high-alert medications (Table 14-2). More than 350 practitioners responded. Nurses and pharmacists did not always agree on which drugs should be considered high-alert medications (Table 14-3). Nurses more often identified IV adrenergic antagonists and agonists, oral and IM narcotics, and liposomal forms of drugs as high-alert medications, whereas pharmacists more often identified hypertonic sodium chloride, warfarin, and subcutaneous insulin as high-alert medications.

The survey revealed gaps between respondents' identification of high-alert drugs and the adoption of precautions to mitigate errors and harm involving these drugs. This difference between perception and practice, as well as the differing responses of nurses and pharmacists, illustrates the need for interdisciplinary discussion of error potential and for commitment to error reduction strategies.

TABLE 14-2   Medications Considered High-Alert by Practitioners[1]

Drug or Category	%[a] (n = 364)
Injectable cancer chemotherapy agents	98
IV potassium chloride	96
Neuromuscular blocking agents (e.g., succinylcholine)	94
Hypertonic sodium chloride injection	91
Insulin, IV	90
Potassium phosphate, IV	90
Heparin, IV	87
Thrombolytics/fibrinolytics, IV (e.g., tenecteplase)	82
Inhaled and IV general anesthetic agents (e.g., propofol)	77
Conscious sedation agents, IV (e.g., midazolam)	75
Opioids, IV	74
Oral cancer chemotherapy agents	73
Warfarin	73
Cardioplegic solutions	62
Calcium gluconate, IV	61
High-concentration dextrose injection	58
Total parenteral nutrition	57
Oral/IM opioids	52
Adrenergic antagonists, IV (e.g., propranolol)	51
Low molecular weight heparin	50
Theophylline, IV	50
Benzodiazepines in patients over 65 (e.g., alprazolam)	47
Liposomal forms of drugs (e.g., amphotericin B)	45
Dialysate	34
Oral hypoglycemic agents (e.g., glipizide)	23

[a] Percentage of respondents who agreed with high-alert designation.

of a medication, and removing high-alert drugs from clinical areas. No experimental data are needed to prove that if a product is not present, it cannot be substituted for something else.[5]

TABLE 14-3   Differences in Drugs Considered High-Alert by Nurses and Pharmacists[1]

	% Considering It High-Alert	
Drug or Category	**Nurses** **(n = 60)**	**Pharmacists** **(n = 232)**
Benzodiazepines in patients over 65 (e.g., alprazolam)	71	40
Cardioplegic solutions	86	58
Dialysate	66	26
Glycoprotein IIb/IIIa inhibitors (e.g., tirofiban)	76	63
Inhaled and IV general anesthetic agents (e.g., propofol)	88	75
Adrenergic agonists, IV (e.g., epinephrine)	92	63
Adrenergic antagonists, IV (e.g., propranolol)	81	43
Calcium chloride, IV	79	63
Inotropic medications, IV (e.g., digoxin, milrinone)	77	64
Opioids, IV	83	70
Liposomal forms of drugs (e.g., amphotericin B)	68	39
Oral conscious sedation agents for children (e.g., chloral hydrate)	84	66
Oral/IM opioids	69	46

A successful application of this principle has been the removal of all concentrated potassium chloride from floor stock,[6] which has reduced errors associated with inadvertent intravenous administration of high-concentration potassium. Another example is the use of tall-man lettering in the labels of dobutamine and dopamine (i.e., DOBUTamine, DOPamine) to reduce the chance of errors resulting from their look-alike and sound-alike names and similar packaging.

A third example is the proactive use of information about external errors to prevent internal errors. If an incident happens in one health care setting, there is a strong likelihood that it will recur elsewhere. The biweekly *ISMP Medication Safety Alert!* newsletter communicates error advisories based on reports from practitioners that are submitted to ISMP and the U.S. Pharmacopeia Medication Errors Reporting Program (USP-ISMP MERP). This information should be constantly monitored and proactively used for error prevention.

Principle 2: Make Errors Visible

When errors do occur, making them visible can help prevent patient harm. An example of this is having two individuals independently check infusion pump settings for high-alert drugs. If an incorrect rate of infusion is programmed into a device, a second, independent check prior to initiation of the infusion should make the error visible. Another example is the use of bar code systems to verify that the correct drug, dose, and administration route are being used at the correct time—for the correct patient.

Principle 3: Minimize the Consequences of Errors

Practices can be changed to reduce the adverse effects of errors that do occur. For instance, fatal errors have occurred when the contents of 50 mL vials of lidocaine 2% were injected instead of mannitol, which was packaged in a vial of similar appearance. Had lidocaine been available only in 10 mL vials, the overdose would have been less likely to be fatal (and less likely to happen, since the vial sizes are different). Also, closer monitoring could improve early detection of errors and prompt remedial action.

SAFEGUARDING HIGH-ALERT DRUG USE

Strategies based on these three principles can be incorporated into medication-use systems to help ensure safe use of high-alert drugs, as discussed below.

Use Fail-safes

Features should be included in the design of medical equipment to compensate automatically for deficiencies in human knowledge and performance, and to ensure that equipment does not become dangerous when one part fails. For example, infusion pumps traditionally required that, when removing the administration set, the operator close a clamp to prevent gravity flow of the solution. When personnel failed to clamp the tubing, patients were harmed by free-flow of solutions containing potentially toxic medications.[7] After years of advocacy by ISMP[8] and ECRI[9] and a 2003 Joint Commission on Accreditation of Health Care Organizations (JCAHO) National Patient Safety Goal (NPSG) addressing the problem, electronic infusion devices now use intravenous sets with an automatic fail-safe clamping mechanism to prevent accidental free-flow of solutions. Safe medication use dictates that all IV pump sets have built-in free-flow protection that cannot be overridden.

Other examples of fail-safes are devices that default to a predetermined safe state in the event of malfunctioning or unintentional operation. For instance, a patient-controlled analgesia (PCA) pump should be programmed with default settings of zero, or the highest possible concentration of opioids used. This way, if a malfunction occurs, the patient receives no medication or a subtherapeutic dose.

Although the concept of fail-safes is usually associated with device design, it can also be applied to technology and processes of care. For example, computer applications may require confirmation before high-risk actions (e.g., deleting patient records, selecting a product name that looks like another) can be performed. Fail-safes can be built into care processes to detect an error and interrupt or pause the sequence of events to allow human intervention.

Use Forcing Functions

Forcing functions are techniques that eliminate or reduce the possibility that a medication can be prescribed, dispensed, or administered in a potentially lethal manner. A case in point is the use of "lock-and-key" designs to prevent the interchange of parts from different systems. For example, device design should prevent liquid in a syringe intended for oral use from being injected into an IV line. Syringes designed for the measurement and administration of oral liquids have tips that are incompatible with and cannot be attached to the standard Luer connection of IV systems or needles. Similarly, the use of epidural tubing without injection ports makes it impossible for a practitioner to accidentally inject a medication into that line once it is connected to the epidural catheter.

Computerized medication order entry programs can be configured with a forcing function to prohibit the ordering of medications if key information, such as allergies and patient weight, has not been entered. The user cannot proceed until a specified condition—entry of the key information—has been met.

Forcing functions are a valuable means of reducing errors, but in rare instances they have failed. Personnel have succeeded in connecting components purposely designed to disallow connection. For example, nurses have managed to administer oral liquids into needleless IV ports. Another example is described on page 322.

Some error-reduction strategies incorporate several different safety elements, including "soft" forcing functions. In contrast to a lock-and-key design, a soft forcing function directs

FATAL GAS LINE MIX-UP

A patient died when a usually effective forcing function failed. A system of uniquely designed connecting pins for medical gases (air, oxygen, nitrous oxide) ensures that regulators designed for a particular gas will fit only in designated wall outlets. All gas cylinders, flow meters, and wall outlets have safety features such as a pin index or diameter index to prevent accidental use of the wrong source or component (Figures 14-1 and 14-2).

In this case, the pin index system was broken, allowing the oxygen flow meter to be forced into a nitrous oxide wall outlet adjacent to the oxygen outlet in a radiology suite. Furthermore, in the dim light, the technician was unable to distinguish the blue outlet (nitrous oxide) from the green outlet (oxygen). Instead of receiving oxygen, the patient died of nitrous oxide poisoning. Similar cases of hypoxic injury have been reported, even though index safety systems and color coding for medical gases have been in use for years.

It may be feasible to reduce the availability of nitrous oxide in some locations, but anesthetics are often given in locations outside the operating room (e.g., for invasive procedures in radiology, endoscopy and bronchoscopy units, cardiac catheterization labs, plastic surgery clinics). Even if nitrous oxide were less available, mix-ups between other gases accessible through wall outlets, including air, as well as inadvertent connection to vacuum outlets, would still be possible.

The wrong gas has also been administered when the patient's tubing is connected to the wrong flow meter, especially when color-coded "Christmas tree" adapters are used between the flow meter and tubing. Green adapters are meant for oxygen and yellow adapters for air. Because the threading for connecting the adapter to the flow meter is universal, it is possible to use the wrong color adapter. If staff rely on the color of the adapter to guide connections, the oxygen tubing could be misconnected to an air flow meter if a green adapter has been used in error.

Safety measures to prevent patient harm from medical gas mix-ups include the following:

- ❑ Standardize the type of flow meters, regulators, and connectors used throughout the facility, and use only those with intact index safety systems to help prevent misconnection.
- ❑ Ensure that gas connections are observable (not hidden under a table or behind a drape) and that the labeling of all gas connections and sources is prominent and visible under the existing conditions (e.g., dim lighting, crowded spaces).
- ❑ If a patient does not respond as expected to treatment with supplemental oxygen, consider the possibility that the wrong gas (or no gas) is being administered and check the flow meter and tubing connections.
- ❑ Consider using clear Christmas tree adapters, forcing the user to look at the flow meter and wall connection.
- ❑ Use an oxygen saturation monitor during invasive procedures, including those performed outside the operating room, to provide early warning of hypoxia, thereby reducing the risk of a bad outcome from a mix-up between nitrous oxide and oxygen.
- ❑ Require biomedical engineering experts to perform regular preventive maintenance on gas wall outlets, gas cylinders, flow meters, and other related equipment to ensure that all connections and connectors are intact and in good working condition. Only trained and certified personnel should be allowed to service, maintain, and use this equipment.
- ❑ Consider whether new standards are needed. The index safety system has worked reasonably well, but adverse events like the one described here suggest the need for standards that make gas line misconnections impossible. Changing the materials used to manufacture pins and attachments so they are less likely to break or wear out is one improvement that could be made. A committee of the Association for the Advancement of Medical Instrumentation has been formed to develop national standards for tubing connectors and will address this safety issue.

Matthew B. Weinger, MD, of the San Diego (California) Center for Patient Safety; Allan Frankel, MD, of Partners HealthCare and the Institute for Healthcare Improvement, Boston, Massachusetts; and John Gosbee, MD, of the Department of Veterans Affairs National Center for Patient Safety, Ann Arbor, Michigan, offered input for this sidebar.

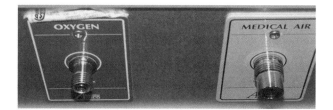

FIGURE 14-1 (also in color section following page 120) The compressed-gas outlets for oxygen and air illustrate the diameter index safety system. The threaded connector for the oxygen outlet is much smaller than that needed for the air outlet, making it physically impossible to attach the oxygen hose to the air outlet. Source: Gaba DM. Thin air. AHRQ WebM&M (Morbidity and Mortality Rounds on the Web), October 2004. Available at: www.webmm.ahrq.gov/case.aspx?caseID=76.

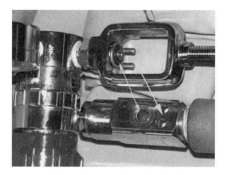

FIGURE 14-2 Pin index system on an oxygen cylinder. The photograph shows the pins on the regulator that fit in matching holes on the cylinder. Other gases have different pin positions. Source: Gaba DM. Thin air. AHRQ WebM&M (Morbidity and Mortality Rounds on the Web), October 2004. Available at: www.webmm.ahrq.gov/case.aspx?caseID=76.

staff to follow a specific pathway that lessens the risk of an error. Such a forcing function, however, is more easily circumvented than a lock-and-key design.

In hospitals and community pharmacies, the way in which products are arranged and shelved can be a soft forcing function. Pharmacy staff should separate potentially dangerous drugs with similar names or similar packaging, forcing the user to physically move to a different area for certain products. If a drug is moved that would normally be stored next to one with which it could be confused, a reminder note should be left in its place to indicate its current location.

Preprinted order forms and computer screens for medication order entry also serve as soft forcing functions. They direct clinicians to choose from a limited list of medications and dosages. Another example is automated dispensing cabinets (ADCs) that require pharmacy screening of orders before allowing nurses access to the drug. Since nurses can easily override this safety feature, it is a soft forcing function.

Use Constraints

Constraints that limit access to or use of medications and related devices can make it hard for practitioners to make mistakes. An example is limiting nonpharmacy staff access to the full array of products when the pharmacy is closed. As discussed in Chapters 10 and 11, it is ideal for hospital pharmacies to be open and staffed by pharmacists 24 hours a day, 7 days a week. In the absence of 24-hour pharmacy services, many hospitals limit the formulary of drugs available to staff after the pharmacy is closed and stock the available medications in small quantities and in the smallest drug containers.

Even during pharmacy hours of operation, access to certain medications should be limited on patient care units. The removal of concentrated electrolytes from patient care areas has reduced the number of deaths from accidental administration. Restricting access to other products, such as neuromuscular blocking agents, hypertonic saline and dextrose, and concentrated insulin products (U-500), would help prevent erroneous use of these high-alert medications. Medications stocked on nursing units should be reviewed frequently and should include only those drugs, concentrations, and quantities considered safe and necessary for emergency use. The quantity of certain products in unit stock, including products in ADCs, should be limited. This not only helps prevent errors but also can make errors visible before they reach the patient. For example, in the event of a 10-fold calculation error, a nurse would need to request additional medication from the pharmacy if only a small quantity of the drug was available on the unit.

For certain error-prone or potentially toxic products, use can be limited to specially trained or credentialed staff. Consultation by a specialist can be required for prescribing certain medications. The dose or duration of therapy can be limited through the use of automated alerts or automatic stop orders.

Externalize or Centralize Error-Prone Processes

As described in Chapter 11, services are available in which pharmacists at a remote location perform functions such as order entry. When the hospital pharmacy is closed, access to the remote support center is available through a secure Internet connection from a computer at the nurses' station. The remote pharmacist can review an order and the patient's record, verify the accuracy of the order, and enter it into the system before the medication is administered.

Another example of externalizing an error-prone process is the use of commercially available IV admixtures. Most high-alert drugs given by IV infusion are available in premixed form. The commercial admixtures are prepared by manufacturers that use automation effectively and follow strict quality control standards.

If commercial forms are not available, IV admixture preparation should be centralized in the pharmacy. When admixtures are prepared in patient care areas, distractions, nonstandard concentrations, lack of nursing expertise, and erroneous calculations can lead to errors. Centralizing this task in the pharmacy helps ensure that admixtures are prepared in a distraction-free environment by staff with expertise, and that appropriate quality control steps (e.g., sterility measures, double checks) are followed. Pharmacy preparation of IV admixtures also facilitates compliance with legally enforceable sterile compounding standards described in Chapter 797 of the *United States Pharmacopeia*,[10] which apply in all settings. These standards are intended to prevent harm from microbial contamination, excessive bacterial endotoxins, errors in the strength of ingredients, and use of incorrect ingredients.[11]

Outsourcing the preparation of complicated parenteral solutions is another way to reduce error potential. Some hospitals have outside pharmacies prepare cardioplegic solutions, total parenteral nutrition (TPN) solutions, dialysate, and IV antibiotics. This can relieve congestion in the hospital pharmacy and ensure the use of appropriate quality assurance steps. Outside facilities used for compounding must certify that they use good manufacturing practices as defined by the Food and Drug Administration (FDA).

Improve Access to Information

Accurate information about the patient and prescribed therapies should be readily accessible to all health care providers at the time they are performing critical tasks related to medication use. Up-to-date information about patients, including height and weight, allergies, pregnancy or lactation status, age, laboratory test results, diagnoses, comorbid conditions, and concomitant drug therapy, should be available to all practitioners in any area of a health care facility, including the pharmacy. Similarly, up-to-date information about medications needs to be quickly available to practitioners at the points of prescribing, transcribing, preparation, dispensing, and administration.

Computerized order entry systems that are interfaced with electronic databases of drug information and patient information (both demographics and clinical information such as diagnostic study results) can provide immediate warnings if unsafe medication orders are entered. Such clinical decision support is discussed in Chapter 15. Although automated decision support systems can bring the most crucial information to the attention of clinicians, the information is provided only when the clinician is actively using the system. For example, if an antibiotic is ordered early in the day, before the patient's lab results are available, the prescriber may not be alerted to an elevated serum creatinine level and the need for a dose adjustment until the next day, when he again logs into that patient's profile. New data monitoring technology is making it possible to notify clinicians of important information as soon as it is available, however.

Nontechnologic approaches can also improve access to information:

- Making pharmacists available in patient care units for immediate consultation when needed;
- Including the medical librarian on patient rounds to follow through with dissemination of patient and staff education materials;
- Ensuring that available drug information texts are up-to-date;
- Displaying charts with information about compatibility, equianalgesic doses, maximum doses, special precautions, and so on;
- Placing lab reports and medication administration records (MARs) at the patient's bedside (secured);
- Using colored wristbands to alert practitioners to patients' allergies. This approach should be used with caution, because the meaning of armband colors in clinical environments is not standardized; confusion can occur, especially when personnel work in more than one location;[12]
- Accelerating laboratory turnaround time.

Patients should be active participants in their care (see Chapter 13), and this is not possible without systems for consistently providing information about their medications, both in clinical settings and at home. An informed patient, or patient representative, may be the final safeguard preventing a harmful error.

Standardize and Simplify

Standardization reduces reliance on human memory and vigilance. It also allows new staff to carry out unfamiliar processes safely. Simplification of processes can reduce the load on working memory, planning, and problem solving. Each additional step in a process adds to the cumulative risk of making an error. If each step is 99% reliable, the probability of error is 1% in a 1-step process, 22% in a 25-step process, 39% in a 50-step process, and 63% in a 100-step process.

Standardization and simplification of medication use means creating and following streamlined, clinically sound, uniform processes and models of care, thereby reducing variation and complexity. It also means reducing options for drug products, doses, and administration techniques.

Using standard concentrations and volumes for high-alert medications decreases the overall drug formulary and pharmacy stock, reduces options available in floor stock medications, and limits options for prescribing. Without a standard concentration for heparin infusions, for example, prescribers could order a wide variety of concentrations: 20,000 units/250 mL, 20,000 units/500 mL, 25,000 units/500 mL, and so forth. Errors in prescribing, dispensing, and administration are less likely with a standard concentration. In addition, the use of dosing and infusion rate charts can be implemented only when standard concentrations for infusions are established. Standardizing pharmacy processes for mixing IV solutions that are not available commercially (e.g., TPN solutions, chemotherapy, cardioplegic solutions) also helps reduce the risk of error.

Standardizing the care of patients with specific diseases, injuries, or conditions can reduce errors and patient harm. Health care organizations can gain consensus among physicians who treat patients with similar problems and establish an order set reflecting each standardized care process. Preprinted order forms, computerized order sets, and clinical pathways are most effective in standardizing care processes when they have undergone rigorous multidisciplinary review.[13]

A standardized and controlled vocabulary in which the use of error-prone abbreviations, symbols, and dose expressions is prohibited is particularly important to patient safety, as discussed in Chapter 8. A JCAHO National Patient Safety Goal has helped health care organizations identify error-prone abbreviations and other expressions that should be not be used.

All health care providers should have access to the same information, for example, through a common, shared database containing standard elements (e.g., height, weight, allergies, pregnancy or lactation status, age, lab values, diagnoses, comorbid conditions, drug therapy). In addition, standard elements should be communicated during handoff when patients are transferred to a different area or level or care; Chapter 9 describes the medication reconciliation process as defined in a 2006 JCAHO National Patient Safety Goal.

Consider Affordances and Natural Mapping

The design of equipment, supplies, and work spaces should help communicate their correct use. The actions involved in using equipment or operating within work spaces should be intuitive: Pushing a button should turn a piece of equipment on or off; turning a knob to the right should produce a corresponding movement to the right (or clockwise). Known as affordances and natural mapping,[14,15] these characteristics take advantage of generally held knowledge of how things work. For example, the manufacturers of some infusion pumps have arranged the numerical keypads in the same pattern as computer and calculator keypads to facilitate proper programming.

An example of failure to consider affordances is confusion between esmolol ampuls and vials. Clinicians usually associate ampuls with ready-to-use single doses, not concentrated products that require dilution. However, single-dose ampuls of esmolol contain a concentrated product, and 10 mL vials contain the more dilute product intended for direct injection. The wrong concentration has often been chosen, and harmful errors have occurred.

Use Differentiation

Look-alike and sound-alike product names and look-alike packaging and labeling offer the most common examples of the need to draw attention to differences between products.

Removing one of a pair of look-alike products from the formulary can reduce confusion, but this may not be an option. Purchasing one of the products from a different manufacturer is another way of reducing packaging and labeling similarity.

Auxiliary warning labels can be used to help differentiate products. For example, labels might be affixed to hydralazine containers stating, "Caution—Read Label Carefully:

Look-Alike or Sound-Alike Drug," because this product has frequently been confused with hydroxyzine. Color can also be used to draw attention to label warnings, and a pen or marker can be used to circle important information on medication labels or MARs.

The appearance of look-alike product names can be changed by using color, boldface type, or tall-man letters.[16,17] For instance, dobutamine and dopamine can be written as DOBUTamine and DOPamine. In 2001, at the urging of ISMP, FDA requested that the manufacturers of 16 look-alike and sound-alike generic name pairs (see Table 6-1) incorporate tall-man lettering in labeling and packaging.[18] Health care providers can use tall-man letters when listing drug names on labels, storage units, preprinted orders, computerized order entry screens, ADC screens, and MARs.

For name pairs known to be problematic, using both the generic and brand names on orders, storage shelves and product labels, computer screens, and MARs can help prevent confusion. Matching the prescribed therapy to the patient's medical condition can also help differentiate products with look-alike names.

Use Reminders

Auxiliary labels on medication packaging and highlighted notes on MARs can remind staff of precautions for safe preparation and administration: "Warning—Highly Concentrated Drug—Must Be Diluted," "For Oral Use Only," "For External Use Only," "IM only," and so on. Label manufacturers can custom-design other reminders and warnings.

Checklists can be used to ensure that complex processes are carried out safely and effectively. Reminders about special precautions or patient monitoring can be embedded into preprinted order sets and protocols.

Computerized systems (e.g., drug inventory databases, order entry systems, ADCs) can be programmed to flash reminders and warnings during operation. Reminders can be built into the screens of ADCs (e.g., "Measure dose using only dropper provided," "Cross allergy to aspirin").

Apply System Redundancies

Although everyone makes mistakes, the probability that two individuals in the same institution will make the same error in association with the same medication for the same patient is quite small. For this reason, a system of redundancies (check systems) in which one person independently checks the work of another is essential. Compare, for example, the following two systems of drug distribution:

1. In the outdated floor stock system, still prevalent in some countries, a nearly complete pharmacy is maintained on every unit in a hospital or nursing home. Acting alone, the nurse interprets and transcribes a physician's order, chooses the proper container from hundreds available on the shelves, prepares the correct amount, places the dose in a syringe or cup, labels it, takes it to the patient, administers it, and verifies that the dose has been administered. (Certain ADCs would be considered floor stock systems.)
2. Unit dose and IV admixture systems in which most medications are dispensed as prescribed for individual patients incorporate many checks and redundant steps before products leave the pharmacy.[6] In addition, nurses perform an independent double check to verify accurate dispensing before each drug is administered.

Redundancies such as independent double checks by several individuals (see Chapter 11) have been shown to reduce accident rates.[19] People are better at finding others' mistakes than their own. A pharmacist or nurse may not recognize that he or she has selected the wrong drug, in part because of confirmation bias (see Chapter 7). Patients can be involved in a double-check system, if they are knowledgeable about the medications they take.

One critical process in which independent double checks are valuable is setting pump rates and concentrations for PCA and infusions of high-alert drugs. All pediatric, geriatric, and chemotherapy dosages should be checked independently by at least two persons. Maximum doses should be established for high-alert medications. If an order exceeds the maximum dose, timely peer review should be used to confirm the safety of the order before the drug is dispensed or administered.

Double checks should be limited to situations that involve certain high-alert drugs, complex processes, and high-risk patients; having too many checkpoints dilutes their effectiveness. Manual double checks are not always the optimal error reduction strategy and may not be practical for all high-alert medications in all circumstances. Although double checks make mistakes visible, they do not prevent them, as would system changes. Bar coding systems, smart infusion pumps (see Chapter 15), and other forms of technology offer automated double checks.

In addition to double checks, other forms of redundancy can be used to reduce the risk of an error:

- Listing both brand and generic names on orders, computer screens, MARs, and labels to help differentiate look-alike drug names,
- Redundant personnel, cross-trained and tested for continued competency to perform critical functions in various patient care areas or pharmacies,
- Implicit verification systems, such as matching the prescribed drug's indication to the patient's condition or reading back a spoken order for verification.

Monitor Patients

Particularly with high-alert drugs, patients should be closely monitored to determine the efficacy of their medications and quickly detect adverse reactions. At set intervals, parameters such as vital signs, quality of respirations, neurological signs, and laboratory results should be evaluated. Automated electronic monitoring and feedback systems are now available (see Chapter 15).

For patients receiving high-alert medications, monitoring parameters should be included in protocols and order sets. They should also be listed on flow sheets kept at the bedside for quick reference and documentation; this is useful for detecting subtle but clinically important changes in patients' response to medications over time. Keeping antidotes and resuscitation equipment close by helps ensure a timely response to life-threatening conditions detected through this monitoring.

Use Failure Mode and Effects Analysis

To reduce the risk of harmful errors, health care providers should proactively identify the ways in which a process or medication-related equipment could fail, why it might fail, how it might affect patients, and how it could be made safer. This process, failure mode and effects analysis (FMEA), is covered in Chapter 21.

SPECIFIC SAFETY IMPROVEMENTS

The remainder of this chapter gives examples of problems that have occurred and system improvements that can be made in the use of each category and specific drug on ISMP's list of high-alert medications (Table 14-1). Table 14-4 summarizes actions for safe use of these medications. Error-reduction strategies such as bar-coded drug dispensing and administration and computerized prescriber order entry are not included; these technological applications will reduce the risk of errors with all drugs, including high-alert medications.

TABLE 14-4 Safety Measures for High-Alert Drugs

Key Changes	Adrenergic Agonists, IV	Adrenergic Antagonists, IV	Anesthetic Agents, Inhaled and IV	Antineoplastics/ Chemotherapy
Fail-safes and Forcing Functions				
Use flow control pumps for continuous IV infusions	X	X	X	X
Use epidural tubing without side ports			X	
Use oral syringes for administration of oral liquid products				
Constraints				
Remove drug from floor stock and dispensing cabinets	X (1:10,000 epinephrine)		X (except approved areas)	X
Sequester drugs if stored on units			X	X
Separate like products when using or storing	X		X (IV lipids/ propofol)	X
Dispense the drug from pharmacy only	X (atypical and nonemergency doses)	X (metoprolol IV as needed)	X	X
Use smallest size package, concentration, and dose for floor stock	X	X	X	
Formulary drug restrictions or criteria for use	X	X	X	X
Switch from IV to oral (or subcutaneous) use as soon as possible		X		
Certify/privilege staff to order, prepare, or administer drug			X	X
Restrict drug administration to designated areas			X	X
Externalize or Centralize Error-Prone Processes				
Move drug preparation off units to pharmacy	X	X	X	X
Use commercially available premixed IV solutions/outsource preparation	X	X	X	X

TABLE 14-4 Safety Measures for High-Alert Drugs (continued)

Key Changes	Adrenergic Agonists, IV	Adrenergic Antagonists, IV	Anesthetic Agents, Inhaled and IV	Antineoplastics/ Chemotherapy
Access to Information				
Post drug information charts	X (infusion rate charts)	X (infusion rate charts)		X
Obtain and communicate laboratory values via guidelines				X
Standardize and Simplify				
Eliminate use of specific abbreviations/drug name stems/acronyms	X (e.g., "epi")	X (e.g., "amp")		X (all)
Use standardized drug/dose expressions	X	X		X
Use preprinted order forms or ordering protocols	X (ordering protocols)	X (ordering protocols)	X (moderate sedation)	X
Order by metric weight, not by volume or ampul	X	X	X	X
Include dose formula with calculated dose		X		X
Use drug preparation guidelines	X	X		X
Use dosing/infusion rate charts	X	X	X	
Standardize and limit drug concentrations/formulations	X	X	X	
Use drug administration protocols	X	X	X (propofol use outside the OR)	X
Dispense medications in unit dose/unit-of-use packages/kits	X	X		X (oral)
Differentiate/Use Warnings and Reminders				
Apply warning labels and/or distinguish drug names/concentrations	X	X	X	X
Establish dose limits and screen orders	X	X	X	X

Use different container size/manufacturer/outer wrap	X	X	X (IV lipids and propofol)	X
Use checklists for complex processes	X		X	X
Label infusion lines, syringes, containers, cups	X	X	X	X
Use tall-man lettering for look-alike names	X (e.g., DOPamine, DOBUTamine)			X (various look-alike products)
Build reminders into order sets, MARs*, protocols, and dispensing cabinets	X		X	X
Redundancies/Independent Double Checks				
Recalculate the dose	X	X		X
Verify drug and/or drug preparation	X	X	X	X
Use peer review process for unusual drug, dose, regimen	X	X		X
Verify patient diagnosis/indication for drug	X	X	X	X
Double-check pump rate, drug, concentration, and line attachments	X	X	X	X
Bar coding and/or "smart" pumps	X	X	X	X
Involve the patient (family) through education	X	X	X (pre-op)	X
Monitor Patients and Respond to Drug Effects				
Require cardiac monitoring (cm)/pulse oximetry (po)/capnography (CO_2)	X (cm for most)	X (cm for most)	X	
Require close observation/vital sign monitoring	X	X	X	X
Have antidotes and/or resuscitation equipment close at hand	X	X	X	X (for extravasations)
Failure Mode and Effects Analysis			X (nurse-administered IV propofol)	X

*MAR = medication administration record.

TABLE 14-4 Safety Measures for High-Alert Drugs (continued)

Key Changes	Cardioplegic Solutions	Colchicine IV	Dextrose 20% or Greater	Dialysis Solutions
Fail-safes and Forcing Functions				
Use flow control pumps for continuous IV infusions	X			X
Use epidural tubing without side ports				
Use oral syringes for administration of oral liquid products				
Constraints				
Remove drug from floor stock and dispensing cabinets		X	X	
Sequester drugs if stored on units				
Separate like products when using or storing		X	X	X
Dispense the drug from pharmacy only	X	X		X (peritoneal/CVVHD*)
Use smallest size package, concentration, and dose for floor stock	X	X	X	X
Formulary drug restrictions or criteria for use	X		X	X
Switch from IV to oral (or subcutaneous) use as soon as possible		X		
Certify/privilege staff to order, prepare, or administer drug	X			X
Restrict drug administration to designated areas	X			X
Externalize or Centralize Error-Prone Processes				
Move drug preparation off units to pharmacy	X	X	X	X
Use commercially available premixed IV solutions/outsource preparation	X		X	X
Access to Information				
Post drug information charts				
Obtain and communicate laboratory values via guidelines		X	X	X
Standardize and Simplify				
Eliminate use of specific abbreviations/drug name stems/acronyms			X	
Use standardized drug/dose expressions			X (not "amp")	

Use preprinted order forms or ordering protocols				X
Order by metric weight, not by volume or ampul			X (not "amp")	
Include dose formula with calculated dose	X			X
Use drug preparation guidelines	X			
Use dosing/infusion rate charts				
Standardize and limit drug concentrations/formulations	X		X	X
Use drug administration protocols	X		X	X
Dispense medications in unit dose/unit-of-use packages/kits		X	X	
Differentiate/Use Warnings and Reminders				
Apply warning labels and/or distinguish drug names/concentrations	X	X	X	X
Establish dose limits and screen orders		X (including cumulative doses)		
Use different container size/manufacturer/outer wrap				
Use checklists for complex processes	X			X
Label infusion lines, syringes, containers, cups	X	X	X	X
Use tall-man lettering for look-alike names				
Build reminders into order sets, MARs, protocols, and dispensing cabinets		X (e.g., max. dose; start/stop dates)		
Redundancies/Independent Double Checks				
Recalculate the dose		X		X
Verify drug and/or drug preparation	X	X	X	X
Use peer review process for unusual drug, dose, regimen		X		X
Verify patient diagnosis/indication for drug		X		
Double-check pump rate, drug, concentration, and line attachments	X			X
Bar coding and/or "smart" pumps		X	X	X
Involve the patient (family) through education		X		X

TABLE 14-4 Safety Measures for High-Alert Drugs (continued)

Key Changes	Cardioplegic Solutions	Colchicine IV	Dextrose 20% or Greater	Dialysis Solutions
Monitor Patients and Respond to Drug Effects				
Require cardiac monitoring (cm)/pulse oximetry (po)/capnography (CO_2)	X			
Require close observation/vital sign monitoring	X		X	X
Have antidotes and/or resuscitation equipment close at hand	X			X
Failure Mode and Effects Analysis				
	X			

* CVVHD = Continuous veno-venous hemodialysis.

Key Changes	Epidural & Intrathecal Medications	Glycoprotein IIb/IIIa Inhibitors	Heparin, Low Molecular Weight	Heparin, Unfractionated
Fail-safes and Forcing Functions				
Use flow control pumps for continuous IV infusions	X	X		X
Use epidural tubing without side ports	X			
Use oral syringes for administration of oral liquid products				
Constraints				
Remove drug from floor stock and dispensing cabinets	X	X (except ED*/cardiac procedure areas)		
Sequester drugs if stored on units				
Separate like products when using or storing	X		X	X
Dispense the drug from pharmacy only	X		X	
Use smallest size package, concentration, and dose for floor stock			X	X
Formulary drug restrictions or criteria for use	X	X	X	X
Switch from IV to oral (or subcutaneous) use as soon as possible				X (warfarin)

Strategy				
Certify/privilege staff to order, prepare, or administer drug			X	X
Restrict drug administration to designated areas			X	X
Externalize or Centralize Error-Prone Processes				
Move drug preparation off units to pharmacy			X	X
Use commercially available premixed IV solutions/outsource preparation	X		X	X
Access to Information				
Post drug information charts			X	X
Obtain and communicate laboratory values via guidelines	X		X	X
Standardize and Simplify				
Eliminate use of specific abbreviations/drug name stems/acronyms	X ("U" for units; also never use < or > signs for dose/aPTT*)	X ("U" for units)	X	X
Use standardized drug/dose expressions	X	X	X	X
Use preprinted order forms or ordering protocols	X	X	X	X
Order by metric weight, not by volume or ampul	X	X	X	X
Include dose formula with calculated dose	X (dose by weight)		X	X
Use drug preparation guidelines			X	X
Use dosing/infusion rate charts			X	X
Standardize and limit drug concentrations/formulations		X	X	X
Use drug administration protocols		X	X	X
Dispense medications in unit dose/unit-of-use packages/kits	X (bolus/flushes)	X (prefilled syringes)	X (bolus/loading dose)	X
Differentiate/Use Warnings and Reminders				
Apply warning labels and/or distinguish drug names/concentrations	X (e.g., for epidural use only)		X	X
Establish dose limits and screen orders		X	X	X

TABLE 14-4   Safety Measures for High-Alert Drugs (continued)

Key Changes	Epidural & Intrathecal Medications	Glycoprotein IIb/IIIa Inhibitors	Heparin, Low Molecular Weight	Heparin, Unfractionated
Differentiate/Use Warnings and Reminders				
Use different container size/manufacturer/outer wrap	X (to differentiate from IV products)			X
Use checklists for complex processes	X	X		
Label infusion lines, syringes, containers, cups	X	X		X
Use tall-man lettering for look-alike names				X (hEParin, HeSpan)
Build reminders into order sets, MARs, protocols, and dispensing cabinets	X	X	X (check for duplicate therapy)	X
Redundancies/Independent Double Checks				
Recalculate the dose		X	X (according to weight)	X
Verify drug and/or drug preparation	X	X		X
Use peer review process for unusual drug, dose, regimen	X	X		
Verify patient diagnosis/indication for drug	X	X	X	
Double-check pump rate, drug, concentration, and line attachments	X	X		
Bar coding and/or "smart" pumps	X	X	X	X
Involve the patient (family) through education	X	X	X	X
Monitor Patients and Respond to Drug Effects				
Require cardiac monitoring (cm)/pulse oximetry (po)/capnography (CO_2)	po/CO_2	cm		
Require close observation/vital sign monitoring	X	X		
Have antidotes and/or resuscitation equipment close at hand	X	X		X
Failure Mode and Effects Analysis				
	X			

* ED = emergency department; aPTT = activated partial thromboplastin time.

Key Changes	Hypoglycemics, Oral	Insulin, IV & Subcutaneous	IV Inotropes	IV Lidocaine (cardiac)
Fail-safes and Forcing Functions				
Use flow control pumps for continuous IV infusions		IV	X	X
Use epidural tubing without side ports				
Use oral syringes for administration of oral liquid products				
Constraints				
Remove drug from floor stock and dispensing cabinets		X (U-500 strength)		X (except ED, critical care, cardiac procedure units)
Sequester drugs if stored on units				
Separate like products when using or storing	X	X	X	X
Dispense the drug from pharmacy only		X (IV)		
Use smallest size package, concentration, and dose for floor stock	X	X		
Formulary drug restrictions or criteria for use		X	X	
Switch from IV to oral (or subcutaneous) use as soon as possible			X	
Certify/privilege staff to order, prepare, or administer drug				
Restrict drug administration to designated areas				X
Externalize or Centralize Error-Prone Processes				
Move drug preparation off units to pharmacy		X (IV)		
Use commercially available premixed IV solutions/outsource preparation				X
Access to Information				
Post drug information charts		X		
Obtain and communicate laboratory values via guidelines	X	X	X	
Standardize and Simplify				
Eliminate use of specific abbreviations/drug name stems/acronyms	X	X ("U" for units)	X (e.g., "dig")	X ("amp")

TABLE 14-4 Safety Measures for High-Alert Drugs (continued)

Key Changes	Hypoglycemics, Oral	Insulin, IV & Subcutaneous	IV Inotropes	IV Lidocaine (cardiac)
Standardize and Simplify				
Use standardized drug/dose expressions		X		
Use preprinted order forms or ordering protocols		X		X
Order by metric weight, not by volume or ampul			X	
Include dose formula with calculated dose			X (peds)	
Use drug preparation guidelines		X (IV)		
Use dosing/infusion rate charts		X		X
Standardize and limit drug concentrations/formulations		X	X	X
Use drug administration protocols		X		X
Dispense medications in unit dose/unit-of-use packages/kits	X	X	X	
Differentiate/Use Warnings and Reminders				
Apply warning labels and/or distinguish drug names/concentrations	X	X	X	X
Establish dose limits and screen orders	X	X	X	
Use different container size/manufacturer/outer wrap	X	X (vials)		
Use checklists for complex processes				
Label infusion lines, syringes, containers, cups		X	X	X
Use tall-man lettering for look-alike names	X (e.g., chlorproMAZINE/chlorproPAMIDE)	X (e.g., humaLOG, humuLIN)		
Build reminders into order sets, MARs, protocols, and dispensing cabinets	Verify diagnosis	X	X	
Redundancies/Independent Double Checks				
Recalculate the dose		X (IV)	X (peds)	
Verify drug and/or drug preparation	X	X	X	X

Key Changes	Liposomal Drug Forms	Magnesium Sulfate Injection	Methotrexate, Oral	Moderate Sedation, IV
Use peer review process for unusual drug, dose, regimen			X	
Verify patient diagnosis/indication for drug		X	X	X
Double-check pump rate, drug, concentration, and line attachments	X	X	X	X
Bar coding and/or "smart" pumps		X	X	X
Involve the patient (family) through education		X	X	
Monitor Patients and Respond to Drug Effects				
Require cardiac monitoring (cm)/pulse oximetry (po)/capnography (CO_2)			X	X
Require close observation/vital sign monitoring		X	X	X
Have antidotes and/or resuscitation equipment close at hand	X	X		
Failure Mode and Effects Analysis		X		

Key Changes	Liposomal Drug Forms	Magnesium Sulfate Injection	Methotrexate, Oral	Moderate Sedation, IV
Fail-safes and Forcing Functions				
Use flow control pumps for continuous IV infusions	X	X		X
Use epidural tubing without side ports				
Use oral syringes for administration of oral liquid products				
Constraints				
Remove drug from floor stock and dispensing cabinets	X	X (larger vial sizes)	X	
Sequester drugs if stored on units		X		X
Separate like products when using or storing	X			
Dispense the drug from pharmacy only	X	X	X	
Use smallest size package, concentration, and dose for floor stock		X		X
Formulary drug restrictions or criteria for use	X	X	X (non-oncologic)	X
Switch from IV to oral (or subcutaneous) use as soon as possible		X		

TABLE 14-4 Safety Measures for High-Alert Drugs (continued)

Key Changes	Liposomal Drug Forms	Magnesium Sulfate Injection	Methotrexate, Oral	Moderate Sedation, IV
Constraints				
Certify/privilege staff to order, prepare, or administer drug				X
Restrict drug administration to designated areas				X
Externalize or Centralize Error-Prone Processes				
Move drug preparation off units to pharmacy	X	X		
Use commercially available premixed IV solutions/outsource preparation		X		
Access to Information				
Post drug information charts				
Obtain and communicate laboratory values via guidelines		X	X	
Standardize and Simplify				
Eliminate use of specific abbreviations/drug name stems/acronyms	X	X (MgSO$_4$)	X (MTX)	
Use standardized drug/dose expressions	X	X		
Use preprinted order forms or ordering protocols		X		X
Order by metric weight, not by volume or ampul	X	X ("amp")		X
Include dose formula with calculated dose				
Use drug preparation guidelines				
Use dosing/infusion rate charts		X		
Standardize and limit drug concentrations/formulations	X	X		X
Use drug administration protocols		X	X (weekly/non-oncologic use)	X
Dispense medications in unit dose/unit-of-use packages/kits	X	X	X	X

Differentiate/Use Warnings and Reminders

Strategy			
Apply warning labels and/or distinguish drug names/concentrations	X	X (weekly dosing)	X (e.g., Doxil, LIPOSOMAL doxorubicin)
Establish dose limits and screen orders	X	X	X
Use different container size/manufacturer/outer wrap			
Use checklists for complex processes			
Label infusion lines, syringes, containers, cups	X		X
Use tall-man lettering for look-alike names			
Build reminders into order sets, MARs, protocols, and dispensing cabinets	X	X (weekly dosing)	X

Redundancies/Independent Double Checks

Strategy			
Recalculate the dose			X
Verify drug and/or drug preparation	X	X	X
Use peer review process for unusual drug, dose, regimen	X	X	
Verify patient diagnosis/indication for drug	X	X	X
Double-check pump rate, drug, concentration, and line attachments	X		
Bar coding and/or "smart" pumps	X	X	X
Involve the patient (family) through education	X	X	X

Monitor Patients and Respond to Drug Effects

Strategy			
Require cardiac monitoring (cm)/pulse oximetry (po)/capnography (CO_2)	X		
Require close observation/vital sign monitoring	X		X
Have antidotes and/or resuscitation equipment close at hand	X		X

Failure Mode and Effects Analysis

Strategy			
	X		X

TABLE 14-4 Safety Measures for High-Alert Drugs (continued)

Key Changes	Moderate Sedation, Oral (peds)	Nesiritide	Neuromuscular Blocking Agents	Nitroprusside Sodium
Fail-safes and Forcing Functions				
Use flow control pumps for continuous IV infusions		X	X	X
Use epidural tubing without side ports				
Use oral syringes for administration of oral liquid products	X			
Constraints				
Remove drug from floor stock and dispensing cabinets			X (except ED, PACU*, OR*, critical care)	
Sequester drugs if stored on units	X		X	
Separate like products when using or storing			X	X
Dispense the drug from pharmacy only		X	X (except ED, PACU, OR, critical care)	
Use smallest size package, concentration, and dose for floor stock	X			
Formulary drug restrictions or criteria for use		X	X	
Switch from IV to oral (or subcutaneous) use as soon as possible				
Certify/privilege staff to order, prepare, or administer drug	X		X	
Restrict drug administration to designated areas	X (also, never in the home)	X		X
Externalize or Centralize Error-Prone Processes				
Move drug preparation off units to pharmacy		X		X
Use commercially available premixed IV solutions/outsource preparation				
Access to Information				
Post drug information charts				
Obtain and communicate laboratory values via guidelines				X

Standardize and Simplify

Strategy	Col 1	Col 2	Col 3	Col 4
Standardize and Simplify				
Eliminate use of specific abbreviations/drug name stems/acronyms	X ("nitro")			
Use standardized drug/dose expressions			X	
Use preprinted order forms or ordering protocols	X	X	X	
Order by metric weight, not by volume or ampul			X	
Include dose formula with calculated dose			X	
Use drug preparation guidelines	X		X	
Use dosing/infusion rate charts	X		X (from manufacturer)	
Standardize and limit drug concentrations/formulations	X	X	X	X
Use drug administration protocols	X	X	X	X
Dispense medications in unit-dose/unit-of-use packages/kits			X (bolus dose)	X
Differentiate/Use Warnings and Reminders				
Apply warning labels and/or distinguish drug names/concentrations	X (keep protected from light)	X (paralyzing agent; causes respiratory arrest)	X	
Establish dose limits and screen orders	X	X	X	
Use different container size/manufacturer/outer wrap	X	X		
Use checklists for complex processes				
Label infusion lines, syringes, containers, cups	X	X	X	
Use tall-man lettering for look-alike names				
Build reminders into order sets, MARs, protocols, and dispensing cabinets		X (paralyzing agent; causes respiratory arrest)	X	X (dose limits)
Redundancies/Independent Double Checks				
Recalculate the dose			X	X
Verify drug and/or drug preparation	X	X	X	X

TABLE 14-4 Safety Measures for High-Alert Drugs (continued)

Key Changes	Moderate Sedation, Oral (peds)	Nesiritide	Neuromuscular Blocking Agents	Nitroprusside Sodium
Redundancies/Independent Double Checks				
Use peer review process for unusual drug, dose, regimen	X			
Verify patient diagnosis/indication for drug		X	X	X
Double-check pump rate, drug, concentration, and line attachments		X	X	X
Bar coding and/or "smart" pumps		X	X	X
Involve the patient (family) through education	X	X	X	X
Monitor Patients and Respond to Drug Effects				
Require cardiac monitoring (cm)/pulse oximetry (po)/capnography (CO_2)	X (po/CO_2)	X (cm)	X	cm
Require close observation/vital sign monitoring	X	X	X	X
Have antidotes and/or resuscitation equipment close at hand	X	X	X	X
Failure Mode and Effects Analysis				

* PACU =postanesthesia care unit; OR = operating room.

Key Changes	Opioids, IV, Epidural, Oral	Potassium Phosphates Injection	Potassium Chloride Injection	IV/Intrathecal Radiocontrast Agents
Fail-safes and Forcing Functions				
Use flow control pumps for continuous IV infusions	X (IV, epidural)	X	X	
Use epidural tubing without side ports	X (epidural)			
Use oral syringes for administration of oral liquid products	X (oral)			

Constraints				
Remove drug from floor stock and dispensing cabinets	X (concentrated oral forms)	X	X	
Sequester drugs if stored on units	X		X	
Separate like products when using or storing	X	X	X	X (ionic/nonionic)
Dispense the drug from pharmacy only	X (IV/epidural infusion)	X	X	
Use smallest size package, concentration, and dose for floor stock	X	X	X	
Formulary drug restrictions or criteria for use	X (selected opioids)	X	X	X (ionic/nonionic)
Switch from IV to oral (or subcutaneous) use as soon as possible	X	X	X	X
Certify/privilege staff to order, prepare, or administer drug	X	X		X
Restrict drug administration to designated areas			X	X
Externalize or Centralize Error-Prone Processes				
Move drug preparation off units to pharmacy	X (IV, epidural)	X	X	
Use commercially available premixed IV solutions/outsource preparation	X (IV, epidural)		X	X
Access to Information				
Post drug information charts		X		
Obtain and communicate laboratory values via guidelines	X		X	X
Standardize and Simplify				
Eliminate use of specific abbreviations/drug name stems/acronyms	X (e.g., MSO$_4$)			
Use standardized drug/dose expressions	X (use mmol, not "amp" or "vial")	X		
Use preprinted order forms or ordering protocols	X		X	X
Order by metric weight, not by volume or ampul	X	X	X	X

TABLE 14-4 Safety Measures for High-Alert Drugs (continued)

Key Changes	Opioids, IV, Epidural, Oral	Potassium Phosphates Injection	Potassium Chloride Injection	IV/Intrathecal Radiocontrast Agents
Standardize and Simplify				
Include dose formula with calculated dose	X (peds)	X		
Use drug preparation guidelines		X		
Use dosing/infusion rate charts	X			
Standardize and limit drug concentrations/formulations	X	X	X	X
Use drug administration protocols	X (PCA*, epidural, IV infusions)	X	X	X
Dispense medications in unit-dose/unit-of-use packages/kits	X		X	X
Differentiate/Use Warnings and Reminders				
Apply warning labels and/or distinguish drug names/concentrations	X (e.g., concentrated solutions)	X (content of potassium and phosphorus in vial)	X	X (ionic/nonionic)
Establish dose limits and screen orders	X	X	X	X (also avoid metformin)
Use different container size/manufacturer/outer wrap	X (PCA)			X
Use checklists for complex processes	X			
Label infusion lines, syringes, containers, cups	X	X	X	X
Use tall-man lettering for look-alike names	X (e.g., HYDROmorphOne, to differentiate from morphine)			
Build reminders into order sets, MARs, protocols, and dispensing cabinets	X	X	X	X
Redundancies/Independent Double Checks				
Recalculate the dose	X (peds)	X		

Key Changes	Sodium Chloride Injection, Hypertonic	IV Thrombolytics/ Fibrinolytics	Total Parenteral Nutrition Solutions	Warfarin
Fail-safes and Forcing Functions				
Use flow control pumps for continuous IV infusions	X (infusions should never exceed 3% sodium chloride)	X	X	
Use epidural tubing without side ports				
Use oral syringes for administration of oral liquid products				
Constraints				
Remove drug from floor stock and dispensing cabinets	X (except dialysis unit)	X (except ED, critical care units, cardiac units)		X
Verify drug and/or drug preparation	X	X	X	X
Use peer review process for unusual drug, dose, regimen	X	X	X	
Verify patient diagnosis/indication for drug	X	X	X	
Double-check pump rate, drug, concentration, and line attachments	X	X	X	
Bar coding and/or "smart" pumps	X	X	X	X
Involve the patient (family) through education	X		X	X
Monitor Patients and Respond to Drug Effects				
Require cardiac monitoring (cm)/pulse oximetry (po)/capnography (CO_2) (e.g., pc/CO_2 for PCA)	X	X (cm as necessary)	X (cm as necessary)	
Require close observation/vital sign monitoring	X		X	X
Have antidotes and/or resuscitation equipment close at hand	X	X	X	
Failure Mode and Effects Analysis	X		X	X

* PCA = patient-controlled analgesia.

TABLE 14-4   Safety Measures for High-Alert Drugs (continued)

Key Changes	Sodium Chloride Injection, Hypertonic	IV Thrombolytics/ Fibrinolytics	Total Parenteral Nutrition Solutions	Warfarin
Constraints				
Sequester drugs if stored on units	X	X		
Separate like products when using or storing	X	X	X	
Dispense the drug from pharmacy only	X		X	X
Use smallest size package, concentration, and dose for floor stock		X		
Formulary drug restrictions or criteria for use	X	X	X	
Switch from IV to oral (or subcutaneous) use as soon as possible			X	X
Certify/privilege staff to order, prepare, or administer drug	X	X	X	
Restrict drug administration to designated areas	X	X		
Externalize or Centralize Error-Prone Processes				
Move drug preparation off units to pharmacy	X	X	X	
Use commercially available premixed IV solutions/outsource preparation	X		X	
Access to Information				
Post drug information charts		X (dose and preparation)		
Obtain and communicate laboratory values via guidelines	X	X	X	X
Standardize and Simplify				
Eliminate use of specific abbreviations/drug name stems/acronyms		X (e.g., TNK, t-pa)	TPN	
Use standardized drug/dose expressions		X	X	X (never use < or > signs for dose/INR*)
Use preprinted order forms or ordering protocols	X	X	X	X
Order by metric weight, not by volume or ampul		X	X	
Include dose formula with calculated dose		X (dose by weight)		

Strategy				
Use drug preparation guidelines		X		X
Use dosing/infusion rate charts		X		X
Standardize and limit drug concentrations/formulations		X		X
Use drug administration protocols	X	X	X	X
Dispense medications in unit dose/unit-of-use packages/kits	X	X		X
Differentiate/Use Warnings and Reminders				
Apply warning labels and/or distinguish drug names/concentrations		X	X	
Establish dose limits and screen orders	X	X		X
Use different container size/manufacturer/outer wrap				
Use checklists for complex processes		X	X	
Label infusion lines, syringes, containers, cups		X	X	
Use tall-man lettering for look-alike names				
Build reminders into order sets, MARs, protocols, and dispensing cabinets	X	X	X	X
Redundancies/Independent Double Checks				
Recalculate the dose		X	X	
Verify drug and/or drug preparation		X	X	
Use peer review process for unusual drug, dose, regimen		X	X	
Verify patient diagnosis/indication for drug		X	X	
Double-check pump rate, drug, concentration, and line attachments	X	X	X	X
Bar coding and/or "smart" pumps		X	X	X
Involve the patient (family) through education	X	X	X	X
Monitor Patients and Respond to Drug Effects				
Require cardiac monitoring (cm)/pulse oximetry (po)/capnography (CO_2)			X (cm)	
Require close observation/vital sign monitoring		X	X	
Have antidotes and/or resuscitation equipment close at hand			X	
Failure Mode and Effects Analysis		X		

* INR = international normalized ratio.

Intravenous Adrenergic Agonists

Problems

Concentration errors

- Adrenergic agonists are often available in varying concentrations, which has led to accidental mix-ups. In addition, the two concentration of epinephrine are expressed as ratios, 1:1,000 and 1:10,000. This is inconsistent with the usual expression of concentration in milligrams per milliliter (mg/mL); it has confused many health care practitioners and contributed to harmful and fatal errors.

Unlabeled containers

- In operating rooms (ORs), adrenergic agonists have been drawn up into unlabeled syringes or put into unlabeled or incorrectly labeled cups or pans, leading to harmful or fatal mix-up of medications and solutions.

"Titration" without limits

- These drugs are often ordered "to titration" (i.e., the dose or rate is to be increased until the desired effect is achieved); a lack of limits on the amount or rate has led to severe vasoconstriction, necrosis, and permanent disability.

Dosing errors

- Isoproterenol has been available in the past in 1 mg and 0.2 mg ampuls. If the dose ordered is "1 amp," the wrong amount may be administered.

Calculation errors

- IV flow rates have been miscalculated because some medications are based on micrograms per kilogram per minute dosing.

Look-alike drug names

- Dopamine and dobutamine, and epinephrine and ephedrine, are subject to mix-ups because of similarities in their names. Dopamine and dobutamine are used in similar settings (e.g., intensive care units) for similar types of patients (e.g., cardiac patients), which contributes to mix-ups. Problems also occur because dopamine and dobutamine are administered in similar doses, are provided in similar concentrations, and, if from the same manufacturer, have similar packaging.

Extravasation

- Extravasation can cause problems if dopamine is given via peripheral veins.

Key Improvements

Constraints

- Remove phenylephrine (Neo-Synephrine) and other adrenergic agonists from the formulary if there is no need for them.
- Store concentrated epinephrine only in crash carts, when possible.

Centralize

- Have pharmacy prepare all infusions and bolus doses of these drugs.

Standardize

- Establish maximum and minimum doses for all titration drugs.
- Use preprinted order sets and standard concentrations.
- Communicate orders in a standard fashion; refer to IV doses in terms of metric weight (i.e., milligrams) rather than concentration, ampuls, or volume. (Note: The concentration may be important for drugs used topically or injected locally.)

Simplify

- Purchase premixed solutions.
- Use prefilled syringes whenever possible.
- Use dosing charts instead of calculating infusion rates.

Differentiate

- Differentiate critical parts of the drug names (on computer screens, shelf or bin labels, MARs, and so on) using tall-man lettering (e.g., DOBUTamine/DOPamine, and EPINEPHrine/ePHEDrine) or another method of differentiation (e.g., color). (Dopamine and dobutamine are on the list of FDA drug name pairs that use tall-man lettering to differentiate the names. ISMP has petitioned USP to require the same action for epinephrine and ephedrine.)
- When possible, use prefilled syringes of epinephrine.
- Purchase available vials and premixed solutions from different manufacturers to ensure that the labels look different.
- Differentiate packaging; for example, purchase dobutamine in 250 mL bags and dopamine in 500 mL bags.
- Store drugs with similar names separately.

Reminders

- Label all containers, including syringes and cups into which drugs are placed.
- Label both sides of containers of drug solutions for IV infusion.
- Label IV bags and delivery pumps with dosage charts and infusion rates for standardized dosages.
- Program alerts concerning look-alike names into ADC screens.
- Program ADC screens to caution users about error-prone conditions (e.g., dose confusion, concentrations, look-alike confusion).

Redundancies

- Perform independent double checks before administering adrenergic agonists. (Have a second nurse independently check dose, pump settings, drug concentration, line attachments, and patient identity.)

Patient monitoring

- Use cardiorespiratory monitors for patients receiving infusions of adrenergic agonists through a central IV line.

IV Adrenergic Antagonists

Problems

Concentration errors

- The more concentrated esmolol (1 to 2.5 g per mL) intended for IV admixture preparation has been confused with the less concentrated product (10 mg/mL) intended for administration as bolus doses. Patients who inadvertently receive the higher concentration may develop bradycardia, electromechanical dissociation, or asystole that may be irreversible.

Dosing errors

- With propranolol and metoprolol, the most common error is the accidental administration of an IV dose equal to the standard oral dose when a patient is being switched from oral to IV therapy. The IV dose is much smaller than the oral dose.

Look-alike containers

- In the past, health care providers confused amiodarone with amrinone, a drug with opposite pharmacologic effects. In July 2000, the nonproprietary name amrinone was officially changed to inamrinone. Amiodarone solutions prepared in glass bottles of 5% dextrose injection have also been confused with nitroglycerin.

Key Improvements

Constraints

- Remove esmolol (ampuls and vials) from patient care areas, night cabinets, emergency kits, and ADCs; store only in the pharmacy. Use available manufacturers' premixed containers.
- Minimize the need for esmolol by selecting alternative agents.

Centralize

- Prepare IV infusions and syringes of beta-blockers only in the pharmacy.

Standardize

- Standardize the units of measure for prescribing esmolol; do not accept orders for an "amp" of esmolol.
- Standardize solution concentrations.

Simplify

- Purchase premixed solutions of esmolol.

Differentiate

- Apply pharmacy labels on glass bottles of 5% dextrose injection (D5W) to distinguish between plain D5W and premixed nitroglycerin or amiodarone.
- Order products from a different manufacturer to maximize differences in labeling and packaging.

Redundancies

- Have routine orders for IV propranolol and metoprolol reviewed by a pharmacist or second nurse before administration.
- Double-check the strength when preparing loading doses and infusions of esmolol.

Patient monitoring

■ Administer esmolol only where resuscitation equipment, including a suitable pacemaker, is available.

Inhalational and IV General Anesthetics

Problems

Look-alike drugs

■ Propofol, a white, opaque drug, has been confused with nutritional IV lipid emulsions.

Medical tubing mix-ups

■ Propofol can make IV tubing appear similar to white pneumatic blood pressure cuff tubing on patient monitors. This has led to rare fatal events in which dislodged tubing, thought to contain propofol, was attached to the patient's IV line; air embolism resulted when the monitor cycled to inflate the cuff.

Use by untrained staff

■ Propofol has been administered as sedation for procedures outside the OR in inappropriate doses and with too rapid titration, leading to respiratory arrest and deaths.

■ Staff (nurses and physicians) administering propofol or other induction agents for procedural sedation have not always been trained to monitor patients and rescue them from deep sedation or general anesthesia.

Lack of preparation for emergencies

■ Patients have received propofol or other induction agents to sedate them for procedures performed in ambulatory surgery centers or physician offices unequipped to handle emergency intubation, ventilation, oxygen enrichment, and cardiovascular resuscitation.

■ Unlike other sedation agents (e.g., midazolam, morphine), there is no reversal agent for propofol. Adverse effects must be treated until the drug is metabolized.

Inadequate patient monitoring

■ Propofol dosing and titration is variable, depending on the patient's tolerance to the drug. Profound changes can occur rapidly. Even with low doses, a patient can go from breathing normally to full respiratory arrest in seconds, without warning from typical assessment parameters.

■ Occasionally, a physician has administered propofol himself or herself while performing an outpatient procedure and has been unable to properly monitor the patient while focused on the procedure.

Dosing errors

■ General anesthetics are available in different concentrations; this can lead to inadvertent subtherapeutic or excessive doses.

■ Mathematical errors in converting milligrams (mg) to micrograms (mcg) have led to serious overdosages.

Unlabeled syringes

- Drugs used during the induction and maintenance of anesthesia have been drawn into unlabeled syringes, or the needle attached to an unlabeled syringe has been left in a medication vial but not properly labeled.

Key Improvements

Constraints

- Permit only licensed medical or nursing staff to connect and reconnect tubing associated with the use of medications (including propofol).
- Permit the use of general anesthetics only in the OR or other areas that are under the direct supervision of anesthesiologists.
- Permit the administration of propofol to nonventilated patients only by persons who are (1) trained in the administration of drugs that cause deep sedation and general anesthesia, (2) able to intubate the patient if necessary, and (3) legally allowed to administer the medication under state practice acts (some states consider propofol administration not within the scope of professional nurse practice), and (4) not involved simultaneously in the procedure itself.
- Determine the qualifications of professionals who can administer propofol to nonventilated patients during procedures. Specify the circumstances, the education and supervised practice required beforehand, and the competencies that must be evaluated and met periodically. (Certification in advanced cardiac life support alone is not sufficient.)
- Limit locations where patients may receive propofol to those that meet all safety criteria, including the presence of staff with expertise in intubation, which is unlikely in physician office settings.

Standardize

- Stock only the weakest concentration and smallest volume of general anesthetics available.

Simplify

- Use dosing charts for unit conversions between milligrams and micrograms.

Differentiate

- Use flexible plastic containers for lipid solutions to differentiate them from the glass bottles that contain propofol.

Reminders

- Label all IV tubing at both ends (patient and pump).
- Affix warning labels: "To be administered only by staff certified to manage deep sedation and anesthesia."

Redundancies

- Require independent double checks for all general anesthetic agents administered outside the OR, regardless of the intended level of sedation (light, moderate, or deep).

Patient monitoring

- Establish a continuous monitoring process and assessment criteria (e.g., vital signs, oxygen saturation, and ideally, capnography) for nonventilated patients who are receiving propofol.
- Ensure that equipment is readily accessible at the point of care to maintain a patent airway, provide oxygen, intubate, ventilate, and offer circulatory resuscitation.

Failure mode and effects analysis

- If nurses are legally permitted to administer propofol, have an interdisciplinary team perform FMEA and remedy risks of patient harm before use; if serious safety hazards cannot be remedied, do not allow nurses to administer propofol. (Legal permission does not automatically qualify nurses to administer propofol.)

Oral and Injectable Cancer Chemotherapy

Problems

Calculation errors

- Doses have been miscalculated when decimal points are involved.

Dosing errors

- Doses intended to be given on distinct days within a course of therapy (e.g., vincristine IV 2 mg days 4 and 11) have been administered daily between the two dates because a dash was used in expressing the protocol or order (e.g., vincristine IV 2 mg days 4–11).
- Prescribers have reordered the drugs as "renew same chemotherapy," which has resulted in dosing errors because the wrong set of orders was referenced.
- Drug doses ordered as a total cycle or course dose have been misunderstood and administered as a single daily dose. (Agents used in cancer chemotherapy are highly toxic and have a narrow range of use; thus, many dosing errors have resulted in catastrophic harm or death.)
- Unsafe doses have been dispensed by pharmacy because dose-range checking was not available within the order entry system, pharmacists did not have the patient's height and weight to calculate the body surface area, or protocols were not readily accessible in the pharmacy for reference and verification of doses.
- Decimal points in precise doses (e.g., 25.4 mg) have been overlooked, leading to 10-fold errors (e.g., 254 mg).

Miscommunication of drugs

- Many cancer chemotherapy regimens are referred to with acronyms (e.g., DAT, DAV, CHOP, COPP), which have been misunderstood as the wrong drugs.
- The liposomal form and conventional form of doxorubicin have been mixed up, resulting in serious dosing errors.

Look-alike drug names and packages

- Some products with similar names (e.g., mitoxantrone and methotrexate; doxorubicin and daunorubicin; cisplatin [Platinol] and carboplatin [Paraplatin]; vincristine, vinblastine, and vinorelbine) have been mixed up in oral and written orders and administered in inappropriate, often harmful doses.

Accidental intrathecal administration

■ Vincristine has been administered intrathecally because the syringe was mixed up with another drug intended for intrathecal administration.

Inappropriate timing of therapy

■ Chemotherapy has been administered under conditions that are not optimal, such as when the patient's white blood cell count is dangerously low.

Key Improvements

Forcing functions

■ Configure the computer system to require entry of the patient's height, weight, age, and allergies before allowing entry of chemotherapy orders.

Constraints

■ Prohibit spoken orders for cancer chemotherapy.
■ Allow only specially trained pharmacy staff to prepare and check cancer chemotherapy before dispensing.
■ Allow only certified nurses to administer cancer chemotherapy.
■ Separate liposomal doxorubicin (Doxil) from conventional doxorubicin.

Improve access to information

■ Establish dose limits for cancer chemotherapy as defined below, and program these into computerized systems where possible:
  – Ceiling for dose of a single drug
  – Daily dose ceiling
  – Ceiling for total dose for a course of therapy
  – Ceiling for total lifetime dose
■ Ensure that nurses and pharmacists have drug references, ready access to chemotherapy protocols, and Internet access to reliable oncology support sites.
■ Educate all patients and their families and caregivers about the prescribed chemotherapy, and provide written information for reference.

Standardize

■ Spell out all antineoplastic chemotherapy orders. Do not use acronyms in prescribing chemotherapy, and avoid potentially confusing terminology (e.g., prescribing "platinum," which may refer to cisplatin or carboplatin).
■ Use preprinted order sets with daily doses and cycles listed and prompts for documenting the reason for dose adjustments, or use a standardized order template for chemotherapy that prompts prescribers to document this information.
■ Never use a dash (–) in communicating distinct days of therapy.

Simplify

■ Round doses of more than 10 mg to eliminate tenths of a milligram and prevent potential misinterpretation of the decimal point. If doses cannot be rounded safely, be sure all decimal points are clear and obvious, and not obscured by fax "noise" or lines on order forms.

Differentiate

- Identify look-alike and sound-alike pairs of chemotherapy drugs, and develop methods of distinguishing between them.
- Segregate intrathecal medications and dispense them at different times, and to different locations, than other medications.
- Dispense IV vincristine in packaging that distinguishes it from other injectable medications (e.g., distinctive outer wrap, dilution in 20–50 mL).

Reminders

- Use checklists for chemotherapy preparation and administration processes.
- Dispense chemotherapy in distinctive bags that are labeled "chemotherapy."
- Add auxiliary labels to liposomal doxorubicin (Doxil) that distinguish it from conventional doxorubicin.

Redundancies

- Require all doses to be ordered with both the total daily dose and the dosage in milligrams per kilogram or milligrams per square meter of body surface area, so that nurses and pharmacists can verify the calculated daily dose.
- Have nurses and pharmacists verify all chemotherapy doses through recalculation and checking against the corresponding protocol or regimen.
- Have two individuals independently check all chemotherapy drugs and doses, pump settings, line attachments, and patients' identity before the drug is administered.
- Develop protocols that require peer review in cases of disagreement between prescribers and clinical personnel.
- Do not accept orders to resume the same chemotherapy. Require prescribers to provide a complete set of new orders for each cycle of chemotherapy, or every 30 days if the cycle runs longer than 1 month.

Patient monitoring

- Establish processes to ensure that patients' laboratory results and clinical assessments (e.g., weight, nausea, side effects) are reviewed and considered before chemotherapy is dispensed and administered.

See Chapter 16 for more detailed information about preventing errors in cancer chemotherapy.

Cardioplegic Solutions

Problems

Compounding errors

- Extemporaneous compounding of cardioplegic solutions has occasionally resulted in improperly mixed solutions. Hypotonic or superconcentrated solutions have been administered, resulting in brain injuries or fatalities.
- Math errors can be made in manual calculation of the amounts of component ingredients.
- Automated compounders can malfunction or be misused.
- The wrong solution or concentration may be placed on the automated compounder, resulting in mixing errors.

Look-alike containers

- Nearly identical computer-generated pharmacy labels on containers have led to confusion between cardioplegic solutions and TPN solutions.
- Labeling on the manufacturer-supplied dextrose containers has contributed to mix-ups between cardioplegic solutions and other injectable medications.

Key Improvements

Constraints

- Allow only specially trained individuals to compound cardioplegic solutions, or outsource preparation to a qualified external IV lab.

Externalize error-prone processes

- Take advantage of manufacturer-prepared cardioplegic solutions, or outsource preparation to a qualified external IV lab.

Standardize

- In conjunction with surgical staff, establish a single, standard concentration of cardioplegic solution.

Differentiate

- Affix a specialized label to cardioplegic solutions to reduce the similarity of their appearance to other injectable solutions.

Redundancies

- Establish and implement stringent quality control standards for preparing and checking the automated equipment and solutions used to mix cardioplegic solutions.
- Require independent double checks of all base and electrolyte solutions, calculations, measurements, and compounder settings by at least two individuals, and document the checks. Automated equipment with bar code capability can contribute to overall safety.
- Require pharmacists to calculate and verify the expected weight of the final product on the basis of the specific gravity of ingredients and the final volume. Weigh each bag to ensure that it is within 5% of the calculated weight.

Colchicine Injection

Problems

Dosing errors

- Deaths have been reported from overdoses when maximum single doses or cumulative doses were exceeded.
- Prescribing the drug prn (as needed) "until symptoms are relieved" has resulted in administration of amounts exceeding the safe cumulative dose.
- Doses have not always been adjusted for geriatric patients with compromised renal and hepatic function, and toxicity has resulted.

Masked signs of toxicity

■ Gastrointestinal symptoms are a poor indicator of toxicity when the drug is administered IV.

Look-alike drug names

■ Oral and handwritten orders for Cortrosyn (cosyntropin) and clonidine have been misheard or misread as colchicine, sometimes leading to patient harm.

Key Improvements

Constraints

■ Orders should include a specific stop date or time and a cumulative dose that should not be exceeded.

Improve access to information

■ Establish maximum daily (4 mg) and cumulative (4 mg/week) doses.
■ Program the order entry computer system to alert the user if a daily dose exceeds safe limits.
■ Program the computer to automatically alert the pharmacist (and prescriber, if using computerized prescriber order entry) if a dose adjustment is needed for hepatic or renal impairment.

Reminders

■ Program reminders into ordering systems about daily and cumulative doses and hepatic and renal precautions.
■ Add reminders about stop dates and maximum cumulative doses to MARs.

Redundancies

■ Verify the patient's diagnosis before dispensing and administering colchicine, to help prevent misinterpreted orders with look-alike or sound-alike drugs.
■ Read back spoken orders, spelling the drug name.

Forcing function

■ If the cumulative dose is reached, the system should not allow continuation of the order.

Hypertonic Dextrose (20% or greater)

Problems

Look-alike drug names and containers

■ Confusion between 5% and 50% solutions in 1 liter bags has led to fatalities from administration of high-concentration dextrose.

Instability

■ 50% dextrose has limited stability and shelf life, once opened.
■ 50% dextrose solution can be problematic as a diluent; it causes precipitation with certain drugs.

Key Improvements

Constraints

- Stock dextrose in concentrations of 20% or higher in the pharmacy only. (Exception: vials or syringes of 50% dextrose for treating hypoglycemia.)

Centralize error-prone processes

- Allow only pharmacy to prepare any dextrose solutions that are not commercially available.

Improve access to information

- Consult pharmacy before administering high-concentration dextrose solutions used alone or in dialysis.

Reminders

- Apply warning labels to high-concentration dextrose solutions or mixtures.

Dialysis Solutions

Problems

Concentration errors

- Commercially available dialysates contain varying standard concentrations of electrolytes, which has led to serious errors.
- Physicians have prescribed nonstandard, tailor-made dialysates, leading to mixing errors.

Compounding errors

- The wrong drugs or concentrations have been used in mixing dialysates to correct electrolyte imbalances, causing serious or fatal outcomes.
- Electrolyte supplements have been added in the wrong quantities to premixed dialysates.
- The wrong base solution has been used to prepare dialysates.
- Precipitates from adding calcium carbonate and sodium bicarbonate have clogged dialysis access sites.

Use by untrained staff

- Nurses and pharmacists unfamiliar with the concepts of osmosis, diffusion, and electrolyte balance have failed to capture harmful errors involving inadvertent preparation of superconcentrated dialysates before they reached the patient.

Improper pharmacy labeling

- Premixed dialysates with additional electrolytes added have been labeled with just the additives listed, not the total amount of the electrolytes and other additives in the solution, which makes detection of potential mixing errors difficult.
- Labels applied to containers in the pharmacy after addition of the prescribed electrolytes have obscured the manufacturer's label that states the electrolyte content in the base solution.

Medical tubing mix-ups

- Peritoneal dialysis tubes and ports have been confused with gastric tubes, leading to administration of gastric feeding into the vascular system.

Key Improvements

Constraints

- Limit preparation and administration of dialysates to practitioners who demonstrate understanding of the physiology of dialysis.

Externalize error-prone processes

- Use commercially available dialysates when possible.

Improve access to information

- Request that pharmacy place labels so that they do not cover the manufacturer's original label listing electrolyte composition.
- Prepare dialysate solutions in the pharmacy, using recipe cards.
- Include the total amount of electrolytes in the bag of dialysate on pharmacy-prepared labels for compounded solutions (i.e., include any added electrolytes plus the electrolyte content of the base solution).

Standardize

- Use preprinted order sets for dialysate that list the typical ranges of electrolytes per liter and prompts for prescribers to clearly indicate the base solution and total electrolytes prescribed.
- Use a standard base solution when compounding dialysates.

Reminders

- Label all tubing connected to dialysis access sites to prevent misconnections with other medical tubing.

Redundancies

- Require independent double checks of all dialysate solutions before dispensing and administration.

Patient monitoring

- Closely monitor patients undergoing peritoneal dialysis or hemodialysis.

Epidural and Intrathecal Medications

Problems

Accidental intrathecal or epidural administration of IV drugs

- IV drugs have been given inadvertently via epidural and intrathecal lines, often causing harm or death, particularly with vinca alkaloid products.
- Ionic contrast media have been injected intrathecally instead of nonionic water-soluble agents; often, this has involved look-alike vials (e.g., Hypaque [diatrizoate meglumine], used for cerebral angiography, and nonionic Omnipaque 300 [iohexol], used for myelography).

Dosing errors

- Attempts to refill an implanted infusion pump reservoir with opioids or baclofen have resulted in direct injection of the entire reservoir contents into the catheter access port in the intrathecal space.
- Unsafe doses of epidural analgesia have been prescribed by practitioners who are not trained in epidural analgesia.

Injection of drug with preservatives

- Poorly visible or ambiguous labeling about preservatives has led to intrathecal and epidural administration of drugs with preservatives. For example, the front label panel on Faulding's morphine vial states, "No bacteriostat added," making it appear that the product is safe for epidural or intrathecal use. However, a statement in small print on the side label panel states, "Not for epidural or intrathecal use. Contains sodium metabisulfite."

Key Improvements

Constraints

- Never dispense an IV medication in a way that allows its entry into the physical location where an intrathecal medication is being administered.
- Establish a list of drugs that can be administered intrathecally (or epidurally), and ban all other injectable drugs from rooms where intrathecal medication is being administered (or lumbar punctures are performed).
- Have pharmacy prepare intrathecal medications immediately before they are needed and deliver the drugs to a specific location that is different from the delivery time and location of the patient's remaining therapy, only after confirmation that all IV drugs have been administered.
- Limit prescribing of fentanyl for epidural PCA to anesthesia staff, pain management teams, or critical care prescribers.
- Store nonionic contrast media in a separate location, away from ionic media and other products, or prepare separate kits for myelograms that include the proper contrast media for intrathecal use.
- Use tubing designed for epidural infusions without any side injection ports for all epidural lines.
- Dilute IV vincristine in 20–50 mL of solution and package the drug in an IV piggyback bag, because intrathecal drugs are usually prepared in volumes less than 10 mL.[20]

Externalize error-prone processes

- If usage of implantable intrathecal infusion devices is low, consider referring patients to another provider that handles implantable pumps more frequently.

Standardize

- Create standardized order sets for the use of implantable pumps, such as for implanting, reprogramming, refilling, and other possible modalities (e.g., myelography).
- Administer intrathecal medications in a designated location (e.g., a treatment room) and at a standard time (e.g., early morning or late evening) only.

Differentiate

- Separate implantable pump access and refill kits to ensure use of the proper template for refilling the reservoir.
- Differentiate intrathecal medications from IV medications by wrapping them in a sterile sheath or bag for distribution.

Reminders

- Label all IV and epidural tubing at both ends (patient and pump).
- Apply warning labels—"FATAL if given intrathecally. IV USE ONLY"—to vinca alkaloid products before dispensing.
- Place prominent auxiliary labels on ionic media that should not be used for myelography.

Redundancies

- Require independent double checks (at least two clinicians independently verifying the patient's identity, medication, infusion rate, infusion pump settings, and line attachment) for all epidural and intrathecal infusions.

Patient monitoring

- Establish written guidelines for early recognition of an error (e.g., symptoms specific to the drug) and prompt treatment in the event an inappropriate drug or substance has been administered intrathecally. This may include an immediate process for active irrigation and drainage of the cerebrospinal fluid, respiratory support, treatment of seizures, and small incremental doses of reversal agents if available.

Failure mode and effects analysis

- Have an interdisciplinary team perform FMEA on the processes used to prescribe, dispense, and administer all forms of intrathecal or epidural drug therapy, and remedy risks that could harm patients.

Glycoprotein IIb/IIIa Inhibitors

Problems

Calculation errors

- Calculation errors have occurred during conversion from micrograms per kilogram (or micrograms per kilogram per minute) to milligrams because some drugs (e.g., eptifibatide) are available in milligrams per milliliter concentrations.

Dosing errors

- Dosing errors have occurred because of complicated and nonstandard dosing schedules and variations in the way the drugs are dosed and administered, especially if multiple products are on the formulary and protocols are absent or poorly designed.
- Bolus doses have been inadvertently omitted.
- Doses have not been adjusted for patients with renal function impairment.

- The term "bolus" or "bolus vial" appears on some product vials (e.g., eptifibatide); this has contributed to errors in which the full vial has been administered as a bolus dose, rather than the prescribed bolus dose.
- Dosing errors have occurred when nurses prepare the drugs in areas for which pharmacy typically does not dispense unit doses for specific patients.

Look-alike drug names

- The trade name of tirofiban (Aggrastat) has been confused with argatroban because both are used in similar patients.

Key Improvements

Centralize error-prone processes

- Have pharmacy prepare all infusions when possible.

Standardize and simplify

- Establish protocols for drug dosing, preparation, mixing of infusions, and drug administration (infusion and bolus).
- Establish dosing charts for use with standard concentrations of infusions, to reduce the risk of calculation errors.

Reminders

- Add warning labels on packaging to guide the proper dosing schedule.
- Program drug name alerts for Aggrastat and argatroban into computerized ordering systems.

Redundancy

- Require an independent double check of the drug, dose calculations, concentration, patient identity, line attachment or access site, and pump settings (for infusions).
- Require all orders to be written with the indication so practitioners can better match the drug therapy to the patient's condition; this reduces the risk of misidentifying a drug.

Patient monitoring

- Develop and follow protocols that require verification of laboratory test values (e.g., blood cell and platelet counts, liver and renal function tests) before prescribing, dispensing, and administering these products.

Low Molecular Weight (LMW) Heparin Injection

Problems

Dosing errors

- Dosing errors have occurred with Lovenox (enoxaparin) prefilled syringes because the barrel lacks sufficient milliliter gradations for accurate measurement of doses.

Duplicate or concurrent therapy

- Fatal errors have occurred from unrecognized concomitant use of LMW heparin and unfractionated heparin or other anticoagulants, most often after hospitalized patients have received one of the products in the emergency department (ED) or other outpatient area.

Spinal hematoma

- When used concurrently with spinal puncture procedures, LMW heparin increases the risk of epidural or spinal hematoma, which has led to permanent paralysis.

Look-alike syringes

- Mix-ups have occurred between heparin flush syringes and LMW heparin syringes.

Look-alike drug names

- Orders for fondaparinux (Arixtra) have been confused with orders for lab tests for anti-factor Xa, or "Anti-Xa."

Key Improvements

Limit access or use

- Limit floor stock of LMW heparin to EDs. Dispense all other LMW heparin from the pharmacy as prescribed for each patient, or make it available in ADCs only after pharmacy screening.

Standardize

- Require consistent documentation of medications administered in the ED and cardiac catheterization lab in a single, standardized place (not embedded within nursing notes) to facilitate review of all drug therapy before a heparin product is prescribed or administered.
- Use protocols, guidelines, and standard order forms to ensure that current and recent drug therapy is considered before any heparin product is ordered, dispensed, and administered.

Reminders

- Include reminders on protocols, guidelines, and standard order forms for heparin, warfarin, and fibrinolytics to assess all drug therapy to avoid concomitant use of heparin products.
- Place an alert on the chart of any patient who has received thrombolytics or is changing from one anticoagulant to another.

Improve access to information

- Establish a process for immediate communication to the pharmacy, upon a patient's admission to the hospital, of all medications administered in the ED (e.g., LMW heparin) or other outpatient settings (e.g., cardiac catheterization lab), to ensure that these medications are in the pharmacy computer system and will generate an automated alert for duplicate therapy or interactions with medications prescribed upon admission. With many pharmacy computer systems, a one-time drug order becomes inactive as soon as it is dispensed, and only active orders are checked for duplicate therapy and drug interactions. To bypass this problem, some pharmacists enter one-time doses of LMW heparin as a set of two "orders": (1) one order for the LMW heparin as prescribed and administered in the ED and (2) a note that the patient has received LMW heparin, along with the National Drug Code number that triggers an interaction alert and a suggested frequency that keeps the order active for about 12 hours. Thus, an interaction message will occur if another heparin product is prescribed within that time frame. Modifications for different computer systems may be necessary, but many systems allow such a safety net to be built.

■ Ensure that computer alerts for duplicate therapy are fully functional for all heparin products.

Differentiate

■ Stock LMW heparin syringes away from look-alike heparin flush syringes.

Unfractionated IV Heparin

Problems

Dosing errors

■ A temporary increase in the heparin pump rate to deliver a bolus dose has caused dosing errors because staff have forgotten to reset the pump after delivery of the bolus.
■ Abbreviating heparin units as "U" has led to numerous 10-fold overdoses.
■ Pump setting errors involving either concentration or rate of infusion have resulted in dosing errors.
■ Dosing errors have occurred after the lab receives a new batch of thromboplastin that changes the therapeutic range for activated partial thromboplastin time (aPTT), if the IV heparin nomogram used for dose adjustments is not changed accordingly.
■ Unverified weights (e.g., as stated by the patient or estimated by a practitioner or family member) have been used to initiate heparin therapy, leading to subtherapeutic or excessive dosing.

Calculation errors

■ Mathematical errors in determining the volume of heparin to administer for a bolus dose, or the rate of infusion of a maintenance heparin solution, have resulted in overdosage or underdosage, sometimes leading to bleeding or clot formation.
■ Practitioners, particularly pharmacy staff, have miscalculated the volume of heparin to be added to TPN or other electrolyte solutions.

Concentration errors

■ Various concentrations of IV heparin bags and heparin vials have been mixed up, in part because of look-alike vials and bags.

- Mix-ups have occurred between heparin 1,000 units/500 mL bags used for maintenance of adult arterial lines and 25,000 units/500 mL bags for IV use.
- Solutions of heparin may be available (or extemporaneously prepared) in various concentrations, leading to occasional errors if the concentration expressed in the order does not match the concentration supplied, or if staff select the wrong concentration.

IV admixture errors

- In settings where a standard concentration of commercially available heparin is not in use, nurses and pharmacists have made errors when mixing heparin solutions.

Duplicate or concurrent therapy

- The preceding section on low-molecular weight heparin describes problems associated with concurrent administration of more than one heparin product, and key improvements.

Improper manufacturer labeling

- Labeling of small-volume injectable products from some manufacturers prominently displays the concentration (e.g., 10,000 units/mL) but not the total volume (10 mL), which can lead practitioners to believe the container holds 10,000 units, not 100,000, units.

Look-alike drug names and packages

- Look-alike vials of heparin (flush solution) and insulin (both dosed in units) are often found together on top of medication carts or counters, resulting in occasional mix-ups.
- Heparin has been confused with other medications (e.g., vaccines) because both are supplied as prefilled syringes or cartridges that look alike and may be stored near one another.
- Large-volume bags of heparin solution have been confused with look-alike bags of lidocaine solution, as well as with look-alike bags of Hespan (hetastarch), which also has a similar name (the letters "h-e" "p-a" and "n" appear in the same order in both names).

Adverse drug reactions

- Heparin therapy has induced thrombocytopenia, which may not be detected early and treated appropriately.
- Porcine heparin is often associated with allergic reactions.

Injection of drug with preservatives

- In newborns, administration of IV heparin that is not preservative free has caused benzyl alcohol toxicity.

Contamination

- Practitioners have accidentally reentered multiple-dose vials of heparin with a contaminated needle, leading to disease transmission. (Although this is poor practice, a single vial of heparin flush solution often is accessed repeatedly within a short time for various patients.)

Incompatibilities

- While reteplase and heparin are incompatible, both have been administered together through the same IV line, forming a mass that stopped the infusion.

Key Improvements

Fail-safes

- Use only free-flow protected pumps to administer heparin infusions.

Constraints

- Do not store heparin vials (flush solution) on top of medication carts and counters, or under laminar flow hoods in the pharmacy. Return the vials to the proper storage area immediately after use.
- Do not store heparin solutions used for arterial lines near other injectable solutions.

Externalize error-prone processes

- Use commercially available premixed solutions.

Improve access to information

- Have the pharmacy place a label on both sides of the bag, taking care not to obscure the manufacturer's label.
- Affix dosing charts (printed on labels) to heparin infusion bags.
- Use the patient's actual weight in kilograms (kg) as the basis for determining heparin doses.

Standardize

- Do not abbreviate units as "U."
- Limit the variety of heparin concentrations in vials or syringes that are available in patient care units; whenever possible, allow only one concentration of vials for bolus doses (and use prefilled syringes for all heparin flushes, as noted below).
- Standardize the concentration used for all therapeutic IV heparin infusions.
- Develop and follow standard, weight-based heparin protocols for specific indications (e.g., deep vein thrombosis, stroke).

Simplify

- Use weight-based heparin infusion charts or nomograms to determine bolus doses and infusion rates.
- Do not deliver a bolus by temporarily modifying the rate of a maintenance heparin infusion; administer the bolus directly from a syringe connected to an IV access port.

Differentiate

- Use unit dose syringes for heparin flushes to differentiate them from other injectable products that are packaged in vials (e.g., insulin, normal saline) and to avoid potential contamination of vials.
- Separate the storage of heparin syringes from look-alike syringes of other medications.

- Separate heparin and insulin, which are both measured in units and may have a similar 100 unit/mL concentration, adding to potential for confusion.
- Separate Hespan, lidocaine, and heparin infusions.
- Use tall-man letters on auxiliary labels and order entry screens to differentiate HeSpan and hEParin.

Reminders

- Affix to infusion bags a reminder to perform an independent double check before starting the infusion.
- Build alerts into order entry systems to remind pharmacists to dispense preservative-free heparin for neonates.
- Add reminders about incompatibility between reteplase and heparin to protocols as appropriate, and provide directions for proper administration.

Redundancies

- Require an independent double check of the drug, concentration, dose calculations, rate of infusion, pump settings, line attachment, and patient identity before the start of a heparin infusion and with each change of the bag or rate of infusion.
- Have infusion pump rate settings independently checked by two persons.
- Have line placement on dual-channel pumps independently checked by two persons.
- Require an independent double check of all admixtures involving heparin in the pharmacy (including the addition of heparin to TPN or other electrolyte solutions).

Patient monitoring

- Develop and follow a standard format for communicating to the pharmacy dose adjustments based on laboratory values.
- Develop and follow a standard process for obtaining aPTT values at required intervals and communicating the results to prescribers.
- Establish and follow a protocol for detecting heparin-induced thrombocytopenia, treating patients who develop signs of this adverse drug reaction, and communicating this information.

Failure mode and effects analysis

- Have an interdisciplinary team perform FMEA for all forms of heparin therapy (including flushes), and remedy risks that could harm patients.
- Evaluate the packaging and labels on all heparin products to identify any potential for confusion and remedy problems by repackaging, affixing auxiliary labels, or switching manufacturers to improve distinction and clarity of labeling and packaging.

Oral Hypoglycemics

Problems

Look-alike and sound-alike names and packages

- Chlorpropamide has been confused with chlorpromazine (an antipsychotic); in some cases this has led to permanent central nervous system impairment and death related to hypoglycemia. Often, the two are stored near one another in alphabetically placed bins, and both are available and prescribed in similar doses (e.g., 100 mg). In addition, unit dose packages of both products may look similar.

■ Potentially serious mix-ups between metronidazole and metformin have been linked to look-alike packaging (both bulk bottles and unit dose packages) and to selection of the wrong product after entering "MET" as a mnemonic.

■ Mix-ups between Avandamet (rosiglitazone maleate and metformin hydrochloride) and Anzemet (dolasetron mesylate) have occurred when the spoken names were misheard.

■ Lethal errors have occurred when the diuretic acetazolamide (Diamox) was confused with the oral hypoglycemic acetohexamide (Dymelor).

■ Glyburide has been confused with glipizide.

■ Glucotrol has been confused with Glucotrol XL.

Drug interactions

■ Drug interactions are common, particularly with warfarin, digoxin, thyroid medications, and beta-blockers, which may worsen hypoglycemia and alter the physiological response to it, thereby masking the symptoms.

Adverse drug reactions

■ Lactic acidosis is a rare but potentially life-threatening condition associated with metformin, with a fatality rate as high as 50%. In nearly all cases of lactic acidosis, the drug has been prescribed when contraindicated.

Key Improvements

Improve access to information

■ Provide pharmacists with easy access to laboratory results needed for patient monitoring. Ideally, lab data should be interfaced with the pharmacy computer system so that an alert appears automatically when a dose adjustment may be needed.

■ Provide pharmacists with the patient's comorbid conditions to facilitate proper screening when these drugs are prescribed.

Differentiate

■ To reduce packaging similarity, purchase look-alike medications from different manufacturers.

■ Consider stocking metronidazole in 250 mg tablets only. (Metformin is not available as 250 mg tablets.)

■ Because chlorpropamide is likely a low-use item, consider repackaging the 100 mg tablets; alternatively, eliminate unit dose packages of chlorpromazine 100 mg and use 2 × 50 mg instead.

■ Use tall-man letters to highlight the differences in look-alike product names (e.g., chlorproMAZINE and chlorproPAMIDE), or underline or highlight the unique characters in look-alike names to make the differences stand out.

■ Separate the storage of products with look-alike names or packages.

Reminders

■ Include metformin on order sets or checklists used to screen patients who will be receiving IV radiographic contrast agents, to remind staff to discontinue the drug 48 hours before the procedure.

Redundancies

- Program the order entry computer to display both brand and generic names of products that would appear on the screen whenever the MET stem is used as a mnemonic (e.g., metronidazole [Flagyl] and metformin [Glucophage]).
- During the dispensing process, use both the order or prescription and the computer-generated label for verification (even with refills).
- Match the prescribed drug's indication to the patient's condition. For example, metformin is used to treat a chronic condition and metronidazole is more likely used for an acute condition; outpatient refills for metronidazole are less common and, therefore, should require a manual double check to ensure that the drug is appropriate for the patient's condition.
- Require a pharmacist to review the patient's full medical history before dispensing metformin to ensure there are no relative contraindications that could lead to lactic acidosis (e.g., patients at risk for drug accumulation because of renal failure; patients with liver disease or excessive alcohol use, whose lactate clearance may be impaired; acutely ill patients at risk of developing tissue hypoperfusion, which could lead to acidosis).
- Write down and read back all spoken orders for verification.

Monitor patients

- Establish a reliable system for monitoring patients taking oral hypoglycemics for interactions with other necessary medications and, when an interaction is recognized, for adjusting the dose or recommending changes in diet or exercise to prevent hypoglycemia from the drug interaction.
- Require pharmacists to monitor patients on metformin for renal or hepatic impairment and signs of lactic acidosis.

Insulins

Problems

Dosing errors

- Incorrect rates have been programmed into infusion pumps, leading to subtherapeutic or excessive doses of insulin.
- Insulin is available in multiple concentrations (100 units/mL, 500 units/mL, pharmacy or nurse-prepared concentrations for pediatric use [e.g., 10 units/mL]). Dosing errors have occurred when the wrong concentration of insulin was used to prepare a dose, or when an insulin syringe was used to prepare a nonstandard concentration. (Insulin syringes are accurate for only the most common concentration, 100 units/mL.)
- Confusion has led to dosing errors with premixed rapid-acting and intermediate-acting insulins offered in varying strengths (Humulin 50/50 or 70/30, Humalog and Humalog Mix 75/25).
- The availability of insulin infusions in more than one concentration has led to dosing errors.
- Diabetic patients with poor eyesight have self-administered the wrong dose or the wrong type of insulin.

Improper mixing

- Incompatible insulins have been drawn into the same syringe and administered.

■ Eighty percent of insulin can be adsorbed to plastic bags and tubing.[21] Even if the tubing is primed, the amount of insulin delivered can vary.

Inappropriate combination therapy

■ Lantus (insulin glargine) has been prescribed without a postprandial or short-acting insulin to treat hyperglycemia after meals, or in combination with long-acting oral hypoglycemics that have inappropriate pharmacokinetic profiles for mealtime coverage, exposing patients to an increased risk of developing diabetic complications.[22,23]

Look-alike syringes

■ Ten-fold overdoses have occurred when nurses accidentally used a tuberculin syringe to prepare an insulin dose. The plunger tip of some tuberculin syringes with 25-gauge needles (e.g., VanishPoint syringes from Retractable Technologies) is orange, a color clearly associated with insulin syringes.

Look-alike names and packaging

■ Similar-looking vials of insulin and heparin (flush solution) have been mistaken for one another, most often when stored near each other or placed on medication carts or countertops together.
■ Similar-looking vials of Lantus and regular insulin (both clear) have led to mix-ups in preparing single doses and insulin infusions; profound hypoglycemia has resulted from erroneously prepared infusions.
■ There are a dozen different types of insulin and several dozen brands, many with look-alike and sound-alike names or look-alike packages that have been confused with one another, especially
  – Lantus and Lente insulin
  – Humalog Mix 75/25 (75% insulin lispro protamine suspension and 25% insulin lispro injection [rDNA]) and Humulin 70/30 (70% human insulin isophane suspension [NPH] and 30% human insulin injection [regular] [rDNA]); prescribers have erroneously ordered Humulin 75/25 or Humalog 70/30.
  – Novolog Mix 70/30 (70% insulin aspart [rDNA origin] protamine suspension and 30% insulin aspart [rDNA] injection) and Novolin 70/30 (70% NPH, human insulin isophane suspension and 30% regular, human insulin injection [rDNA]); "Novolog 70/30" has been prescribed without including "Mix" in the product name.
■ New forms of insulins are becoming available, including intranasally administered products such as Exubera (insulin human [rDNA origin]) Inhalation Powder. This increases the potential for confusion, particularly in the conversion of prior insulin doses in units to doses of the inhalation product in milligrams.

Similar dosing units

■ Mental slips have resulted in mistaking insulin and heparin for one another because they may be stored near each other and both are administered in units.

Miscommunication of insulin orders

■ The abbreviation "SSRI" (for sliding-scale regular insulin) has been interpreted as "selective serotonin-reuptake inhibitor."

- Overdoses have occurred when "U" has been used as an abbreviation for "units" in orders; the "U" has been mistaken for a zero (0), the number 4, or "cc."
- "NPH 10/12 regular insulin" has been confused with 10 units of NPH and 112 of regular insulin when the slash mark was read as the numeral one (1).
- Physicians have sometimes prescribed doses of U-500 insulin (which is five times more concentrated than U-100 insulin) by citing the measurement level that would be used to draw the dose into a U-100 syringe (e.g., prescribing "25 units" of U-500 insulin when 125 units of the U-500 insulin is the intended dose). Patients have received too little insulin when the nurse administered the dose exactly as written (e.g., U-500 insulin measured to the 5 unit mark on a U-100 syringe to equal a "25 unit" dose as in the prior example).
- Insulin orders have not been discontinued or adjusted when enteral feeding was stopped, when a patient was ordered NPO, or when TPN was discontinued (or the infusion rate lowered) while a separate insulin infusion was running, often resulting in significant hypoglycemia.

Wrong patient errors

- Insulin has been mistakenly administered to patients who are not diabetic, leading to profound hypoglycemia.

Unsafe IV administration

- Intravenous insulin is lethal if it is given in substantially excessive amounts or in place of other medications.
- Humalog, Novolog, and Lantus have been administered IV in error, mostly because of the outdated idea that clear insulins could be administered IV.

Confusion about onset of action

- Patients have developed hypoglycemia because they have not eaten within a specified time, especially after receiving insulin analogs such as ultrashort acting insulin lispro (Humalog) or insulin aspart (Novolog). Hypoglycemia has also occurred when short-acting insulins were ordered for administration "every morning" or "every evening," not at a specified mealtime.
- It is no longer true that all clear insulins are short acting (e.g., Lantus is clear but long acting).

Complex dosing regimen

- Patients often receive widely varying doses and more than one type of insulin concurrently. Patients' confusion between different insulins and failure to discontinue previously prescribed insulin when switching to a new product has led to errors and harm. The nonprescription availability of most insulin (except some ultrashort acting or long-acting products) may contribute to the problem.
- The benefits of prescribing sliding-scale insulin coverage for hospitalized patients are not well supported in the literature. Furthermore, physicians have prescribed according to a sliding scale that is not standardized within the organization. Variation in patients' sliding scales, depending on prescribers' preferences, has led to dosing errors.

Expired drug

- Open insulin vials have not been discarded according to the manufacturer's recommendation (e.g., 30 days if stored at room temperature [which limits local irritation at the injection site]).

Poorly trained patients

- Improper mixing has led to clumps of aggregated insulin flowing out of insulin pens, followed by symptoms of hypoglycemia, or to less than 5% of the prescribed dose flowing from the pen, leading to hyperglycemia.[24]

Failure to properly adjust insulin therapy

- Blood glucose concentrations have not been prescribed or measured at defined intervals.
- Blood glucose concentrations have been miscommunicated, leading to the administration of higher or lower doses than actually required.

Key Improvements

Constraints

- Remove atypical concentrations (e.g., Humulin R U-500, 500 units/mL) from patient care areas and dispense these products in prefilled syringes from the pharmacy as prescribed for specific patients.
- Store heparin and insulin separately, particularly in areas where they are used to prepare individual doses or IV solutions (e.g., under pharmacy compounding hoods in IV admixture areas, on countertops). Do not store them together on tops of medication carts.
- When possible, do not store tuberculin syringes on patient care units. Except on pediatric units, tuberculin syringes are used primarily for skin tests or small subcutaneous doses of medications (including U-500 insulin) that can be dispensed in a syringe from the pharmacy.
- Store insulin syringes separately from all other syringes, perhaps near a refrigerator where insulin is stored, to prevent mix-ups with tuberculin syringes with orange plunger tips.
- Avoid using U-500 insulin for doses less than 100 units; this form of insulin should be used only for patients with marked insulin resistance who require doses above 200 units a day, since these larger doses can be administered subcutaneously in a smaller volume of fluid.
- Limit the insulin analog 70/30 mixtures on hospital formularies to a single product (e.g., Humalog Mix 75/25 or Novolog Mix 70/30).
- In hospitals, have pharmacy prepare and dispense prefilled syringes for once-daily doses of long-acting insulin (e.g., Lantus).
- In hospitals where dual-channel pumps are in use, consider using only single-channel pumps for insulin infusions to prevent programming the wrong channel. In addition, keeping the insulin line physically apart from other IV lines may reduce the possibility of adjusting the rate of the wrong medication.
- Require documentation of the date an insulin vial was first entered, and conduct drug storage safety rounds to ensure disposal of insulin vials kept at room temperature after 30 days.

Improve access to information

- Provide patient education by certified staff in a well-structured clinical setting; include both spoken and written material.
- Have nurses inform all alert patients that they are receiving insulin to treat their diabetes. (Questions from patients not expecting insulin can help avert a potential error.) Always tell the patient the full name of the insulin and the dose before administering the drug. If applicable, also tell patients their blood glucose concentration.
- Educate patients about their insulin therapy and how to prevent and treat hypoglycemia. Reinforce how physical activity and snacks affect glucose levels and how to handle circumstances such as travel and illness.
- Ask patients to demonstrate glucose monitoring skills and insulin administration, including measuring the correct dose.
- Ensure that patients who take U-500 insulin know how to communicate their doses correctly in terms of the type of insulin, the dose in units, and the volume in milliliters needed for each dose when using a tuberculin syringe.
- Post educational charts with insulin names; concentration; onset, peak, and duration of action; acceptable routes of administration; time of administration in relationship to meals; appropriate drug delivery devices; and special precautions (e.g., measuring the proper dose, mixing instructions, more frequent patient glucose monitoring). Pictures of the boxes in which insulin is packaged are also helpful.
- Do not place an insulin vial back in the carton after use; if a vial is returned to the wrong box (e.g., a vial of regular insulin is placed in a box for NPH insulin), a staff member may automatically select the wrong product.
- Establish pharmacy-managed diabetes clinics to better monitor and educate patients to manage their diabetes and self-administer insulin safely.
- Obtain an accurate history of insulin therapy from patients and follow up with questions to detect confusion between the many look-alike and sound-alike insulin products. Whenever possible, encourage patients or families to bring in the insulin for validation.
- Encourage patients to review nonprescription insulin with a pharmacist before purchase.

Standardize and simplify

- Standardize and simplify prescriptions for insulin, as follows:
  - Do not abbreviate "units"; use "units" instead of "U."
  - Do not use "SSRI" as an abbreviation for sliding-scale regular insulin, because it may be interpreted as "selective serotonin-reuptake inhibitor."
  - Do not use slash marks to separate NPH and regular insulin doses.
  - Require a standard format for prescribing insulin, preferably using preprinted order forms or electronic order sets that list specific products, ingredients, and component ratios.
  - Use a single concentration for adult IV insulin infusions. If a nonstandard insulin concentration is needed, list the concentration and the patient's dose in units and volume.
  - Consider the patient's usual times for meals and specify a clear relationship between insulin administration and the meals.
  - Prescribe U-500 insulin doses in terms of both units and volume (e.g., 200 units, 0.4 mL).

- Use spoken orders only when necessary, and spell back the name to avoid confusion with sound-alike insulin products.
- Standardize the preparation and administration of insulin, as follows:
    - Never prepare U-100 insulin doses in tuberculin syringes. The metric scale may be confused with the apothecary scale (minims) on disposable syringes.
    - Use only a tuberculin syringe (with only a volumetric scale) for U-500 insulin. If a U-100 syringe is used, doses may be incorrectly referred to on the basis of the U-100 scale. (A U-500 scale syringe is not available in the United States.)
    - For outpatients, encourage prescribers to order insulin pens and cartridges when appropriate (if insurance coverage is available) to simplify self-administration.
    - For neonates, use insulin 100 units/mL for doses of 5 units or more, with a U-100 insulin syringe. For doses less than 5 units, have pharmacy prepare and prominently label a 10 units/mL concentration and use a 1 mL tuberculin syringe with 0.01 mL graduations (1 unit equals 0.1 mL). Otherwise, consider IV infusion for insulin delivery.
- Standardize the insulin dilution used to prepare all neonatal solutions.
- Eliminate the use of sliding insulin dosage scales; if a sliding scale is used, standardize it through the use of a protocol and preprinted order form or computer order set that clearly designates the specific increments of insulin coverage.
- Establish a standard process for alerting physicians, pharmacists, and nurses that insulin doses must be adjusted or discontinued when changes occur in the patient's carbohydrate intake (e.g., changes in enteral feedings, TPN, NPO status). Include a notation on the patient's MAR to adjust or discontinue insulin under these conditions.
- Prepare solutions with insulin in glass bottles, and establish and follow procedures that minimize the degree of insulin absorption by plastic tubing.

Differentiate

- Help diabetic patients with poor eyesight to properly identify their insulin using tactile cues (e.g., place tape or a rubber band around regular insulin vials to differentiate them from NPH insulin).
- Accentuate differences in look-alike insulin product names by using tall-man letters (e.g., NovoLIN, NovoLOG MIX) on all drug selection screens, or underline or circle the distinguishing parts of names before dispensing the vials.
- For drug selection screens, emphasize the word "mixture" or "mix" along with the name of insulin product mixtures.
- Label pharmacy-prepared vials of diluted insulin for neonatal intensive care units with bold warnings, "NICU only," to clearly distinguish them from insulin vials containing standard concentrations. An empty vial, different in size from standard insulin vials, should be used to further distinguish the diluted neonatal insulin.

Reminders

- Place reminders about confusion between look-alike insulin products in storage locations and in computer systems.
- If the concentration of an insulin vial or syringe is not 100 units/mL, apply bold warning labels that clearly state the concentration and explicit instructions for measuring the proper dose in units and volume with a specified type of syringe.

Redundancies

- Require an independent double check before dispensing insulin from the pharmacy.
- Require an independent double check of the drug, concentration, dose, pump settings, route of administration, and patient identity before administering all IV insulin. ("Smart" infusion pumps with set dose limits also can serve as a double check for all except the route of administration and the patient's identity.)
- With selected high-risk populations, use independent checks of the drug, dose, route of administration, and patient identity for subcutaneous insulin doses before administration.
- Require an independent double check of all IV pump rate changes for insulin infusions.
- Write down and read back the transcription of all spoken orders for insulin, expressing the dose in single digits (e.g., say "one-six units" instead of "16 units"; otherwise, "sixteen" may sound like "sixty").
- Caution patients that pharmacies have dispensed the wrong type of insulin and that they should double-check their medication when filling prescriptions.
- If Lantus has been prescribed, have pharmacists confirm that a short-acting insulin has also been prescribed to control postprandial glucose.
- Require verification of the patient's diagnosis of diabetes, hyperglycemia, or other suitable condition before dispensing insulin.
- Before dispensing an insulin pen, require patients to perform a return demonstration of mixing and drug administration technique.

Patient monitoring

- When prescribing insulin, include or refer to defined standards for laboratory testing and clinical monitoring of patients.
- Increase patient monitoring through more frequent home visits or home testing of blood glucose concentration.
- Use diabetic flow sheets to track and trend blood glucose values, carbohydrate intake, and insulin administration (kept at the bedside or otherwise readily accessible when patients are hospitalized; maintained by the patient or home health care provider when patients are home). Remind patients to take their diabetic flow sheets to each physician office and hospital visit.
- Implement standardized procedures for communicating, both orally and in writing, point-of-care or lab-drawn glucose values from those who obtain the results to those who prescribe and administer the insulin; procedures should include read-back after spoken reports of test results and designation of a standard place, such as the MAR or diabetic flow sheet, for recording lab values.
- Monitor more closely patients at risk for hypokalemia and hypoglycemia (e.g., people who are fasting or have autonomic neuropathy, those taking potassium-lowering drugs). Patients with these electrolyte imbalances and renal or hepatic impairment may require reduction in the total daily doses of all insulin.

Failure mode and effects analysis

- Proactively anticipate and address problems with insulin use in both inpatient and outpatient settings through FMEA and by discussing insulin errors that have happened in other practice sites.
- Conduct FMEA before adding a new insulin product to the formulary or purchasing a new insulin administration device (e.g., insulin pen, different syringes, inhaled insulin).

IV Inotropic Drugs

Problems

Dosing errors

- A temporary increase in the pump rate to deliver a bolus dose of milrinone has caused dosing errors when staff have forgotten to reset the pump after delivery of the bolus.
- Doses have not been appropriately adjusted for elderly patients and those with renal impairment, in part because pharmacists have not been aware of the patient's comorbid conditions and lab results. (Digoxin has a narrow therapeutic index.)

Concentration errors

- Infants have received the adult concentration of digoxin (0.25 mg/mL) instead of the pediatric concentration (0.1 mg/mL), especially when the prescriber orders the dose in milliliters, not milligrams (or micrograms).

Drug interactions

- Most drugs in this class are associated with significant drug interactions (e.g., digoxin and calcium, digoxin and quinidine) as well as drug–herbal interactions (e.g., digoxin and ginseng).

Look-alike drug names and packages

- Digoxin has been confused with Desogen in handwritten prescriptions.
- Prefilled syringes of digoxin have been confused with other medications in prefilled syringes, especially if they are from the same manufacturer (e.g., Carpuject syringes).
- Inamrinone (formerly amrinone) has been mixed up with amiodarone.
- Inamrinone vials have been confused with azathioprine vials. After reconstitution, both drugs are yellow solutions.

Insufficient patient monitoring

- Failure to monitor patients carefully (e.g., serum drug levels, signs of toxicity) has resulted in adverse effects, particularly in elderly patients receiving high doses (both oral and IV).

Key Improvements

Constraints

- Store only pediatric concentrations of digoxin on units that serve pediatric patients. If both pediatric and adult strengths are needed, store them in separate locations, place reminders on storage bins or containers of each product, and alert staff that multiple concentrations are available.
- Separate injectable digoxin storage from look-alike syringes of other medications.
- Do not deliver a bolus dose of these drugs via a maintenance infusion by temporarily modifying the infusion rate; administer the bolus directly from a syringe connected to an IV access port.

Improve access to information

- Program dose limits for drugs in this class in the order entry computer system so an alert will appear for prescribed dosages outside the specified range.
- Provide pharmacists with easy access to laboratory results needed for patient monitoring. Ideally, lab data should be interfaced with the pharmacy computer system so that an alert appears automatically when a dose adjustment may be needed.
- Provide pharmacists with the patient's comorbid conditions to facilitate proper screening when these drugs are prescribed.
- Provide pharmacists with a complete list of medications the patient has been taking at home, including herbals, so proper screening for drug interactions can occur.
- Build alerts into the pharmacy computer system to warn staff about look-alike drug names, particularly inamrinone and amiodarone.

Standardize

- Require prescribers to include the milligrams per kilogram or micrograms per kilogram dose of these drugs along with the patient-specific dose for all pediatric patients.
- Do not accept orders for medications without a specified dose in metric weight, not volume.

Reminders

- For pediatric-strength medications, change the computer inventory description so that "pediatric" is part of the drug name, if possible, to help practitioners select the correct strength when entering orders.
- Include the designation "pediatric" on labels to ensure that the appropriate drug strength is selected during product preparation.

Redundancies

- Require an independent double check of all pediatric doses.
- Match the prescribed drug's indication to the patient's condition.

Patient monitoring

- Educate patients and caregivers about the importance of compliance with lab testing and the signs of toxicity and how to respond to them.
- Ensure adequate patient monitoring through regular clinic or office visits and lab or home testing of serum drug concentrations.
- Assist patients with scheduling follow-up lab studies for drug concentrations before the patient leaves the provider's facility.

IV Lidocaine (and Local Anesthetics)

Problems

Dosing and calculation errors

- Lidocaine is available in a variety of formulations and concentrations, which are expressed as a dilution ratio or percentage (1%, 2%, 10%, 20%). Studies show that knowledge about converting ratio or percentage concentrations to doses in milligrams or micrograms is inadequate, even among physicians.[25-27] Errors due to confusion between concentrations have been reported.

Unlabeled containers and syringes

- Lidocaine has been prepared in unlabeled syringes and basins, leading to mix-ups with other medications and solutions, especially in the OR and ED.

Look-alike or ambiguous labeling and packaging

- Mix-ups have occurred when lidocaine and heparin have been obtained from a single manufacturer and have similar labeling. Confusion between premixed heparin and lidocaine IV solutions has been reported. Errors have also occurred when 50 mL vials of lidocaine were confused with other drugs available in 50 mL vials (e.g., sodium bicarbonate, mannitol, and 50% dextrose).
- The labels on polypropylene ampuls of lidocaine (e.g., Xylocaine MPF 10 mg/mL Polyamp DuoFit, 10 mL ampuls) are difficult to read; this has led to errors in which the wrong drug or wrong dose was selected.

Possible contamination

- Economic constraints may force hospitals to use multidose containers in patient care areas. Multidose vials of lidocaine used as a local anesthetic have become contaminated as a result of poor aseptic technique.[28]
- Refrigerating lidocaine multidose vials after initial use can worsen contamination by prolonging the survival of any bacterial contaminants.[28]

Use by untrained staff

- Toxicity, occasionally leading to seizures or death, has occurred when health care providers failed to consider the systemic absorption of topical lidocaine and the potential for neurotoxicity or cardiac toxicity. Lidocaine is extensively absorbed (up to 35%) after topical administration to mucous membranes. This can lead to toxic plasma levels if large amounts are used, such as during bronchoscopy.[29]

Adverse drug reactions

- Methemoglobinemia, a serious and sometimes fatal adverse drug reaction, may occur with use of lidocaine.[30]
- The use of topical (viscous) lidocaine in the oral cavity for painful mouth lesions has caused aspiration due to oropharyngeal anesthesia and loss of sensation of food bolus that may be present in the oral cavity.

Nursing IV admixture errors

- Nurses have occasionally added lidocaine to IV potassium chloride solutions to reduce discomfort during infusion. However, this practice has led to errors, including the addition of an excessive dose of lidocaine and addition of the wrong drug (e.g., insulin instead of lidocaine). The practice could also mask infection or vein injury that presents as phlebitis, or mask symptoms of a potassium chloride overdose by preventing the burning sensation that characteristically occurs along the vein.

Improper storage or disposal

- Pets or small children who chew on a new or used lidocaine patch (e.g., Lidoderm, 5% lidocaine patch used to treat postherpetic neuralgia) may ingest a fatal amount.

Key Improvements

Constraints

- Do not place vials that hold more than 500 mg in patient care areas.

Centralize error-prone processes

- When the addition of lidocaine to potassium chloride infusions is warranted, require pharmacy to add the lidocaine and dispense the solution to patient care units as needed for specific patients.

Improve access to information

- Create a dose conversion chart reflecting lidocaine concentrations available in the facility; post it on code carts and in other areas where emergency medications may be prepared. Review the dose chart for emergency drugs during annual certification in cardiopulmonary resuscitation.
- Provide staff education on the use of topical lidocaine and the potential for toxicity from systemic absorption.

Standardize and simplify

- Specify maximum doses in protocols for the use of topical and IV lidocaine.
- Use prefilled syringes or single-dose vials to reduce the risk of overdose and eliminate the risk of contamination.
- If multidose vials are used, follow the manufacturer's recommended storage guidelines and do not refrigerate the vials after initial use.
- Use premixed, properly labeled IV solutions for all cardiology patients.
- Store a single concentration of lidocaine, where possible, on units for use in cardiac resuscitation.

Reminders

- Label all syringes and basins on and off the sterile field.
- Add warning labels to lidocaine patches and MARs to remind patients and staff to dispose of patches properly, and to apply patches only to intact skin surfaces to minimize the potential for increased absorption of lidocaine.

Patient monitoring

- Extra care and monitoring are needed when lidocaine is used in infants, the elderly, and patients with hepatic or cardiac impairment.

Failure mode and effects analysis

- Conduct FMEA to determine whether the benefits of adding lidocaine to potassium chloride infusions outweigh the risks. Consider alternatives such as optimizing oral potassium replacement, increasing IV potassium dilution, slowing the infusion rate, lowering the solution's osmolality, splitting and administering the dose in less concentrated solution via two veins simultaneously, and using a safe, rational, standardized protocol for replacement that includes access via a large-bore vein as appropriate.

Liposomal Drug Forms

Problems

Dosing errors and look-alike drug names

■ Name similarity between conventional and liposomal forms of drugs has led to administration of the wrong formulation. Such mix-ups are often harmful because of the vast differences between doses of liposomal and conventional forms. For example
  - Doses of the liposomal form of amphotericin B (Abelcet, Amphotec, Ambisome) are higher than the conventional form but vary from product to product. Giving the conventional form of amphotericin B at a higher liposomal dose has led to deaths.
  - Although both are given at 3 to 4 week intervals, conventional doxorubicin hydrochloride (Adriamycin) and liposomal doxorubicin (Doxil) are dosed differently and administered differently. Giving the liposomal form of the drug IV push, without further dilution, can cause serious harm.
  - Liposomal daunorubicin (Daunoxome) is typically dosed at 40 mg/m^2 every 2 weeks, while doses of conventional daunorubicin hydrochloride vary greatly and may be administered more frequently. Giving the conventional form at a dose appropriate for the liposomal form has led to patient harm.

Use by untrained staff

■ Staff unfamiliar with the differences between liposomal and conventional forms of drugs have prescribed, dispensed, and administered the wrong formulation, sometimes leading to patient harm from significant overdoses.

Key Improvements

Constraints

■ Dispense all antineoplastics and other products available in both liposomal and conventional forms from the pharmacy after required preparation and labeling to preserve a nurse–pharmacist double-check system. Storage in patient care areas and automated dispensing equipment is discouraged.
■ In the pharmacy, do not store conventional and liposomal products together.

Improve access to information

■ In hospitals, have pharmacy provide a list of drugs for which there are both liposomal and conventional forms, with notations about dosing differences.
■ Educate staff, at the time of new employee orientation and during continuing education programs, about the risk of patient harm if these products are confused.

Differentiate

■ Encourage physicians to include the brand name when prescribing liposomal products. (Various brands of liposomal amphotericin B are dosed quite differently.)

Encourage staff to refer to the lipid-based products by their brand names. Reinforce this safety measure in hospital and medical staff newsletters, or use other available methods of communication.

- List both the brand and generic names of liposomal products on protocols, preprinted orders, MARs, computer screens, labels, and other forms of communication about drug therapy.
- When listing generic names, place the words "liposomal form" with the drug name to enhance recognition.

Reminders

- Use cautionary labels or another mechanism to remind staff about the differences between conventional and liposomal products (e.g., "Doxil, LIPOSOMAL doxorubicin"). Also add these prominent statements to MARs.
- Program name alerts into computer systems to reduce the risk of confusing conventional and liposomal products.

Redundancies

- Require an independent double check before dispensing and administering products that are available in both liposomal and conventional forms.
- Stop and verify that the correct drug is being used if staff, patients, or family members notice a change in the solution's appearance from previous infusions. Lipid-based products may appear milky rather than clear.

Magnesium Sulfate Injection

Problems

Miscommunication of medication orders

- Errors have resulted from mix-ups between the abbreviations "MS" or "MSO$_4$" for morphine sulfate and "MgSO$_4$" for magnesium sulfate.

Dosing errors

- On occasion, "mg" (milligrams) and "mL" (milliliters) have been confused, as have "mg" and "mEq" (milliequivalents), resulting in serious dosing errors.
- Infusion pump programming errors and free-flow incidents have led to fatal overdoses.
- Staff have accidentally restarted a previously discontinued solution of magnesium sulfate used during labor instead of starting a newly hung bag of oxytocin after delivery.
- Staff have accidentally programmed a magnesium sulfate solution at the rate intended for a maintenance infusion of lactated Ringer's solution, leading to serious overdosage.

Concentration errors

- Nurse preparation of magnesium sulfate solutions has resulted in erroneous concentrations, often due to misreading the label of magnesium sulfate vials.
- Dosing errors have occurred with double-strength concentrations of magnesium sulfate for fluid-restricted obstetrical patients when the infusion pump was programmed at a rate for a standard-strength solution.

Use by untrained staff

- Patients have suffered respiratory arrest because of staff's unfamiliarity with safe dosage ranges and signs of toxicity, and inadequate monitoring.

Patient transfer

- Among the most common factors in fatal magnesium sulfate errors are transfer of obstetrical patients to units with lower staffing levels and chaotic environments with changing nursing assignments.[31]

Key Improvements

Fail-safe

- Always require that magnesium sulfate infusions be administered via an infusion pump with protection from solution free-flow when the tubing is removed from the pump (preferably, a "smart" pump with operational dose range alerts).

Constraints

- Store drug containers holding more than 2 mL of 50% magnesium sulfate only in the pharmacy.
- If IV magnesium sulfate has been discontinued, immediately remove the infusion bag and tubing from the patient's access site, pump, and IV pole to prevent later accidental infusion, and dispose of the bag properly. If the drug is discontinued temporarily, remove its tubing from the IV tubing Y-site.

Externalize or centralize error-prone processes

- Use a standard concentration of commercially available premixed solutions for bolus doses and maintenance infusions.

Improve access to information

- Educate staff during orientation and in-service training about proper dosing and signs of toxicity.

Standardize

- Standardize the concentration of magnesium sulfate solutions used in obstetrical settings.
- Establish dosing and administration protocols and standard order sets for magnesium sulfate that reference a maximum dose.
- Standardize the units of measure used for prescribing magnesium sulfate (e.g., grams or milliequivalents) and for reporting lab values (e.g., milligrams per deciliter, milliequivalents per liter, millimoles per liter).
- Prohibit the use of "$MgSO_4$" and "MSO_4" or "MS" as abbreviations for magnesium and morphine, respectively.
- Establish standard procedures for responding to emergencies caused by overdosage.
- Use 20 g/500 mL premixed solutions (not 40 g/L) to reduce harm in the event of free-flow.

Simplify

■ Administer bolus doses using separate premixed piggybacks, not from the maintenance infusion.

Reminders

■ Label all IV tubing connected to IV magnesium sulfate solutions.
■ Establish and publicize maximum doses (e.g., post wall charts in pharmacy, enter dose maximums in computer).

Redundancies

■ Require independent, redundant checks of all calculations, dose preparations, and infusion pump settings.
■ When infusions are started or the rate is adjusted, trace the tubing by hand from the IV bag to the pump, and then to the patient for verification.
■ Teach patients and families the signs of toxicity to report.
■ When transferring patients, have the receiving and transferring nurse check the drug, concentration, line attachment, and pump settings at the bedside against the original order.

Patient monitoring

■ During magnesium sulfate infusions, frequently monitor patients' vital signs, oxygen saturation, deep tendon reflexes, and level of consciousness (also fetal heart rate and maternal uterine activity if the drug is used for preterm labor).
■ Assess patients for signs of toxicity (e.g., visual changes, somnolence, flushing, muscle paralysis, loss of patellar reflexes) or pulmonary edema and notify the physician if these are observed.
■ When giving a bolus dose, remain at the bedside to monitor the patient continuously, and subsequently assess the patient at intervals of 15 minutes for the first hour, 30 minutes for the second hour, and then hourly.
■ Ensure that staffing patterns on antepartum and postpartum units allow time for proper monitoring.
■ Stock calcium gluconate on the unit, with directions for use during respiratory depression.

Oral Methotrexate for Nononcologic Use

Problems

Miscommunication of medication orders

■ Patients have taken methotrexate daily instead of once a week for nononcologic diagnoses (e.g., rheumatoid arthritis, asthma, psoriasis, inflammatory bowel disease, myasthenia gravis, inflammatory myositis), leading to fatalities and permanent disabilities. Accidental prescribing of the medication daily instead of weekly, mistaken directions on prescription labels to take the drug daily, and patients' misunderstanding of the frequency of administration all have resulted in this error.
■ Prescribers, pharmacists, and patients are more familiar with daily than with weekly dosing of medications, which contributes to occasional errors.

- "MTX," an error-prone abbreviation for methotrexate, has been misinterpreted as mitoxantrone, resulting in dispensing errors.
- Some patients have taken extra doses of methotrexate in an attempt to control their symptoms.

Look-alike names

- Handwritten orders for medications with similar-appearing names have been mistaken as orders for methotrexate and dispensed with directions to take the drug daily (e.g., an order for minoxidil 2.5 mg four times daily was dispensed as methotrexate).

Key Improvements

Improve access to information

- Include a specific clinical indication (e.g. rheumatoid arthritis, psoriasis) in the prescription directions for methotrexate. (The drug can be prescribed daily for some indications in oncology, with proper patient monitoring.)
- Establish a system to ensure that a pharmacist counsels all patients who receive weekly doses of methotrexate before each prescription is dispensed. Explain to patients that taking extra doses is dangerous. Encourage feedback to ensure that the patient understands the weekly dosing schedule and that the medication should not be used "as needed" for symptom control.
- Provide patients with printed drug information leaflets containing clear instructions about the dosing schedule.
- Prepare instructions in large print for patients with poor eyesight.

Standardize

- Avoid the use of drug name abbreviations, particularly MTX for methotrexate.

Simplify

- Provide patients with clear written instructions that name a specific day of the week for taking the tablet(s). Avoid choosing Monday, since it could be misread as "morning."
- Prescribe and dispense the drug as a dose pack (e.g., Rheumatrex by Stada Pharmaceuticals), which helps to reinforce the weekly dosing schedule.

Reminders

- Program alerts into pharmacy and prescriber computer systems to warn clinicians to verify the indication and dosing frequency whenever oral methotrexate is entered. (If the purpose of the medication is unknown to community pharmacists, they should speak directly with the prescriber to determine the reason for use and verify the proper dosing schedule.)
- Apply auxiliary labels to prescriptions to alert pharmacy staff that patient education and counseling is needed.

Redundancy

- As a final quality control check, pharmacists should always review the prescription label with the patient or caregiver before dispensing weekly methotrexate.

IV Moderate Sedation Agents

Problems

Confusion about onset of action

- Misunderstanding about the onset of midazolam's sedative effect has led to serious dosing errors. Although some clinicians believe the onset of action is immediate, the drug takes 5 to 10 minutes to reach its peak effect. Additional doses have been given in the meantime, resulting in respiratory arrest and, occasionally, death.

Dosing errors

- Overdoses have been associated with confusing labels. In some cases the concentration of the drug has been displayed on the front panel as "1 mg/mL" or "5 mg/mL." Users may erroneously believe these numbers refer to the total amount in the vial. Depending on package size, the amount actually varies from 2 mg (1 mg/mL in a 2 mL container) to 50 mg (5 mg/mL in a 10 mL container).

Titration without limits

- Overdosage has occurred when staff have continued to increase the dose or rate to achieve the desired effect, without considering maximum dose limits.

Lack of preparation for emergencies

- Staff administering midazolam have sometimes been unprepared to treat emergency conditions related to respiratory depression and arrest.

Key Improvements

Constraints

- Restrict use of moderate sedation agents to locations where staff are specifically trained to administer these drugs and monitor the patients. For example, do not use midazolam for preoperative sedation except in the OR, since appropriate monitoring equipment and trained staff may not be available.

Standardize

- Stock only one concentration of moderate sedation agents. When possible, stock the lowest concentration (e.g., 1 mg/mL of midazolam, not 5 mg/mL) to allow slow adjustment of the dose.
- Establish guidelines promoting slow administration of IV midazolam (not as a bolus or by rapid infusion), since the drug may take longer than expected to reach full effect.
- Remind adult patients who receive moderate sedation agents (including oral agents) to avoid driving or handling hazardous equipment for 24 hours after drug administration.

Patient monitoring

- Provide appropriate supportive treatment and monitoring (e.g., supplemental oxygen, pulse oximetry, capnography, automated blood pressure readings, sedation scale assessments) during the administration of moderate sedation and for an adequate period of time after the procedure.

■ Ensure that resuscitation equipment and reversal agents (when available) are readily accessible in areas where moderate sedation is administered.

Oral Moderate Sedation Agents for Children

Problems

Concentration errors

■ Oral chloral hydrate is often used for sedation in ambulatory care, particularly for pediatric patients. The drug has been available at times in two concentrations (250 mg/5 mL and 500 mg/5 mL), which has led to accidental overdosage when the higher concentration was administered in error.

■ With two concentrations available, overdosage has occurred when physicians have ordered chloral hydrate in terms of volume (e.g., teaspoonfuls) rather than in milligrams.

Dosing errors

■ Chloral hydrate may be ordered as a sedative as needed for agitated children. A child may receive multiple doses before the drug reaches its full effect, resulting in overdosage.

■ Maximum pediatric doses in current drug information compendia are unclear, which has led to accidental overdoses.

Duplicate therapy

■ Nurses have mistakenly given duplicate doses because there was confusion about the actual dose given to the child at home before the procedure.

Administration by untrained staff and parents

■ Chloral hydrate has been administered by technicians or parents who are unfamiliar with proper dosing, particularly in outpatient settings and in the patient's home; this has led to serious dosing errors.

Lack of preparation for emergencies

■ Chloral hydrate is often used as premedication before procedures, and parents, who are unfamiliar with proper dosing, are responsible for administering the drug before the designated appointment. Dosing errors at home have led to serious harm and death because proper equipment and trained staff were not available to rescue the patient.

■ Despite the recognized safety hazard, many health professionals favor administration of chloral hydrate at home because of its delayed onset of action.

Key Improvements

Constraints

■ Allow only properly trained licensed clinicians to administer oral chloral hydrate or midazolam.

■ Do not allow parents to administer sedation at home prior to a procedure. Have licensed clinicians administer the drug only after the child has arrived in a patient care area of the health care facility. (Official labeling for midazolam states that the syrup is intended for use only in monitored settings, never the home.)

- Do not order on an as-needed basis. If such an order is essential, limit the total allowable dosage (e.g., "up to 1 g").
- Limit access to bulk supplies of these medications by requiring pharmacy to dispense oral moderate sedation agents for each patient as prescribed in labeled unit dose oral syringes or unit-of-use cups.

Standardize

- Stock and prescribe only one concentration of oral moderate sedation agents.
- Prescribe and express doses in milligrams, not by volume or concentration.
- Calculate pediatric doses by weight, preferably in milligrams per kilogram.

Redundancies

- Include a milligrams per kilogram dosage along with the patient-specific dose when prescribing these medications so nurses and pharmacists can perform an independent double check of the calculated dose before dispensing or administering these drugs.

Patient monitoring

- Monitor all children who have received chloral hydrate for preoperative sedation before, during, and after the procedure.
- Have age- and size-appropriate resuscitation equipment and reversal agents available wherever the medications are administered, and where procedures under sedation are performed.

Nesiritide

Problems

Dosing errors

- This drug, used to treat congestive heart failure, is in a relatively new medication class (human peptides), with novel infusion preparation and dosing guidelines. Failure to follow these guidelines can lead to serious patient harm. Overdoses result in extreme, prolonged hypotension.
- Errors have been made when calculating infusion rates.
- Bolus doses have been incorrectly drawn directly from the vial of the drug, not from the infusion bag after mixing.

Key Improvements

Constraints

- Pharmacy should mix all infusions.
- Administer the drug only in locations where detailed cardiac monitoring, blood pressure support agents, and trained staff are available.

Improve access to information

- Provide education to nurses who will be administering the drug and monitoring its effects.

Standardize and simplify

- Follow the manufacturer's weight-based infusion table for bolus and continuous-infusion doses.

Reminders

- Add auxiliary labels to remind staff to draw the bolus from the infusion bag, not the vial.

Neuromuscular Blocking Agents

Problems

Administration to unventilated patients

- Neuromuscular blocking agents have been inadvertently administered to patients who were not receiving proper ventilator assistance. Because the respiratory muscles were paralyzed, some patients have died or sustained serious, permanent injuries. While some errors have occurred in the OR, most have taken place outside this setting, in EDs, interventional radiology departments, intensive care units (ICUs), and other medical, surgical, and psychiatric units.

Look-alike names, packages, and labels

- Vials of neuromuscular blocking agents have been mixed up with look-alike vials of products such as normal saline, heparin, and vaccines, especially when both are stored in the refrigerator.
- Infusions or syringes of neuromuscular blocking agents prepared for specific patients have been mixed up with other infusions or syringes and erroneously administered to a patient who was not being mechanically ventilated.
- Handwritten orders for vancomycin have been misread as vecuronium, leading to dispensing errors.
- Neuromuscular blocking agents have been left in the patient's medication supplies after extubation and accidentally administered instead of a medication in a look-alike infusion bag.

Unlabeled syringes

- Unlabeled syringes containing neuromuscular blocking agents have been mistaken as saline flushes and administered to unventilated patients.

Unsafe storage

- Erroneous administration of neuromuscular blocking agents has occurred when vials of the drug (which resemble vaccine vials) were unexpectedly available in the refrigerator on units where the drug was previously not stocked. (Neuromuscular blocking agents were available as floor stock outside the OR in 80% of hospitals responding to the 2004 ISMP Medication Safety Self-Assessment; 59% of respondents said that when available outside the OR, these drugs were not sequestered from other floor stock items or labeled with auxiliary warnings.)
- In one high-profile event, a neuromuscular blocking agent (mivacurium), packaged in foil overwraps, was purchased by anesthesia staff without pharmacy knowledge. The bags were subsequently delivered to the pharmacy and accidentally dispensed instead of metronidazole, another drug packaged in foil overwraps, leading to the death of a patient.

Use by untrained staff

- Neuromuscular blocking agents have been erroneously entered into the wrong patient's chart or profile and subsequently administered by staff who did not recognize that patients receiving these drugs must be ventilated.

- Patients have been extubated while an order for one of these agents still exists, occasionally leading to continued administration by staff who did not realize the patient required mechanical ventilation. (This problem has occurred upon transfer from ICU to a medical unit if an order for a neuromuscular blocking agent has not been discontinued after extubation, especially if the drug is prescribed for "agitation.")
- Nurses have occasionally administered neuromuscular blocking agents (prescribed for subsequent intubation) too soon, before the patient has been intubated.

Key Improvements

Constraints

- Allow floor stock of these agents only in the OR, ED, and critical care units, where patients can be properly ventilated and monitored.
- When these agents must be available as floor stock, have pharmacy assemble the vials in a sealed box with warnings affixed as noted below. Sequester the boxes, in both refrigerated and nonrefrigerated locations.
- Require bedside attendance of a licensed practitioner who has experience with intubation and airway management during initial administration of a neuromuscular blocking agent.
- Promptly remove discontinued neuromuscular blocking agents. Place vials, bags, and syringes of neuromuscular blocking agents in a sequestered bin for immediate pharmacy pickup after the patient has been extubated or the drug has been discontinued.

Externalize and centralize

- When possible, dispense neuromuscular blocking agents from the pharmacy as prescribed for specific patients.

Improve access to information

- Build alerts into the pharmacy computer to verify the patient's location when neuromuscular blocking agents are entered. If the patient is not in a critical care unit, ED, OR, or invasive procedure area, question the order and verify ventilatory assistance before dispensing the drug. If possible, establish computerized cross-checking of the patient's location when entering neuromuscular blocking agents (and other drugs limited to administration on a specific unit).

Standardize

- Do not accept neuromuscular blocking agent orders for "use as needed for agitation."
- Establish order sets to prevent misinterpretation of handwritten orders. Include the need for ventilation support during and after administration, and a protocol that stipulates automatic discontinuation of these agents after extubation and removal of the patient from a ventilator.
- Never accept orders to "resume the same medications" upon patient transfer.
- Never refer to neuromuscular blockers as "relaxants."

Differentiate

- Use brands of neuromuscular blockers that clearly differentiate the vials from other products through warnings on the package label, vial cap, and metal ferrule around the rubber stopper. (As of October 1, 2005, USP requires all manufacturers of these agents to provide this cautionary labeling.[32])

Reminders

- Affix commercially available fluorescent red labels that state, "Warning: Paralyzing Agent—Causes Respiratory Arrest" to each vial, syringe, bag, and storage box of neuromuscular blocking agents.
- Sequester and affix warning labels to vials of neuromuscular blocking agents stocked in the pharmacy. Be sure the labels do not obscure the vial label in any way.
- Cautionary messages reminding staff that the patient must be mechanically ventilated should appear on ADC screens when applicable. A pop-up box stating, "Ensure that the patient is intubated and ventilated" may also be helpful.

Redundancies

- Before dispensing and administering these agents, require an independent double check of the drug against the actual order.

Nitroprusside Sodium for Injection

Problems

Dosing errors

- Serious dosing errors have occurred because of miscalculated rates of infusion, misprogrammed pumps, and accidental free-flow of infusions. Excessive doses can cause severe hypotension as well as cyanide toxicity.

Titration problems

- During titration, even small boluses of the drug have resulted in severe hypotension.

Concentration errors

- Some nurses and pharmacists have mixed solutions of the drug for pediatric and neonatal patients using the "rule of 6," resulting in nonstandard concentrations and subsequent dosing errors when the dose was adjusted.

Miscommunication of drug

- Nitroprusside infusions have been administered in error instead of nitroglycerin infusions when the prescriber ordered a "nitro drip."

Look-alike labels and packages

- Nitroprusside vials have been mixed up with look-alike vials of dexamethasone.

Instability

- Exposure to light, including during administration, can alter the drug's stability.

Key Improvements

Standardize

- Avoid using the name stem "nitro" for nitroprusside or nitroglycerin.
- Standardize the concentration of nitroprusside infusions, including those administered to pediatric patients and neonates.
- Establish a protocol and preprinted orders to help guide the prescribing, preparation, administration (including wrapping IV bags in foil), and monitoring of the drug.

Simplify

- Use preprinted dosing charts to obtain infusion rates for standard concentrations of nitroprusside infusions.

Differentiate

- Stock and dispense nitroprusside vials in their original containers, because the carton packaging can help distinguish the drug from other medications. This also protects the drug from light.

Reminders

- Apply primary and important auxiliary labels to both the immediate container and the outer opaque wrapping.

Redundancies

- Require an independent double check of nitroprusside solutions before administration.

Patient monitoring

- Check the patient's blood pressure every 5 minutes at the start of the infusion and every 15 minutes thereafter.
- If possible, place an arterial pressure line and regulate drug flow to achieve the desired pressure.

Opioids, IV, Epidural, Transdermal, and Oral

Problems

Redundancies bypassed

- Narcotic accidents are among the most frequent of all serious incidents reported. One reason for errors with these drugs is that injectable narcotics are usually kept in nursing areas as floor stock items. Doses are often identified, prepared, and administered by the same nurse; no redundant safety checks are performed, as would be done if pharmacy dispensed these products as prescribed for each patient.

Look-alike drug names

- Mix-ups between hydromorphone and morphine are common; most often they are related to the look-alike product names and some practitioners' misconception that hydromorphone is the generic name for morphine. Hydromorphone is approximately five times as potent as morphine.

■ Opioids are often stored side by side in secured storage areas. This has contributed to selection of the wrong medication, as have the look-alike syringes, vials, and minibags of various opioids.

Dosing errors

■ Misprogramming of infusion pumps has led to serious opioid overdoses.

■ Fentanyl patches have not been removed prior to application of a new patch, leading to overdoses. The clear backing of some patches makes them difficult to see once applied to the skin.

■ Fentanyl has sometimes been improperly prescribed for episodes of acute pain, such as postoperative pain or pain from dental surgery.

■ Patients who have not been educated about the use of fentanyl patches have applied multiple patches to the site of their pain, leading to serious overdoses and fatalities.

■ Physicians have prescribed fentanyl patches in doses that were too high for opioid-naïve patients, leading to overdoses and fatalities.

■ Opium tincture has been dispensed and administered instead of paregoric (camphorated tincture of opium), leading to fatal overdoses. (Paregoric has just 0.4 mg/mL of morphine, whereas opium tincture contains 10 mg/mL.)

Miscommunication of drugs

■ DTO (as an abbreviation for deodorized tincture of opium) has been used to mean diluted opium tincture (1:25) or paregoric, leading to confusion about the actual dose and to serious dosing errors.

■ The abbreviations MSO_4 (for morphine sulfate) and $MgSO_4$ (for magnesium sulfate) have been confused, leading to administration of morphine when magnesium was intended.

Concentration errors

■ Concentrated forms of oral liquid morphine (20 mg/mL) have often been confused with the standard solution (2 mg/mL), leading to serious errors and fatalities.

■ Overdoses of oral liquid morphine have resulted when physicians prescribe the medication by volume rather than by metric weight and nurses use the more concentrated form to prepare the dose.

■ Pharmacists and nurses have selected the 5 mg/mL morphine concentration instead of the 1 mg/mL concentration for PCA use.

■ Extended-release and immediate-release morphine products have been confused.

PCA by proxy

■ Delivery of opioid doses via PCA devices by nurses or family members has led to serious and fatal dosing errors.

■ Improper patient selection for PCA has led to unsafe use in unresponsive adults, young children, and neonates, who cannot activate the pump themselves.

Accidental epidural administration

■ PCA and epidural lines are sometimes confused, leading to errors in route of administration.

PCA infusion pump design flaws

- Several manufacturers' PCA pumps have unsafe default settings. For example, an Abbott PCA pump defaults to a 0.1 mg/mL setting, which has been misread as 1 mg/mL during programming for morphine infusion. A Deltec PCA pump (CADD-Prizm PCS Pain Control System) defaults to a preexisting concentration if the current setting is not confirmed by pressing "Enter" within a short period of time. Both design flaws have resulted in fatal overdoses.

Adverse drug reactions

- Allergic reactions to opioids are common.
- Meperidine use, especially in the elderly, has led to toxic levels of its metabolite, normeperidine, which, in turn, may induce irritability and nervousness, agitation, twitching, tremors, and even generalized tonic-clonic seizures.

Inadequate pain control

- Some patients have not received adequate pain control because they do not know how to use the PCA device.

Patient monitoring problems

- Insufficient monitoring of patients receiving opioids has resulted in respiratory arrest.

Unintended use

- Fentanyl patches prescribed for adults have been applied by young children because of unsecured storage or disposal (used patches still contain significant amounts of the drug).

Key Improvements

Constraints

- Limit oral liquid opioids available in floor stock to conventional concentrations. Avoid stocking concentrated morphine solutions in patient care units; this includes the ED, since the drug is used primarily to treat chronic pain.
- Dispense concentrated oral morphine solutions only when ordered for a specific patient (not as unit stock).
- Separate morphine and hydromorphone in drug storage areas.
- Avoid the use of meperidine for pain control, especially in the elderly.
- Consider deleting paregoric and opium tincture from the hospital formulary; there are more effective medications for treating pain and controlling diarrhea. In neonatal abstinence syndrome due to opioid withdrawal, some pediatricians recommend opium tincture in a 1:25 dilution. This is similar to the amount of morphine in paregoric, but paregoric contains 45% alcohol and other potentially harmful ingredients, so pharmacy should prepare an aqueous oral solution of morphine from morphine injection.
- Do not store opium tincture on patient care units, including in automated dispensing units.
- Dispense opium tincture for individual patients in a small dropper bottle or unit dose package.

■ Return unused supplies of concentrated liquid morphine to the pharmacy immediately after patient discharge.

■ Instruct patients who use fentanyl patches to store and dispose of the patches in a secure manner to avoid unintended access by children, pets, or drug-seeking adults.

Improve access to information

■ Educate staff about the possibility of mix-ups between hydromorphone and concentrated morphine.

■ Post equianalgesic charts for opioid-to-opioid conversions on all patient care units for reference by prescribers and nurses.

■ Include the brand name Dilaudid along with the generic name hydromorphone when prescribing, transcribing, and dispensing (on labels) this drug.

■ Educate patients and families about PCA preoperatively, preferably before admission when patients are alert, not after they have received anesthesia. Teach patients how to use PCA, and warn against dosing by proxy.

■ Before applying a fentanyl patch to a newly admitted patient, ask about patches that may have been applied at home. If the patient is unable to be questioned, inspect the skin before applying the patch.

■ Establish appropriate dose ranges for opioids by weight, and build alerts into the order entry system for exceeding a maximum dose.

Standardize

■ Establish one standard concentration for each opioid in use.

■ Prohibit MSO_4 (morphine sulfate) and $MgSO_4$ (magnesium sulfate) as abbreviations.

■ Use only generic names, except for hydromorphone, which can be more easily distinguished by using the brand name Dilaudid followed by the generic name.

■ Reduce the variety of opioids and other analgesics prescribed for patients, through applicable protocols and various standard order sets.

■ Always prescribe or dispense liquid medications with the dose specified in milligrams.

■ Establish protocols and preprinted orders for PCA.

■ In establishing patient selection criteria for PCA, consider this safety feature: A sedated patient will not press the button.

■ Standardize to a single drug, morphine, as the opioid of choice for PCA.

■ Do not refer to paregoric by its dangerous synonyms, camphorated tincture of opium or DTO for diluted solutions. If the product is available, paregoric, the official name for camphorated tincture of opium, should be used in prescribing and for listing on formularies, in computer systems, and on labels.

Differentiate

■ Stock morphine and hydromorphone in different strengths or forms (e.g., 1 mL prefilled syringes of hydromorphone 1 mg/1 mL; 2 mL prefilled syringes of morphine 2 mg/mL).

■ Use tall-man lettering, HYDROmorphone, on pharmacy labels, auxiliary labels, MARs, and drug listings in computer order entry systems and ADC screens. It may also be helpful to emphasize the final "o" in the name (HYDROmorphOne).

- Affix an auxiliary label to concentrated solutions to avoid confusion with standard concentrations.
- Apply auxiliary labels to prefilled syringes of opioids that look similar to help differentiate them.

Reminders

- Label the distal ends of all access lines to distinguish IV from epidural lines.
- Apply auxiliary labels to concentrated forms of morphine or other opioids noting that the drugs are highly concentrated.
- Place auxiliary labels on all containers stating the strength of morphine per milliliter (10 mg/mL), as well as labels stating, "WARNING! Do NOT use opium tincture in place of paregoric."
- Build alerts into the computer system to warn staff about the differences between paregoric and opium tincture.
- If concentrated morphine is available on patient units, affix an auxiliary label to the bottle and segregate the concentrated solution from the other concentrations.

Redundancies

- Implement protocols for the use of PCA and other opioids that ensure independent double checks of the appropriateness of the drug, dose, pump setting, and line placement.
- Question all patients about allergies and sensitivities to opioids before administration.

Patient monitoring

- Ensure that oxygen and naloxone or an equivalent are available in areas where narcotics are administered.
- Establish guidelines for appropriate monitoring of patients who are receiving opioids.
- In patients receiving opioids, frequently monitor the quality of respirations and be alert to signs of oversedation.
- If providing nurse-delivered PCA to confused adults or young children, establish strict requirements for enhanced observation and monitoring.
- Do not rely on pulse oximetry readings alone to detect opioid toxicity. Use capnography to detect respiratory changes caused by opioids, especially for patients who are at high risk (e.g., patients with sleep apnea, obese patients).

Failure mode and effects analysis

- Conduct FMEA for PCA to uncover risks and take action to reduce the chance of harmful errors (see Chapter 21 for an example).

Phosphate Salts (Sodium and Potassium)

Problems

Dosing errors

- Physicians, pharmacists, and nurses have not considered the amount of potassium in potassium phosphate; excessive oral or IV potassium from potassium phosphate has resulted in serious harm, including fatalities.

Calculation errors

■ Errors have occurred in converting a dose ordered in milligrams to the dosing unit that is stated on the product label or required for entry into the pharmacy system.

Miscommunication of drug doses

■ Prescribers occasionally order phosphate in terms of "amps" or "vials" rather than the amount (expressed in millimoles [mmol]), leading to dosing errors if the vial used to prepare the dose contains more than the physician intended.

Improper manufacturer labeling

■ Commercially available vials have been labeled as "single dose." This is misleading because the vials come in various sizes and some contain several doses. Such confusion has led to dosing errors.
■ Some commercial products are poorly labeled, making it difficult to interpret the contents of a vial. Practitioners have confused milliliter (mL), millimole (mmol), milliequivalent (mEq), and milligram (mg) amounts listed on labeling.

Look-alike vials

■ Vials of sodium phosphate and potassium phosphate have been mixed up on automated compounders.

Use by untrained staff

■ Undiluted potassium phosphate has been administered IV, leading to cardiac arrest.

Key Improvements

Constraints

■ Store IV potassium phosphate solutions only in the pharmacy, except in controlled-access night cabinets where 24-hour pharmacy service is not available.
■ Administer phosphate replacement therapy by the oral route whenever possible.
■ Use sodium phosphate instead of potassium phosphate when possible.

Improve access to information

■ Add auxiliary labels to any vials that are stored outside the pharmacy (e.g., in a night cabinet), highlighting the contents expressed in the standard dosing units.
■ Program alerts for potassium and phosphate into computer ordering systems to warn of excessive doses or of dose adjustments that may be indicated by the patient's most recent laboratory results.

Standardize

■ Use guidelines for potassium phosphate administration based on the patient's level of inorganic phosphate and other clinical factors (e.g., weight or age). The normal dose should not exceed 0.32 mmol/kg over 12 hours, repeated until serum phosphate is greater than 2 mg/dL.

- Assess the appropriateness of orders for potassium phosphate in terms of phosphorus and potassium content. If possible, enter the dose of each component into the pharmacy computer system.
- Establish a standard dosing unit to be used for all potassium phosphate orders (e.g., millimoles). Do not accept orders if the dose is not specified.
- Establish standard criteria for delivery rates of IV phosphate. Use a pump to administer all solutions.

Redundancies

- Require quality control checks of all solutions added to pharmacy compounders before use of the equipment.
- Require an independent double check of any dose calculations and dose preparation before potassium phosphate administration.

Patient monitoring

- Assess the patient's most recent serum potassium and phosphate levels before prescribing, dispensing, or administering potassium phosphate; assess recent sodium and phosphorus levels before prescribing, dispensing, or administering sodium phosphate.
- Monitor patients' electrolytes before, during, and after replacement therapy; perform electrocardiography as indicated.

Potassium Chloride for Injection
Problems
Miscommunication of drug therapy

- Some physicians use the term "bolus" when ordering potassium at a rapid rate to treat acute hypokalemia. Such orders have been misunderstood to mean that the dose should be given by IV push, using a syringe.

Dosing errors

- Simultaneous infusion of multiple potassium chloride-containing products has resulted in overdoses.

Nursing IV admixture errors

- Nurses have improperly added potassium chloride to IV solutions, resulting in dosing errors as well as inadvertent rapid administration of large doses because the potassium chloride additive and the IV solution were not properly mixed.

Mental slip

- Nurses who know that concentrated potassium chloride cannot be administered IV have inadvertently selected a vial of potassium chloride and administered it along with, or instead of, furosemide, in large part because they have made a mental slip and quickly associated potassium loss from diuretics with potassium chloride.

Unsafe storage

- Vials of concentrated potassium chloride have been available in patient care units, contributing to mix-ups with look-alike vials.

Look-alike vials

- On patient care units, vials of potassium chloride have been mixed up with look-alike vials (e.g., insulin, heparin, sterile water, sterile saline), leading to serious errors and harm.
- Vials of potassium chloride have been mixed up with other vials, particularly sodium chloride vials, in the pharmacy during the compounding of electrolyte solutions, including adult and infant TPN, and dialysate.
- Bulk supply cartons of potassium chloride and sodium chloride have been mixed up, leading to later compounding errors.

Use by untrained staff

- Undiluted potassium chloride has been administered IV, leading to cardiac arrest.
- Diluted potassium chloride has been infused too rapidly (i.e., at a rate exceeding 10 mEq of potassium chloride per hour), leading to cardiac arrest.
- Some clinicians erroneously believe IV potassium chloride replacement therapy must be started immediately; thus, they may not want to await pharmacy dispensing of the solution.

Key Improvements

Constraints

- Do not store concentrated potassium chloride vials on patient care units, including in automated dispensing modules, except in controlled-access night cabinets where 24-hour pharmacy service is not available.
- Potassium chloride should never be given by IV push, and initiation of an infusion is never an emergency. Therefore, there is no need to store concentrated potassium chloride outside the pharmacy, especially if premixed solutions are available.
- In pharmacies, store bulk supplies and immediate inventory of concentrated potassium chloride (and other concentrated electrolytes) in areas totally segregated from other drugs and distinctly separated by product.
- Validate the competency of staff engaged in medication-use processes that involve concentrated electrolytes (including potassium replacement therapy).

Externalize or centralize error-prone processes

- Purchase premixed solutions in 10, 20, and 40 mEq strengths in 50 or 100 mL minibags and large-volume bags.
- Centralize the preparation of IV potassium chloride solution in the pharmacy, and dispense solutions to patient care units in a timely manner.

Improve access to information

- Program alerts into computer systems to warn of excessive doses or of the need for dose adjustment as indicated by the patient's most recent laboratory results.

Standardize

- Medical staff should work to standardize available solutions and ensure that premixed solutions maintained in the pharmacy or in patient care areas match the ordering preferences of prescribers.

- Do not compound electrolyte solutions that are available commercially.
- Establish and follow standard protocols for potassium replacement therapy; include the following:
  - Indications for IV potassium chloride (example: patient's serum potassium is <2.8 meq/L, patient is on diuretics or other potassium-wasting medications),
  - Maximum rate of IV delivery,
  - Maximum allowable concentration,
  - Guidelines for when continuous cardiac monitoring is necessary,
  - Stipulation that potassium chloride be given via a pump or other suitable infusion control device,
  - Prohibition of IV administration of multiple simultaneous potassium chloride solutions (e.g., no IV potassium chloride while receiving TPN; Ringer's solution contains 4 mEq of potassium per liter),
  - Automatic substitution of oral potassium chloride for IV potassium by pharmacy when appropriate,
  - Use of preprinted order forms for potassium replacement therapy,
  - Standardized terminology for prescribing the electrolyte; the term "bolus" is not to be used in reference to potassium chloride, and
  - Frequency of laboratory studies to monitor electrolyte levels.

Differentiate

- Purchase concentrated electrolytes from different vendors if possible, to avoid packaging similarities.

Redundancies

- When concentrated electrolytes are delivered to the pharmacy, require two individuals to independently verify that the correct product has been received and that it has been placed in the proper storage area.
- Require a pharmacist to perform a final independent check of all IV admixtures of electrolyte solutions (containing potassium chloride), including batch solutions.
- Perform quality control checks for automated compounders used to prepare electrolyte solutions (containing potassium chloride).

Failure mode and effects analysis

- Inventory all concentrated electrolytes in the pharmacy and perform FMEA, paying particular attention to errors that may originate in the pharmacy. Be sure to include evaluation of the look-alike potential of product containers. Take the necessary steps to reduce the risk of errors.

Radiocontrast Agents, IV

Problems

Accidental intrathecal administration

- Inadvertent intrathecal injection of ionic water-soluble contrast media has led to severe neurotoxicity and death.

Drug interactions

- Orders for radiocontrast media are not routinely screened by pharmacy, and significant interactions between radiocontrast media and current patient medications have been missed.

Adverse drug reactions

- Patient allergy information may not be readily available to radiology staff, which increases the risk of preventable allergic reactions.

Complications of IV administration process

- Extravasation and air emboli have occurred during administration of contrast media.

Delayed onset of symptoms from an error

- Symptoms of accidental administration of ionic water-soluble contrast media are often delayed 1 to 6 hours after administration, which reduces the opportunity to recognize the error and treat the patient quickly.

Ineffective manufacturer label warning

- FDA-required warnings on the labels ("Not for Intrathecal Use," "Not for Myelography") of ionic water-soluble contrast media have not been wholly effective; some warning statements are not prominent or centered on the vial.

Look-alike containers

- Mix-ups have occurred between look-alike vials of contrast media, especially if the products are from the same manufacturer. (For example, Hypaque [diatrizoate meglumine, used for cerebral angiography] has been confused with nonionic Omnipaque 300 [iohexol, used for myelography] from the same manufacturer.)

Key Improvements

Constraints

- Store each type of contrast medium separately, according to use.
- Store nonionic products used strictly for intrathecal procedures in a locked box in an exam room reserved only for intrathecal procedures.

Improve access to information

- Label all syringes of contrast media, even if only one product is in use.
- Post educational charts about the use of each contrast agent in areas where the drugs are used.
- Provide radiology with a list of medications that may cause serious interactions with radiocontrast media.
- Provide radiology staff and nurses who may be caring for patients after myelography with a written list of symptoms associated with inadvertent use of an ionic water-soluble contrast agent, to promote timely recognition of errors and treatment.

Simplify

- Package kits for myelograms that include the proper contrast agent.

Reminders

- Affix prominent auxiliary labels to ionic contrast media, noting that they should not be used for myelography.

Redundancies

- If radiology manages the procurement of contrast media, a pharmacist (rather than a technician or the purchasing department) should evaluate all requisitions and double-check all products before they are dispensed to the radiology department.
- Independent double checks of the contrast medium, or a "time out" like those used with surgical procedures (i.e., JCAHO's universal protocol for preventing wrong site, wrong procedure, or wrong person surgery), should precede administration.

Failure mode and effects analysis

- Perform FMEA on the use of radiocontrast media and address the hazards uncovered, including inadvertent intrathecal administration of ionic contrast media, allergic reactions, extravasation, and air emboli during administration. Ensure that all areas where contrast media are stored (e.g., radiology, OR, cardiac catheterization lab) are represented.
- During FMEA, also evaluate pharmacy's role in the distribution of contrast media. These products are not just standard floor stock items; they should be given as much attention as other injectable drugs.

Sodium Chloride Injection (Hypertonic)

Problems

Dosing errors

- Accidental IV administration of hypertonic sodium chloride solution has caused rapid changes in serum sodium concentration, resulting in serious harm and death.

Unsafe storage

- Infusion of hypertonic sodium chloride injection is rarely necessary; nonetheless, this product has been available on patient care units, contributing to mix-ups with look-alike vials and IV bags.

Look-alike packages

- Bags of 5% sodium chloride injection have been confused with 5% dextrose and sodium chloride injection.
- Bags of 3% sodium chloride injection may be confused with 0.3% sodium chloride injection, which may be ordered as a nonstandard concentration. (Standard concentrations are dextrose with 0.2% sodium chloride injection, and 0.45% and 0.9% sodium chloride injection alone or in combination with dextrose.) Even the 3% product has 512 mEq/L, or 0.5 mEq/mL, of sodium.
- Vials of hypertonic sodium chloride in 23.4% or 14.6% concentrations (sometimes found in pediatric ICUs for use in preparing enteral feedings) have been mixed up with other vials, particularly 0.9% sodium chloride vials.

Improper manufacturer labeling

- Regulatory authorities have not established labeling standards with appropriate highly visible warnings to help reduce medication errors associated with hypertonic forms.

Key Improvements

Constraints

- Allow only commercially available standard concentrations of sodium chloride injection outside the pharmacy. (One exception follows.)
- In dialysis units, stock a single concentration of hypertonic saline. Store it in a locked area, limit access, and affix special hazard labeling. (Dialysis units may use hypertonic solutions to increase blood volume and reduce cramping.)
- Do not stock 5% sodium chloride injection in the facility; stock the 3% concentration because it is less likely to be confused with 5% dextrose solutions.
- In pharmacies, store bulk supplies and immediate inventory of concentrated sodium chloride (and other concentrated electrolytes) in areas totally segregated from other drugs.
- Validate the competency of staff engaged in medication-use processes that involve concentrated electrolytes (including sodium chloride).

Centralize error-prone processes

- Limit the mixing of enteral feedings to pharmacy if periodic adjustments in sodium content are needed.
- Centralize IV admixture of electrolyte solutions that contain sodium chloride.

Improve access to information

- Program alerts into computerized systems to warn of excessive sodium chloride doses or of dose adjustments that may be indicated by the patient's most recent laboratory results.

Standardize

- Establish and follow standard protocols for treatment of hyponatremia; include the following:
  - Indications that clearly specify when to use isotonic or hypertonic sodium chloride solutions,
  - Maximum rate of IV delivery,
  - Maximum allowable concentration,
  - Stipulation that sodium chloride solutions used to treat hyponatremia be given via a pump or other suitable infusion control device, and
  - Frequency of laboratory studies to monitor electrolyte levels.

Differentiate

- Purchase concentrated electrolytes from different vendors if possible, to avoid packaging similarities.

Redundancies

- When concentrated electrolytes are delivered to the pharmacy, require two individuals to independently verify that the correct product has been received and that it has been placed in the proper storage area.
- Require a pharmacist to perform a final independent check of all IV admixtures of electrolyte solutions (containing sodium chloride), including batch solutions.
- Perform quality control checks for automated compounders used to prepare electrolyte solutions (which use concentrated sodium chloride).

Failure mode and effects analysis

- Inventory all concentrated electrolytes in the pharmacy and perform FMEA, paying particular attention to errors that may originate in the pharmacy. Be sure to include evaluation of the look-alike potential of product containers. Take the necessary steps to reduce the risk of errors.

Thrombolytics and Fibrinolytics, IV

Problems

Miscommunication of drugs

- Alteplase has been called "t-PA." This drug designation has been confused with TNKase (tenecteplase), which has been called TNK-t-TPA. Each fibrinolytic has its own dosing regimen, so confusion has resulted. Serious dosing errors and hemorrhage have occurred when TNKase was given instead of Activase.
- "t-PA" has been confused with "t-RA" (oral tretinoin [Vesanoid], an antineoplastic), and with "r-PA" (reteplase [Retavase], another thrombolytic).

Used by untrained staff

- Nurses have confused the different thrombolytics and fibrinolytics and administered the wrong drug to patients, especially when multiple agents were available.

Lack of preparation for emergencies

- Delayed administration has resulted in less than optimal results.

Nursing IV admixture errors

- Nurses have improperly prepared the solutions, primarily in the ED, leading to subtherapeutic effects or to overdosage and subsequent hemorrhage.

Incompatibilities

- Heparin and reteplase can be given simultaneously but never mixed within the same container or administered through the same IV line. Together, the drugs react to form a mass of solid or semisolid material, which can stop the infusion.

Key Improvements

Constraints

- Remove thrombolytic and fibrinolytic agents from unit stock where possible, and have pharmacy dispense the solutions as prescribed in a timely manner. (Although an increasing number of hospitals can accomplish this with satellite pharmacies, clinical pharmacists, "clot-buster" teams, or 24-hour pharmacy service, most sites still store thrombolytics in the ED to decrease "door-to-needle" time.)
- If pharmacy cannot prepare all solutions, create "heart attack" (acute myocardial infarction) and "brain attack" (stroke) boxes that contain the correct agent, related protocol, and clear instructions for preparing, dosing, and administering the drug and monitoring the patient. (Alternatively, some facilities have affixed stickers to the opening of each carton, describing how to prepare and dose the drug for specific indications.)

Standardize

- Establish protocols for use of each agent for each indication. Include dosing instructions and administration precautions, including incompatibilities.
- Limit the variety of agents on the formulary, and select one to manage heart attacks and one to manage brain attacks. (Some have chosen Activase and Retavase because they are dosed in milligrams and units, respectively, which helps differentiate them.)
- Prescribe the drugs using preprinted order sets (one for each drug) that list both the brand and generic name.
- Avoid the use of "t-PA" to describe any of the tissue plasminogen activators, "TNK" for TNKase, "r-PA" for reteplase, and "t-RA" for tretinoin.

Reminders

- Display warnings on ADC screens about the potential for mix-ups among the different agents available.

Redundancies

- Require an independent double check of all drugs and doses, including loading bolus and pump settings.

Total Parenteral Nutrition Solutions
Problems
Compounding errors

- Errors made in preparing TPN (particularly with the dextrose content) have resulted in serious and permanent neurological effects and death.
- Errors have occurred when pharmacy technicians have manually added medications to TPN, particularly insulin in neonatal TPN, since a different concentration (10 units/mL) is often required. If the pharmacist checks only the volume of drug added to the TPN (as marked by the used syringe) without verifying the concentration, accidental use of insulin in a standard concentration (100 units/mL) may not be detected before the solution is dispensed.

Order entry errors

- Doses of electrolytes in TPN have been entered into the pharmacy computer incorrectly; this occurs especially with orders for pediatric TPN when the amounts of some additives are on a per liter basis and the amounts of others are on a per container basis.

Dosing errors

- Errors in infusion rates have led to overdoses and rapid infusions of dextrose.

Look-alike containers

- Since enteral feeding bags can be spiked with an IV administration set, they have been mistaken for three-in-one TPN solutions, which can look similar, and administered IV. TPN and cardioplegic solutions often look alike because of the multiplicity of electrolytes in both and the similar volumes, labels (including computer-generated pharmacy labels), and containers.

Miscommunication of drugs

- TPN has been used as an abbreviation for Taxol/Platinol/Navelbine in oncology; this meaning could be confused with total parenteral nutrition.

Key Improvements

Constraints

- Segregate products used to prepare neonatal TPN solutions from products used to prepare adult TPN.
- Allow only specially trained pharmacy staff to prepare all TPN solutions.

Externalize or centralize error-prone processes

- Outsource the preparation to a reputable company.

Standardize

- Use preprinted order sheets or computerized order sets for all TPN orders.
- Standardize the way additives should be prescribed; use a single, consistent dosing method (e.g., amount per liter, amount per 24-hour container).
- Standardize the insulin dilution used in the preparation of neonatal TPN.
- Spell out all chemotherapy orders to avoid any confusion with TPN.
- When mixing neonatal TPN with insulin, use a standard dilution of insulin, clearly labeled as "NICU only."

Differentiate

- Affix a special label to cardioplegic solutions to reduce the similarity of their appearance to that of other solutions.

Simplify

- Many consider it best practice to treat hyperglycemia in patients on TPN with a separate insulin infusion that can be adjusted independently according to the patient's blood glucose level. (If the insulin is being delivered separately, it can also be discontinued temporarily if the patient's serum glucose concentration is low, while the TPN solution continues to deliver essential nutrition. However, if the TPN infusion is slowed or discontinued but the insulin infusion is accidentally left at the same rate, hypoglycemia could occur; therefore, directions to adjust or discontinue the insulin infusion under these conditions should be tied to the TPN order and listed prominently on the MAR.)

Reminders

- Label enteral feedings with "WARNING—For enteral use only, not for IV use."

Redundancies

- Require an independent double check before infusing TPN.
- Employ end-product testing of TPN (e.g., refractometry) to verify the base glucose solution.

Warfarin

Problems

Duplicate or concurrent therapy

- Injuries and fatalities have occurred from unrecognized concomitant use of warfarin and other anticoagulants or thrombolytics.
- Confusion about the generic and brand names has led consumers to take both warfarin and Coumadin, leading to dangerous duplicate therapy and bleeding.

Accidental stoppage of therapy

- Automatic stop orders for patients taking the drug for alternative purposes (e.g., atrial fibrillation) can cause unintended discontinuation.
- Prescribers have occasionally forgotten to resume warfarin therapy after holding a dose or doses because of an elevated international normalized ratio (INR). Failure to resume therapy has resulted in thrombosis.

Look-alike names

- Handwritten orders for Avandia (rosiglitazone), a diabetes drug, have been confused with orders for Coumadin (warfarin).

Patient monitoring problems

- Failure to verify the most recent laboratory values before administering warfarin has resulted in preventable bleeding episodes.
- Improper monitoring of prothrombin time (PT) or INR has resulted in preventable bleeding.
- Clinicians may adjust doses too frequently without assessing downward or upward trends in INR values, potentially resulting in labile anticoagulation levels.
- Lab-related errors have resulted in incorrect INR calculations. Changes in the thromboplastin reagent without requisite changes in equipment calibration have led to erroneously low INR values and rare fatalities from overdoses of warfarin. The amount and concentration of sodium citrate in blood collection tubes and overfilling the tube with blood can also produce artificially prolonged or shortened clotting times.

Dosing errors

- Directions to take different doses on alternate days have confused patients and led to errors.
- Frequent dose adjustments on the basis of lab results have led to confusion and subsequent patient self-administration errors, especially since dose adjustments are usually made by telephone and the directions on the patient's prescription bottle may be different from what is currently prescribed.
- If prescribers have used phytonadione to reverse the effects of warfarin in preparation for a procedure (e.g., cardiac catheterization), they may resume therapy and continue to increase the warfarin dose for days, not realizing that the phytonadione administered before the procedure is still blocking the effects of warfarin. When the effects subside, the warfarin dose may be dangerously high, increasing the risk of bleeding.

Drug and food interactions

- Clinically significant drug, herbal, and food interactions with warfarin have been overlooked, leading to subtherapeutic or excessive anticoagulation.

Key Improvements

Improve access to information

- Encourage patients to keep a medication diary or home MAR to document all doses administered and better track alternating or changing doses.
- Provide patients with oral and written information about dietary effects on warfarin and how to maintain a diet to reduce fluctuations in INR.
- When giving patients dose changes over the telephone, ask them to
  - Retrieve a pen and paper,
  - Document the information as received and date the entry,
  - Read back the dose and instructions to verify understanding, and
  - Keep the new information with the prescription bottle for reference.
- Provide patient education by certified staff in a structured setting.
- Have pharmacists investigate all orders for phytonadione doses of 10 mg or higher. If phytonadione is being used to reverse the effects of warfarin before a procedure, recommend a dose lower than 10 mg and ensure that the prescriber understands that the effects of phytonadione will linger after the procedure. If warfarin is restarted, it may take a few days to reach a therapeutic dosage.
- Ensure that computer alerts for duplicate therapy are fully functional for anti-coagulants and related antithrombotic medications.
- Do not automatically discontinue warfarin according to automatic stop policies (if applicable) without verifying the drug's indication and contacting the physician.

Reminders

- Program the pharmacy computer system for alerts to impending drug interactions. For the most clinically significant alerts, require pharmacists to document a reason before bypassing the alert.

Patient monitoring

- Establish protocols for the frequency of laboratory monitoring for patients beginning and continuing warfarin therapy.
- Establish a reliable tickler system for patients whose warfarin has been placed on hold; these patients should be contacted within a designated time frame (e.g., 24 hours after lab testing) to advise them about the resumption of warfarin therapy.
- If warfarin doses are based on frequent lab testing, the pharmacy profile and nursing MAR should reflect this as an ongoing active order, listing the drug, route, and frequency and noting that a dose must be prescribed each day.
- If warfarin is held for a procedure, the order should be rewritten fully after the procedure.
- Implement pharmacy monitoring of inpatients on warfarin and pharmacy-run outpatient anticoagulation clinics to improve patient monitoring and education.
- Use process control charts to track INR values in order to clearly visualize trends and ensure minimal variation. Set upper and lower limits that signal the need

for a dose adjustment, especially if the threshold is breached two or more consecutive times.

- Clinical staff should ask the lab to investigate if INR results do not appear to correlate with the clinical status of the patient. (Centralized pharmacy monitoring of patients on warfarin will help identify possible lab errors.)

REFERENCES

1. Institute for Safe Medication Practices. Survey on high-alert medications. Differences between nursing and pharmacy perspectives revealed. *ISMP Medication Safety Alert!* October 16, 2003;8(21).
2. Tubman M, Majumdar SR, Lee D, et al. Best practices for safe handling of products containing concentrated potassium. *BMJ.* 2005;331:274–7.
3. Leape LL, Berwick DM, Bates DW. What practices will most improve safety? Evidence-based medicine meets patient safety. *JAMA.* 2002;288:501–7.
4. Smith GCS, Pell JP. Parachute use to prevent death and major trauma related to gravitational challenge: systemic review of randomized controlled trials. *BMJ.* 2003;327:1459–61.
5. Hyland S, Senders J, Perri D, et al. Potassium chloride issue needs clarification. *BMJ.* Rapid Response August 5, 2005. Available at: http://bmj.bmjjournals.com/cgi/eletters/331/7511/274#114016#114016.
6. Cohen MR, Senders J, Davis NM. Failure mode and effects analysis: a novel approach to avoiding dangerous medication errors and accidents. *Hosp Pharm.* 1994;29:319–24, 326–8, 330.
7. Infusion Pumps: Preventing Future Adverse Events. *Sentinel Event Alert.* No. 15. Oakbrook Terrace, Ill: Joint Commission on Accreditation of Healthcare Organizations. November 30, 2000. Available at: www.jointcommission.org/SentinelEvents/SentinelEventAlert/sea_15.htm.
8. Cohen MR, Davis NM. Free flow associated with electronic infusion devices: an underestimated danger. *Hosp Pharm.* 1992;27(May):384–90.
9. *ECRI Special Report SR0018.* Plymouth Meeting, Pa: ECRI; March 21, 2003.
10. *The United States Pharmacopeia, 27th rev, and The National Formulary, 22nd ed*; First Supplement. Rockville, Md: U.S. Pharmacopeia; February 2004.
11. Kastango ES, Bradshaw BD. *USP* chapter 797: establishing a practice standard for compounding sterile preparations in pharmacy. *Am J Health Syst Pharm.* 2004;61:1928–38.
12. Commonwealth of Pennsylvania. Patient Safety Authority. Use of Color-Coded Patient Wristbands Creates Unnecessary Risk. *Patient Safety Advisory.* 2005;2 (December 14).
13. Institute for Safe Medication Practices. Designing preprinted order forms that prevent medication errors. *ISMP Medication Safety Alert!* April 23, 1997.
14. Norman DA. *The Design of Everyday Things.* New York: Doubleday/Currency; 1988.
15. Kohn LT, Corrigan JM, Donaldson MS, eds. *To Err Is Human: Building a Safer Health System.* Washington, DC: National Academies Press; 2000.
16. Grasha A. Cognitive systems perspective on human performance in the pharmacy: implications for accuracy, effectiveness, and job satisfaction. Executive Summary Report. Alexandria, Va: National Association of Chain Drug Stores; October 2000. Report No. 062100.
17. Filik R, Purdy K, Gale A, et al. Drug name confusion: evaluating the effectiveness of capital ("Tall Man") letters using eye movement data. *Soc Sci Med.* 2004;59:2597–601.
18. U.S. Food and Drug Administration. Center for Drug Evaluation and Research, Office of Generic Drugs. FDA Name Differentiation Project. May 8, 2002. Available at: www.fda.gov/cder/drug/MedErrors/nameDiff.htm.
19. Leape LL. Error in medicine. *JAMA.* 1994;272:1851–7.
20. Trissel LA, Zhang Y, Cohen MR. The stability of diluted vincristine sulfate used as a deterrent to inadvertent intrathecal injection. *Hosp Pharm.* 2001;36:740–5.
21. Fuloria M, Friedberg MA, DuRant RH, et al. Effect of flow rate and insulin priming on the recovery of insulin from microbore infusion tubing. *Pediatrics.* 1998;102:1401–6.
22. Reinhart L, Panning CA. Insulin glargine: a new long-acting insulin product. *Am J Health Syst Pharm.* 2002;59:643–9.
23. Parkin C, Brooks N. Is postprandial glucose control important? Is it practical in primary care settings? *Clin Diabetes.* 2002;20:71–6.
24. Jehle DR, Breitig D, Boehm BO. Inadequate suspension of NPH insulin in pens. *Lancet.* 1999;354:1604–7.
25. Rolfe S, Harper NJ. Ability of hospital doctors to calculate drug doses. *BMJ.* 1995;310:1173–4.
26. Jones SJ, Cohen AM. Confusing drug concentrations. *Anaesthesia.* 2001;56:195–6.
27. Nelson LS, Gordon PE, Simmons MD, et al. The benefit of houseofficer education on proper medication dose calculation and ordering. *Acad Emerg Med.* 2000;1311–6.

28. Kirschke DL, Jones TF, Stratton CW, et al. Outbreak of joint and soft-tissue infections associated with injections from a multiple-dose medication vial. *Clin Infect Dis.* 2003;36:1369–73.

29. Micromedex Healthcare Series, Version 2.00.000, Volume 127. Greenwood Village, Colo: Thomson Micromedex. Edition expires March 31, 2006.

30. Moore TJ, Walsh CS, Cohen MR. Reported adverse event cases of methemoglobinemia associated with benzocaine products. *Arch Intern Med.* 2004;164:1192–6.

31. Simpson KR, Knox GE. Obstetrical accidents involving intravenous magnesium sulfate. *Am J Maternal Child Nurs.* 2004;29:161–71.

32. *The United States Pharmacopeia, 28th rev, and The National Formulary, 23rd ed.* Rockville, Md: U.S. Pharmacopeia; 2006.

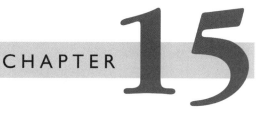

CHAPTER 15

USING TECHNOLOGY TO PREVENT MEDICATION ERRORS

Matthew Grissinger, Hedy Cohen, and Allen J. Vaida

For more than a decade, the Institute for Safe Medication Practices (ISMP) and the National Academy of Sciences Institute of Medicine (IOM) have been promoting the use of technology to enhance patient safety. In its 1991 book *The Computer-Based Patient Record*,[1] IOM called for the elimination of paper-based records within 10 years. The 1999 IOM report *To Err Is Human: Building a Safer Health System*[2] estimated the annual costs of drug-related morbidity and mortality at $77 billion. IOM's 2002 report *Crossing the Quality Chasm*[3] urged health systems to place greater emphasis on the adoption of technology. This was followed in 2004 with *Patient Safety: Achieving a New Standard for Care*,[4] which presented a detailed plan for the development of data standards for collecting and classifying patient safety information. The 2004 report called for immediate access to complete patient information and decision support tools (e.g., alerts, reminders) for clinicians and their patients. The 2006 IOM report *Preventing Medication Errors*[5] strongly supports greater use of information technologies. It recommends enhanced point-of-care use of drug references via the Internet or personal digital assistant, full electronic prescribing by 2010, widespread use of computerized monitoring systems that detect medication-related problems, and improved consumer drug information on the Internet.

In 2000, ISMP issued a white paper supporting electronic prescribing and calling for the elimination of handwritten prescriptions within 3 years.[6] A follow-up report in 2002 called for manufacturers to include machine-readable codes on medications and advocated point-of-care bar coding for drug administration.[7]

Other organizations have joined IOM and ISMP in promoting the role of technology in patient safety. A consortium of health care providers, suppliers, information technology (IT) vendors, payers, and others, the National Alliance for Health Information Technology (NAHIT), formed in 2002. One of its first efforts was to support the Food and Drug Administration (FDA) final rule, issued in 2004, on the use of bar codes in the labeling of certain human drugs and biological products. Acknowledging that the federal government needed to play a role in expanding IT in the health care community, President George W. Bush created the position of National Health IT Coordinator in 2004.

The ISMP Medication Safety Self Assessment for Hospitals was released in 2000, in partnership with the American Hospital Association. The 200 items in this tool included more than a dozen on the use of technology. An updated version was released in 2004. Comparing the results from 2000[8] and 2004 (unpublished) revealed that many hospitals had made progress in the use of technology, or at least had begun discussing it. For example, the percentage of hospitals that had not seriously discussed the implementation of point-of-care bar coding dropped from 61% in 2000 to 21% in 2004. By 2004, 6% had fully

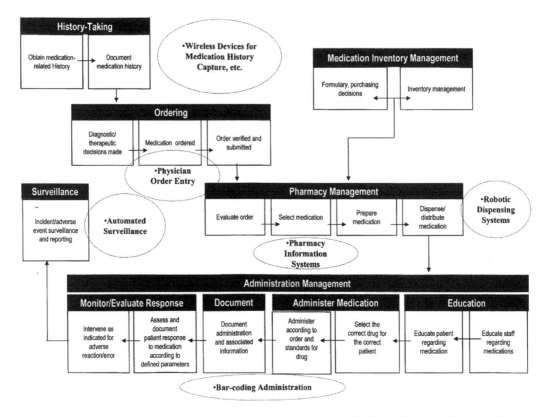

FIGURE 15-1 Medication-use processes in acute care with roles for technology. Reprinted with permission from reference 9.

implemented point-of-care bar coding and 7% had partially implemented it, compared with 1% and 2% in 2000. Progress may seem slow, but it reflects the overall lag in the adoption of technology for patient safety compared with its adoption for financial systems and to meet regulatory requirements.

New technology will not be a panacea for medication errors, but it can provide safeguards not possible with fully manual processes. Chapter 14 presents a number of error reduction strategies for high-alert medications, including the use of forcing functions, electronic alerts, and other strategies in which technology is integral. This chapter describes applications of technology in the medication-use process and discusses their potential to prevent errors. It also notes new errors that technology may introduce and provides recommendations for appropriate integration of technology into practice.

GETTING STARTED

Figure 15-1 illustrates a typical medication management process in an acute care setting and the points in the process where technology can play a role. Kilbridge and Classen[9] used this model to detail each process, where failures can occur, and how technology can help to address the failure points. Many organizations have used such models to perform failure mode and effects analysis (FMEA) on their medication-use systems. In looking at the traditional components of medication use and where errors occur, a study by Leape and colleagues[10] is often used as a reference. In that study, 39% of errors occurred during the prescribing phase, 12% during transcription, 11% during dispensing, and 38% during administration. Close to half of the errors that occurred during prescribing were intercepted before they reached the patient; in contrast, only 2% of errors during the administration phase were intercepted. In the absence of labor-intensive double-checking of all medications or the use of technology such as point-of-care bar coding, practitioners administering medications have no additional lines of defense against error.

Despite the greater likelihood that prescribing errors will be intercepted, much emphasis has been placed on the use of technology in prescribing. There are good reasons for this, including the many errors that involve misinterpreted handwriting or error-prone abbreviations, the prescribing of inappropriate doses, and the occurrence of interactions and allergic reactions. Eliminating handwritten orders and activating medication-checking software with decision support in prescribing systems can prevent such errors. However, the goal of every health care organization should be to incorporate technology across the whole medication management spectrum. Realistically, this cannot be accomplished all at once. This chapter examines the separate "layers" of technology presented in Figure 15-1, beginning with pharmacy computer systems, the foundation for all drug-related information in a hospital.

PHARMACY COMPUTER SYSTEMS

In 1998, practitioners were asked to test whether their pharmacy computer systems detected 10 fatal errors that had been reported to the U.S. Pharmacopeia (USP)–ISMP Medication Errors Reporting Program (MERP). Participants were to enter these orders (for fictitious patients) and check whether the system alerted them to an error or prohibited them from processing the order (i.e., a hard stop). The results (Table 15-1)[11] were surprising.

Only 4 out of 307 systems detected all the unsafe orders in the test. In most of the participants' systems, orders that alerted the pharmacist to a problem did not require staff action (such as entering a password or documenting a reason for bypass of the message) to ensure that warnings were acknowledged. Warnings could be bypassed simply by pressing the Enter key, and could easily be overlooked by staff working under pressure. Most participants said their systems did not detect orders that exceeded a maximum dose, including lethal overdoses of cisplatin and vincristine in children and intravenous colchicine in adults.

A majority of the participants (69%) said their systems allowed them to build alerts (Table 15-2). Vendors market their pharmacy and prescriber order entry systems by promoting their ability to detect unsafe orders. Often, however, a system's full capabilities are not used because of the complex and time-consuming programming that is required of practitioners for maximum system performance. Vendors' claims about a system's

TABLE 15-1 Unsafe Medication Orders Used in 1998 Test of Pharmacy Computer Systems[11]

Order (Patient Description)	% of Systems	
	Unsafe Order Not Detected	Can Override without Note
Cephradine oral suspension IV	61	36
Ketorolac 60 mg IV (aspirin-allergic patient)	12	64
Vincristine 3 mg IV for one dose (2-year-old)	62	56
Colchicine 10 mg IV for one dose (adult patient)	66	55
Cisplatin 204 mg IV for one dose (26 kg child)	63	62
Nizatidine 300 mg hs (patient on famotidine)	18	71
Colchicine 1 mg IV q4h for 8 doses	70	62
Ketoconazole 200 mg daily (patient on cisapride)	15	67
Tobramycin 120 mg IV q8h (creatinine clearance = 10 mL/min)	87	73
Acetaminophen (patient on Percocet)	35	68

TABLE 15-2   1998 Computer System Capabilities[11]

Statement or Question	% Positive Responses
1. The system allows you to build alerts for error-prone situations (i.e., look-alike names, labeling problems).	69
2. The system is capable of providing management with regular reports of drug warning overrides by staff.	79
3. Drug interaction alerts without clinical significance are not present or are easily eliminated.	74
4. The system produces computer-generated or electronic MARs.	88
4a. Would nursing staff give the MARs a positive rating?	74
5. The system is directly interfaced with the laboratory system.	43
5a. The system automatically screens orders and alerts staff according to current laboratory values.	20
6. The system integrates inpatient and outpatient records.	37
7. The system currently allows for direct physician order entry.	13
8. The vendor is readily available to assist staff with questions and software support.	74

capabilities are meaningless unless the applications are user friendly and maximum functionality can be easily achieved at a cost that is not prohibitive. It is crucial to maximize system capabilities by incorporating alerts and clinical decision support based on known safety recommendations and new information from the literature and practitioners' own experience.

The findings of this practitioner survey by ISMP echoed those in an earlier study that was widely publicized. A Georgetown University study on the state of pharmacy computer systems was featured in *U.S. News & World Report* in 1996. The cover story, "Danger at the Drugstore," concluded that pharmacy computer systems in this country are of limited reliability for detecting and correcting prescription errors, most notably serious drug interactions.[12]

The results of ISMP's survey prompted hospitals to check the safety features of their computer systems. The Leapfrog Group[13] used the results as evidence that computerized prescriber order entry (CPOE), which would address handwriting problems, should be supported by alerts and decision rules to ensure safe medication prescribing. In many pharmacy systems and CPOE systems today, however, the capability to detect the same errors ISMP tested in 1998 is still absent or is not utilized or maintained.

ISMP conducted a similar computer survey in 2005, and the results showed minimal improvement in the safety of pharmacy computer systems (Table 15-3).[14] Only 4 of 182 systems were able to detect all the errors tested. For example, fewer than half of the systems detected a serious overdosage of carbamazepine for an adult; only one-third detected an overdose of this drug for a 4-year-old child. Only 1 in 4 systems detected a significant overdose of lomustine based on the patient's body surface area (BSA) and a potentially fatal overdose of methotrexate for a patient being treated for rheumatoid arthritis. Fewer than half of the systems detected a potentially deadly order for conventional amphotericin B dosed according to the drug's liposomal form. Compared with the systems tested in 1998, fewer systems tested in 2005 offered dose alerts based on the patient's age, weight, or BSA. This is surprising, since most current systems offer weight-based dosage checking; it suggests that the software is being inactivated or that patient weight is not being routinely entered.

Although most of the pharmacy computer systems tested in 1998 were able to intercept orders for drugs to which patients were allergic, in 2005 fewer than half of the systems alerted staff when an order for Fluzone (influenza virus vaccine) was entered for a patient allergic to eggs. In addition, little improvement from 1998 to 2005 was seen in detecting

TABLE 15-3 Unsafe Medication Orders Used in 2005 Test of Computer Systems[14]

Order	Patient Description	% of Systems		
		Unsafe Order Detected	Able to Override Warning	Able to Override Warning if Reason Noted
Methotrexate 7.5 mg PO daily	Rheumatoid arthritis	29	87	77
Wellbutrin XL 300 mg PO daily	Seizure disorder	18	85	85
Percocet (any strength) PO q4h prn	Also on Tylenol 650 mg po q4h prn	72	91	85
Fluzone 0.5 mL IM	Allergy to eggs	44	85	79
Zyban 150 mg PO b.i.d.	Also on Wellbutrin SR 150 mg PO b.i.d.	81	96	81
Lovenox 60 mg subcutaneously q12h	Also on heparin 1,000 units/hour IV	85	94	86
Sporanox 100 mg PO daily	Congestive heart failure	14	89	84
St. John's wort 300 mg PO t.i.d.	Also on indinavir 800 mg PO q8h	24	83	76
Varivax 0.5 mL subcutaneously	Pregnant	18	88	75
Metformin 500 mg PO b.i.d.	Serum creatinine 2.1 mg/dL	45	88	80
Neutra-Phos-K 2 packets PO t.i.d.	Serum potassium 6.1 mEq/L	31	89	76
Rifampin 600 mg PO daily	Also on saquinavir 1,200 mg PO t.i.d.	74	92	91
Lomustine 190 mg PO daily for 6 weeks	Body surface area 1.46 m^2	24	75	71
Carbamazepine 400 mg PO b.i.d.	4-year-old child	32	89	76
Carbamazepine 1,300 mg PO b.i.d.	Not applicable	45	88	75
Lantus 25 units IV now	Diabetes	30	61	51
Vincristine 2 mg intrathecally today	Acute leukemia	35	60	43
Amphotericin B 260 mg IV daily	Not applicable	42	88	78

errors involving the wrong route of administration. Slightly more than one-third of the systems in 2005 flagged a potentially fatal order for intrathecal vincristine; in 1998 a similar proportion of systems failed to detect an order to give an oral suspension by the IV route.

In 2005 the systems did poorly in an area not tested in 1998; only 1 in 5 systems intercepted the entry of a drug contraindicated on the basis of the patient's diagnosis or condition (pregnancy). Diagnosis checking is available in many vendors' software, but first the diagnoses or conditions must be entered into the system (e.g., using International Classification of Diseases [ICD] codes). Adding a diagnosis or condition as free text will not activate the software. Pharmacists and IT personnel are well aware of a similar situation with allergy alerts; if allergies are not properly coded and are entered as free text, alerts will not activate.

Safety Features

Pharmacy computer systems should contain a number of safety features. They should have a drug information database that provides alerts for allergies, interactions, duplications, maximum doses, and disease or diagnosis contraindications. They should be integrated or interfaced with the laboratory information system. It should be easy to add alerts and warnings. The system should have fields requiring the entry of allergies and patient weight before medications can be entered. The system should allow the font to be changed so tall-man letters can be used in look-alike medication names. Verification of all orders by a pharmacist should be required before orders can be activated for drug dispensing or administration (e.g., when profiled automated dispensing cabinets [ADCs] or a point-of-care bar code administration system is used). The system should contain hard stops (forcing functions) for designated unsafe orders that require the user to supply a reason for an override. The system should default to a review of current orders before new orders are entered. The system should be able to generate customized medication administration records (MARs), unless a pharmacy-generated electronic MAR is used.

Alerts and Warnings

Only 31% of respondents to the 2004 ISMP Medication Safety Self Assessment for Hospitals said their pharmacy computer systems performed dose range checks to warn practitioners about overdoses and underdoses for all high-alert drugs. Most respondents (84%) said their systems could automatically screen for allergies and provide clear warnings, but 59% indicated that the listing and coding of allergies before medication entry was not a required field. Almost all respondents (91%) said patient weight was not a required field in their systems. Dosages of many medications (e.g., heparin, including low molecular weight heparin; thrombolytics; and cardiac, oncology, and antiseizure medications) are weight based. Without knowing a patient's weight, a pharmacist cannot check—either electronically or manually—whether the correct dose has been prescribed.

Furthermore, weight and allergies must be updated during a patient's stay in the hospital and with each new admission. In a case reported to ISMP, the pharmacy system required that allergies be listed before medications were dispensed, but patients' allergies from a prior admission automatically populated the new admission history, with no notification to verify current allergies. Since his last admission, this patient had had an allergic reaction to cefazolin, not documented in the pharmacy system. The allergy screen listed several allergies from the previous admission, so the required field was populated and new medications could be entered. The patient was ordered cefazolin and became hypotensive and unresponsive after receiving the drug. Diphenhydramine was immediately administered, and the patient recovered. Because the MAR was generated by pharmacy, it did not warn the nurse of the new allergy before cefazolin administration.

The computer system must have the ability to warn practitioners when allergies, weights, or diagnoses are automatically received from a prior admission but have not been verified as current information. Some systems highlight the information, flash the information, or provide other warnings in this situation. A hard stop in the system is the best mechanism for ensuring this verification step.

Presentation of Information on Labels, MARs, and Screens

Pharmacy systems must be able to generate medication labels and MARs (either printed or electronic) that are clear to nurses and contain recommendations for ensuring that the correct medication is administered properly. The presentation of information on labels and MARs should be reviewed prospectively by frontline pharmacists and nurses who will be using the information. Labels and MARs should be free of error-prone abbreviations (see Chapter 8). The format should allow the use of tall-man lettering to distinguish look-alike names, a safety strategy that has been shown to reduce drug selection errors by 35% in a simulated pharmacy dispensing environment.[15] Tall-man lettering is recommended in look-alike drug names that appear in alphabetized lists and on computer

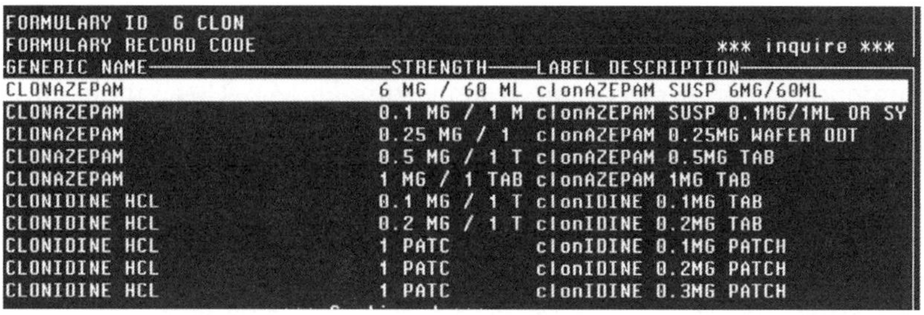

```
FORMULARY ID   G CLON
FORMULARY RECORD CODE                                              *** inquire ***
GENERIC NAME————————————————STRENGTH————LABEL DESCRIPTION————
CLONAZEPAM                          6 MG / 60 ML  clonAZEPAM SUSP 6MG/60ML
CLONAZEPAM                          0.1 MG / 1 M  clonAZEPAM SUSP 0.1MG/1ML OR SY
CLONAZEPAM                          0.25 MG / 1   clonAZEPAM 0.25MG WAFER ODT
CLONAZEPAM                          0.5 MG / 1 T  clonAZEPAM 0.5MG TAB
CLONAZEPAM                          1 MG / 1 TAB  clonAZEPAM 1MG TAB
CLONIDINE HCL                       0.1 MG / 1 T  clonIDINE 0.1MG TAB
CLONIDINE HCL                       0.2 MG / 1 T  clonIDINE 0.2MG TAB
CLONIDINE HCL                       1 PATC        clonIDINE 0.1MG PATCH
CLONIDINE HCL                       1 PATC        clonIDINE 0.2MG PATCH
CLONIDINE HCL                       1 PATC        clonIDINE 0.3MG PATCH
```

FIGURE 15-2   Screen from a pharmacy computer system that accommodates tall-man lettering.

screens (Figure 15-2). Vendors should incorporate the ability to use tall-man lettering into medication dispensing and prescribing systems as well as pharmacy computer systems.

Technology used in the medication process should also allow the use of commas in the strength field and ensure proper spacing between the drug dose and strength. Without the use of a comma, a heparin dose of 1000 units can easily be misread as 10000 units. This could occur during pharmacy order entry when medications are selected from drop-down screens; when nurses read pharmacy-generated MARs, medication labels, and ADC screens; or when prescribers select medications in a CPOE system.

A common question is how to shorten the expression of large numbers (e.g., 10,000, 100,000, and 1,000,000) on computer screens, labels, and printed information. The safest way is to use the words "million" and "thousand," which have nearly as many digits as the corresponding numbers but are less likely to be misread than a number with many zeros. Abbreviations for "million" and "thousand" should be avoided. The letter M has been used for million, but it could also be interpreted as the Roman numeral for 1,000— which could lead to a 1,000-fold error.[16]

The use of mnemonics to select drugs during pharmacy computer entry has led to errors. For example, the oral antidiabetic agent Actos (pioglitazone hydrochloride) 30 mg daily was ordered for a newly admitted diabetic patient, but Actonel (risedronate) 30 mg, indicated for osteoporosis or Paget's disease, was dispensed and administered for 16 days before the error was noticed. In processing the order, the pharmacist had entered the first four letters of the drug name, ACTO, into the computer and then accidentally selected Actonel instead of Actos from the screen. For more than 2 weeks, the nurses failed to notice the dispensing error. The label of prepackaged Actonel tablets listed both the brand and generic names. The handwritten MAR correctly stated "Actos." At quick glance, the nurses had repeatedly misread Actonel on the label as Actos. The patient's blood glucose levels remained high throughout this period, peaking at over 400 mg/dL. A pharmacist finally noticed the error while reviewing the orders upon the patient's transfer to a rehabilitation unit. Errors in the selection of metronidazole and metformin have occurred when the mnemonic MET is used; these drugs also have similar dosage strengths. If the first few letters of a drug name are used during order entry, practitioners should use caution in selecting the correct drug from multiple choices on the screen. When available, both the brand and generic names of the medication should be matched to confirm that the correct drug has been selected.

Information Sharing across Systems

The availability of drug information in a facility's pharmacy system and other electronic systems used in the medication process should be considered. Some computer system vendors use a specific vendor for drug information updates, and the hospital's ability to use other vendors for drug information may not be considered. In evaluating computer systems, the presentation of drug information and the ability to change it with ongoing updates should be explored. ISMP, with the assistance of practitioners, compiled methods for safe communication in electronic systems (appendix). This guide can be used in evaluating the presentation of drug information in pharmacy systems, ADCs, bedside bar coding systems, CPOE systems, and electronic medical records.

A lack of integration or seamless interface between the pharmacy computer system and other hospital information systems is a leading cause of preventable patient harm due to medication prescribing, dispensing, and administration. A patient's allergies, height and weight, diagnosis and comorbid conditions, and laboratory information may be available in electronic format, but often the systems that contain this information cannot easily transfer it to the pharmacy system. Such patient information must be coded correctly in order to activate safety warning software. Without interoperability of the total system, it is impossible to maximize the use of automatic alerting mechanisms during medication order entry.

Schiff and colleagues[17] reported on the importance of linking laboratory and pharmacy information in a seamless fashion. They cited examples of hyperkalemic patients receiving potassium supplements, patients receiving medication doses too high for their renal or hepatic status, and patients receiving the wrong antibiotic for the organism shown in their blood cultures. In the ISMP 2004 Medication Safety Self Assessment, only 19% of respondents said the computer system used for medication order entry was directly interfaced with the laboratory system to automatically alert practitioners to the potential need for drug therapy changes. Table 15-4[17] lists ways laboratory and pharmacy information can be linked to improve care.

The need for information sharing extends beyond the acute care setting. To cite an example, a physician telephoned an order for Pamelor (nortriptyline) 75 mg for a patient whose regimen already included Zoloft (sertraline) 150 mg. A pharmacy technician received the telephone order (in a state where this is allowed) and misheard Pamelor as "Tambocor." The patient received Tambocor, an antiarrhythmic, took it for 1 month, and called the physician's office for a refill. The physician's office staff realized that a dispensing error had occurred because of the similar sounding names. The patient complained of fatigue but had no specific cardiovascular symptoms. At the suggestion of a cardiologist, the medication was stopped, with no permanent harm expected. The error might have been prevented if the technician had read back what he thought he heard, but ambulatory care pharmacies' typical lack of access to clinical information, including diagnosis and laboratory data, was a contributing factor.

System Maintenance and Support

Pharmacy computer systems must be continually maintained and upgraded when new versions become available. Failure to update technology may be one explanation for the general lack of improvement in performance between the 1999 and 2005 ISMP pharmacy computer system surveys. More than half (56%) of the participants in the 2005 survey were using a pharmacy computer system at least 5 years old, with no recent upgrades to new versions available; 38% had been using the same system for 8 years or more without upgrades. If a hospital, health system, or standalone community pharmacy expects technology to improve medication safety, a financial commitment to maintenance and upgrades is imperative. Furthermore, money must be budgeted yearly not just for hardware and software upgrades but also for internal personnel responsible for testing the current system, orienting new employees to correct use of the system, working with vendors to provide customized enhancements as necessary, and continually interacting with all users of the system and the information it provides (e.g., physicians, nurses, patients).

TABLE 15-4 Ways Lab and Pharmacy Can Be Linked to Improve Care

Concept	Example (Drug–Lab Pair)[a]	Role for Computer Linkage
Drug Selection		
Lab finding contraindicates drug	+Pregnancy test–ACE inhibitor ↑ SUN/Cr–metformin hydrochloride	Prevents prescription writing or dispensing
Lab finding suggests indication for drug	↑ TSH–levothyroxine sodium ↑ Cholesterol–lipid-lowering treatment	Generates timely reminders, tracking intervention
Dosing		
Lab finding affects drug dose	↑ Creatinine–digoxin, vancomycin hydrochloride	Performs dose calculations based on age, sex, lab value, weight
Drug requires lab measure for titration (dose determination)	Warfarin sodium–PT/INR Anticonvulsants–drug levels	Statistical process control dosing adjustment charts
Monitoring		
Abnormal lab value signals toxicity	Liver enzymes–isoniazid, glitazones ↓ HCT, WBC–chloramphenicol	Triggers alert, assesses likelihood
Drug warrants lab monitoring for toxicity	Clozapine–WBC Amphotericin B–creatinine	Oversees scheduling of both baseline and serial monitoring tests
Lab Interpretation		
Drug influences or interferes with lab finding	Carbamazepine–free thyroxine Quinolones–false-positive urine opioids	Warns against/interprets false-positives and false-negatives
Drug affects response to lab finding	Insulin–↓ or ↑ glucose Penicillin– + RPR	Resets alarm threshold for treated patients
Improvement		
Surveillance for drug toxicity/effects	Detects signals of previously undocumented reaction (e.g., hepatotoxicity)	Data mining of lab and drug data to generate new hypotheses of drug effects
Quality oversight	Treatment delay after abnormal results (↑ TSH, ↑ K+, + blood culture) and initiation of appropriate treatment	Monitors time interval between lab testing and prescription change, adequacy/appropriateness of lab monitoring

Abbreviations: ACE = angiotensin-converting enzyme; Cr = creatinine; HCT = hematocrit; INR = international normalized ratio; K^+ = potassium; lab = laboratory; PT = prothrombin time; RPR = rapid plasma reagin; SUN = serum urea nitrogen; TSH = thyrotropin; WBC = white blood cell count.

[a] Plus sign indicates positive.

Source: Adapted with permission from reference 17.

AUTOMATED DISPENSING CABINETS

Most hospital pharmacies in the past few decades provided scheduled and as-needed medications by manually filling patient-specific cassettes with a 24-hour supply of unit dose medications and delivering the cassettes to nursing units for storage in medication carts. Supplies of narcotics were normally stored in double-locked cabinets on the unit or in the medication cart, and drugs needed in an emergency were contained in storage cabinets in medication rooms or carts on the unit. Paper forms were used for tracking and documenting the use of narcotics and stock medications.

The introduction of ADCs in the 1980s changed the method of dispensing, storing, and documenting narcotics and stock medications.[18] The adoption of this technology started slowly. Only 49.2% of hospitals were using ADCs in 1999, but by 2005, perhaps because of mounting safety concerns, 71.8% were using the technology.[19]

ADCs are designed to control the storage and documentation of medications in patient care areas. As used initially, for narcotics and emergency floor stock medications, they were a valuable safety enhancement. Nurses no longer had to search for the keys to a narcotic cabinet and manually document medication use on paper forms. Furthermore, ADCs offered automated charge capture and inventory control. To access medications in the device, staff must log in with a unique password or fingerprint identification. Various levels of access can be assigned to staff members, depending on their role in the medication-use process. For example, respiratory therapists can have access to storage areas that contain only medications that they administer. Once logged into the system, the practitioner can obtain medications from drawers or bins that open after a drug is chosen from a list of medications that is contained as a separate drug data repository in the system or is interfaced with the existing pharmacy drug data repository. The devices provide a report directly to the pharmacy on drug usage, who removed each dose and when, and inventory replacement needs.

In many hospitals, ADCs are now used for other medications as well as narcotics and emergency floor stock, because newer systems have advanced features, such as

- Direct interfaces with pharmacy computer systems to limit access until pharmacy has screened and profiled medication orders. This is probably the most important safety enhancement.
- Display screen alerts for practitioners obtaining medications, such as warnings on drug–drug interactions, drug–allergy interactions, drug–lab interactions (requires a laboratory interface), drug–drug duplications, monitoring parameters that should be checked or recorded before administering the medication, and other safety alerts (look-alike or sound-alike drug names, monitoring recommendations).
- Bar-code scanning capability for verifying the stocking and removal of medications.
- Medication-specific storage cubicles, including patient-specific cubicles.

Because of these upgrades, some health care facilities have replaced their patient-specific medication cassette exchange system with large ADCs that contain most medications patients will require. (A problem with this is that many existing systems lack the pharmacy review software enhancements or allow nurses to bypass the system.) Additional reasons hospitals have switched to ADCs for complete drug storage on patient care units include the following:

- *Improved productivity within the pharmacy.* Using ADCs streamlines the dispensing and delivery process. Filling a centralized station containing most medications requires fewer steps than filling each patient's individual medication cassette. ADC use also has the potential to reduce the time for obtaining first doses and the number of phone calls between nurses and pharmacists to locate or obtain missing medications. Use of these systems can give pharmacists more time to spend reviewing new orders and ensuring that the prescribed medications are correct for the patient. It also eliminates the need to return unused or discontinued medications from each patient cassette to pharmacy stock. It is not necessary to credit unused or discontinued medications to specific patient accounts, since charges are captured when the medication is obtained from the cabinet for the patient.

- *Improved nursing and pharmacy productivity.* If most medications are stored in ADCs, nurses can spend less time collecting medications from various delivery or storage sites on patient care areas (e.g., pharmacy drop-off area, pneumatic tube, patient cassette, floor stock area). Newly ordered medications can be obtained faster, with less pressure on the pharmacy to make timely deliveries.
- *Cost reduction.* ADC use can increase nursing and pharmacy productivity and thus reduce the number of staff needed. Supplying and storing prn medications for multiple patients in one location decreases the inventory expense of supplying each medication in individual patients' own cassettes. As mentioned, ADC use eliminates the need to retrieve discontinued medications from a patient's cassette—a task that can add to inventory costs if delayed.
- *Improved charge capture.* Even the most basic ADCs are usually interfaced with the hospital's accounting system, which allows for the capture of all patient charges associated with the medications removed from storage.

Limitations of ADCs

Limitations of ADC use beyond narcotics and emergency supplies must be considered. These systems cannot improve or enhance medication safety unless an adequate number of cabinets are available for each patient care area and their design and use is carefully planned and implemented. Financial and space considerations may cause facilities to overlook the importance of this. When nurses must wait in line to obtain medications for their patients, storage of medications outside the ADCs is often the result. If there are only one or two cabinets to hold most medications for all the patients on the unit, nurses cannot be expected to obtain only one patient's medications at a time and comply with any warnings and alerts on the screen. They are likely to revert to using old medication carts with patient cassettes to store all the medications they need for a work shift. The time saved in the pharmacy is transferred to nursing personnel, and the availability of medications outside the ADCs makes errors likely when medications are discontinued or dosages are changed. (In a properly maintained patient cassette exchange system, pharmacy personnel replace changed medications and retrieve discontinued ones throughout the day.) Making sure that enough ADCs are in strategically placed areas throughout the nursing unit will avoid such opportunities for error. Before a hospital makes systemwide changes in drug storage and delivery, it is important to compare notes with other organizations that have implemented ADCs and to test one patient care unit at a time to find out how many cabinets are needed for safe and efficient workflow.

Lack of pharmacy screening of routine (i.e., nonemergency) orders before a medication can be obtained from an ADC is another limitation that increases the chance for error. Bypassing pharmacy screening eliminates an independent double check of the original order and does not meet standards of accrediting bodies such as the Joint Commission on Accreditation of Healthcare Organizations (JCAHO). At a minimum, medication orders should be screened by the pharmacy for the appropriateness of the drug, dose, frequency, and route of administration; therapeutic duplication; allergies or sensitivities; interactions between the prescription and other medications, food, and laboratory values; and other contraindications. This is particularly important for high-alert medications stored in ADCs.

Choosing the wrong medication from an alphabetic pick list in ADCs is a common contributing factor in medication errors, often involving look-alike names. One organization reported several mix-ups between diazepam and diltiazem removed from the ADC in the intensive care unit (ICU). In one case, diazepam was given at the ordered diltiazem dose. In another case, a physician noted the amber color of the diazepam vial as the nurse was drawing up the dose (thinking it was diltiazem). The organization concluded that once the wrong drug was chosen, the ADC seemed to confirm that the choice was correct by opening the drawer containing the medication selected on the screen. In these cases, nurses relied on their ability to choose the right drug from the pick list; no physical check of the product or reading of the label took place. If the cabinet had contained profile capability and an override of the device had not been chosen, the nurse would have been alerted that the patient had no order for the incorrectly selected medication and strength. Since diazepam had been entered on the patient's pharmacy profile, the cabinet would not have allowed entry if diltiazem had been picked from the screen display. Similar mix-ups have involved incorrect selection of hydromorphone from the screen display instead of morphine. If the patient's correct medications have not been entered in the pharmacy profile and an incorrect choice is made, the individual compartment containing the incorrect drug (e.g., hydromorphone) may open, resulting in administration of the wrong drug. Many hospitals have added screen alerts for look-alike and sound-alike medications such as these, but it is important that all ADCs have the capability to require pharmacy review of orders prior to drug access.

Even ADCs that have pharmacy review capability also have an override feature for emergency access to drugs—and the override is often misused. When any technology requires extra steps for practitioners, "work-arounds" are common. In most cases, people are trying to perform their job functions according to policy and procedure but are forced to work with ineffective or inefficient systems. Often, the interaction of users with technology and the capability of systems to perform under a variety of working conditions are not fully considered when organizations purchase systems such as ADCs. Users are likely to find work-arounds if the device does not respond as expected or appears to hamper patient care. In several of the errors described in this section, overrides were used to obtain medications before orders were reviewed. In most such errors reported to ISMP, the override function was used because of inefficiencies in the system such as lag time for order review, inadequate training of personnel in use of the ADC, and lack of policy on what constitutes an emergency. The override function of ADCs should be used in emergency situations only. A list of medications that can be obtained without pharmacy review is not recommended as a remedy; this would give the false impression that certain medications could always be obtained without review, rather than promoting understanding that only medications needed in a true emergency should be obtained via override. Prescribers, nurses, and pharmacists should institute a policy on what is considered an emergency and have the policy approved by the hospital's pharmacy and therapeutics (P&T) committee.

A common misconception is that because ADCs are automated they must be safe. This reasoning has led to stocking large quantities of medications in the cabinet, a practice that contributed to a fatal 10 mg IV dose of colchicine. The colchicine order had been written with a trailing zero (1.0 mg), and a nurse obtained and administered 10 ampuls containing 1 mg each. The availability of 10 ampuls of the medication in the ADC was a factor in the error, along with misinterpretation of the order and the lack of a profile system on the ADC (a review by pharmacy could have instructed the nurse to remove one vial). Before ADC implementation, the hospital had never kept 10 ampuls of colchicine on a patient care unit. Another reported case involved an order for "calcium gluconate 1 g IV," written after the pharmacy was closed. A nurse misread the vial label and believed that 10 vials of 10% calcium gluconate (each 10 mL vial containing 93 mg of elemental calcium) were needed for the ordered dose. The ADC contained only six vials, so the nurse contacted a pharmacist at home and the error was discovered. This fatal error and near miss highlight the importance of limiting stock in ADCs, especially where pharmacy screening of orders is not available 24 hours a day, 7 days a week.

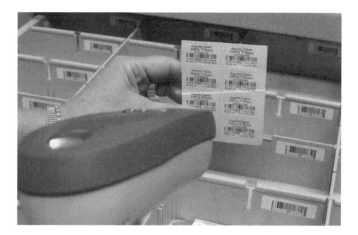

FIGURE 15-3   Bar-coded drawers of an automated dispensing cabinet. (Used with permission of Omnicell, Inc.)

ADC Stocking

Pharmacy is responsible for restocking medications in ADCs. Some cabinets have bar-code identification capability (Figure 15-3). Where this is absent, individual vigilance or double checks involving two staff members must be relied upon to minimize errors in restocking. One hospital reported that tizanidine, a muscle relaxant, was placed in one of the matrix drawers instead of tiagabine, an anticonvulsant. Both the generic names and the doses of these drugs are similar, and the error was not noticed for several days. One patient received four doses of the incorrect drug but suffered no ill effects. In another hospital, a nurse found a Carpuject syringe of digoxin 0.25 mg/mL in the drawer for ketorolac 30 mg. Many of the Carpuject syringes look similar and could be mixed up during stocking. In another case, a similar-appearing ampul of dicyclomine was found in the digoxin matrix. Probably an ampul of dicyclomine was returned to pharmacy stock, placed accidentally in the adjacent digoxin storage bin, and not detected during ADC restocking. Until bar codes are fully utilized, a checking process after ADC restocking is just as important as the checking process before stock medications leave the pharmacy. ISMP recommends that nurses never return unadministered medications to ADC stock. Many errors have been reported in which medications were returned to the wrong storage compartment and subsequently administered. It is preferable for unused medications to be placed in a central return bin in the ADC for restocking by pharmacy.

Of practitioners responding to an ISMP survey in 1999, 56% said a pharmacist always checked medications to be used in restocking ADCs before they were placed in the compartments, 15% said this check process never took place, and 54% said correct drug placement in cabinets was never verified after restocking.[20] Some respondents said medications could be stocked or returned to stock by nursing personnel. Most respondents (96%) said bar code technology was not used to verify that medications were placed in the correct bins in the ADC.

ADC-Related Errors

In one reported case, a patient had orders for both MS Contin (morphine sulfate controlled release) 15 mg tablets and morphine sulfate immediate release 15 mg tablets. A pharmacy technician loaded both medications in the ADC on the patient care unit, inadvertently placing MS Contin in the pocket for morphine sulfate immediate release and morphine sulfate immediate release in the pocket for MS Contin. Nurses administered several doses of each medication, but the patient suffered no apparent adverse effects. Another nurse discovered the error when removing the medication for the next dose. At most hospitals, nursing personnel and pharmacy delivery personnel perform a double check of narcotics put into ADCs.

An error in restocking furosemide 40 mg/4 mL vials in an ADC was caught before administration of the drug. A pharmacy technician obtained what he thought were vials of furosemide 40 mg/4 mL from the stock in a satellite pharmacy and, without a pharmacist double check, left the pharmacy and filled the ADC. A nurse went to the cabinet to obtain a dose of furosemide 240 mg. She took six vials out of the ADC and drew the contents into a syringe. After drawing up the sixth vial, the nurse noticed precipitation and checked the vials. She had used five vials of furosemide 40 mg/4 mL and one vial of phenylephrine 1% 5 mL. Both medications were in amber vials of a similar size with very little label differentiation.

Storing medications with look-alike names or packaging close to one another in ADCs has contributed to more than half of the errors reported through MERP that involved ADCs. A common cause of these mix-ups is what human factors experts call "confirmation bias" (see Chapters 1, 7, and 11). Confirmation bias can occur both during ADC restocking and during removal of medications from the cabinet. For example, when a physician asked for ephedrine, a hurried nurse picked epinephrine from the ADC, drew it into a syringe, and handed it to the primary nurse, who administered it. The patient suffered hypertension and chest pain but eventually recovered. In another example, a physician ordered morphine to be administered via patient-controlled analgesia (PCA) pump. By using the ADC override feature, the nurse inadvertently removed a PCA syringe containing meperidine. The error was discovered the next morning during review of the override report generated by the ADC. The meperidine cartridge was still in the PCA pump, with the infusion parameters set for morphine administration; thus, the patient had received an inappropriate dose of analgesia throughout the night.

Another error involved a physician's request for heparin 2,000 units during a procedure. A nurse retrieved two vials of heparin from an ADC that was normally stocked with heparin 1,000 units/1 mL vials. A pharmacy technician had accidentally stocked the cabinet with heparin 10,000 units/1 mL. Both concentrations, manufactured by American Pharmaceutical Partners, are in the same size vial with similar orange-brown labels and vial caps, and the nurse did not catch the stocking error. Shortly after the patient received heparin 20,000 units, the nurse noticed the mistake. The patient was given protamine, and no harm resulted. In the pharmacy, the 10,000 units/mL concentration was stored next to the 1,000 units/mL concentration, making it easy to choose the wrong vials for restocking the cabinets. The omission of commas, discussed earlier, can also contribute to selection errors, as can the use of "U" for units (1000U) on ADC screens.

When ADCs are used to provide most of patients' medications, there is a tendency to stock only certain strengths of some medications because of space limitations. If the ordered dose of a drug is 50 mg, for example, and only the 25 mg strength is stocked, the screen will direct the nurse to take more than one tablet to make up a dose. This is an unsafe practice if the medication is available in the needed strength. Nurses should not be expected to make up doses of medications when the ordered strength is available. An even greater concern is the expectation that nurses split tablets to make the ordered dose; ADC screens will not direct the nurse to take a partial dose (because the device cannot account for the return of partial doses to its compartments, which is not an approved practice). Instead the screen will prompt the nurse to take one tablet. This is extremely risky with high-alert medications such as warfarin and cardiac medications. A drug such as warfarin should be dispensed in the strength ordered whenever possible.

Control by Off-Site Pharmacists

Small and rural hospitals where pharmacists are not on site 24 hours a day have been using ADCs and telepharmacy services to provide after-hours order review. Pharmacists at an off-site location receive new orders by fax, electronic scanning, or transmission from a CPOE system. They access the hospital pharmacy system via a secure Internet connection, review orders against the patient's medication profile, and authorize release of the medication from the ADC for administration. Some institutions using this process have added video capability; the off-site pharmacist can view a nurse obtaining the medication and displaying it for an additional check. This is especially important if the on-site nurse or other qualified health care professional must prepare an IV medication or admixture in an emergency. The use of technology for remote order review is expected to expand. An increasing number of health systems are offering this capability for their small and rural hospitals, and several outsourcing companies also provide the service.[21]

ADC Safety Steps

Organizations purchasing and implementing ADCs should take the following steps to ensure the safe use of this technology:

- Purchase an adequate number of cabinets for each patient care area.
- Purchase only systems that allow for patient profiling (pharmacist review of new orders against the patient's existing medication regimen) to ensure order review prior to drug removal and administration.
- Purchase a system that uses bar-code technology during the stocking, retrieval, and drug administration processes. When using an older system, develop checks to ensure accurate stocking of the cabinets until an upgrade can be made.
- Carefully select the drugs and quantities that will be stocked in the cabinets. Consider the needs of each patient care unit, as well as the age and diagnoses of patients being treated on the units. Avoid bulk supplies of medications, and stock drugs, including oral solutions, only in ready-to-use unit doses.
- Place different medications and different strengths of the same medication in individual matrix bins.
- If possible, use individual cabinets to separate pediatric and adult medications; for areas serving patients of all ages, such as operating rooms, recovery rooms, and emergency departments (EDs), place adult and pediatric medications in separate drawers.
- Periodically reassess the drugs stocked in each unit-based cabinet. As appropriate, remove seldom-used medications.
- Remove only a single dose of the medication ordered. If the dose is not administered, return it to the pharmacy or ADC return bin and allow pharmacy to replace it in the cabinet.
- Incorporate screen alerts for certain medications (look-alike products, IV/IM/oral use only, dosage forms that should not be crushed).
- Incorporate a system of documenting why an override occurred and requiring a double check of the order and the medication before it is removed.
- Routinely run and analyze override reports to help track and identify problems.
- Develop and test a downtime procedure for use in the event of a power outage or mechanical problem with the ADC.

When these recommendations are followed, ADCs help safeguard medication storage, retrieval, and documentation. ADCs also offer a way of identifying and collecting information on adverse drug events (ADEs). Romero and Malone[22] reported on the use of tracer drugs (50% dextrose, naloxone) obtained from ADCs that required the selection of reasons from a drop-down box before products could be removed. Several of the reasons identified possible ADEs. Information collected in this way can be used to further analyze ADEs.

COMPUTERIZED PRESCRIBER ORDER ENTRY

Electronic entry of medication orders by prescribers (CPOE) has been promoted as an essential technology for health care settings.[23-25] The use of technology was among the performance expectations for health systems outlined in IOM's *Crossing the Quality Chasm*.[3] The federal government's Quality Interagency Coordination Task Force promoted the use of technology, and some health systems (e.g., the Veterans Health Administration) and purchasers have mandated it. The Leapfrog Group, representing large purchasers of health care, identified CPOE as one of three safety initiatives it expects hospitals to implement.[13] The 2006 IOM report *Preventing Medication Errors*[5] notes the potential for computerized prescribing to eliminate problems with illegible handwriting and, when combined with decision-support tools, to alert prescribers to potential safety issues. With the prescribing system linked to the patient's history, prescribers are alerted to allergies, interactions, duplicate therapy, contraindications based on diagnosis, and unsafe or subtherapeutic doses. The report also suggests that an electronic prescription can follow the patient from the hospital to other care settings, including physician offices, thus avoiding problems associated with handoffs in care. The report calls for prescribers to have plans in place by 2008 for electronic prescribing; by 2010, it calls for all prescribers to order medications electronically and for all pharmacies to receive electronic prescriptions.

Reports of the challenges encountered in implementing CPOE[26,27] have made some health care organizations reluctant to adopt it. Early adopters reported significant barriers to successful implementation, new sources of error, and unanticipated needs for major infrastructure changes.[28,29] Most of the negative experiences were due to poor planning and implementation.

Health care organizations must carefully analyze which technology to invest in first and how to implement it in their facilities. Changes in the medication-use system involve many departments and disciplines, all of which must be involved in the planning. Organizations often use FMEA to identify potential roadblocks and proactively address them.[30] Of all the technologies discussed in this chapter, CPOE probably requires the most painstaking planning. It has the greatest effect on physicians' practice, and physician leadership must be involved from the earliest stages. Medical staff champions must be identified and compensated for their time commitment during the planning and implementation phase.

Two documents from the First Consulting Group provide guidance for health systems planning CPOE implementation: Computerized Physician Order Entry: Costs, Benefits and Challenges: A Case Study Approach[31] and Computerized Physician Order Entry in Community Hospitals: Lessons from the Field.[32] A consensus statement outlining nine considerations for successful CPOE implementation[33] emphasizes the importance of devoting enough financial resources to "people issues" involved in the process: replacement staff for current employees who will be involved in the implementation, around-the-clock availability of training personnel to assist users, and ongoing staff devoted to maintaining the system. If staff training is inadequate, the display of information is inappropriate for the users, or implementation occurs before the system itself is ready, the result will be that physicians will not use the system as intended and more errors may be introduced.[28]

Integrate or Interface?

Too often, hospitals have tried to interface a CPOE system with an out-of-date pharmacy computer system. If the CPOE and pharmacy systems are not integrated or seamlessly interfaced, orders entered electronically by prescribers may be received in the pharmacy as a paper printout for manual entry into the pharmacy system. This not only adds a step to the process (orders must be reentered in the pharmacy computer) but also increases the opportunity for error.[24] If the drug data repositories are different for the CPOE system and the pharmacy system, extra effort is needed to maintain two or even more (e.g., point-of-care bar coding, smart pumps) drug databases and ensure their ongoing functionality. When the CPOE system is from the same vendor as the hospital information system, which includes the pharmacy system, laboratory system, point-of-care bar coding, and other systems, there is a single database of medications, integrated with clinical information components. Organizations that choose to interface systems from various vendors (i.e., the "best of breed" approach) should be prepared to devote more effort to initial implementation and ongoing maintenance.

MAR Support

The CPOE system and pharmacy system, whether from the same or different vendors, need to support the MAR. Pharmacy and nursing must work together closely in formatting the drug information contained on the print or electronic MAR. Pharmacy should have the ability to provide nurses with important drug administration information and warnings when necessary. Also, the information on the MAR should closely match what is contained on medication labels, especially for IV solutions. ISMP recommends that information flow electronically in only one direction: from the CPOE system to the pharmacy system to the MAR. The various systems should be able to interact in these ways. Merely sharing coded electronic information is not enough; its full context should be easily passed within the system or between systems.[34–36]

Staff Involvement

An important component of successful CPOE implementation is team commitment by all health care practitioners who will be affected in the process.[31] A multidisciplinary team should investigate all systems available, thoroughly analyze workflow and changes that may be needed, identify the capabilities of the software and the ease of developing new rules, establish policies and procedures, "sell" the benefits and objectives of the technology to the affected staff, develop an implementation plan, and review the implementation. The team should address in advance who will be responsible for maintaining and updating the system and who will provide ongoing education and orientation of current and new staff—considerations often overlooked in budgeting.

It is beneficial to include several current members of the P&T committee on the CPOE implementation team. The P&T committee or a new or existing subcommittee will have to be involved in the initial setup and ongoing maintenance of standardized order sets, clinical decision support rules, and policies and procedures that govern medication prescribing, dispensing, and administration. Pharmacy and nursing are usually well represented on the implementation committee, and their role in vendor selection, implementation, and maintenance of the medication components of CPOE is paramount. If the implementation team consists mainly of P&T committee members, it is important to ensure that respiratory, laboratory, and other departments are also represented on the team.

The team should review existing technology used in the health system's medication process. Does the current pharmacy system provide computer-generated MARs, and are they functional? If not, is time being allotted to refine the MAR printout to include user-friendly information for nurses, such as standardized order sets for chemotherapy administration, sliding-scale insulin doses, anticoagulant protocols, preoperative medications, and other complicated administration displays? Has the use of dangerous abbreviations, trailing zeros, and spacing between the medication name, dose, and strength been addressed to eliminate error-prone expressions identified by ISMP, JCAHO, and other organizations?

These preparatory steps are crucial. If nurses' first look at an electronic MAR is concurrent with CPOE implementation, the refinements that may be needed in physician, pharmacist, and nursing displays of electronic information will likely be overwhelming. Nurses, physicians, and pharmacists must participate in refining electronic printouts and displays of medication profiles and MARs before the introduction of CPOE.

Drug versus Lab Orders

A CPOE system may allow physicians to view options for all types of orders on the same screen. Options for laboratory tests, especially for assays and serum drug levels, may be expressed so that they look like drug names. For example, "acetaminophen" might indicate a lab test for acetaminophen level, or the drug itself. Prescribers who see "acetaminophen" could order the lab study by mistake and fail to notice that they have not finished ordering the drug by indicating dose, route, and frequency. The same could happen with other lab tests, such as a digoxin level, although prescribers would be less likely to forget to order the dose, route, and frequency for nonroutine medications. It may be safest to establish different pathways for ordering drugs and lab studies so that options for both cannot be viewed on the same screen. Also, the nomenclature for medications and laboratory studies should be selected carefully to reduce the risk of confusion.

Clinical Decision Support

The CPOE team must realize at the outset that building and maintaining clinical decision support (CDS) software requires a great deal of ongoing effort. Even when the system vendor offers rules for CDS, the team must decide which components will be used immediately and which will be added incrementally. Medications and the way they are used, administered, and monitored change constantly, so an ongoing committee and budgeted time for clinical practitioners are always needed after CPOE implementation. Establishing an ad hoc group or special task force to begin CPOE and disbanding it once the real work of support and maintenance begins is a setup for failure. An ongoing CDS team must be established.

A study by Nebeker et al.[37] showed that high rates of ADEs may continue after CPOE implementation if the system lacks CDS for drug selection, dosing, and monitoring. The CPOE system must contain standardized order sets and automated corollary orders for prophylaxis and drug therapy monitoring.[38] For example, in Figure 15-4, a warning is displayed on the screen because a chemotherapy order exceeded the daily dose limit. As another example, when warfarin is ordered the system should immediately check the patient's lab orders for an international normalized ratio (INR) and display the results for the prescriber. If no INR has been ordered, the system would suggest it and an easy-to-activate order would be displayed. As discussed in Chapters 9 and 10, the immediate availability of patient and drug information to the prescriber can prevent a large portion of medication errors.

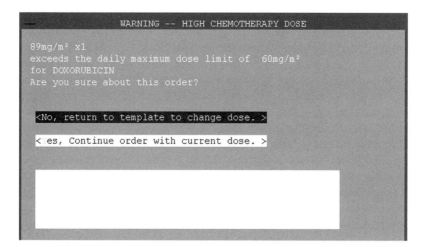

FIGURE 15-4 Alert screen for computerized prescriber order entry.

In designing CDS for CPOE systems, deciding how much information will automatically appear to the user and how it will be displayed is crucial.[39-42] The effects of excessive "noise" (alert overload) must be considered. The results of ISMP's pharmacy computer system testing (Tables 15-1 and 15-3) could be partially attributable to system alerts being turned off. CDS must be introduced judiciously during CPOE implementation. For example, many systems have the ability to categorize allergies into at least three levels of severity; prescribers could be alerted only to allergic reactions that are considered serious. If CDS is not well planned, practitioners will begin to bypass even the most serious alerts.[43] Bates et al.[44] believe electronic CDS will move clinicians toward the practice of evidence-based medicine, which has the potential to improve quality and safety while simultaneously reducing health care costs.

POINT-OF-CARE BAR CODE MEDICATION ADMINISTRATION

The use of bar codes to automate grocery checkout was first described in the 1930s. In the 1970s, with the creation of the Universal Product Code (UPC), most retail industries began using point-of-sale bar code systems.[45] Health care practitioners took notice and began experimenting with the use of this technology for medication distribution and administration.[46-49] The ADE Prevention Study[10] revealed that 38% of medication errors occur during drug administration and that only 2% of these errors are intercepted. Another study using the direct observation method in 36 health care facilities found that medication administration errors occurred in almost 20% of doses administered.[50] The 1999 IOM report *To Err Is Human*[2] noted that point-of-care bar coding offers a simple way to ensure that the identity and dose of the drug are as prescribed, that it is being given to the right patient, and that all of the steps in the dispensing and administration processes are checked for timeliness and accuracy. Since the late 1990s and into this century, the use of bar coding in drug administration has picked up momentum. Bar code medication administration (BCMA) is used in all Department of Veterans Affairs (VA) health care facilities. Studies have shown that BCMA can reduce medication errors by 65–86%.[51-53] In 2004 FDA issued a rule requiring bar code labels on most commercial human drug and biological products by April 2006.[54]

The VA has published 15 best practice recommendations for BCMA.[55] Consensus documents, readiness assessment tools, and primers are also available for hospitals to refer to in planning for BCMA.[56,57] Poor design of systems, inadequate training, and lack of attention to hardware needs can introduce error when BCMA is implemented.[58]

BCMA can improve medication safety through several levels of functionality. At the most basic level, the system helps to verify that the right drug is being administered to the right patient in the right dose by the right route and at the right time. On admission, patients are issued a bar-coded identification wristband. Nurses or other practitioners administering medications scan their bar-coded employee identifier and the patient's bar-coded wristband. Then, using an electronic MAR, the practitioner checks the patient record and scans the bar code on the medication to be administered. The system generates an approval if the correct match is made and a warning if not. The system may also display administration instructions, information on the drug, monitoring parameters to be followed, and other information as described below.

An electronic MAR is likely to be more accurate than traditional handwritten MARs. All orders should be profiled by the pharmacy before listing on the MAR, and all medication doses should contain a bar code. This may entail changes in the way pharmacy receives orders and dispenses medications. Bar code scanning at the point of administration records the time each dose is administered on the electronic MAR.

BCMA systems can provide the following:

- Increased accountability and capture of charges for items such as unit-stock medications.
- Up-to-date drug reference information from online medication reference libraries. This could include pictures of tablets or capsules, usual dosages, contraindications, adverse reactions and other safety warnings, pregnancy risk factors, and administration details.
- Customizable comments or alerts (e.g., allergies, exceeding maximum daily dose limits for opioids or acetaminophen-containing products) and reminders of actions to be taken when administering certain medications.
- Data capture for analysis of trends in patient misidentification, wrong drug or dose, doses administered late, omitted doses, or other information that could suggest the need for system changes. It is important that this information be used to improve the system, rather than to punish individual employees.
- Identification of laboratory specimens and blood for transfusions.

Frontline staff members, especially nurses, must be involved in all decisions related to the purchase of, education for, and implementation of bar code technology. Before embarking on BCMA implementation, facilities must anticipate failures and develop contingency plans for unexpected results. It is helpful to study reports appearing in the literature as more hospitals adopt this technology.

Workflow Changes

One VA hospital discovered time-consuming changes in nurses' workflow when BCMA was first introduced.[58] The nurses were not prepared for the automated actions programmed into the BCMA software. For example, medications were automatically removed from the patient's drug profile list 4 hours after the scheduled administration time, even if the medication was never administered. Therefore, if the patient returned from a procedure more than 4 hours after a scheduled administration time, the nurse could not see whether the dose had been administered. The software was changed to keep unadministered medications in the system beyond 4 hours.

Also, changing to an electronic MAR (eMAR) decreased coordination of patient information between prescribers and nurses. Before implementation of the eMAR and BCMA, prescribers could quickly review the handwritten or printed MAR at the patient's bedside or in the unit's medication room. This problem could be addressed by having more terminals for use by prescribers.

With the new system, nurses found it more difficult to document deviations from routine medication administration. If a patient refused a medication, the nurse had to spend time manually documenting this, since the medication had already been documented as given when it was originally scanned. The software was revised so nurses could document such changes by selecting the medication and choosing a drop-down menu option.

BCMA required the nurses to type in an explanation when medications were given outside established administration time frames. To avoid this, nurses scanned medications beforehand and held them for later administration. Particularly in long-term care settings, some nurses scanned and poured medications for patients who were unavailable so that the computer record would show on-time administration. Thus, the nurses had to rely on memory to administer opened, unlabeled medications in an unlabeled cup when the patient returned to the unit. Nurses may think one of the main purposes of BCMA is to track the timeliness of their medication administration. Organizations must review their administration time windows to ensure that they are compatible with the system they use for transferring new orders to the pharmacy and delivering medications to the unit.

Work-arounds

To save time, the nurses used work-arounds that circumvented the safety features of BCMA. Some nurses routinely typed the patient's Social Security number (which was used as a patient identifier) into the system rather than scanning the patient's wristband. This avoided difficulties in scanning the wristband (e.g., because of a damaged bar code or the curvature of the band on patients with small wrists). Such work-arounds are common; often a second set of patient wristbands is printed and kept on a ring, or the patient wristband is kept at the bedside rather than on the patient to expedite scanning (e.g., when a new IV bag is hung and the patient is asleep).

One work-around that led to an error involved an order for digoxin elixir, which was stocked on the patient unit as a 60 mL (0.05 mg/mL) multidose bottle (the usual dose is 0.125–0.25 mg [2.5–5 mL]). The nurse misinterpreted the dose of digoxin elixir as 60 mL, accidentally retrieved a bottle of doxepin (an antidepressant) from unit stock, and attempted to administer a 60 mL dose of what she thought was digoxin. Scanning the bar code on the bottle of doxepin had generated an error window on the electronic MAR screen stating "drug not on profile," but the nurse did not investigate the warning. Instead, she manually entered the doxepin national drug code (NDC), overriding the digoxin NDC that had been entered by the pharmacy. The result was administration of doxepin 60 mL to the patient.

Alerts and Overrides

Like ADCs, BCMA systems allow overrides in case medications need to be administered in an emergency. All caregivers administering medications must understand that using an override bypasses the important step of order verification by a pharmacist. BCMA systems should have additional features to prevent harm from overrides. In the digoxin–doxepin example, a maximum dose warning incorporated in the software would have displayed on the MAR. Automated redundancies such as this (alerts for the prescriber, pharmacist, and nurse) should be incorporated in CPOE, pharmacy, and BCMA systems. The number of alerts should not be overwhelming, but alerts for high-severity allergic reactions, incorrect doses or routes of administration, and other errors that can cause patient harm should be displayed for all practitioners involved in medication use.

Bar Codes on All Doses

Unit dose packaging would have decreased the magnitude of the digoxin–doxepin error; multidose bottles should never be stocked outside the pharmacy. The availability of manufacturer-supplied, bar-coded unit dose medications is a concern to hospitals implementing BCMA. Although FDA now requires bar codes on containers, it does not require that unit dose containers be available for all medications. Unit dose packaging of some established products has been discontinued. Hospitals that are planning to implement BCMA must be prepared to repackage many medications and relabel each dose with a bar code. This will entail the purchase of automated repackaging equipment, an increase in technical staff in the pharmacy, and adequate space within the pharmacy to prepare these medications. Still, the safety features of BCMA far outweigh the additional costs.

Important considerations in preparing medications for use with BMCA are as follows:

- The orientation of the bar code on the product. Bar codes on curvatures of vials and infusion bags are hard to scan. Placing bar codes vertically on products helps to avoid this.
- Pharmacies should verify that the bar code on a manufacturer's product is readable and matches the product in the drug database.
- The pharmacy computer system should print readable bar codes for multiproduct IVs that match the components of the product.
- Bar codes should be affixed to the end product container, not just to the outer container (e.g., package that contains the insulin vial).
- Patient-specific doses with bar codes should be dispensed whenever possible. This includes half tablets, oral syringes that contain the exact dose of an oral solution, and IV syringes that contain the patient's exact dose.
- Bar-code label equipment, including printers, must be continually checked for accuracy and readability and undergo routine preventive maintenance by IT or biomedical staff.

Additional Considerations

Hospitals implementing BCMA should inform their patients about how the system works and how it helps ensure that they receive the correct medications. Patients can be uneasy about the scanning process if they have never experienced it. They should be told about the process when entering the hospital and asked to participate by displaying their wristband and verifying the medications they are receiving when possible. Informed patients will appreciate the value their hospital places on safety.

As hospitals consider BCMA, they should watch the maturation of another technology: radio frequency identification (RFID). As with bar coding, health care is behind other market segments in applying RFID. RFID tags are commonly used on clothing, electronic equipment, and other merchandise to track inventory and prevent theft. A key chain with RFID can be used to pay at a gasoline pump, and a tag can be mounted on a car window to pay tolls. FDA, the pharmaceutical industry, wholesalers, and retailers are using RFID technology to combat the shipment of counterfeit drugs.[59] This technology is also being used in clinical drug studies to track and record the medications participants are taking. Hospitals are using it to track inventory; track, document, and confirm the administration of blood products and IV solutions; and trace the movement of equipment such as IV pumps within the facility. For most applications in the health care environment, the cost of RFID is still prohibitive but is expected to decrease. Privacy concerns have been raised about tagging individual medications and tracking specific patients' compliance, but this technology will continue to develop. Hospitals should not hesitate to move ahead with BCMA while awaiting the refinement and economic feasibility of RFID.

"SMART" PUMPS

CPOE can decrease the number of prescribing errors, especially when it is integrated with a pharmacy computer system and both systems have CDS software. Where most medications are dispensed in patient-specific doses with bar codes, BCMA can decrease administration errors. Similarly, IV drug administration errors can be decreased through the use of "smart" infusion pumps, a term ISMP coined because they incorporate medication safety software. An incorrect pump setting can lead to a catastrophic error, even if the drug is ordered and dispensed correctly and administered to the right patient. Many high-alert medications are administered intravenously, and errors with these drugs often cause serious patient harm.[60]

Infusion pumps are designed with the flexibility to be used in multiple clinical areas. The same pump used for a 100 kg patient in the adult ICU may also be used on a 10 kg child in the pediatric unit. Most infusion devices are capable of delivering medications at rates ranging from 0.01 mL/hr to 1,000 mL/hr. Given this range, programming errors are fairly common and may go undetected until patient harm has occurred. Many infusion devices are programmed to calculate a rate when patient information or other parameters (e.g., mcg/kg/minute, units/hr) are entered.

An error in pump programming results in an error in the infusion rate, as in the following examples[61]:

- A 67 kg patient was about to receive an insulin infusion at 7 units of insulin/kg/hr, when the ordered dose was 7 units/hr.
- For an infusion to a neonate, a mistake in pressing a zero instead of a decimal point changed the rate to 304 mL/hr when the ordered rate was 3.4 mL/hr.
- An infusion rate for heparin was entered as 800 mL/hr rather than the correct dose of 800 units/hr.

Since most pumps allow such a wide range of infusion rates, safe use is reliant on perfect programming by the individual practitioner or an independent double check by another practitioner.

Even when infusion pumps are programmed correctly, unlimited changes in the rate can lead to patient harm. A Levophed (norepinephrine) infusion was ordered to start at 1 mcg/min, with adjustment of the rate to maintain systolic blood pressure above 90 mm Hg. Similar orders are not unusual for ICU patients receiving pressor medications such as epinephrine, phenylephrine, and dopamine. In this case a nurse gradually increased the dose of norepinephrine to 38 mcg/min to maintain systolic blood pressure above 90 mm Hg. This rate was maintained throughout the night, resulting in so much peripheral vasoconstriction that irreversible ischemia occurred in several of the patient's toes, leading to gangrene and eventual amputation.

To help prevent errors like this, device manufacturers have introduced "smart" pumps with medication safety software. These pumps have a comprehensive library of drugs, usual concentrations, dosing units (e.g., mcg/kg/min, units/hr), and dose limits (minimum/maximum) that can be set according to institution-established parameters. The software can also be configured by patient type or location in the organization (e.g., adult

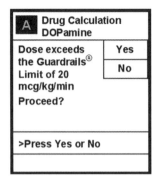

FIGURE 15-5 Sample screen of "smart" infusion pump (Alaris System with Guardrails software). (Photo courtesy of Cardinal Health.)

ICU, pediatric ICU, ED). Such systems can provide additional verification at the point of care to help prevent IV infusion errors. A nurse programs the pump by selecting the appropriate care area or patient type and entering the patient parameters, followed by the drug, concentration, and desired dose. Programmed doses are automatically checked to determine whether they are within the ranges established by the institution. If the dose is below or above the organization's established limits, the nurse receives an alert (Figure 15-5). Depending on the drug and the software configuration by the hospital, alerts may be warnings that can be overridden (soft limits) or hard stops that must be confirmed or that require reprogramming for a different infusion rate.

A smart pump averted the continuation of an error when an ED physician wrote an order for Integrilin (eptifibatide) but inadvertently prescribed a dose appropriate for Reopro (abciximab). The Integrilin infusion was initiated at the ordered rate and continued for 36 hours after the patient's transfer to a medical–surgical unit. During this time, the patient's mental status deteriorated. The hospital was in the process of switching to the Alaris Medley system, which performs a "test of reasonableness" before allowing an infusion to begin. As the nurse was transferring the patient's infusion parameters to the new system, the safety software alerted the nurse that there was a "dose out of range." The pump would not allow the nurse to continue until a pharmacist was called and the mistake was corrected. In another case, a hospital's heparin protocol called for a loading dose of 4,000 units followed by a continuous infusion of 900 units/hour. The loading dose was administered correctly, but the nurse inadvertently programmed the continuous dose as 4,000 units/hour. Since the pump limit for heparin as a continuous infusion was set at 2,000 units/hour, the infusion device would not start until the dose was corrected.

The use of a smart pump with maximum rate limits by patient type and care area might have averted another error reported to ISMP. For a baby receiving total parenteral nutrition, a nurse attempted to program the infusion pump at 13.0 mL/hour. The decimal point key on the pump was worn and difficult to engage. Without realizing it, the nurse programmed a rate of 130 mL/hour. The error was discovered within 1 hour, and although the baby's blood glucose concentration rose to 363 mg/dL, no permanent harm occurred.

Smart pump software also provides access to transaction data from the infusion device for use in quality-improvement efforts. Reports can be generated on near misses (programming errors that were corrected), warnings that were bypassed, and warnings that required the practitioner to enter a notation before proceeding. This information can be used to assess current practices and identify ways of improving medication safety.

As with any technology, smart pumps can improve patient care only to the extent that their safety features are fully used. Rothschild et al.[62] found that the use of smart pumps in a cardiac surgical intensive care and stepdown unit had no measurable impact on the rate of serious medication errors. This was due in part to poor compliance with the safety features on the pumps; nurses were able to easily override alerts in the system.

Institutions implementing smart pump technology should establish a multidisciplinary team to determine best practices. IV-related policies and procedures, concentrations, dosing units (e.g., mcg/min versus mcg/kg/min), and drug nomenclature should be standardized and consistent with usage in the MAR, the pharmacy computer system, and other technology used in the institution.

Drug references usually provide information on the maximum dose per 24-hour period but may not provide the minimum and maximum doses that can be administered over 1 hour. The team should determine dosage limits for infusions and bolus doses on the basis of current policy and practice, the literature, and consensus among the group. The team also should decide which dose limits require a hard stop versus a soft stop.

Unit-based dosage limits should be developed (e.g., for adult ICU, adult general care, pediatric ICU, pediatric general care, labor and delivery, and anesthesia). A procedure should be developed for nurses to follow when a drug is not in the software library or a nonstandard concentration must be used.

Bates et al.[63] reviewed data from 100 hospitals that were using smart pump technology and found wide variation in the nomenclature used for drugs, dosage units, concentrations, and minimum and maximum rate limits. They concluded that reaching national or international consensus on usage could substantially improve IV medication safety.

Smart pump technology has been incorporated into PCA pumps. Many errors related to PCA have involved incorrect programming of the drug concentration, leading to 10-fold overdoses, or programming a rate that is outside the safe limits for most opioid-naïve patients (e.g., misprogramming a morphine rate for a hydromorphone infusion).

Smart infusion systems can also integrate point-of-care bar code technology for an additional check. With this added step, the patient, drug, and correct infusion rate can be matched and immediately programmed into the pump.

STANDALONE DATA-MONITORING TECHNOLOGY

A lack of information about patients or their prescribed medications contributes to more than half of all serious, preventable ADEs.[10] Today, automated CDS systems can offer clinicians the crucial information they need to provide the best care. For example, a physician prescribing an antibiotic can be alerted to adjust the dose on the basis of the patient's most recent laboratory values. A pharmacist entering a diuretic order into a pharmacy computer system integrated with the laboratory system can be alerted to the patient's low potassium level.

These systems help give clinicians the right information to make the right decisions, but most systems cannot ensure that clinicians receive crucial information at the right time. Most CDS systems provide information only when the clinician is actively using the system. For example, if an antibiotic is ordered early in the day, before the patient's lab results are available, the prescriber may not be alerted to an elevated serum creatinine level and the need for a dose adjustment until the next day, when he again logs into the system or that patient's profile. New data-monitoring technology is making it possible to notify clinicians of important information as soon as a potential problem is detected.

The new standalone CDS systems can "listen" to a wide variety of information sources across the organization, "watch" for specific problems predefined by the organization, and "notify" clinicians of situations that may represent a risk to their patients as soon as this information becomes available. Some of the components of these systems are being integrated into existing health care IT systems, including CPOE.

Standalone data-monitoring technology is available commercially (e.g., from Misys [Insight], VigiLanz [Dynamic PharmacoMonitoring], and Cerner [Discern Expert for Cerner Millennium and Classic systems]). It uses computer industry data-compatibility standards (HL7 compliant) to constantly communicate information from various hospital clinical departments' computer systems (e.g., radiology, laboratory, pharmacy, nutrition), tying it to the hospital's patient information database and proprietary software in a central system server. Each piece of data is then checked to see if a relationship exists among pre-established clinical rules to trigger an alert.

If an imminent or existing adverse clinical or drug event is detected, the system sends a message via personal digital assistant, pager, cell phone, e-mail, or fax to alert the appropriate clinician(s) to the problem. Alerts can be sent to a department or designated individuals (e.g., physicians, clinical pharmacists, nurses), as determined by the professional staff in each hospital. Notification can be provided in real time for situations deemed critical. Alternatively, the system can allow a specified time interval before notification while it scans to see if appropriate action has been taken.

The power of these clinical data-monitoring systems is great. Hundreds of rules can be designed to alert clinicians immediately to safety issues such as elevated liver enzymes in a patient receiving a drug metabolized in the liver, an abnormal potassium level in a patient taking digoxin, a decreased platelet count in a patient receiving heparin, or signs that an allergic response or drug interaction may be occurring.

The system could notify staff about a patient with pneumonia who did not receive the first dose of antibiotic within 8 hours of admission, or prompt a change in antibiotic for a patient on vancomycin whose culture and susceptibility report did not support its continued use. Failure to act on such data in a timely fashion can have serious consequences for both patients and staff. A case in point from a hospital that uses this technology was the rapid notification of a positive lab test for acid-fast bacilli, which led to the immediate isolation and treatment of the patient and significantly reduced staff exposure to tuberculosis.

The use of rapid response teams for such acute situations has been advocated,[64] and most hospitals have had a call system in place for these types of "panic" values. But nonautomated call systems are more likely to fail. The appropriate clinician may not receive the information in a timely fashion. Meaningful changes in a patient's physiological state due to disease or drug therapy may not be noticed quickly if staff relies only on "panic" lab values or relies on a practitioner to notice a problem.

When nurses, pharmacists, and physicians are relied upon to detect problems, they must navigate massive charts, sets of daily lab results, and multiple computer systems to collect information. Even when all records are in electronic form, the information must be accessed before it can be acted upon. The success of this labor-intensive process in preventing medication errors is threatened by staffing shortages and budget constraints.

The key to using automated decision-support systems to prevent errors is making sure the system provides timely advice tailored to the needs of each individual patient, and that the advice is provided unobtrusively to the clinician best able to quickly fix the problem. The use of clinical data-monitoring technology is not limited to health systems that use computerized prescribing. This technology has the potential to vastly improve patient outcomes, at a cost affordable to most hospitals. These systems will likely pay for themselves through savings realized by preventing adverse events and improving drug utilization and staff efficiency.[65]

CONCLUSION

Total integration of the technologies described in this chapter into existing electronic medical records will help health systems prevent ADEs, but the implementation of any new technology requires adequate planning and preparation of the staff to properly use the safety features and not devise work-arounds. The process requires total commitment from the organization's executive and medical leadership as well as all staff members who will be affected by the implementation. Leaders need to send a clear message that the goal is improved patient safety.

Technology cannot eliminate all errors, but the use of CDS and automated redundancies can help prevent errors from reaching patients. The goal should be to move the 2% of intercepted errors in the administration process identified by Leape et al.[10] to nearly 100%. This will be achievable only through devoting time and resources to the planning, implementation, and continued maintenance of the technology, and to analyzing the data collected in the light of current information on error prevention.

REFERENCES

1. Dick RS, Steen EB, Detmer DE, eds. *The Computer-Based Patient Record: An Essential Technology for Health Care.* Washington, DC: National Academies Press; 1991.
2. Kohn LT, Corrigan JM, Donaldson MS, eds. *To Err Is Human: Building a Safer Health System.* Washington, DC: National Academies Press; 2000.
3. Committee on Health Care in America. Institute of Medicine. *Crossing the Quality Chasm: A New Health System for the 21st Century.* Washington, DC: National Academies Press; 2001.
4. Aspden P, Corrigan JM, Wolcott J, et al., eds. *Patient Safety: Achieving a New Standard for Care.* Washington, DC: National Academies Press; 2004.
5. Committee on Identifying and Preventing Medication Errors; Aspden P, Wolcott J, Bootman JL, et al., eds. *Preventing Medication Errors.* Washington, DC: National Academies Press; 2006. Prepublication copy available at http://darwin.nap.edu/books/0309101476/html/R2.html. Accessed July 21, 2006.
6. Institute for Safe Medication Practices. A call to action: eliminate handwritten prescriptions within 3 years! Huntingdon Valley, Pa: Institute for Safe Medication Practices; 2000.
7. Institute for Safe Medication Practices. A call to action: safeguard drug administration within 2 years! Huntingdon Valley, PA: Institute for Safe Medication Practices; 2002.
8. Smetzer JL, Vaida AJ, Cohen MR, et al. Findings from the ISMP Medication Safety Self Assessment for Hospitals. *Jt Comm J Qual Saf.* 2003;29:586–97.
9. Kilbridge P, Classen D. A Process Model of Inpatient Medication Management and Information Technology Interventions to Improve Patient Safety. VHA's 2001 Research Series (Volume 1). Irving, Tex: VHA; 2001. Available at: https://www.vha.com/portal/server.pt/gateway/PTARGS_0_2_38373_0_0_18/medication management.pdf. Accessed March 6, 2006.
10. Leape LL, Bates DW, Cullen DJ, et al. Systems analysis of adverse drug events. *JAMA.* 1995;274:35–43.
11. Institute for Safe Medication Practices. Overreliance on pharmacy computer systems may place patients at great risk. *ISMP Medication Safety Alert!* February 10,1999;4(3).
12. Headden S, Lenzy R, Kostyu P, et al. Danger in the drugstore: too many pharmacists fail to protect consumers against potentially hazardous interactions with prescription drugs. *US News & World Report.* August 26, 1996:46–53.
13. The Leapfrog Group. Computer Physician Order Entry; Fact Sheet: 2003. Washington, DC: The Leapfrog Group; 2004. Available at: www.leapfroggroup.org/media/file/Leapfrog-Computer_Physician_Order_Entry_Fact_Sheet.pdf. Accessed March 6, 2006.
14. Institute for Safe Medication Practices. Safety still compromised by computer weaknesses; comparing 1999 and 2005 pharmacy computer field test results. *ISMP Medication Safety Alert!* August 25, 2005; 10(17).
15. Grasha A. Cognitive systems perspective on human performance in the pharmacy: implications for accuracy, effectiveness, and job satisfaction. Executive Summary Report. Alexandria, Va: National Association of Chain Drug Stores; 2000 Oct. Report No. 062100.
16. Institute for Safe Medication Practices. A million abbreviations. *ISMP Medication Safety Alert!* March 11, 2004;9(5).
17. Schiff GD, Klass D, Peterson J, et al. Linking laboratory and pharmacy: opportunities for reducing errors and improving care. *Arch Intern Med.* 2003;163:893–900.
18. Murray MD. Automated medication dispensing devices. In: Shojania KG, Duncan BW, McDonald KM, et al. *Making Health Care Safer: A Critical Analysis of Patient Safety Practices.* Rockville, Md: Agency for Healthcare Research and Quality; 2001:111–6.

19. Pedersen CA, Schneider PJ, Scheckelhoff DJ. ASHP national survey of pharmacy practice in hospital settings: dispensing and administration—2005. *Am J Health Syst Pharm.* 2006;63:327–45.

20. Institute for Safe Medication Practices. Survey of automated dispensing shows need for practice improvements and safer system design. *ISMP Medication Safety Alert!* June 16, 1999;4(12).

21. Keeys CA, Dandurand K, Harris J, et al. Providing nighttime pharmaceutical services through telepharmacy. *Am J Health Syst Pharm.* 2002;59:716–21.

22. Romero AV, Malone DC. Accuracy of adverse-drug-event reports collected using an automated dispensing system. *Am J Health Syst Pharm.* 2005;62:1375–80.

23. Bates DW, Cullen DJ, Laird N, et al. Incidence of adverse drug events and potential adverse drug events: implications for prevention. ADE Prevention Study Group. *JAMA.* 1995;274:29–34.

24. Bates DW, Cohen M, Leape LL, et al. Reducing the frequency of errors in medicine using information technology. *J Am Med Inform Assoc.* 2001;8:299–308.

25. Bates DW, Leape LL, Cullen DJ, et al. Effect of computerized physician order entry and a team intervention on prevention of serious medication errors. *JAMA.* 1998;280:1311–6.

26. Kilbridge P. Computer crash—lessons from a system failure. *N Engl J Med.* 2003;348:881–2.

27. Manthous CA. Leapfrog and critical care: evidence- and reality-based intensive care for the 21st century. *Am J Med.* 2004;116:188–93.

28. Koppel R, Metlay JP, Cohen A, et al. Role of computerized physician order entry systems in facilitating medication errors. *JAMA.* 2005;293:1197–1203.

29. Han YY, Carcillo JA, Venkataraman ST, et al. Unexpected increased mortality after implementation of a commercially sold computerized physician order entry system. *Pediatrics.* 2005;116:1506–2.

30. American Society of Health-System Pharmacists. *Improving Medication Safety in Health Systems through Innovations in Automation Technology.* Proceedings of symposia and educational sessions held during the 2004 ASHP Midyear Clinical Meeting. Available at: http://ashpadvantage.com/website_html/ce_pubs.htm. Accessed March 6, 2006.

31. First Consulting Group. *Computerized Physician Order Entry: Costs, Benefits and Challenges, A Case Study Approach.* Commissioned by the American Hospital Association and the Federation of American Hospitals. Chicago, January 2003.

32. California Healthcare Foundation and First Consulting Group. *Computerized Physician Order Entry in Community Hospitals: Lessons from the Field.* Oakland, Calif: California Healthcare Foundation; 2003. Available at: www.chcf.org/topics/view.cfm?itemID=20729. Accessed March 6, 2006.

33. Ash JS, Stavri PZ, Kuperman GJ. A consensus statement on considerations for successful CPOE implementation. *J Am Med Inform Assoc.* 2003;10:229–34.

34. Walker J, Pan E, Johnston D, et al. The value of health care information exchange and interoperability. *Health Aff* Web Exclusive; January 19, 2005. Available at: http://content.healthaffairs.org/webexclusives/index.dtl?year=2005.

35. Brailer DJ. Interoperability: the key to the future health care system. *Health Aff* Web Exclusive; January 19, 2005. Available at: http://content.healthaffairs.org/webexclusives/index.dtl?year=2005.

36. Hammond WE. The making and adoption of health data standards. *Health Aff.* 2005;24:1205–13.

37. Nebeker JR, Hoffman JM, Weir CR, et al. High rates of adverse drug events in a highly computerized hospital. *Arch Intern Med.* 2005;165:11–6.

38. Kaushal R, Shojania KG, Bates DW. Effects of computerized order entry and clinical decision support systems on medication safety: a systematic review. *Arch Intern Med.* 2003;163:1409–16.

39. Weingart SN, Toth M, Sands DZ, et al. Physicians' decisions to override computerized drug alerts in primary care. *Arch Intern Med.* 2003;163:2625–31.

40. Hsiech TC, Kuperman GJ, Jaggi T, et al. Characteristics and consequences of drug allergy alert overrides in a computerized physician order entry system. *J Am Med Inform Assoc.* 2004;11:482–91.

41. Payne TH, Nichol WP, Hoey P, et al. Characteristics and override rates of order checks in a practitioner order entry system. *Proc AMIA Symp.* 2002;602–6.

42. van der Sijs H, Aarts J, Vulto A, et al. Overriding of drug safety alerts in computerized physician order entry. *J Am Med Inform Assoc.* 2006;13:138–47.

43. Galanter WL, DiMomenico RJ, Polikaitis A. A trial of automated decision support alerts for contraindicated medications using computerized physician order entry. *J Am Med Inform Assoc.* 2005;12:269–74.

44. Bates DW, Kuperman GJ, Wang S, et al. Ten commandments for effective clinical decision support: making the practice of evidence-based medicine a reality. *J Am Med Inform Assoc.* 2003;10:523–30.

45. Neuenschwander M, Cohen MR, Vaida AJ, et al. Practical guide to bar coding for patient medication safety. *Am J Health Syst Pharm.* 2003;60:768–79.

46. Hokanson JA, Keith MR, Guernsey BG, et al. Potential use of barcodes to implement automated dispensing quality assurance programs. *Hosp Pharm.* 1985;20:327–37.

47. Nold EG, Williams TC. Bar codes and their potential applications in hospital pharmacy. *Am J Hosp Pharm.* 1985;42:2722–37.

48. Lefkowitz S, Cheiken H, Barhart MR. A trial of the use of bar code technology to restructure a drug distribution and administration system. *Hosp Pharm.* 1991;26:239–42.

49. Meyer GE, Brandell R, Smith JE, et al. Use of bar codes in inpatient drug distribution. *Am J Hosp Pharm.* 1991;48:953–66.

50. Barker KN, Flynn EA, Pepper GA, et al. Medication error observed in 36 health care facilities. *Arch Intern Med.* 2002;162:1897–903.

51. Malcolm B, Carlson RA, Tucker CL, et al. Veterans Affairs: eliminating medication errors through point-of-care devices. Paper presented at: Healthcare Information and Management Systems Society Conference; April 200; Dallas, Tex. Vol. 2 (Session 73): 218–26.

52. Puckett F. Medication management component of a point of care information system. *Am J Health Syst Pharm.* 1995;52:1305–9.

53. Johnson CL, Carlson RA, Tucker CL, et al. Using BCMA software to improve patient safety in Veterans Administration Medical Centers. *J Healthc Inf Manage.* 2002;16(1):46–51.

54. Department of Health and Human Services. Food and Drug Administration. 21 CFR Parts 201, 606, and 610 [Docket No. 2002N–0204] Bar Code Label Requirement for Human Drug Products and Biological Products. February 25, 2004. Available at: www.fda.gov/cber/rules/barcodelabel.pdf. Accessed March 6, 2006.

55. Patterson ES, Rogers ML, Render ML. Fifteen best practice recommendations for bar-code medication administration in the Veterans Health Administration. *Jt Comm J Qual Saf.* 2004;30:355–65.

56. Cummings J, Bush P, Smith D, et al. Bar-coding medication administration review and consensus recommendations. *Am J Health Syst Pharm.* 2005;62:2626–9.

57. Assessing Bedside Bar-Coding. Pathways for Medication Safety. Available at: www.ismp.org/Tools/pathways.asp.

58. Patterson ES, Cook RI, Render ML. Improving patient safety by identifying side effects of introducing bar coding in medication administration. *J Am Med Inform Assoc.* 2002;9:540–53.

59. FDA embraces RFID to protect drug supply [news]. *Am J Health Syst Pharm.* 2004;61:2612–5.

60. Hicks RW, Cousins DD, Williams RL. Summary of Information Submitted to MEDMARX in the Year 2002. Rockville, Md: USP Center for the Advancement of Patient Safety; 2003.

61. Vanderveen T. Medication safety: averting highest-risk errors is first priority. *Patient Saf Qual Healthc.* 2005;2:16-21.

62. Rothschild JM, Keohane CA, Cook EF, et al. A controlled trial of smart infusion pumps to improve medication safety in critically ill patients. *Crit Care Med.* 2005;33:533–40.

63. Bates DW, Vanderveen T, Seger D, at al. Variability in intravenous medication practices: implications for medication safety. *Jt Comm J Qual Saf.* 2005;31:203–10.

64. Institute for Healthcare Improvement. Establish a rapid response team. Available at: www.ihi.org/IHI/Topics/CriticalCare/IntensiveCare/Changes/EstablishaRapidResponseTeam.htm. Accessed April 26, 2006.

65. Institute for Safe Medication Practices. New data monitoring technology offers real-time reporting of impending adverse events. *ISMP Medication Safety Alert!* June 26, 2003; 8(13).

66. Institute for Safe Medication Practices. It's time for standards to improve safety with electronic communication of medication orders. *ISMP Medication Safety Alert!* February 20, 2003;8(4). Available at: www.ismp.org/Newsletters/acutecare/articles/20030220.asp. Accessed March 6, 2006.

APPENDIX

DRAFT GUIDELINES FOR THE ELECTRONIC PRESENTATION OF INFORMATION ABOUT PRESCRIBED MEDICATIONS[66]

Safe presentation of drug nomenclature and dose expressions in electronic systems

1. List all products by generic name (use lowercase letters, unless using tall-man letters as mentioned in item 7) as the primary drug nomenclature, ensuring that each matches FDA-approved nomenclature so that all package labels agree with medication records.

2. Do not include the salt of the chemical when expressing a generic name unless multiple salts are available (e.g., hydroxyzine hydrochloride and hydroxyzine pamoate). If the salt is used as part of the name (e.g., USP-approved abbreviations such as K, Na, HBr, and HCl), it should follow the drug name, not precede it (e.g., warfarin Na, not Na warfarin, which can look like "no warfarin").

3. As appropriate, list associated brand names in a requisite field. When used, present brand names in uppercase letters (e.g., LANOXIN, LASIX) to differentiate them from generic names (use of all uppercase letters is a standard for trademarks throughout the pharmaceutical industry). Trademark symbols (e.g., ™ or ®) should not be used.

4. Express suffixes that are part of the brand name (e.g., SR, SA, CR) within both the generic name field and the brand name field (e.g., diltiazem XT and DILTIA XT).

5. Avoid use of all potentially dangerous abbreviations and dose expressions (see Table 8-3), including the following:
   a. Do not use trailing zeros (5 mg, never 5.0 mg).
   b. Use leading zeros for doses less than one measurement unit (0.3 mg, never .3 mg).
   c. Spell out the word "units." If adequate space is not available (see item 10), use the abbreviation UT (never U, which easily can be mistaken as a zero, causing a 10-fold overdose).
   d. Include properly spaced commas for dose numbers expressed in thousands (e.g., 5,000 units). Avoid using M as an abbreviation for thousands (e.g., 5 M units), which has been mistaken as million. Use the word "thousand" for larger doses in the hundreds of thousands (e.g., 150 thousand rather than 150,000). Use the word "million" for doses expressed in millions (e.g., 1 million units) to avoid possible misplacement of commas and misreading of the dose if the commas are not seen correctly with such large numbers.
   e. Express weights and measures in a standard fashion, and use USP standard abbreviations for dosage units, as follows:
      (1) m (lowercase) = meter
      (2) kg = kilogram
      (3) g = gram
      (4) mg = milligram
      (5) mcg = microgram (do not use the Greek letter mu, which has been misread as mg)
      (6) L (uppercase) = liter
      (7) mL (lowercase/uppercase) = milliliter (do not use cc, which has been misread as U or the number 4)
      (8) mEq = milliequivalent
      (9) mmol = millimole

6. To avoid confusion, do not abbreviate drug names (e.g., MTX for methotrexate has been misunderstood as mitoxantrone; MSO_4 for morphine sulfate has been misinterpreted as magnesium sulfate).

7. Use tall-man letters (e.g., hydrOXYzine and hydrALAZINE) to help distinguish look-alike products on screens and reports and minimize the risk of selecting the wrong product when medication names appear alphabetically in look-up lists (Table 6-1 lists generic drug names for which the FDA has required the use of tall-man lettering by pharmaceutical manufacturers).

8. When the drug name, strength, dosage form and dosage units appear together, list the generic name first, followed by brand name, strength, dose (if different from strength) and dosage form (e.g., timolol [TIMOPTIC] 0.5% ophthalmic solution; diazepam [VALIUM] 5 mg tablet). When the strength and dose differ, also list the amount needed for the dose (e.g., propranolol [INDERAL] 5 mg [½ × 10 mg] tablet).

9. When the drug name, strength, dosage form, and dosage units appear together, avoid confusion by providing a space between them (e.g., propranolol20 mg has been misread as 120 mg and 10Units has been misread as 100 Units).

Design features for electronic order entry systems (pharmacy and prescriber) that support safe communication of orders

10. Provide adequate space for items in data fields used to communicate drug names, dosing units, routes of administration, and frequencies. Two- or three-character fields force use of potentially dangerous abbreviations (QD for daily, often misread as QID; QOD for every other day, often misread as QID; U for units, often misread as a 0 or 4). Seeing the use of dangerous abbreviations in electronic formats may encourage practitioners to use them.

11. Provide a field that requires entry of the *purpose* for the following types of medication orders: all prn medications; look-alike products that are known to be problematic (few look-alike name pairs are used for the same purpose); and medications that have different dosing for varying indications or have multiple indications not in approved labeling (e.g., most prescriptions for gabapentin are for off-label uses such as neuropathic pain syndrome, generalized anxiety, social phobia, migraine therapy). Communicating the drug's indication reduces the risk of improper drug selection and offers clues to proper dosing when a medication has an indication-specific dosing algorithm.

12. Provide users with ways to emphasize medication- or patient-related warnings or other important clinical notes related to prescribed medications (e.g., uppercase and lowercase letters, contrasting color, boldface or italic type, flashing information, choice of fonts, audible alerts).

13. Provide users with the ability to search by brand name, generic name, synonym, or mnemonic, and link all means of accessing a name to a generic name default. Also, organize generic and brand names by dosage form in look-up tables (e.g., multiple gentamicin products should be organized as injectable, ophthalmic solution, cream, and other dosage forms).

14. Provide the ability to clearly communicate medications prescribed for specific, nonroutine administration times or under certain conditions (e.g., with dialysis, while NPO, until tolerating liquids, prior to surgery).

15. Provide a field that requires entry of the product's dosage form (e.g., tablets, capsules).

16. Provide the capability for users to link medications only to the appropriate routes of administration available for each drug. For example, vincristine injection should link only to the IV route of administration.

17. Provide required dose fields for users to designate the actual prescribed dose after product strength has been selected (e.g., selection of NPH insulin 100 units/mL requires a dose field to enter the prescribed dose in units).

18. Provide the generic name on all computer-generated labels and reports, including computer-generated MARs. Provide the option for listing brand names.

19. Provide a mechanism to facilitate safe order entry of complex medication regimens (e.g., chemotherapy, sliding-scale insulin) and medications that require a tapering dose schedule (e.g., corticosteroids) so that the orders appear clearly and in a logical order for those who dispense and administer the medications.

20. Provide the capability for clinicians to select the time or date to begin drug administration, regardless of when the order was entered, so that it appears on profile screens and computer-generated MARs on the correct date/time (e.g., a daily medication order entered after the typical 0900 administration time could appear on the current day's records).

21. Provide the capability to link all closely associated drug therapies so that they appear sequentially together on medication profile screens and computer-generated MARs (e.g., orders for PCA should be linked to corresponding orders for nausea, itching, and break-through pain) and to facilitate discontinuation of associated therapies when the primary therapy is discontinued.
22. Provide a mechanism for placing medication orders on hold under specified conditions, and for alerting users at specified times while a medication is on hold.
23. To prevent the risk of misinterpretation, limit the potential for free-text entries in CPOE systems. Allow full capability for free-text entries in the pharmacy computer system to facilitate communication of important information among pharmacists (via pharmacy computer screens) and nurses (via computer-generated MARs).

Other communication-related topics for which further investigation and standards are needed

24. Standards are needed for mnemonics or short names that allow practitioners to access a particular medication listing without entering the full name.
25. Standards are needed for the use of fonts (size and style) and colors that facilitate clarity of information presented on computer screens and in printed materials derived from electronic databases (e.g., labels, reports).
26. Consideration must be given to the role that symbols and certain letter characters may play in creating errors during electronic communication. For example, slash marks and hyphens have been misread as the number 1, and symbols for more than and less than have been misinterpreted as the opposite of what was intended. Also, the letter O can be misread as a zero (0), the letter z as the number 2, and a lowercase L (l) as the number 1 or the letter i (I).

CHAPTER 16

PREVENTING MEDICATION ERRORS IN CANCER CHEMOTHERAPY

Michael R. Cohen

From 1993 to 1998, 5,366 medication errors were reported through the Food and Drug Administration (FDA) Adverse Event Reporting System; 469 of those errors were fatal. Of those fatalities, 72 (15.4%) involved an antineoplastic agent.[1] More recently, it has been estimated that 500 deaths occur annually from medication errors associated with cancer chemotherapy and that only 3% of those errors are reported.[2] In a survey of 186 oncology nurses, 63% said chemotherapy errors had occurred in their workplace.[3] Errors involving anticancer drugs can be devastating because these drugs typically have narrow therapeutic ranges. At the same time, dosages of some chemotherapeutic agents vary widely depending on what condition is being treated, how the drug is used, and the use of rescue therapy. Furthermore, chemotherapy regimens have become increasingly complex and intensive as supportive therapies (antiemetics, colony-stimulating factors, and bone marrow and stem cell transplantation) have improved. These newer chemotherapy regimens carry greater risks of injury.

Events at a comprehensive cancer center in 1994 may have been a turning point in the battle against medication errors because of the unprecedented publicity.[4] Betsy Lehman, a 39-year-old health care reporter for the *Boston Globe*, died of a drug overdose during treatment for metastatic breast cancer. According to the investigational protocol, the cyclophosphamide dose was "4 g/m^2 over four days." This ambiguous order was misinterpreted by a number of health care professionals. What should have been ordered was a daily dose of 1 g/m^2 for 4 consecutive days. Instead, the patient received cyclophosphamide 6.52 g per day for 4 consecutive days, for a total of 26.08 g instead of a total of 6.52 g. The error was not recognized, and Lehman's death was attributed to cardiotoxicity.

The Lehman case and others prompted me to review the literature on medication errors, summarize how measures to prevent errors may apply to cancer chemotherapy, and invite a panel of experts to discuss the resultant document at a meeting held by the Institute for Safe Medication Practices (ISMP) in conjunction with the 1995 American Society of Health-System Pharmacists (ASHP) annual meeting. Comments by the panelists and audience were incorporated into the original document, appropriate literature citations were added, and revisions were made on the basis of guidelines developed by the Royal College of Physicians and the Royal College of Radiologists.[5] For this chapter, the original article[6] was updated to reflect English-language reports on chemotherapy-related errors published between 1996 and January 2005, as well as published advice on error prevention.[7-13] The recommendations at the end of the chapter are based in part on the document that originated with the ISMP–ASHP panel discussion.

As with all medications, the goal of drug administration in cancer chemotherapy is to ensure delivery of the right drug to the right patient in the right dose and dosage form via the right route at the right time. Achieving this goal requires a comprehensive, systematic approach. Drug manufacturers, regulatory agencies, prescribers, unit clerks, nurses or other professionals responsible for drug administration and documentation, pharmacists and other pharmacy personnel, and patients all play important roles. This chapter addresses the following error-prevention measures as they relate to cancer chemotherapy: educating health care providers, verifying the dose, establishing dosage limits, standardizing the prescribing vocabulary, working with pharmaceutical manufacturers, educating patients, and improving communication. The need to increase pharmacists' involvement throughout these steps is discussed.

EDUCATING HEALTH CARE PROVIDERS

The single most important reason medication errors reach patients is that information about the patient and the medication is not available when it is needed.[14] Ideally, each institution should provide a computerized system that makes important patient-specific information available. However, few hospitals have institutionwide computer systems that make patient-specific and general information available to practitioners at the time of prescribing, dispensing, preparing, and administering chemotherapy. Most practitioners must rely on electronic drug information databases and traditional educational materials for information.

At the Children's Hospital of Philadelphia, distractions and interruptions were identified as contributors to chemotherapy errors.[15] As a result, two rooms adjacent to the oncology inpatient unit were set aside for chemotherapy ordering and were equipped with protocol books, reference materials, and a computer terminal. At the National Institutes of Health (NIH) Clinical Center (an intramural hospital for NIH research), an interdisciplinary task force implemented the following enhancements to the computerized prescriber order entry (CPOE) system: automatic chemotherapy dosage calculations based on the height and weight entered in the patient's record, automatic addition of protocol-specific laboratory parameters to computer-generated orders, and instant access to drug information and investigational drug sheets from any computer terminal.[16]

Educational Process

Education should be tailored to the health care provider's function: prescribing, dispensing, preparing, or administering antineoplastic drugs. All providers should undergo orientation and competency testing on the mechanisms involved in documented cases of serious medication errors.[7,9,10] The need for such testing is supported by standards of the Joint Commission on Accreditation of Healthcare Organizations (JCAHO). At the NIH Clinical Center, all physicians must complete a training module before being credentialed to prescribe chemotherapy. All hospital personnel who prescribe, prepare, or administer chemotherapy attend a lecture on the serious nature of chemotherapy errors.[16] Annual assurance of the competency of staff involved in chemotherapy has been suggested.[7,9,10] Pharmacists and pharmacy technicians should undergo testing before they are permitted to prepare and dispense antineoplastic drugs.[17] Education is needed when a new agent is added to the formulary and when an institution becomes involved in an investigational drug protocol. Information about the new agent could be provided through a traditional newsletter, guidelines, or a checklist;[18] staff members' signatures would indicate that they understand the appropriate use of a new agent.

Pharmacy education about antineoplastic drugs should not be limited to clinical specialists or oncology hospitals. Despite efforts to restrict administration times to periods of optimal staffing, cancer chemotherapy may be needed in the evenings or on weekends. To ensure competent 24-hour coverage, all staff pharmacists must be educated in the use of these drugs. Pharmacists who practice in community hospitals encounter unique problems because of a lack of standardization. A patient may begin chemotherapy in an oncology hospital, where specialists familiar with investigational regimens prescribe and administer the initial dose, but may receive subsequent doses in the community. In such a case, doxorubicin was inadvertently administered by the intrathecal route.[19] In a survey at small rural hospitals in Australia, staff members identified the information they need for continuing chemotherapy: patient details, diagnosis, chemotherapy protocol, dosages and method of confirmation, interval between cycles, supportive care, contact information for the prescriber, availability of premixed cytotoxics, methods of administration, and possible adverse effects.[20]

Community-based oncologists not participating in cooperative group studies may vary in the way they write orders. For example, an oncologist may try a new regimen after reading about it or may modify an existing protocol. Another complexity of therapy is that different protocols may specify different administration methods. For example, in April 1998 at the Dana-Farber Cancer Institute, there were 14 active pediatric oncology group protocols in which 23 unique cyclophosphamide regimens were specified.[21] A multidisciplinary group at Children's Hospital of Philadelphia also found that different protocols had different methods of administration for cyclophosphamide and cisplatin.[15] Another obstacle to standardization is the use of both body surface area and patient weight in dosage calculations.[15]

Pharmacists should initiate and participate in educational sessions for other health care providers. Pharmacists are uniquely qualified to instruct new house staff and attending physicians about institutional policies on prescribing and administering antineoplastics.[7] Oncology pharmacy specialists at the NIH Clinical Center and clinical research pharmacists at the Pharmaceutical Management Branch of the Division of Cancer Treatment and Diagnosis, National Cancer Institute (NCI), collaboratively developed guidelines for describing cancer chemotherapy regimens in treatment protocols, order forms, and product labels.[22]

Describing actual medication errors, especially consequences of nonstandard prescribing practices that have occurred within the institution or that have been published, can be highly effective. The use of an automated intervention program initiated by pharmacists allows errors to be presented and discussed by the pharmacy and therapeutics committee in a nonthreatening, evaluative manner.[23] Memorial-Sloan Kettering Cancer Center has a successful and nonpunitive quality assurance program, in which trends in potentially harmful chemotherapy orders are identified and discussed with the staff; it has resulted in increased reporting and detection of error-prone practices.[24] Institutions can share their preventive measures and standardized prescribing practices with other institutions and can monitor error "alerts" from JCAHO and ISMP.[10]

Reference Materials

Reference materials should be developed and made readily available to all health care providers involved in prescribing, dispensing, preparing, and administering antineoplastic drugs. They should cover appropriate uses of these agents (FDA-approved and investigational uses), precautions, adverse effects, dose-limiting effects, solution preparation and infusion methods, usual adult and pediatric doses, and doses for single and multiple courses of therapy. Excellent resources have been published.[25–27] However, textbooks rapidly become outdated and can contain errors.[28–30] Institution-specific resources, especially in cancer research centers, should be developed, preferably in forms that can be easily updated, such as summary sheets, notebooks, and computerized databases. These reference materials should be placed in all pharmacy locations (including all satellites) and at strategic locations throughout the institution (e.g., nursing stations). In the 2004 ASHP national survey of pharmacy practice, 60.4% of the hospitals reported having an electronic drug information service or product (e.g., AHFSfirst or Micromedex) to provide objective drug information.[31] In addition, complete copies of treatment protocols, along with the patient's informed-consent sheet, should be readily available in all pharmacies that dispense antineoplastic agents.

PDQ (Physician Data Query), a database provided by NCI, contains information on different cancer therapies, along with current information on many active and closed protocols. The database can be accessed free of charge at www.nci.nih.gov/cancertopics/pdq/cancerdatabase. CancerNet (http://cancernet.nci.nih.gov/), also run by NCI, provides access to PDQ and clinical trial results. The Micromedex (www.micromedex.com/) computerized drug information service provides information about specific agents and has charts with dosing and other important information. Another resource is the annual Guide for the Administration and Use of Cancer Chemotherapeutic Agents (www.oncologyse.com/articles/7319/pdf/7319.pdf?CFID=441510&CFTOKEN= 46542611).[32]

VERIFYING THE DOSE

Although computerized dose-verification systems are available, many practice sites have yet to acquire and properly utilize them. Each institution should develop its own dose-verification process with several independent double checks. The process should specify how the prescribing physician, unit clerk, nurse, dispensing pharmacist, clinical pharmacist, pharmacy technician, and staff responsible for drug administration will interact. A detailed checklist covering prescribing, transcribing, dispensing, and administration is needed. For example, do house staff physicians have independent prescribing privileges, or must orders be cosigned by an attending physician?

In 2002 CPOE was not available in 524 (83.7%) of 626 U.S. hospitals; it was fully or partially available in 9.6% and 6.5%, respectively.[33] In the 2004 ASHP national survey of pharmacy practice, only 4.2% of hospitals reported CPOE systems.[31] The low rate of CPOE implementation is surprising, since studies have shown CPOE to reduce medication errors.[34,35] At one academic institution, CPOE combined with electronic medication administration records (MARs) eliminated all physician and nursing transcription errors.[36] Another academic institution reported a significant increase in voluntarily reported medication errors after CPOE implementation.[37] A trend toward fewer prescribing errors and a significant increase in reported pharmacy order-processing errors per patient discharge were noted. It is possible that pharmacy order-processing errors could be decreased by enabling the pharmacy computer system to communicate electronically with the CPOE system. Although CPOE is believed to reduce medication errors, a cisplatin overdose (760 mg) has been attributed to the characteristics of prescription software.[38]

Institutions have reported their experiences with CPOE for cancer chemotherapy.[15,16,36,39] The CPOE system at the NIH Clinical Center automatically calculates chemotherapy dosages based on the height and weight that are entered in the patient's record.[16] IntelliDose, a software program with error-checking routines for single, multiple, and cumulative dosing, was developed in an office and cancer center setting; no errors in calculations or chemotherapy prescribing occurred during a 3-year study period.[40] In Germany, a computer-aided therapy planning system in pediatric oncology (CATIPO) was developed to generate a printed, patient-specific, protocol-guided therapy plan that contains all drugs (cytostatic and supportive care) to be administered during a single chemotherapy cycle.[41] This computer-generated document is used for ordering drugs from the pharmacy and documenting drug administration. CATIPO can help avoid mistakes because all cytostatic drug dosages are calculated at least twice; physicians entering the patient-specific information also use conventional calculations to double-check dosages. Medication errors were reduced in a bone marrow transplant unit in Italy when CPOE replaced spoken and handwritten prescribing.[39] As a result of warnings generated during CPOE, about 10% of the drugs selected were not administered; in most cases the dosage was merely adjusted to the patient's renal and hepatic function.

Because spoken orders can easily be misinterpreted, they should not be accepted for antineoplastic agents. An actinomycin overdose resulting from a spoken order was reported to ISMP. The oncologist at a sarcoma clinic had called in an order to the patient's local oncologist's office. The order was for actinomycin D 4 mg over 4 days, but the oncology nurse wrote actinomycin D 4 mg daily for 4 days. Six days after completing the course of therapy, the patient died from bleeding and sepsis secondary to severe thrombocytopenia and leukopenia. A telephone order from an oncologist to a pharmacist for flutamide was misinterpreted as thalidomide, but the error was detected before reaching the patient.[42] Faxed orders may be acceptable under certain circumstances, but faxes should not be accepted unless all of the information is clear. Furthermore, antineoplastic drugs should be ordered only during specified working hours so that adequately trained staff members are on hand to provide necessary clinical review.

All doses should be calculated independently by the physician who writes the order, the pharmacist who checks the order and dispenses the drug, and the nurse who administers it. This is especially important in cancer chemotherapy, because repeating doses within a cycle or during subsequent cycles multiplies any error in calculation. The prescription should specify both the dose according to body surface area or body weight and the calculated amount. When physicians specify chemotherapy doses in this format (e.g., "25 mg/m² [50 mg]" for a patient whose body surface area is 2 m²), the dose calculation can be double-checked. Guidelines developed by the NIH Clinical Center recommend this format for describing cancer chemotherapy regimens.[12]

Dosages may need to be modified because of drug-induced bone marrow suppression, other toxicities, or renal or hepatic dysfunction. Pharmacists must have access to laboratory data and must become familiar with formulas for dosage adjustment. Computer software should link appropriate laboratory test results (e.g., white blood cell counts, platelet counts, and serum creatinine levels) with dosage adjustment criteria so that necessary modifications in the dose can be determined automatically. Relevant lab values should be independently checked by prescribers, nurses, and pharmacists before any doses are administered. The computer system at the NIH Clinical Center automatically adds protocol-specific laboratory parameters to computer-generated orders.[16] Simple dosing tables for all regimens, listing the dose per body surface area, body weight, or both, could serve as a ready reference against which to compare calculated doses. This would help ensure that those responsible for prescribing, dispensing, and administering a drug have properly interpreted the dosage requirements of the protocol.

The dose-verification policy should specify whether the prescriber must identify the protocol (e.g., by listing the protocol number, institutional review board [IRB] number, or a published citation) on the order form. Dose verification steps in the NIH Clinical Center's chemotherapy error-reduction program include checking the dose with the principal investigator or study chairperson.[16] If a regimen is unfamiliar, the pharmacist should verify the dose by reviewing at least two independent literature sources. However, erroneous information can appear in published articles. An overdose resulted because a journal article incorrectly indicated that the dose of vincristine sulfate was 1.4 mg/m² on days 1 through 8 instead of days 1 *and* 8, even though the pharmacist initially recognized a problem.[43,44] Another article listed the dose of vincristine as 1.4 mg/m² on days 1 through 5, when it should have been given only on day 1.[45] Also, an incorrect dose of sodium thiosulfate was published,[46] and an article stated that docetaxel and doxorubicin were given three times a week instead of every 3 weeks.[30]

While chemotherapy overdoses can have devastating consequences, underdoses of chemotherapy can also lead to poor outcomes. Cladribine underdosing in two patients with hairy-cell leukemia has been reported.[47] Both patients failed to respond to therapy. When their records were investigated, it was determined that the portable pump that was to contain 7 days of therapy contained only 1 day's dose. The chemotherapy orders had been written clearly, but the person preparing the medication did not multiply the calculated dose by 7 days.

ESTABLISHING DOSAGE LIMITS

Hospitals should define situations in which pharmacists are not to dispense certain antineoplastic agents without further expert review, for example, when a prescribed dose exceeds a preset maximum single dose, dose per cycle, or cumulative dose. Pharmacists should work with physicians, nurses, and other health care providers to identify dosage limits and to establish a review process (involving individuals other than the prescriber and reviewing pharmacist) to be completed before a drug that exceeds a preestablished limit can be dispensed.

In a national survey conducted by the American Society for Blood and Marrow Transplantation, 15 of the 115 responding transplant centers reported a total of 18 patients who were inadvertently given overdoses of chemotherapy between 1989 and 1994.[48] Thirty percent of those errors were a result of the cumulative drug dose being given as a daily dose. The estimated chemotherapy overdose error rate was 0.06%.

From September 1998 through August 2003, 3,871 errors involving oncology drugs were reported to the United States Pharmacopeia (USP) MEDMARX program.[49] Most of the errors (88%) did not cause harm; 3% caused some type of harm. Improper dose/quantity was selected as the type of error in 25% of the cases. The numbers of errors reported with various chemotherapy agents are listed at www.usp.org/pdf/EN/patient Safety/capsLink 2004-04-01.pdf.

Serious toxicity or death has been attributed to overdoses in patients receiving many antineoplastic drugs as monotherapy, including cisplatin,[38,50–54] carboplatin,[55] cytarabine,[56] irinotecan,[57] melphalan,[58] mitoxantrone,[59] mechlorethamine,[60] methotrexate,[61–65] vinblastine,[66] and vincristine,[67–70] as well as in patients receiving multiple agents.[71] In some of these cases, an excessive dose was recognized during the order-review process. Communication breakdowns, failure of the prescriber to fully consider the clinical implications of the dose in question, and failure of pharmacists and nurses to stand their ground can result in patient harm. With preset limits and a review process for exceptions, the chance that an improper dose will be administered is greatly reduced.

The risk of error is particularly high with the antineoplastic agents methotrexate and lomustine because mistakes in their dosing schedules are common (see the following sidebar).

Each institution should form a committee of oncologists, pharmacists, and nurses to establish maximum doses for all FDA-approved antineoplastic agents. The dosage ceiling should be based on the literature[72] and on clinical studies at the specific institution. At least four types of dosage limits are necessary for antineoplastic agents: (1) the maximum amount for a single dose for each type of schedule (e.g., weekly versus every 3 weeks) and regimen (single-agent versus combination), (2) the maximum amount per 24 hours, (3) the maximum amount per course of therapy (definable for each drug), and (4) the maximum amount per patient lifetime. These limits should be specified in milligrams, units, milligrams or units per square meter of body surface area, or milligrams or units per kilogram of body weight.

METHOTREXATE AND LOMUSTINE

Errors in the dosing schedule have led to dozens of fatalities in patients receiving the cytotoxic agent methotrexate for nonmalignant conditions. Low-dose methotrexate is used for immuno-modulation in rheumatoid arthritis, asthma, psoriasis, inflammatory bowel disease, myasthenia gravis, and inflammatory myositis. For these conditions, it is administered as a weekly dose, but mistakes have occurred because relatively few medications are dosed in this manner and clinicians and patients are more accustomed to daily dosing. One patient died after he misunderstood the directions for use and took methotrexate 2.5 mg every 12 hours for 6 consecutive days, instead of 2.5 mg every 12 hours for three doses each week. Another patient died after he misread the directions on a prescription bottle and took 10 mg every morning instead of every Monday.

Methotrexate errors in hospitalized patients have also been reported. In one case, the physician had properly recorded that the patient had been taking methotrexate 7.5 mg weekly as an outpatient, but when he prescribed three 2.5 mg tablets weekly, the order was transcribed incorrectly as three times daily. When the patient was transferred to another unit, the dose was transcribed incorrectly as three times a week. Both errors were detected during pharmacy review of orders and did not reach the patient.

Similar errors have been reported in other countries. One patient in Australia took extra doses of methotrexate as needed to relieve arthritic symptoms. Three elderly patients took the medication daily despite clearly written instructions to take it weekly. Two cases involved incorrect transcription of the dosing schedule for hospitalized patients. Three of the six patients died as a result of the errors.

A study of errors with oral methotrexate revealed more than 100 cases during a 4-year period, resulting in 25 deaths and 48 other serious outcomes.[62] Most involved patients who accidentally took their dose daily instead of weekly.

The following measures can help reduce the risk of error with oral methotrexate:

❑ Build alerts into electronic prescribing systems and pharmacy computers to warn clinicians whenever doses of oral methotrexate have been entered (and, in a retail setting, remind staff to check the indication with the patient). Configure the systems to avoid default to a daily dosing schedule.

❑ Have a pharmacist conduct drug-use review before dispensing oral methotrexate to deter-mine its indication for use, verify proper dosing, confirm the correct dosing schedule on medication administration records (MARs) and prescription labels, ensure staff and patient education, and promote appropriate monitoring of the patient.

❑ Establish a system to ensure that outpatients receive counseling when picking up new prescriptions and refills (e.g., mark the bag with a red flag to alert clerical staff that counseling is required, not optional).

❑ Provide patients with clear written instructions that name a specific day of the week for taking the tablet(s). Avoid choosing Monday because it might be misread as "morning." Prepare instructions in large print for elderly patients with poor eyesight.

❑ Advise patients to contact their physician if they miss taking a dose. Tell them that a flare-up of the disease because of one missed dose is unlikely.

A similar problem exists with lomustine. A single dose of oral lomustine (130 mg/m^2), used to treat brain cancer and Hodgkin's disease, should be taken only once every 6 weeks. Like methotrexate, lomustine has often been erroneously administered daily. One cancer patient's usual dose of lomustine 140 mg was due the day after she had been admitted to the hospital for a laparoscopic procedure. Her oncologist ordered a single dose of the drug, but the hospital pharmacist mistakenly entered it as a daily dose, and this appeared on the nurse's computer-generated MAR. After the patient received the drug daily for 5 days, routine lab tests detected severe thrombocytopenia, azotemia, and neutropenia. By then, the patient was febrile and had severe bruising and hematuria. The oncologist discovered the error, and the patient recovered after prolonged hospitalization. A recent error occurred when a patient took a prescription for a single 160 mg dose of lomustine to a community pharmacy. The pharmacist decided to offer the patient a full package containing 20 capsules (40 mg each), since the drug was costly and he would likely have to discard the remaining capsules. Although the package directions correctly said to take four capsules, the patient misunderstood and took four capsules daily for 5 days. The error was discovered when the patient attempted to refill the prescription. The pharmacist contacted the oncologist. The patient was admitted to the hospital and apparently recovered, although the full effects of the overdose had not been determined.

In another case, a 24-year-old woman with brain cancer died as a result of a lomustine overdose. The poorly legible prescription was for lomustine 190 mg every 6 weeks. The pharmacist misunderstood the directions as daily for 6 weeks and dispensed a 6-week supply of capsules with directions to take 190 mg daily. The patient's physician had not explained how to take the medication, so she followed the label directions and took 190 mg daily for 21 days. She was hospitalized with severe bone marrow suppression and acute bleeding and died a month later.

Bristol-Myers Squibb has enhanced the labeling and the packaging of its lomustine product CeeNU. "Single Dose Only" is now printed in red on the label, and "Dispense Single Dose Only" is embossed on the cap of stock bottles. However, these warnings have been overlooked in some cases. A boxed warning in the package insert also states that the drug should not be administered more frequently than every 6 weeks, but this warning can be missed because it is embedded within information about the potential risk for bone marrow suppression. Additional safeguards should be considered for this high-alert medication:

❑ Program warning messages such as "single dose only" into order entry systems. Also configure the system to limit the quantity prescribed or dispensed to 300 mg or less for each prescription or order.

❑ Prepare patient prescriptions or doses using unit-of-use dose packs available from the manufacturer. Each 300 mg dose pack contains two 100 mg capsules, two 40 mg capsules, and two 10 mg capsules, with instructions for the pharmacist to select the correct patient dose (within 10 mg), place the capsules in a single vial, and affix the special patient label provided.

❑ When possible, present dosing frequency directions on patient labels and nursing MARs in bold type or all capital letters (e.g., CAUTION: SINGLE DOSE ONLY). Use large print to assist elderly patients with poor eyesight.

❑ Establish a system to ensure that patients receive counseling when picking up new prescriptions and refills (e.g., mark the bag with a red flag to alert clerical staff that counseling is required, not optional). Require the pharmacist to review the prescription label with the patient or caregiver and to ask for confirmation that the patient understands the dosing schedule.

❑ Ensure that patients receive written drug information leaflets that contain clear advice about the "single dose only" schedule.

To reduce the risk of errors, pharmacists, technicians, and nurses who handle oral (and injectable) chemotherapy must have initial and ongoing education in the use of these drugs. Only certified oncology nurses should administer oral or injectable chemotherapy.

Establishing maximum doses may be challenging in community hospitals. Each oncologist should be invited to agree in advance to limits beyond which no drug should be dispensed. Because of the diversity of doses and treatment methods used for different malignancies, it may not be feasible to establish strict limits for all antineoplastic agents. Maximum-dose guidelines, such as those for vincristine,[73] have been questioned. Nevertheless, limits and a review process for dosages that exceed the limits should be established.

Pharmacists should work with computer programmers or software vendors to develop electronic warnings and order-screening routines that will not permit processing of orders when the established dosage limit is exceeded. At the NIH Clinical Center, a multidisciplinary task force recommended that the capability for maximum dose checks be added to the computer's ordering screens.[16] Although such an automated system can help identify doses that surpass established ceilings, a manual verification and tracking program must also be in place. For example, if the maximum single dose of carboplatin in a comprehensive cancer center is determined to be 1,200 mg and the system does not allow another dose to be dispensed for at least 3 weeks, the pharmacist must contact the prescriber if a dose is ordered sooner, to verify the dose and identify the treatment protocol before dispensing. If the pharmacist does not agree with the prescriber's decision and the issue cannot be resolved to the ultimate satisfaction of the pharmacist and the prescriber, a preestablished peer-review committee must make a judgment.

Stating dosage limits in the labeling of drug containers can help reduce the likelihood of errors. All Platinol containers state the dosage limit for cisplatin directly on the packaging,[74] and such labeling may be appropriate for other drugs, such as vincristine. Despite the Platinol labeling, a pediatric patient received a cisplatin dose of 204 mg when a dose of 20.4 mg was misinterpreted.[54] Pharmacists may want to add their own dosage warnings on certain drug containers.

Warnings about dosage limits should not be restricted to the packaging and labeling. Consideration should be given to including dosage limits in chemotherapy protocols and on preprinted order forms. Pharmacists should include maximum doses in summary sheets. The limits must be communicated during employee orientation and in-service programs and placed in locations where these drugs are prescribed, stored, dispensed, and administered. Once limits are identified and endorsed by other health care providers, pharmacists must not become complacent. Although electronic messages and labels are useful tools that augment the dose-verification process, they should not become substitutes for other checks.

Other types of limits related to administration should also be established, such as the minimum duration of infusion and the appropriate route. There have been many reports of patient death after inadvertent intrathecal administration of vincristine;[75-88] survival is rare.[89-93] A patient with Burkitt's lymphoma received vincristine intrathecally instead of methotrexate. He suffered paralysis and agonizing pain and died 10 weeks after a neurologist administered the drug. The vincristine was intended for IV use. Such errors most often occur because a practitioner picks up the wrong syringe.

Reports like this prompted ISMP to ask USP to issue an official dispensing standard.[94] USP requires that when vincristine is not dispensed in its original container, the drug must be packaged in an overwrap that bears the following statement: "Fatal if Given Intrathecally. For IV Use Only. Do Not Remove Covering Until Moment of Injection." Dispensers must apply this warning to all syringes. FDA asked manufacturers to provide overwrap and labeling to facilitate dispensing. Manufacturers must provide a label that can be affixed directly to an extemporaneously prepared syringe. Each syringe must be placed within the overwrap prior to dispensing.

Even when vincristine is properly labeled and packaged, a staff member could remove the drug from its overwrap in advance of IV injection. If a syringe of vincristine is nearby when an intrathecal medication is being administered, a physician, focused on performing a lumbar puncture, maintaining sterility, and preventing patient movement, could overlook the syringe label and administer the wrong medication intrathecally. A neurologist, who might not be familiar with cancer drugs or protocols, may be administering the intrathecal drug. If two syringes are present, the neurologist may believe both are for intrathecal administration.

Suggestions for preventing intrathecal administration of vincristine and other IV drugs also include the following:

1. Restrict the route of administration of vincristine in the pharmacy/prescriber order entry system to IV only.[16]

2. Prepare vincristine for IV bolus administration in a small-volume IV bag instead of a syringe (with USP-required warning label) to prevent confusion with intrathecal syringes.[95–100] Some believe that preparing vincristine in a small-volume bag for administration into a peripheral vein may increase the risk of extravasation, particularly in pediatric patients,[101] but the M. D. Anderson Cancer Center has been preparing vincristine with 25 mL of normal saline in minibags for over 20 years.[100]

3. Use a forcing function in which intrathecal medication is not dispensed until the empty bag of vincristine is returned to the pharmacy.[15]

4. Do not dispense an IV medication in a way that allows its entry into a location where an intrathecal medication is being administered. Intrathecal administration might be restricted to a designated location[98] such as a treatment room and to a standard time (e.g., early morning or late evening). The pharmacy could prepare and deliver intrathecal medications to the specified location immediately before use.[98,102]

5. Never deliver intrathecal and IV medications together.[98,102]

6. Establish a list of drugs that can be administered intrathecally (or epidurally) and ban all other injectable drugs from rooms where lumbar punctures are performed. The list of intrathecal drugs used for any disease is very small. Cytarabine, methotrexate, thiotepa, gentamicin, vancomycin, and hydrocortisone are among those used for cancer patients.

7. Have at least two health care professionals independently verify and document the accuracy of all intrathecal doses before administration.[98] In some cases, such as when a patient will receive both IV vincristine and an intrathecal medication, the patient and family should be asked to participate in the checking and help ensure that vincristine is not injected intrathecally.

8. Develop syringes for intrathecal or epidural use that are not interchangeable with syringes for IV use.[103] Several such devices are in development, and commercial applications are being pursued.[104] A specially designed syringe for IV vincristine, known as the Vincotube System, is readily distinguishable from all other available syringes.[105]

9. Have accrediting and regulatory bodies provide oversight to ensure that facilities where chemotherapy is administered are following policies and procedures to prevent accidental intrathecal injection of IV drugs.

In England, the National Health Service (NHS) has developed guidance on the safe administration of intrathecal chemotherapy (www.dh.gov.uk/assetRoot/04/06/50/49/04065049.pdf). Unlike the USP guidelines, the NHS guidelines state that negative labeling (e.g., "Not for Intrathecal Use") should not be used. Instead, they recommend the following: "For Intravenous Use Only—fatal if given by other routes."[106]

In addition to the errors with intrathecal vincristine administration, the drug has been inadvertently administered intramuscularly[107,108] when confused with a syringe for asparaginase, and intraventricularly[109,110] when mistaken for cytarabine. Interferon alfa-2a has also caused problems after inadvertent administration by the IV route;[111] the drug should be administered by the subcutaneous or intramuscular route.

Another drug that has caused major toxicity after intrathecal administration is doxorubicin.[19] Even drugs that are suitable for intrathecal administration can be highly toxic if the dose intended for systemic use is given intrathecally (e.g., cytarabine,[112] methotrexate[113–118]).

STANDARDIZING THE PRESCRIBING VOCABULARY

Failure to control the prescribing vocabulary is a major cause of chemotherapy errors. Conversations among oncology experts are replete with abbreviations, acronyms, and coined names. Efforts to squeeze large amounts of information into abstracts presented at meetings help perpetuate this problem.

These shortcuts may be convenient for oncology specialists, but they are an obstacle to health care providers less familiar with cancer chemotherapy and can easily be misinterpreted. For example, the abbreviation MTX has been misinterpreted as Mustargen (mechlorethamine).[119] An order for the bisphosphonate Aredia (pamidronate) was misread as Adria, a nickname for the Adriamycin brand of doxorubicin.[120] A vague order for "platinum" led to the substitution of cisplatin for carboplatin.[121] An order for CPT 200 mg was almost misinterpreted as cisplatin, which would have resulted in an overdose; the abbreviation CPT or CPT-11 actually stands for irinotecan.[122] A computer entry for "BUS10" resulted in busulfan 10 mg being dispensed instead of the antianxiety agent BuSpar (buspirone hydrochloride) 10 mg prescribed for a 5-year-old child.[123] Acronyms like COPP and MOPP are other examples of risky shortcuts. The MINE regimen (mesna, ifosfamide, mitoxantrone, and etoposide) has been confused with the MIME regimen (mitoguazone, ifosfamide, methotrexate, and etoposide).[124] These examples illustrate the importance of using only approved generic names (United States Adopted Names [USAN]), not abbreviations, acronyms, or coined names.

The chemoprotective drug leucovorin calcium is a pharmacologically active form of folic acid. It is used as rescue therapy to counteract folate deficiency and toxicity secondary to the administration of folic acid antagonists such as methotrexate, trimetrexate, trimethoprim, and pyrimethamine. It can also enhance the antitumor effects of fluorouracil in colorectal cancer. The British nonproprietary name of this drug, folinic acid, is used occasionally by prescribers in the United States. Since clinicians are familiar with folic acid and often unfamiliar with folinic acid, confirmation bias has led many to misread a folinic acid order as folic acid.

In one case, a prescription for "folinic acid 5 mg weekly" was dispensed as folic acid 1 mg, with directions to take 5 tablets weekly. Four hospital pharmacists with 80 years of combined experience had never seen "folinic acid" used for leucovorin calcium but were familiar with folic acid. A home care nurse noticed the error and called the pharmacy. In other examples, nurses have borrowed folic acid from patient supplies or taken a dose from an automated dispensing unit instead of waiting for pharmacy to dispense the drug. In one case both a nurse and a pharmacist contributed to the error; a pharmacist accidentally entered the physician's order for folinic acid 10 mg daily for a patient being treated with the antimalarial pyrimethamine as folic acid 1 mg daily, and nurses obtained four doses from an automated dispensing unit before the error was recognized.

To avoid such errors, the USAN leucovorin calcium should always be used. Errors with this drug could also occur if the abbreviation "FA" is used for folinic acid and misinterpreted as folic acid or if an order for "leucovorin" (rather than "leucovorin calcium") is interpreted as the anticancer drug Leukeran (chlorambucil).

In addition to misinterpreted names, another important source of error is confusion between patients' individual dose and the total dose over a course of therapy. For example, the order "cisplatin 100 mg/m^2 continuous infusion days 1–4" is ambiguous. The prescriber intended that the patient receive a total of 100 mg/m^2 over the entire 4-day period, a dose well within the usual limit of 120 mg/m^2 per course, which usually is repeated every 4 weeks. The order was misinterpreted, and the drug was dispensed as 100 mg/m^2 daily for 4 days.[15] The patient died. The preferred way to write the order is "cisplatin 25 mg/m^2/day (or "daily") as a 24-hour continuous IV infusion on 7/5/95, 7/6/95,

7/7/95, and 7/8/95." A patient whose chemotherapy dose was ordered to be given over 96 hours was given the entire course dose over 6 hours when the order was misread as q6 hours. In another case, a patient was given the entire 4-day course of therapy with doxorubicin and vincristine for 4 consecutive days. Chemotherapy orders should specify the drug dose to be administered each day, followed by the number of days it is to be administered.[12]

Protocols for study drugs should be written in ways that are not open to misinterpretation. Pharmacists and nurses must be involved in the early stages of protocol development to ensure that dosage regimens are easily understood—that they are written properly and as simply as possible. A pharmacist should be a voting member of the IRB that approves the scientific and ethical treatment of all patients enrolled in a research protocol. The Eastern Cooperative Oncology Group, the Children's Oncology Group, and the Southwest Oncology Group have a pharmacy committee to evaluate protocols; this should be mandatory for all oncology cooperative groups. Once protocols are written, prescribing patterns should be reviewed routinely to ensure compliance. Noncompliance may indicate the need for clarification.

As with all medication orders, caution must be exercised in the use of decimal points in chemotherapy orders. When possible, dosages should be rounded off to avoid the need for decimal points. Missing decimal points were responsible for three of five vincristine overdoses in one study.[67] Whereas leading zeros are mandatory (e.g., vincristine sulfate 0.9 mg), trailing zeros should be eliminated because they can lead to overdosage (e.g., vincristine sulfate 1.0 mg could be read as 10 mg). The absence of a leading zero in an order for vincristine 0.4 mg led to the administration of an overdose of 4 mg. Decimal points that were not seen on the order form accounted for the administration of 204 mg of cisplatin instead of 20.4 mg[54] and 1,695 mg of cytarabine instead of 169.5 mg.

Orders should indicate both the dose according to body surface area and the calculated dose. The method for calculating body surface area should be standardized within an institution. Different formulas can lead to clinically important dosing differences, especially in children. Likewise, formulas for modifying the dose because of drug-induced bone marrow suppression, renal dysfunction, hepatic failure, and other organ toxicity should be standardized.

The use of preprinted chemotherapy order forms helps ensure that the recommendations discussed in this chapter are followed.[45,125] When preprinted forms are used, orders for antineoplastics are physically separated from orders for other medications. Enhancements such as color and shading can be used to further distinguish these forms. This approach is also applicable to CPOE systems.

A standardized chemotherapy order sheet[126] and templated orders[127] have improved the ordering, dispensing, and administration of chemotherapy. For both inpatients and outpatients, computerized preprinted orders that include premedications, antiemetics, drug dosage, dilution, infusion rate, and proper administration sequence have decreased the risk of chemotherapy errors.[128]

One potential problem with preprinted chemotherapy order forms is the incorporation of a list of medications with space beside the drug names for specifying the doses. This practice can lead to errors when the list of drugs is in alphabetical order and single-spaced. For example, an oncologist accidentally wrote a dose for carboplatin in the space next to cisplatin (Figure 16-1).[129] Having vincristine, vinblastine, and vinorelbine so close to each other on this form could also lead to error.

Each facility should create its own form and ensure that it undergoes the appropriate approval process.[130] Pharmacists should contribute to the development of these forms to ensure ease of use and interpretation, completeness, adherence to the ASHP Guidelines on Preventing Medication Errors in Hospitals,[131,7] institutional compatibility, and instructional value to the house staff.

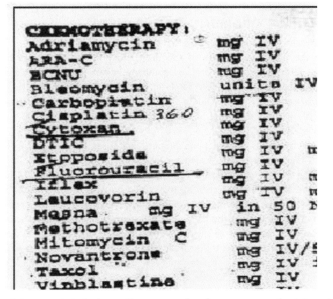

FIGURE 16-1 On this preprinted chemotherapy order form, an oncologist accidentally wrote a dose for carboplatin in the space next to cisplatin.

The pharmacists at NIH and NCI developed and proposed guidelines for clearly and consistently describing chemotherapy drug regimens in treatment protocols, preprinted order forms and templates for computer-based orders, pharmaceutical manufacturers' product packaging information, and labeling of drug products dispensed for patient care.[12] Key points for writing antineoplastic drug orders, based on Memorial Sloan-Kettering Cancer Center guidelines, are listed on page 458.

WORKING WITH MANUFACTURERS

Problems that can occur when drug names look or sound alike are discussed in Chapter 6. A list of names that have been confused can be found at www.ismp.org/tools/confuseddrugnames.pdf. Errors have occurred because of mix-ups in a number of chemotherapy drug names, such as cisplatin for carboplatin, Cytoxan for Cytosar, dactinomycin for daptomycin, Xeloda for Xenical, Neupogen for Neumega, isotretinoin for tretinoin, Taxotere for Taxol, propylthiouracil for Purinethol, Rituxan for Remicade, methotrexate for medroxyprogesterone acetate,[132] and thalidomide for flutamide.[42]

Accidental substitution of vincristine for vinblastine led to a massive overdose and permanent peripheral paresthesia.[69] The labeling of these two chemotherapy drugs was changed to highlight the differing syllables with tall-man letters: vinCRIstine and vinBLAstine.[133] The names mitoxantrone, mitomycin, and Mithracin (plicamycin) are also easily confused.[119]

Substitution of cisplatin for carboplatin led to a massive overdose of cisplatin in the absence of IV hydration. The patient suffered severe myelosuppression, renal failure necessitating a kidney transplant, and permanent deafness.[50] Because of accidental overdosages and confusion with carboplatin, Bristol-Myers Squibb made the following changes to the packaging and labeling: (1) the first three letters of cisplatin are in bold, uppercase red characters, (2) a "stop" sign on the packaging warns health care providers to verify the drug name and dose, (3) the labeling warns that dosages of cisplatin greater than 100 mg/m² every 3 to 4 weeks are rarely used, and (4) the vial seals and closures call attention to the maximum dose.

CHEMOTHERAPY ORDERING GUIDELINES

❑ Always double-check the dose against the protocol.
❑ Use only the full generic name of the drug. Do not refer to drugs by brand names, nicknames, abbreviations, acronyms, or company names. Do not use common drug class names (e.g., does "platinum" mean cisplatin, carboplatin, or oxaliplatin?).
❑ Never allow spoken orders (including telephone orders) for chemotherapy.
❑ Prescribe all drug doses in metric weight (e.g., milligrams or grams) or units. Include the dosage interval.
❑ Do not use dangerous abbreviations in specifying doses (e.g., "U" for units could be read as "0," and the patient could receive a 10-fold overdose).
❑ Use a leading zero when the dose is less than a whole unit (e.g., write "0.1 mg," not ".1 mg").
❑ Do not use a trailing zero (e.g., "10.0 mg" could be read as "100 mg").
❑ Express the dose in milligrams per square meter (mg/m^2) or, when applicable, milligrams per kilogram (mg/kg). Give the daily dose times the number of days; do not list the total course dose (e.g., "cisplatin 25 mg/m^2 [50 mg] daily × 4 days [6/1, 6/2, 6/3, and 6/4]").
❑ Round doses above 5 mg to the nearest whole number (e.g., 6 mg, not 5.8 mg).
❑ Date all orders with the month, day, and year. Add time of day for inpatient orders.
❑ Specify the route of administration and the duration of infusion in hours for all injections.
❑ Record the patient's current body surface area or body weight on the drug order.

Although the USAN Council and FDA are reluctant to change established names, it has been done; "mithramycin" was changed to plicamycin because of confusion with mitomycin. These organizations are receptive to testing names with panels of practitioners before nomenclature is finalized.[134]

In addition to participating in nomenclature decisions, pharmacists need to work with manufacturers and FDA to eliminate ambiguous dosing information from official resources. The following wording appeared in the cyclophosphamide package insert,[135] as well as in many textbooks:

> Although a few instances of cardiac dysfunction have been reported following use of recommended doses of cyclophosphamide, no causal relationship has been established. Cardiotoxicity has been observed in some patients receiving high doses of cyclophosphamide ranging from 120 to 270 mg/kg administered over a period of a few days, usually as a portion of an intensive antineoplastic multidrug regimen or in conjunction with transplantation procedures.

It is not clear whether this means 270 mg/kg was given daily for several days or in divided doses over several days. Although the former is obviously a massive overdose, this information could be misinterpreted, with tragic results like the Betsy Lehman case. Many would argue that 270 mg/kg in divided doses over a few days is also an overdose; the package insert actually refers to the upper limit tested in a dose-ranging study, not the upper limit of a regimen that remains in clinical use.

Three vinorelbine overdosages can be attributed to labeling ambiguity.[136] When the drug was investigational, the computer-generated label indicated that the vial contained vinorelbine (as the tartrate) 10 mg/mL, but the total volume was on a portion of the label far away from the drug name and concentration. Nurses assumed that the vial contained only 10 mg of drug, instead of recognizing that the 5 mL vial contained 50 mg. Another overdosage was reported after the drug was marketed. The nurse in an oncologist's office thought she was preparing a 50 mg dose of vinorelbine from five 10 mg vials but accidentally prepared the dose from two 50 mg vials and three 10 mg vials, for a total dose of 130 mg. The 50 mg and 10 mg vials look very much alike, despite slightly different labels and sizes. This patient recovered after a 2-day hospitalization for abdominal distention and leukopenia. In this situation, no one double-checked the doses prepared by the nurse.

Labeling for Camptosar (irinotecan) caused several overdoses when the 20 mg/mL concentration was assumed to indicate the entire vial's content. Because the vials actually contained 100 mg, the patients received fivefold overdoses. The manufacturer changed the package label to more clearly state the contents as 100 mg/5 mL (20 mg/mL).

Errors in the reconstitution of Taxotere (docetaxel) have occurred. Taxotere is packaged in a carton containing two vials: the concentrated drug and the diluent. Taxotere 20 mg and 80 mg vials actually contain 23.6 mg and 94.4 mg of docetaxel, respectively, and the diluent vials also contain overfill. To ensure that any overfill is taken into account, the concentration is noted as "20 mg/0.5 mL" or "80 mg/2 mL." However, it is unclear whether this refers to the concentration after the diluent is added, which actually is 10 mg/mL. In one case a technician drew up 1.27 mL of the diluted drug for a 51 mg dose, thinking the vial contained 20 mg/0.5 mL after dilution. Personnel who mix chemotherapy must be aware that the drug vial label could easily be mistaken for the final concentration. The pharmacy computer system should provide information about the postdilution concentration of this product along with instructions for IV admixture preparation.

Another reconstitution error was reported when Herceptin (trastuzumab) was initially packaged with a 30 mL vial of bacteriostatic water for injection. Since only 20 mL of the diluent was required, the resulting concentration, if the entire 30 mL was used, was less than intended and patients received subtherapeutic doses. Herceptin is now packaged with a 20 mL vial of bacteriostatic water for injection.[137] Neumega (oprelvekin) also had a diluent problem; it was supplied with a 5 mL vial of sterile water when only 1 mL was required for reconstitution. Neumega is now supplied with 1 mL vials of diluent.[138] The labeling for Mylotarg (gemtuzumab ozogamicin) was originally misleading because it stated that "each 20 mL vial contains 5 mg of Mylotarg," when the 20 mL referred to the size of the container and not the volume after reconstitution. The instructions for reconstitution required that 5 mg be mixed as a 1 mg/mL concentration. The 20 mL description of the vial has now been removed from the product labeling.[139]

These and other nomenclature and labeling problems come under the auspices of manufacturers and regulatory agencies. ISMP works in cooperation with USP in the Medication Errors Reporting Program to bring such information to the attention of authorities as well as practitioners. Practitioners can report errors by telephone (1-800-FAIL-SAFE, or 1-800-324-5723) or via the Internet (https://www.ismp.org/orderForms/reporterrortoISMP.asp).

EDUCATING PATIENTS

Pharmacists have a responsibility to educate patients about their drug therapy and how to protect themselves from errors. The importance of double-checking the details of chemotherapy cannot be overstated. Patients or a family member should be invited to become part of the care team so they can help check doses and request recalculation if the patient's body weight or (in children) height changes. Adverse outcomes have occurred when patients who did not understand their treatment regimens failed to stop taking chlorambucil,[140] lomustine,[141] methotrexate,[61,62] and procarbazine.[142] The death of Betsy Lehman demonstrates that even the best-informed consumers are at risk.[5]

A patient should be informed of the proprietary and generic names of each antineoplastic agent he or she is to receive, the indication, the usual and actual dosages, expected and possible adverse effects, and methods of preventing or managing adverse effects.[143]

Patients can help prevent errors by knowing the regimen prescribed by their oncologist, including hydration therapy and antiemetics; selecting a facility in which a pharmacist prepares the chemotherapy; writing down the names and dosages of every medication in their treatment plan and keeping up-to-date records of all doses received; and having a family member or friend present during their treatments.[144] Inpatients should be sure their armbands are checked before each course of chemotherapy, and outpatients should repeat their names to the professional administering the drugs. When patients are interested in unapproved or alternative therapies, pharmacists should offer educational materials and direct the patients to NCI, relevant Web sites, libraries, or bookstores for further information.

Pharmacists can help ensure that patients undergoing chemotherapy understand the consent forms they sign. Forms should be designed for readability and completeness.[145] Patients should be informed of their right to ask questions and seek satisfactory answers. After the therapeutic plan is described to the patient or family, the patient must be given enough time to understand the treatment and what to expect. Patients should consider enlisting the support of family members or friends who understand the language of medicine. Practice sites should have a formal method for providing assistance to the patient, or a patient advocate when necessary. The American Society of Clinical Oncology (ASCO) policy statement on the oversight of clinical research offers recommendations for the informed consent process (page 461).[146]

IMPROVING COMMUNICATION

Caregivers should take time to listen carefully when patients have questions about their therapy or when they express concern about any aspect of their care. Alert and knowledgeable patients can be the last line of defense against medication errors. Failure to heed patient concerns has led to serious errors that could have been prevented.[147]

Pharmacists should make sure that patients are aware of the pharmacist's important role in their treatment. Patients who understand the benefits of comprehensive pharmaceutical services may decide against receiving chemotherapy in a physician's office without pharmacist involvement.

Poor communication among physicians, pharmacists, and nurses can lead to medication errors. Health care providers from all disciplines should cooperate in identifying potential problems and solutions. Multidisciplinary discussions should take place after a medication error and routinely as part of quality improvement efforts. Pharmacists can direct the discussion by asking, What should the pharmacist do in the event of a disagreement with the prescriber? What are the most effective ways of making this type of inquiry? If the discrepancy cannot be resolved, should the pharmacist refuse to dispense the drug? Such discussion can provide a basis for policy development and can help practitioners learn, through role playing, to handle disagreements. Chapter 9 offers suggestions for resolving conflicts concerning drug therapy.

NEED FOR PHARMACIST INVOLVEMENT IN CHEMOTHERAPY

As suggested throughout this chapter, pharmacists should be involved at all sites where antineoplastic agents are provided. Pharmacists can help establish sound policies for drug administration and provide indispensable safety checks. In a study of pharmacists' interventions in the treatment of hematology–oncology patients between October 1995 and May 1996, 503 interventions were reported, of which 85 (17%) were to correct prescribing errors.[148] Physicians accepted 97% of the pharmacists' recommendations. The absence of a pharmacist has reportedly contributed to three children's deaths from vincristine overdoses[67] and to two deaths and one serious injury from vinorelbine overdoses.[136]

INFORMED CONSENT TO PARTICIPATE IN CLINICAL RESEARCH[146]

1. Clinical investigators should be responsible for providing clear information to educate potential trial participants.
2. Institutional review boards should review the entire informed consent process, not only the informed consent document.
3. Potential trial participants should have a sufficient interval of time to decide about participating in the trial.
4. The consent form should be simplified to increase comprehensibility and clarity.
5. Consent forms should include information about how the clinical investigator is compensated by the research sponsor.
6. The informed consent process should be dynamic and ongoing.
7. A variety of tools (e.g., video, DVD, CD-ROM) can be used to inform the potential participant.

Increasingly, cancer chemotherapy is being provided in outpatient settings because of greater convenience and lower cost. Pharmacists have little involvement in some ambulatory care clinics and most private oncologists' offices. Each organization should establish a minimum acceptable level of pharmacist responsibility in its outpatient settings, for example, prospectively reviewing orders, screening laboratory test results, providing drug information, counseling patients, and reviewing drug storage. Investigational drug protocols should be initiated only at sites where comprehensive pharmaceutical services are available. Prospective review of more than 10,000 orders in three outpatient infusion centers (two adult and one pediatric) at the Dana-Farber Cancer Institute in 2000 found a 3% error rate.[149] Most of the errors (82% in adults and 60% in pediatric patients) had the potential to cause an adverse drug event (ADE). Pharmacists and nurses intercepted 45% of the potential ADEs before they reached patients.

Even in some hospitals, pharmacists need to be more involved in cancer chemotherapy. Some institutions have pharmacy technicians or nurses prepare doses that are not checked by a pharmacist, and this trend could increase as financial pressures cause staffing reductions. The professional and legal implications of pharmacy technicians' preparing chemotherapy without a pharmacist's supervision have been described.[150] An Oncology Nursing Society (ONS) position paper titled Prevention and Reporting of Medication Errors[9] recommends that pharmacists be consulted and included in patient care rounds. An ASCO position statement cautions oncologists about the potential for errors when chemotherapy drugs are prepared or administered by entities not under their control, such as infusion centers or home care agencies.[151]

This chapter has reviewed available guidelines for cancer chemotherapy, as well as suggestions by experienced pharmacists. Pharmacy organizations should use this information as a starting point for developing guidelines on cancer chemotherapy administration. Drafts of such guidelines should undergo review by other health care provider groups (e.g., ASCO, ONS) and the American Cancer Society. After endorsement by multidisciplinary groups, the guidelines could be presented to accrediting agencies such as JCAHO and NCI (which accredits cancer research centers).

CONCLUSION

Tragic accidents involving antineoplastic drugs have generated widespread publicity and concern. Because of their training and experience, pharmacists should take the lead in implementing policies that will minimize the risk of future errors. Institutions should establish dosage limits for antineoplastic agents, set up dose-verification procedures that stress multiple independent checks, and work to standardize the prescribing vocabulary. Patients and health care providers must be educated about cancer chemotherapy.

If caregivers work together, most errors can be kept from reaching patients. All errors should be reported so that practitioners can learn from them. Each error should be reviewed by a multidisciplinary team, with the goal of system improvements.

REFERENCES

1. Phillips J, Beam S, Brinker A, et al. Retrospective analysis of mortalities associated with medication errors. *Am J Health Syst Pharm.* 2001;58(19):1835–41. Erratum in: *Am J Health Syst Pharm.* 2001;58(22):2130.
2. Northfelt DW, Allbritton DW, Parra LS, et al. Medication errors in cancer therapy: review and proposal for systematic study. *Proc Am Soc Clin Oncol.* 2003;22:542. Abstract 2181.
3. Schulmeister L. Chemotherapy medication errors: descriptions, severity, and contributing factors. *Oncol Nurs Forum.* 1999;26(6):1033–42.
4. Knox RA. Response is slow to deadly mixups. Too little done to avert cancer drug errors. *Boston Globe.* June 26, 1995:29,33.
5. United Kingdom Joint Council for Clinical Oncology. *Quality Control in Cancer Chemotherapy. Managerial and Procedural Aspects.* Oxford, England: Royal College of Physicians of London; 1994.
6. Cohen MR, Anderson RW, Attilio RM, et al. Preventing medication errors in cancer chemotherapy. *Am J Health Syst Pharm.* 1996; 53:737–46.
7. American Society of Health-System Pharmacists. ASHP guidelines on preventing medication errors with antineoplastic agents. *Am J Health Syst Pharm.* 2002;59:1648–68.
8. Griffin E. Safety considerations and safe handling of oral chemotherapy agents. *Clin J Oncol Nurs.* 2003;7 (6 Suppl):25–9.
9. Oncology Nursing Society. Prevention and reporting of medication errors. *Oncol Nurs Forum.* 2001;28(1): 15–6.
10. Kloth DD. Prevention of chemotherapy medication errors. *J Pharm Pract.* 2002:15(1):17–31.
11. Muller T. Typical medication errors in oncology: analysis and prevention strategies. *Onkologie.* 2003;26(6): 539–44.
12. Kohler DR, Montello MJ, Green L, et al. Standardizing the expression and nomenclature of cancer treatment regimens. *Am J Health Syst Pharm.* 1998;55(2):137–44.
13. Boyle DA, Schulmeister L, Lajeunesse JD, et al. Medication misadventure in cancer care. *Semin Oncol Nurs.* 2002;18(2):109–20.
14. Leape LL, Bates DW, Cullen DJ, et al. Systems analysis of adverse drug events. *JAMA.* 1995;274:35–43.
15. Womer RB, Tracy E, Soo-Hoo W, et al. Multidisciplinary systems approach to chemotherapy safety: rebuilding processes and holding the gains. *J Clin Oncol.* 2002;20(24):4705–12.
16. Goldspiel BR, DeChristoforo R, Daniels CE. A continuous-improvement approach for reducing the number of chemotherapy-related medication errors. *Am J Health Syst Pharm.* 2000;57(Suppl 4):S4–9.
17. Peters BG, Wilson AL, Lunik MC, et al. Certification program in antineoplastic drug preparation for pharmacy technicians and pharmacists. *Am J Hosp Pharm.* 1994;51:1902–06.
18. Melamed AJ, Nacov CG, Muller RJ. Antineoplastic agents: some preparation and handling considerations. *Pharm Pract News.* 1986;13:18–9.
19. Aricó M, Nespoli L, Porta F, et al. Severe acute encephalopathy following inadvertent intrathecal doxorubicin administration. *Med Pediatr Oncol.* 1990;18:261–3.
20. Gilbar PJ. Preventing medication errors in cancer chemotherapy referred to rural and remote hospitals. *Aust J Rural Health.* 2001;9(1):47–51.
21. Sievers TD, Lagan MA, Bartel SB, et al. Variation in administration of cyclophosphamide and mesna in the treatment of childhood malignancies. *J Pediatr Oncol Nurs.* 2001;18(1):37–45.
22. Kohler DR, Montello MJ, Green L, et al. Standardizing the expression and nomenclature of cancer treatment regimens. *Am J Health Syst Pharm.* 1998;55(2):137–44.
23. Wang Chin JM, Muller RJ, Lucarelli CD. A pharmacy intervention program: recognizing pharmacy's contribution to improving patient care. *Hosp Pharm.* 1995;30:120, 123–6, 129–30.
24. Sklarin NT, Timoney J, Kampel LJ, et al. MSKCC quality assessment (QA) monitoring program for potentially harmful chemotherapy orders. *J Clin Oncol.* 2004;22(14S):Abstract 6078.
25. Finley RS, Balmer CM, Dozier N, et al. *Concepts in Oncology Therapeutics. A Self–Instructional Course.* Bethesda, Md: American Society of Hospital Pharmacists; 1991.
26. Dorr RT, Von Hoff DD, eds. CPT–11. In: *Cancer Chemotherapy Handbook.* 2nd ed. East Norwalk, Conn: Appleton and Lange; 1994:314–6.

27. Perry MC, ed. *The Chemotherapy Sourcebook*. 3rd ed. Baltimore, Md: Williams & Wilkins; 2001.
28. Institute for Safe Medication Practices. Safety briefs. *ISMP Medication Safety Alert!* Huntingdon Valley, Pa: Institute for Safe Medication Practices; August 14, 1996.
29. Institute for Safe Medication Practices. Error in chemotherapy regimen. *ISMP Medication Safety Alert!* Huntingdon Valley, Pa: Institute for Safe Medication Practices; July 2, 1997.
30. Institute for Safe Medication Practices. Textbook errata. *ISMP Medication Safety Alert!* Huntingdon Valley, Pa: Institute for Safe Medication Practices; August 21, 2003.
31. Pedersen CA, Schneider PJ, Scheckelhoff DH. ASHP national survey of pharmacy practice in hospital settings: prescribing and transcribing—2004 . *Am J Health Syst Pharm*. 2005; 62: 378–90.
32. Adams VR, Bence AK. Guide for the administration and use of cancer chemotherapeutic agents 2004. *Oncology*. Special Edition. 2004; 7: 147–63. Available at: www.oncologyse.com/articles/7319/pdf/7319.pdf? CFID=441510&CFTOKEN=46542611. Accessed June 28, 2005.
33. Ash JS, Gorman PN, Seshadri V, et al. Computerized physician order entry in U.S. hospitals: results of a 2002 survey. *J Am Med Inform Assoc*. 2004;11(2):95–9.
34. Bates DW, Leape LL, Cullen DJ, et al. Effect of computerized physician order entry and a team intervention on prevention of serious medication errors. *JAMA*. 1998;280(15):1311–6.
35. Bates DW, Teich JM, Lee J, et al. The impact of computerized physician order entry on medication error prevention. *J Am Med Inform Assoc*. 1999;6(4):313–21.
36. Mekhjian HS, Kumar RR, Kuehn L, et al. Immediate benefits realized following implementation of physician order entry at an academic medical center. *J Am Med Inform Assoc*. 2002;9(5):529–39.
37. Spencer DC, Leininger A, Daniels R, et al. Effect of a computerized prescriber-order-entry system on reported medication errors. *Am J Health Syst Pharm*. 2005;62: 416–9.
38. Pourrat X, Antier D, Crenn I, et al. A prescription and administration error of cisplatin: a case report. *Pharm World Sci*. 2004;26(2):64–5.
39. Krampera M, Venturini F, Benedetti F, et al. Computer–based drug management in a bone marrow transplant unit: a suitable tool for multiple prescriptions even in critical conditions. *Br J Haematol*. 2004;125(1):50–7.
40. DuBeshter B, Walsh C. Automating management of chemotherapy patients utilizing IntelliDose: improved efficiency and error free dosing. *Proc Am Soc Clin Oncol*. 1999; 734. Abstract 734.
41. Knaup P, Wiedemann T, Bachert A, et al. Efficiency and safety of chemotherapy plans for children: CAT-IPO—a nationwide approach. *Artif Intel Med*. 2002;24(3):229–42.
42. Cohen MR. Flutamide or thalidomide? *Nursing*. 2004;34(6):18.
43. Lopez TM, Hagemeister FB, McLaughlin P, et al. Small noncleaved cell lymphoma in adults: superior results for stages I–III disease. *J Clin Oncol*. 1990; 8:615–22.
44. Cohen MR. Misprint in journal article leads to vincristine overdose. *Hosp Pharm*. 1994;29:294,302.
45. Adams VR. Adverse events associated with chemotherapy for common cancers. *Pharmacotherapy*. 2000;20(7, Pt 2):96S–103S.
46. Crookes P, Leichman CG, Leichman L, et al. Systemic chemotherapy for gastric carcinoma followed by postoperative intraperitoneal therapy: a final report. *Cancer*. 1997;79(9):1767–75.
47. Golde DW, Jakubowiak A, Caggiano J, et al. Cladribine underdosing in hairy-cell leukemia: a cause for apparent response failure. *Leuk Lymphoma*. 2002;43(2):365–7.
48. Chen CS, Seidel K, Armitage JO, et al. Safeguarding the administration of high-dose chemotherapy: a national practice survey by the American Society for Blood and Marrow Transplantation. *Biol Blood Marrow Transplant*. 1997;3(6):331–40.
49. U.S. Pharmacopeia. *CAPSLink Electronic Newsletter*. April 2004. Available at: www.usp.org/pdf/EN/ patientSafety/capsLink2004–04–01.pdf. Accessed June 9, 2005.
50. Chu G, Mantin R, Shen Y–M, et al. Massive cisplatin overdose by accidental substitution for carboplatin. *Cancer*. 1993;73:3707–14.
51. Pike IM, Arbus MH. Cisplatin overdosage [letter]. *Am J Hosp Pharm*. 1992;49:1668.
52. Schiller JH, Rozental J, Tutsch KD, et al. Inadvertent administration of 480 mg/m² of cisplatin [letter]. *Am J Med*. 1989;86:624–5.
53. Charlier C, Kintz P, Dubois N, et al. Fatal overdosage with cisplatin. *J Anal Toxicol*. 2004;28(2):138–40.
54. Cohen MR. Medication errors. Cisplatin death. *Nursing*. 1998;28(2):18.
55. Liem RI, Higman MA, Chen AR, et al. Misinterpretation of a Calvert–derived formula leading to carboplatin overdose in two children. *J Pediatr Hematol Oncol*. 2003;25(10):818–21.
56. Trigg ME, Nadkarni V, Chidekel A, et al. Effects of an inadvertent dose of cytarabine in a child with Fanconi's anemia: reducing medication errors. *Paediatr Drugs*. 2002;4(3):205–8.
57. Institute for Safe Medication Practices. Special alert. Important error prevention advisory. *ISMP Medication Safety Alert!* Huntingdon Valley, Pa: Institute for Safe Medication Practices; September 16, 1996.
58. Jost LM. Overdose with melphalan (Alkeran): symptoms and treatment. A review. *Onkologie*. 1990;13: 96–101.

59. Hachimi–Idrissi S, Schots R, DeWolf D, et al. Reversible cardiopathy after accidental overdose of mitoxantrone. *Pediatr Hematol Oncol.* 1993;10:35–40.

60. Zaniboni A, Simoncini E, Marpicati P, et al. Severe delayed neurotoxicity after accidental high-dose nitrogen mustard [letter]. *Am J Hematol.* 1988;27:305.

61. Sosin M, Handa S. Low dose methotrexate and bone marrow suppression. *BMJ.* 2003;326(7383):266–7.

62. Moore TJ, Walsh CS, Cohen MR. Reported medication errors associated with methotrexate. *Am J Health Syst Pharm.* 2004;61(13):1380–4.

63. Harris W. Methotrexate-associated medication errors. *Am J Health Syst Pharm.* 2004;61(24):2635.

64. Institute for Safe Medication Practices. Beware of erroneous daily oral methotrexate dosing. *ISMP Medication Safety Alert!* Huntingdon Valley, Pa: Institute for Safe Medication Practices; April 3, 2002.

65. Institute for Safe Medication Practices. Methotrexate overdose due to inadvertent administration daily instead of weekly. *ISMP Medication Safety Alert!* Huntingdon Valley, Pa: Institute for Safe Medication Practices; December 3, 2002.

66. Conter V, Rabbone ML, Jankovic M, et al. Overdose of vinblastine in a child with Langerhans' cell histiocytosis: toxicity and salvage therapy. *Pediatr Hematol Oncol.* 1991;8:165–9.

67. Kaufman IA, Kung FH, Koenig HM, et al. Overdosage with vincristine. *J Pediatr.* 1976;89:671–4.

68. Kosmidis HV, Bouhoutsou DO, Varvoutsi MC, et al. Vincristine overdose: experience with 3 patients. *Pediatr Hematol Oncol.* 1991;8:171–8.

69. Maeda K, Ueda M, Ohtaka H, et al. A massive dose of vincristine. *Jpn J Clin Oncol.* 1987;17:247–53.

70. Stones DK. Vincristine overdosage in paediatric patients. *Med Pediatr Oncol.* 1998;30(3):193.

71. Kim IS, Gratwohl A, Stebler C, et al. Accidental overdose of multiple chemotherapeutic agents. *Korean J Intern Med.* 1989;4:171–3.

72. DeVita V, Hellman S, Rosenberg M, eds. *Cancer. Principles and Practice of Oncology.* 7th ed. Philadelphia: Lippincott Williams & Wilkins; 2005.

73. McCune JS, Lindley C. Appropriateness of maximum-dose guidelines for vincristine. *Am J Health Syst Pharm.* 1997;54(15):1755–8.

74. Cohen MR. Cisplatin vial seals to carry message on dose limits. *Hosp Pharm.* 1995;30:538–9.

75. Al Fawaz IM. Fatal myeloencephalopathy due to intrathecal vincristine administration. *Ann Trop Paediatr.* 1992;12:339–42.

76. Bain PG, Lantos PL, Djurovic V, et al. Intrathecal vincristine: a fatal chemotherapeutic error with devastating central nervous system effects. *J Neurol.* 1991;238:230–4.

77. Gaidys WG, Dickerman JD, Walters CL, et al. Intrathecal vincristine. Report of a fatal case despite CNS washout. *Cancer.* 1983;52:799–801.

78. Manelis J, Freudlich E, Ezekiel E, et al. Accidental intrathecal vincristine administration. Report of a case. *J Neurol.* 1982;228:209–13.

79. Schochet SS Jr, Lampert PW, Earle KM. Neuronal changes induced by intrathecal vincristine sulfate. *J Neuropathol Exp Neurol.* 1968;27:645–58.

80. Shepherd DA, Steuber CP, Starling KA, et al. Accidental intrathecal administration of vincristine. *Med Pediatr Oncol.* 1978;5:85–8.

81. Slyter H, Liwnicz B, Herrick MK, et al. Fatal myeloencephalopathy caused by intrathecal vincristine. *Neurology.* 1980;30:867–71.

82. Williams ME, Walker AN, Bracikowski JP, et al. Ascending myeloencephalopathy due to intrathecal vincristine sulfate. A fatal chemotherapeutic error. *Cancer.* 1983;51:2041–7.

83. Fernandez CV, Esau R, Hamilton D, et al. Intrathecal vincristine: an analysis of reasons for recurrent fatal chemotherapeutic error with recommendations for prevention. *J Pediatr Hematol Oncol.* 1998;20(6):587–90.

84. Institute for Safe Medication Practices. Pain, paralysis, and knowledge of impending death marks intrathecal vincristine. *ISMP Medication Safety Alert!* Huntingdon Valley, Pa: Institute for Safe Medication Practices; April 5, 2000.

85. Institute for Safe Medication Practices. Worth repeating…again! *ISMP Medication Safety Alert!* Huntingdon Valley, Pa: Institute for Safe Medication Practices; May 1, 2003.

86. Dettmeyer R, Driever F, Becker A, et al. Fatal myeloencephalopathy due to accidental intrathecal vincristine administration: a report of two cases. *Forensic Sci Int.* 2001;122(1):60–4.

87. Kwack EK, Kim DJ, Park TI, et al. Neural toxicity induced by accidental intrathecal vincristine administration. *J Korean Med Sci.* 1999;14(6):688–92.

88. Alcaraz A, Rey C, Concha A, et al. Intrathecal vincristine: fatal myeloencephalopathy despite cerebrospinal fluid perfusion. *J Toxicol Clin Toxicol.* 2002;40(5):557–61.

89. Bleck TP, Jacobsen J. Prolonged survival following the inadvertent intrathecal administration of vincristine: clinical and electrophysiologic analyses. *Clin Neuropharmacol.* 1991;14:457–62.

90. Dyke RW. Treatment of inadvertent intrathecal injection of vincristine. *N Engl J Med.* 1989;321:1270–1.

91. Zaragoza MR, Ritchey ML, Walter A. Neurourologic consequences of accidental intrathecal vincristine: a case report. *Med Pediatr Oncol.* 1995;24:61–2.

92. Al Ferayan A, Russell NA, Al Wohaibi M, et al. Cerebrospinal fluid lavage in the treatment of inadvertent intrathecal vincristine injection. *Childs Nerv Syst.* 1999;15(2–3):87–9.

93. Michelagnoli MP, Bailey CC, Wilson I, et al. Potential salvage therapy for inadvertent intrathecal administration of vincristine. *Br J Haematol.* 1997;99(2):364–7. Erratum in: *Br J Haematol.* 1998;101(2):398.

94. Cohen MR. Warning: vincristine practice standard must be followed by pharmacists and others. *Hosp Pharm.* 1995;30:740–1.

95. Trissel LA, Zhang Y, Cohen MR. The stability of diluted vincristine sulfate used as a deterrent to inadvertent intrathecal injection. *Hosp Pharm.* 2001;36:740–5.

96. Davis NM. The preparation of vincristine in minibags will prevent deadly medication errors [editorial]. *Hosp Pharm.* 2001;36:707

97. Gilbar P, Dooley M, Brien J. Inadvertent intrathecal administration of vincristine: are we fulfilling our role as oncology pharmacists? [editorial]. *J Oncol Pharm Practice.* 2004;10:187–9.

98. Institute for Safe Medication Practices. Fatal reports of intrathecal vincristine continue. *ISMP Medication Safety Alert!* Huntingdon Valley, Pa: Institute for Safe Medication Practices; April 4, 2003.

99. Stefanou A, Dooley M. Simple method to eliminate the risk of inadvertent intrathecal vincristine administration [letter]. *J Clin Oncol.* 2003;21(10):2044.

100. ISMP–Canada. Published data supports dispensing vincristine in minibags as a system safeguard. *ISMP–Canada Safety Bulletin.* October 3, 2001.

101. Womer RB, Bickert B. Simple method to eliminate the risk of inadvertent intrathecal vincristine administration [reply]. *J Clin Oncol.* 2003;21(10):2044.

102. Dyer C. Doctors suspended after injecting wrong drug into spine. *BMJ.* 2001;322:257.

103. Laws D. The time has come for non-interchangeability of spinal and epidural equipment with intravascular access ports. *Br J Anaesth.* 2001;86(6):903.

104. Sheppard I, Morris L, Blackstock D. Medication safety alerts (spinal injection safety system). *Can J Hosp Pharm.* 2004;57:176–9.

105. Palmieri C, Barron N, Vigushin DM. The Vincotube System: a design solution to prevent the accidental administration of intrathecal vinca alkaloids [letter]. *J Clin Oncol.* 2004;22(5):965; author reply 965–6.

106. NHS Health Technology Assessment Programme. Department of Health. The prevention of intrathecal medication errors. April 2001. Available at: www.dh.gov.uk/assetRoot/04/06/50/49/04065049.pdf. Accessed June 9, 2005.

107. Clark BS, Gallegos E, Bleyer WA. Accidental intramuscular vincristine: lack of untoward effects and recommendations for management. *Med Pediatr Oncol.* 1997;28(4):314–5.

108. Olcay L, Safak T. Inadvertent intramuscular administration of vincristine: lack of untoward effects without any treatment except administration of hot compresses. *Pediatr Hematol Oncol.* 2003;20(5):427–8.

109. Lau G. Accidental intraventricular vincristine administration: an avoidable iatrogenic death. *Med Sci Law.* 1996;36(3):263–5.

110. Meggs WJ, Hoffman RS. Fatality resulting from intraventricular vincristine administration. *J Toxicol Clin Toxicol.* 1998;36(3):243–6.

111. Hanson DS, Leggette CT. Severe hypotension following inadvertent intravenous administration of interferon alfa-2a. *Ann Pharmacother.* 1997;31(3):371–2.

112. Lafolie P, Liliemark J, Bjork O, et al. Exchange of cerebrospinal fluid in accidental intrathecal overdose of cytarabine. *Med Toxicol Adverse Drug Exp.* 1988;3:248–52.

113. Ettinger LJ. Pharmacokinetics and biochemical effects of a fatal intrathecal methotrexate overdose. *Cancer.* 1982;50:444–50.

114. Widemann BC, Balis FM, Shalabi A, et al. Treatment of accidental intrathecal methotrexate overdose with intrathecal carboxypeptidase G2. *J Natl Cancer Inst.* 2004;96(20):1557–9.

115. Trinkle R, Wu JK. Intrathecal leukovorin after intrathecal methotrexate overdose. *J Pediatr Hematol Oncol.* 1997;19(3):267–9.

116. Trinkle R, Wu JK. Intrathecal methotrexate overdoses. *Acta Paediatr.* 1998;87(1):116–7.

117. Jardine LF, Ingram LC, Bleyer WA. Intrathecal leucovorin after intrathecal methotrexate overdose. *J Pediatr Hematol Oncol.* 1996;18(3):302–4.

118. Lee AC, Wong KW, Fong KW, et al. Intrathecal methotrexate overdose. *Acta Paediatr.* 1997;86(4):434–7.

119. Davis NM, Cohen MR, Teplitsky B. Look-alike and sound-alike drug names: the problem and the solution. *Hosp Pharm.* 1992;27:95–98, 102–05, 108–10.

120. Cohen MR. "Adria," a dangerous abbreviation for Adriamycin, looks like Aredia. *Hosp Pharm.* 1994;9:141, 158.

121. Cohen MR. Safety alert—overdoses of Platinol (cisplatin) and Paraplatin (carboplatin). *Hosp Pharm.* 1992;27:991–2.

122. Institute for Safe Medication Practices. Warning—extremely dangerous synonym! *ISMP Medication Safety Alert!* Huntingdon Valley, Pa: Institute for Safe Medication Practices; June 18, 1997.

123. Sullivan P, Heaney J. Hospital admits giving wrong drug to sick child. *Boston Herald.* April 6, 1995:7.

124. Institute for Safe Medication Practices. MIME and MINE: safety problems posed by investigational drug name abbreviations and acronyms. *ISMP Medication Safety Alert!* Huntingdon Valley, Pa: Institute for Safe Medication Practices; December 3, 1997.

125. Slimovitz R. Thoughts on a medical disaster [letter]. *Am J Health Syst Pharm.* 1995;52:1464–5.

126. Opfer KB, Wirtz DM, Farley K. A chemotherapy standard order form: preventing errors. *Oncol Nurs Forum.* 1999;26(1):123–8.

127. Dinning C, Branowicki P, O'Neill JB, et al. Chemotherapy error reduction: a multidisciplinary approach to create templated order sets. *J Pediatr Oncol Nurs.* 2005;22(1):20–30.

128. Shaikh BS, Mowatt RB, Parr DD. Chemotherapy ordering process: safety and efficiency considerations. *J Clin Oncol.* 2004;22(14S):Abstract 6110.

129. Institute for Safe Medication Practices. Design of preprinted cancer chemotherapy order forms is critical for patient safety. *ISMP Medication Safety Alert!* Huntingdon Valley, Pa: Institute for Safe Medication Practices; February 14, 1996.

130. Cohen MR, Davis NM. Developing safe and effective preprinted physician's order forms. *Hosp Pharm.* 1992;27:508, 513, 528.

131. American Society of Hospital Pharmacists. Guidelines on preventing medication errors in hospitals. *Am J Hosp Pharm.* 1993;50:305–14.

132. Sweet JM, Holstege CP. Bone marrow failure from medication error: diagnosis by history, not biopsy. *Arch Intern Med.* 2001;161(15):1911–2.

133. Kenagy JW, Stein GC. Naming, labeling, and packaging of pharmaceuticals. *Am J Health Syst Pharm.* 2001;58(21):2033–41.

134. DiDomizio G, Cohen MR. Medication errors: who's at fault and who's counting. *Med Malpract Law Strategy.* 1995;12(5):1–4.

135. Cyclophosphamide [package insert]. Princeton, NJ: Bristol–Myers Squibb; 1995.

136. Cohen MR. Cancer chemotherapy needs improved quality assurance. *Hosp Pharm.* 1995;30:258–9.

137. Herceptin [package insert]. South San Francisco, Calif: Genentech Inc; 2004. Available at: www.gene.com/gene/products/information/pdf/herceptin–prescribing.pdf. Accessed June 9, 2005.

138. Neumega [package insert]. Philadelphia, Pa: Wyeth Pharmaceuticals Inc; 2004. Available at: www.wyeth.com/content/ShowLabeling.asp?id=121. Accessed June 9, 2005.

139. Mylotarg [package insert]. Philadelphia, Pa: Wyeth Pharmaceuticals Inc; 2004. Available at: www.wyeth.com/content/ShowLabeling.asp?id=119. Accessed June 9, 2005.

140. Enck RE, Bennett JM. Inadvertent chlorambucil overdose in adult. *NY State J Med.* 1977;9:1480–1.

141. Hörnsten P, Sundman–Engberg B, Gahrton G, et al. CCNU toxicity after an overdose in a patient with Hodgkin's disease. *Scand J Haematol.* 1983;31:9–14.

142. Hadjiyanni M, Valianatou K, Tzilianos M, et al. Prolonged thrombocytopenia after procarbazine "overdose" [letter]. *Eur J Cancer.* 1992;28A:1299.

143. Muller RJ, Agre P. Patient education: a multidisciplinary approach to influence patient compliance. *Top Hosp Pharm Manage.* 1991;10(4):50–58.

144. Cohen H, Cohen J. How you can help to ensure your safety when receiving cancer treatments. *Coping.* 1998 (September/October). Available at: www.ismp.org/MSAarticles/cancertreatment.html. Accessed June 9, 2005.

145. Grossman SA, Piantodosi S, Cvahay C. Are informed consent forms that describe clinical oncology research protocols readable by most patients and their families? *J Clin Oncol.* 1994;12:2211–15.

146. American Society of Clinical Oncology. American Society of Clinical Oncology policy statement: oversight of clinical research. *J Clin Oncol.* 2003;21(12):2377–86.

147. Knox RA. Doctor's orders killed cancer patient. *Boston Globe.* March 23, 1995:1, 16.

148. Waddell JA, Solimando DA Jr, Strickland WR, et al. Pharmacy staff interventions in a medical center hematology–oncology service. *J Am Pharm Assoc.* 1998;38(4):451–6.

149. Gandhi TK, Bartel SB, Shulman LN, et al. Medication safety in the ambulatory chemotherapy setting. *Cancer.* 2005;104:2477–83.

150. Welch CW, Deffenbaugh JH. Risks of using technicians and not pharmacists to handle antineoplastic drugs. *Am J Health Syst Pharm.* 2000;57(19):1750, 1753.

151. American Society of Clinical Oncology. American Society of Clinical Oncology statement regarding the use of outside services to prepare or administer chemotherapy drugs. Available at: www.asco.org/portal/site/ASCO/menuitem.c543a013502b2a89de912310320041a0/?vgnextoid=72848c393c458010VgnVCM100000ed730ad1RCRD. Accessed June 9, 2005.

152. Muller RJ, Kloth DD. Designing strategies to prevent cancer chemotherapy errors–part 1. *Pharm Practice News.* 2005 (May):83–88.

APPENDIX

RECOMMENDATIONS FOR PREVENTING ERRORS IN CANCER CHEMOTHERAPY[4,152]

1. Educate health care providers
   a. The educational process should be customized according to whether the individual will be involved in prescribing, dispensing, or administering antineoplastic agents.
   b. Consider a certification process to validate knowledge before allowing practitioners to prescribe, dispense, or administer antineoplastics. Competency must be proved.
   c. The pharmacy department should provide informational guidelines or a checklist when a new drug is added to the formulary. The guidelines should include therapeutic indication, usual dosage range (for single and multiple courses), reconstitution instructions (if applicable), infusion guidelines, and a description of adverse effects. Information on solution incompatibilities is helpful.
   d. Pharmacists should participate in educational sessions with prescribers and nurses who administer the drugs. Describing actual medication errors and the consequences of nonstandard prescribing methods can be highly effective. Each institution, especially clinical research centers, should develop specific educational resources.
   e. Distribute *ISMP Medication Safety Alert!* to all practitioners responsible for prescribing, dispensing, or administering chemotherapy. Practitioners should be responsible for, and become knowledgeable about, medication errors involving chemotherapeutic agents and adjunctive medications.
2. Verify the dose
   a. Each institution should develop a dose-verification process with as many independent manual checks as possible. A computer system to verify the dose and route is ideal, but most hospitals do not have this.
   b. All doses should be calculated independently (e.g., by the physician who writes the order, the pharmacist who prepares the dose, and the nurse who administers it).
   c. All health care providers should have ready access to resources for verifying a patient's laboratory test data and body surface area.
   d. Investigational drug doses must be verified by checking the institutional review board protocol number, two independent sources, or both.
3. Establish dosage limits
   a. Maximum single, per course, and lifetime doses should be established at each institution. The limits should be communicated during employee orientation programs and in-service education programs.
   b. Maximum dosage limits should be entered into pharmacy computer systems and listed on preprinted order forms.
   c. Limits should be established for minimum duration of infusion and appropriate route of administration.
   d. Manufacturers should help practitioners avoid medication errors by improving package labeling.
4. Standardize the prescribing vocabulary
   a. Use the full generic name of the drug. Brand names and abbreviations are not acceptable.
   b. Express all drug doses in milligrams or units.
   c. All orders should be dated with the month, day, and year.
   d. Use a leading zero when the dose is less than a whole unit (e.g., write "0.1 mg," not ".1 mg").
   e. Do not use a trailing zero when writing an order ("2.0 mg" looks like "20 mg" if the decimal point is overlooked).
   f. Include the current body surface area with the order.

g. Do not refer to drugs in terms of common drug classes (e.g., does "platinum" mean cisplatin, carboplatin, or oxaliplatin?).

h. The use of preprinted order forms should be encouraged.

i. Prescribing guidelines should be in place at every organization where chemotherapy is prescribed—even in private practice settings.

j. Preprinted chemotherapy order forms should be required except where order entry is computerized.

5. Work with drug manufacturers

a. Errors should be reported to the USP–ISMP Medication Errors Reporting program (www.ismp.org or www.usp.org).

b. Pharmacists should work with manufacturers to eliminate ambiguous dosing information from educational resources (e.g., package inserts, textbooks, company-sponsored educational programs).

6. Educate patients

a. Patients should be informed of the name of the antineoplastic agent, therapeutic indication, usual and actual doses, expected and possible adverse effects, and methods for preventing or managing adverse effects.

b. Patients should be instructed on how they can protect themselves from medication errors. Patients should be informed of their right to ask questions and seek satisfactory answers.

c. Health professionals need to listen carefully to what patients are telling them.

7. Improve communication

a. An interdisciplinary team at each practice site should review medication errors and resolve the miscommunication that is a leading cause of problems.

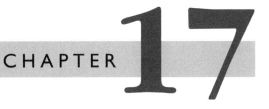

CHAPTER 17

PREVENTING MEDICATION ERRORS IN PEDIATRIC AND NEONATAL PATIENTS

Stuart Levine and Michael R. Cohen

Education in the health professions concentrates mainly on adult patients. Only a small portion of practitioners' training is devoted to the care of pediatric patients, often during residencies and fellowships in facilities that specialize in pediatric and neonatal care.[1] Similarly, most medical research is focused on adults rather than children. More data are needed on medication disposition and dosing in pediatric and neonatal patients. These young patients not only have some unique diseases, but have an increased risk of adverse drug events (ADEs), for several reasons:[2]

1. Pharmacokinetic parameters are different at various developmental stages.[1,3]
2. Multiple calculations are needed to individualize doses on the basis of age, weight, or body surface area.
3. Extemporaneous compounding is common because of the lack of available dosage forms and concentrations for pediatric and neonatal patients.
4. Oral liquid drug preparations are measured inconsistently.
5. Drug delivery systems are not designed for pediatric patients.
6. There is a lack of published information and Food and Drug Administration (FDA)-approved product labeling addressing the dosing, pharmacokinetics, safety, efficacy, and clinical use of medications in pediatric patients.

Furthermore, the pediatric population is diverse; it can be divided into preterm neonates (less than 36 weeks' gestation), full-term neonates (birth to 30 days), infants (1 month to 12 months), toddlers (1 to 4 years), children (5 to 12 years), and adolescents (over 12 years). A 100-fold difference can exist between a medication dosage for an adolescent and that for a preterm neonate. A pediatric dose could be one-tenth of an adult's dose but still be 10 times the appropriate dose for a preterm neonate.

Kaushal et al.[4] and Fortescue et al.[5] have evaluated medication safety and the rates of errors and ADEs (actual, potential, and preventable) in pediatric inpatient settings. Kaushal et al.[4] noted that although the rates of medication errors and preventable ADEs were similar for adults and children, the rate of potential ADEs was three times higher for pediatric patients. The rates of errors and potential ADEs were significantly higher in neonatal intensive care unit (NICU) patients than in any other age group. Most errors (74%) and potential ADEs (79%) originated in the ordering phase. Incorrect dosing accounted for 28% of the medication errors and 34% of the potential ADEs.

TABLE 17-1   Use of Medication Safety Practices in Pediatric Units[6]

Error Prevention Practice	Rating (%)	GPU n = 167	PICU n = 39	NICU n = 72	NUR n = 34	All N = 312
Physicians include both the mg/kg dose and the calculated dose for all drug orders.	Always	1	5	8	6	4
	Frequently	18	23	25	24	21
	Sometimes	53	46	50	50	51
	Never	28	26	17	21	24
Pharmacists verify the mg/kg dose listed in the prescriber's drug orders.	Always	47	67	63	58	54
	Frequently	37	28	23	27	31
	Sometimes	10	3	7	9	9
	Never	6	3	7	6	6
Pharmacists recalculate the patient's actual dose before preparing/dispensing medications.	Always	45	51	60	50	50
	Frequently	36	28	26	31	32
	Sometimes	16	18	10	9	14
	Never	3	3	4	9	4
The patient's weight in kg is entered into the pharmacy computer before medication orders are entered and drugs are dispensed.	Always	45	68	59	71	54
	Frequently	42	32	26	21	34
	Sometimes	9	0	9	6	8
	Never	4	0	7	3	4
The patient's age is entered into the pharmacy computer before medication orders are entered and drugs are dispensed.	Always	80	95	87	91	85
	Frequently	17	5	7	6	12
	Sometimes	2	0	0	3	2
	Never	0	0	6	0	1
Pediatric and neonatal parenteral solutions that are prepared in the pharmacy are independently double-checked by a pharmacist before dispensing.	Always	63	76	70	53	66
	Frequently	16	13	16	28	17
	Sometimes	11	5	7	9	9
	Never	9	5	6	9	8
Pharmacists/technicians who prepare parenteral solutions have undergone specialized training and demonstrated competency in pediatric drugs and dosing.	Always	51	59	67	47	55
	Frequently	22	31	23	28	24
	Sometimes	12	3	1	16	9
	Never	15	8	9	9	12
A clinical pharmacist is physically present on the unit to participate in daily patient rounds and provide input into the selection and administration of drugs.	Always	14	24	31	3	18
	Frequently	18	39	26	12	22
	Sometimes	13	24	7	3	12
	Never	55	13	36	82	48
Nurses who provide care to patients have undergone specialized training and demonstrated competency.	Always	66	89	88	82	76
	Frequently	23	11	11	18	18
	Sometimes	9	0	0	0	5
	Never	2	0	1	0	1
Charts or tables that list infusion rates or doses for typical parenteral solutions or medications are available to minimize the need for mathematical calculations.	Always	35	38	41	39	37
	Frequently	35	33	28	23	32
	Sometimes	21	21	15	6	18
	Never	9	8	15	32	13

TABLE 17-1 Use of Medication Safety Practices in Pediatric Units[6] (continued)

Error Prevention Practice	Rating (%)	GPU n = 167	PICU n = 39	NICU n = 72	NUR n = 34	All N = 312
A second nurse independently double-checks any dose calculations performed on the unit before drugs or solutions are administered.	Always	23	26	49	41	32
	Frequently	30	42	28	31	31
	Sometimes	38	32	23	25	32
	Never	8	0	0	3	5
Before parenteral solutions are administered, a second nurse independently double-checks the solution against the original order and verifies, at the bedside, the line attachment (e.g., IV, UVC, rate of infusion, and the patient).	Always	21	32	43	40	30
	Frequently	21	18	13	10	17
	Sometimes	34	24	23	27	29
	Never	25	26	21	23	24

GPU = general pediatric unit; NICU = neonatal intensive care unit; PICU = pediatric intensive care unit; NUR = level I/II nursery; UVC = umbilical venous catheter.

Fortescue et al.[5] rated the effectiveness of 10 strategies for reducing the rate of pediatric medication errors. The three strategies with the highest potential impact were as follows:

1. Improved communication among physicians, nurses, and pharmacists. This might have prevented 75.5% of medication errors.
2. Unit-based clinical pharmacists making rounds with the health care team. This might have prevented 81.3% of medication errors.
3. Use of computerized prescriber order entry (CPOE) with decision support. This might have prevented 72.7% of medication errors.

The findings of a survey in 2000 by the Institute for Safe Medication Practices (ISMP) and the Pediatric Pharmacy Advocacy Group (PPAG)[6] suggest that such safety practices are not widely implemented during the prescribing, preparation, dispensing, and administration of medications to pediatric patients (Table 17-1).

REASONS FOR INCREASED RISK OF ERROR

Lack of Pediatric Formulations, Dosage Forms, and Guidelines

Health care professionals often cannot use a commercially available formulation to prepare and administer the appropriate medication dose for a pediatric patient.[7] For example, because small children cannot swallow tablets and capsules, tablets may be crushed and capsules may be opened and their contents added to food (e.g., applesauce, ice cream) or beverages (e.g., juices, formula, soda). Such manipulation can not only cause solubility and bioavailability problems but can increase the potential for error.[7-9] Many commercially available dosage forms, such as tablets, capsules, patches, and extended-release products, cannot be reformulated into dosage forms suitable for infants and children. Even if reformulation were possible, problems might arise because of insufficient information about product stability, compatibility, sterility, and bioavailability, not to mention the lack of dosing guidelines for children.

When extemporaneous formulation is necessary, compatibility and stability data should be obtained. The fewer data that are available, the sooner should be the expiration date given to the reformulated product. For some formulations, preparation just before administration may be recommended.

Reasons for the lack of available pediatric formulations and dosing guidelines may be largely economic. Testing drugs in children is complicated, and if the anticipated market for a drug or dosage form is limited, the pharmaceutical industry has little incentive to develop the product.[9] This is unfortunate, because the availability of formulations for pediatric patients could increase medication safety.

The American Academy of Pediatrics (AAP) states that it is unethical to deny children appropriate access to existing and new therapeutic agents.[10] AAP holds that it is the shared responsibility of the pediatric community, pharmaceutical industry, and regulatory agencies to conduct the necessary studies to ensure that all children have access to important medications and receive optimal drug therapy.

To that end, the Pediatric Research Equity Act of 2003 gave FDA the power to require drug companies to conduct pediatric studies on medications that are used in children. If a pharmaceutical company believes children will use its product, pediatric testing must be included in the planning for clinical trials. A federal court barred a similar FDA regulation in 2002, stating that it exceeded the agency's authority. The 2003 legislation should help promote the availability of more pediatric dosage formulations, as well as dosing guidelines, to improve the safety and effectiveness of pediatric medications.[11]

Confusion between Adult and Pediatric Formulations

Even when manufacturers offer both adult and pediatric formulations (e.g., acetaminophen, digoxin, gentamicin), there is potential for error. When a prescriber ordered digoxin by volume instead of by weight and did not specify the strength of the solution, an infant received 1.5 mL of an adult concentration of digoxin (0.25 mg/mL) instead of the pediatric concentration (0.1 mg/mL). The nurse had obtained the dose from an automated dispensing cabinet (ADC) that contained both adult and pediatric concentrations. Another error occurred when an intended gentamicin dose of 7.8 mg (0.78 mL of the pediatric concentration of 10 mg/mL) for an infant was incorrectly prepared from the adult concentration (40 mg/mL) by the pharmacy.

Lupron Depot-Ped (leuprolide acetate for depot suspension) has been confused with the adult formulation Lupron Depot-3 Month because both have an 11.25 mg strength. Several errors occurred when pharmacy staff selected the wrong computer drug record during order entry. Although the product labels use a picture of either an adult or a child to differentiate the dosage forms, a price sticker had been placed over the picture, rendering the visual clue useless. Use of the Lupron Depot-3 Month adult formulation resulted in absorption of the child's dose over 3 months instead of 1 month.

Prescribers should be required to indicate the dose of medication in weight (milligrams), not volume. When possible, ADCs and other storage areas on pediatric units should be stocked with only pediatric concentrations. If both pediatric and adult concentrations need to be stocked, they should be stored in separate locations.

Confusion among Concentrations of Oral Liquids

Errors also occur with oral liquid dosage forms that are available in multiple pediatric concentrations. Overdoses have been reported when Infants' Tylenol drops, concentrated acetaminophen (100 mg/mL), have been administered instead of Children's Tylenol (160 mg/5 mL). The manufacturer, McNeil Consumer Products, redesigned the label of

Infants' Tylenol drops to emphasize the concentrated form. McNeil also developed a special package with floppy "cusps" in the bottle's neck that allow a dropper to be inserted but act as a one-way valve to prevent outward flow of the concentrated suspension. This makes it difficult to pour out teaspoonful amounts. This safety feature is not, however, used in the packaging of generic infants' acetaminophen drops or combination products that contain infants' acetaminophen.

Similarly, since Sudafed Children's Liquid is available as a 15 mg/5 mL concentration and many generic pseudoephedrine liquids are available as 30 mg/5 mL, errors can occur when a physician instructs parents to administer nonprescription Sudafed by volume (e.g., teaspoonfuls, milliliters) instead of by milligrams.

Fatal overdosages of chloral hydrate oral solution, which is used to sedate pediatric patients for diagnostic procedures, have occurred when the two available concentrations, 500 mg/5 mL and 250 mg/5 mL, were confused. Again, prescribing by volume instead of by weight (milligrams) has been a contributing factor.

Errors in concentration can also result from incorrect preparation of medications that require dilution. For example, an error occurred with a prescription for Zoloft (sertraline) Oral Concentrate 20 mg/mL for an 11-year old child. The technician who entered the prescription into the computer did not realize that explicit instructions were on the bottle for the dilution of this medication, and he placed the computer-generated pharmacy label over the instructions. The pharmacy label stated that the patient should take 5 mL per day. The father, unable to read the manufacturer's instructions for dilution, administered the undiluted concentrate to his child, who complained of a burning sensation in his throat.

Switching between two commercially available concentrations (e.g., amoxicillin 125 mg/5 mL and 250 mg/5 mL) has also led to errors in dispensing or administration. A new concentration may be more convenient, but an incorrect dose may be dispensed if the product is prepared in the same way as previous concentrations. When extemporaneous products are prepared, it is important to use one consistent formula or concentration, which should be recorded in a compounding log so that subsequent preparations by other staff members are consistent.

A tragic error in a 5-year-old child, involving the compounding of an imipramine solution, might have been averted if the pharmacy had used a standard concentration and formula. Imipramine was dispensed in a concentration five times greater than prescribed because the technician entered the concentration into the computer as 50 mg/mL instead of 50 mg/5 mL, with directions to administer 2 teaspoonfuls at bedtime. The technician mixed the solution using the incorrect concentration on the computer-generated label. The pharmacist did not check the prescription before it was dispensed to the patient's mother, and the patient died from imipramine poisoning. Strategies that might have averted such an error include (1) the use of fail-safe mechanisms to ensure independent double checks before dispensing and (2) not filling or compounding prescriptions from computer-generated labels.

Prescribers should be required to indicate the dose of medication in milligrams (weight), not volume. Only one concentration of a drug should be stocked; if more than one concentration is needed, their storage should be separated. Parents should be educated about the different formulations and strengths of acetaminophen and other common nonprescription products (e.g., pseudoephedrine). New parents should be required to demonstrate the correct measurement and dosing of acetaminophen for their infant before leaving the hospital. Medications for conscious sedation should be administered to children only by trained health care providers in settings where emergency equipment is available for use if respiratory depression occurs (sidebar, page 474).[12,13]

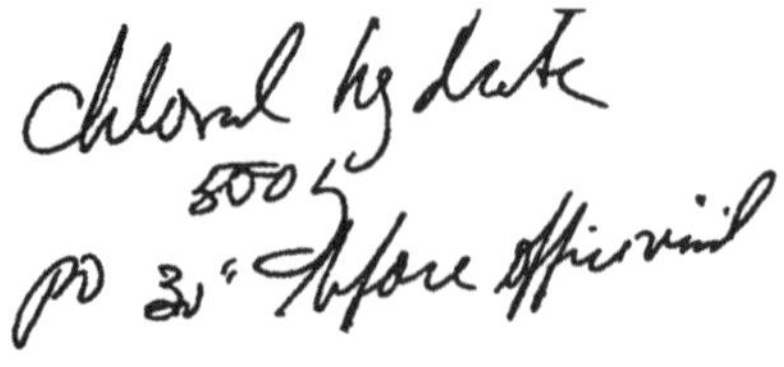

FIGURE 17-1   This order was intended as chloral hydrate 500 mg PO 30 minutes before an office visit for a procedure, but the pharmacist dispensed 30 mL of a 500 mg/mL concentration.

CHILDREN SHOULD NOT RECEIVE PREPROCEDURE SEDATION AT HOME

A physician prescribed chloral hydrate 500 mg for a 17-month-old girl, intending the parents to give the medication prior to the child's office visit for a procedure. As shown in Figure 17-1, he used double hash marks (″) to indicate minutes, although that symbol actually indicates seconds. The pharmacist misinterpreted the double hash marks as "cc" and dispensed 30 mL of a 500 mg/5 mL concentration of chloral hydrate, not realizing the child would receive a 3,000 mg single dose. The child became comatose shortly after her mother gave her the large dose. She was rushed to the hospital, was resuscitated, and recovered.

Other children have died after receiving accidental overdoses of chloral hydrate at home. One error occurred because the dose had been prescribed by volume (teaspoonfuls). The physician assumed that a 250 mg/5 mL concentration would be used to fill the prescription, but the pharmacist filled it using a 500 mg/5 mL concentration. The child received a twofold overdose. In another error, the original prescription instructed the mother to give her child "12 mL" of chloral hydrate, but the pharmacist dispensed a 120 mL bottle labeled with instructions to give the entire bottle before a procedure.

Inpatient and outpatient health care providers should abandon the practice of asking parents to administer sedation to their children at home. According to the American Academy of Pediatrics, children should not receive sedatives (e.g., chloral hydrate, midazolam [Versed]) or anxiolytic medications without supervision and monitoring by skilled medical personnel who have readily available, age- and size-appropriate resuscitation equipment (and reversal agents when applicable). Pursuant to this guideline, one hospital designates an inpatient bed and a pediatric nurse for admitting, medicating, monitoring, and transporting all pediatric outpatients receiving moderate sedation.[12-14]

Look-Alike Packaging and Look-Alike and Sound-Alike Names

Medication names that look and sound alike have led to errors in pediatric patients. For example, mix-ups between Zyrtec (cetirizine) syrup and Zantac (ranitidine) syrup have been reported frequently. One commonly reported error with look-alike packaging involves mix-ups between Cafcit (caffeine citrate) oral solution and the formulation for intravenous use. Both are clear, colorless liquids packaged in single-dose vials. The IV vials have a white cap marked "For Intravenous Use Only," and the oral solution vials have a blue cap marked "For Oral Use Only." However, this difference is easily missed because both products look like vials of injectable drugs. Chapters 6 and 7 discuss strategies for preventing errors caused by look-alike packaging and look-alike and sound-alike drug names.

Multiple Dosing Styles

Continuous IV infusions of medications for pediatric patients usually are prescribed on the basis of weight, but any of the following may be used: micrograms per kilogram per

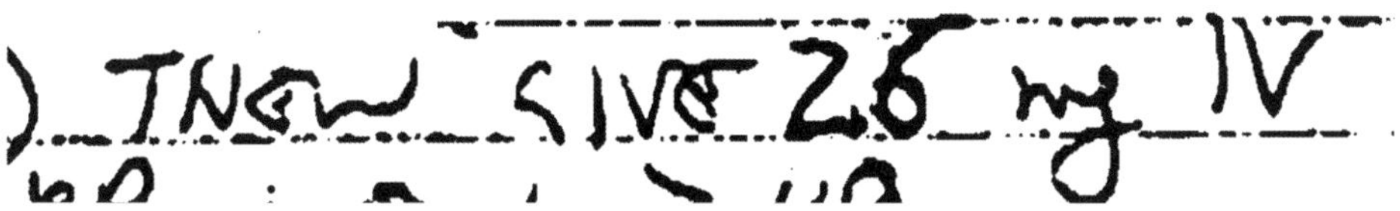

FIGURE 17-2 Order for hydralazine 2.6 mg misread as 26 mg.

minute, milligrams per hour, micrograms per kilogram per hour, milligrams per kilogram per minute, milligrams per kilogram per hour, and micrograms per minute. Although these are all legitimate ways of ordering medications, errors have occurred when prescribers have been allowed to use their own individual styles for expressing doses, rather than one standard. If pharmacists and nurses must work with a number of different prescribing styles, errors are likely to occur. It is safest to set a standard dosing style (e.g., as micrograms per kilogram per minute or milligrams per kilogram per hour) that should always be used in prescribing specific weight-based pediatric medications.

Calculation Errors

Dosages for pediatric patients (those weighing less than 40 kg) are often calculated on the basis of age, status of prematurity, weight, and body surface area (height and weight). Simple errors in computation can have harmful effects. An error at one children's hospital reinforced the importance of communicating orders legibly and developing systems for recognizing errors when orders are not clear. Because of an obscured decimal point, the prn order for hydralazine in Figure 17-2 (top line) for a 9-year-old patient with leukemia was misread as 26 mg. The order was supposed to be for 2.6 mg of hydralazine IV every 4 to 6 hours. An experienced nurse gave the incorrect dose, and the child became hypotensive. He was resuscitated but never regained consciousness and was removed from ventilator support 4 days later. He had been hospitalized to undergo bone marrow transplantation.

In orders for pediatric patients, prescribers should include the dose in milligrams per kilogram and the calculated dose. Pharmacists and nurses should then be responsible for independently double-checking the calculation (recalculating, not just "eyeballing" the math). The child who received the massive hydralazine overdose weighed 57 pounds (25.9 kg). If the physician had written the dose as "2.6 mg (0.1 mg/kg)," the mistake might not have occurred. It is essential that prescribers ensure that their orders are clear and understandable before leaving the patient care unit or before concluding a call, in the case of a telephone order. Prescribers should always take the time to look over their handwritten orders and go over them with key personnel. They should always ask that their spoken orders be transcribed and read back. Rather than work on a pile of patient charts, prescribers should complete them one at a time and hand them off to the individual responsible for transcribing. Then, if the transcriber has questions, the prescriber can answer them immediately.

Errors like the hydralazine overdose are probably more likely to occur when nursing personnel have access to medications before the orders are independently reviewed by a pharmacist. Thus, policies should limit the medications available in clinical areas before pharmacy review. Although CPOE systems solve legibility problems, they cannot always prevent orders for 10-fold overdosages, especially in pediatrics where dose ranges are so variable. Independent review of orders before administration is critical.

Errors in calculating pediatric doses are quite frequent. Potts et al.[15] gave 34 first-year family practice and pediatric residents clinical problems that required conversion of common units and mathematical calculations of maintenance fluids, drug dosages, and rehydration therapy. The mean score was 42% for all residents and 57% for pediatric residents. Only 5 of the 34 residents wrote acceptable fluid orders for a child with dehydration.

Koren et al.[16,17] have described 10-fold computational errors in doses administered to pediatric and neonatal patients. The most frequent error was a misplaced decimal point. The drugs included phenobarbital, pancuronium, digoxin, aminophylline, atropine, and gentamicin; the consequences of the errors included coma, respiratory failure, cardiac arrest, tachycardia, and transient renal failure.

Perlstein et al.[18] reported that 1 of every 12 dosages calculated by 95 registered nurses in a NICU contained an error that would result in 10-fold overdosage or underdosage. Eleven pediatricians made similar errors in 1 of every 26 calculations they attempted. Pharmacists demonstrated far better computational skills than either the nurses or the physicians. Pharmacy recalculation of all pediatric doses before dispensing is an important safety measure. For example, when a pharmacist received an order for oral clonidine 1 mg for a growth hormone stimulation test in an 8-year-old child, he recalculated the dose and determined that the correct dose should have been 0.15 mg/m². After a call to the physician, the order was changed to clonidine 0.1 mg, averting a 10-fold overdose.

These study findings further illustrate the need for prescribers to include the milligram per kilogram dosage along with the calculated dosage. For example, a dosage of amoxicillin for a 15 kg patient should be written as amoxicillin "250 mg (50 mg/kg/day) orally every 8 hours." Then, if the nurse and pharmacist have access to the patient's current weight, they can confirm the accuracy of the dosage. However, unless nurses and pharmacists perform the recalculation to verify accuracy, the prescriber's extra effort is wasted. Pharmacists and nurses should mathematically double-check the calculated dose and initial the order to show that this has been done. Initials should be placed where they cannot be confused with parts of the order.

Calculation errors can also occur during the preparation of a nonstandard strength or concentration of a medication. The pharmacy often must make extemporaneous preparations for children from adult dosage forms. Recipes for extemporaneous preparation should be written and should use a standard concentration to facilitate accurate dosage calculations.

Recommendations for preventing calculation errors can be summarized as follows:

1. Establish a reliable method of making the patient's current weight in kilograms available to physicians, nurses, and pharmacists so that all weight-based doses can be prescribed accurately and verified.
2. Require prescribers to include the calculated dose and the dose per weight (e.g., milligrams per kilogram) or body surface area on medication orders to facilitate an independent double-check of the calculation by a pharmacist, nurse, or both. This should apply to both inpatient and outpatient orders.
3. Establish a procedure for independent double checks in which all calculations are repeated by a second person without influence from the previous health care provider. Pharmacists should double-check the prescriber's calculations before dispensing the medication; nurses should double-check the prescriber's calculations before administering the first dose.
4. To help detect potential calculation errors, structure the pharmacy system and CPOE system to include warnings for doses that are subtherapeutic or exceed established maximum dose guidelines based on body weight or body surface area.
5. For common pediatric medications, use approved dosing charts with precalculated dosages for different weights to avoid the need for dose calculations.

6. For all extemporaneously prepared pediatric medications, provide dosing recipes using a standard concentration.
7. Provide readily accessible standard references for pediatric dosing in areas where prescriptions are written, drugs are dispensed, and medications are administered.
8. Encourage prescribers to round off doses to even numbers when possible.
9. Certify the computational capabilities of all health care personnel who prescribe, prepare, dispense, or administer medications.

Errors with Measuring Devices

Oral medications may be generally regarded as having less potential to cause harm than injectable medications. But oral liquid medications are most often used for pediatric patients, who are quite vulnerable to the effects of an error, and this dosage form is the least likely to be dispensed in unit doses. Special precautions in preparing oral liquid doses, including the use of proper measuring devices, are necessary.

Oral liquids are often prescribed for children as fractions of a teaspoonful. Three decades ago, AAP pointed out that a household spoon is not an accurate measuring device for medications. Still, three out of four Americans rely on teaspoons in their kitchen drawers to measure medicine doses, which often leads to dosing errors in infants and children.[19] A teaspoonful is equivalent to 5 mL, but household teaspoons can hold from 3 to 7 mL.

Droppers, cylindrical spoons, oral dosing syringes, medication cups, or small-volume dosers with attachable nipples should be used instead of household spoons. However, these different measuring devices may express calibration in terms of milliliters (mL), cubic centimeters (cc), fractions of a teaspoonful, or a combination of all three. Also, increments of calibration vary from one device to another; for example, a 1 mL oral syringe is calibrated in increments of 0.1 mL, whereas the calibration of a 5 mL syringe is in 0.2 mL increments. The various units of calibration can confuse parents. One pharmacist labeled metoclopramide syrup for an infant correctly, as 0.7 mL every 6 to 8 hours, but the mother measured out 7 mL of medication and administered a 10-fold overdose to her child.

Numerous errors have resulted from caregivers' unfamiliarity with measurement devices, their calibration scale, and volume equivalents.[20] A mother inadvertently gave her child a fivefold overdose of children's acetaminophen (640 mg instead of 120 mg) because she thought the cup included with the product held exactly one dose.[21] Another parent did not receive instructions or a calibrated dropper to measure the prescribed dose of theophylline for his infant. The infant was hospitalized with seizures because the father measured the doses inaccurately and administered a significant overdose.

When caregivers were asked to demonstrate how they measured and administered the liquid form of albuterol to their children, 22% measured an improper dose and 17% inaccurately measured the intended dose.[22,23] All who used a household teaspoon measured the intended dose incorrectly. Most of these caregivers had a high school education.

The words used in directions can lead to errors. For example, a pharmacist averted a potential error involving the term "dropperful." The physician had ordered "ferrous sulfate 1 dropperful 3 times daily," but a dropperful can be misinterpreted to mean a dropper filled to the upper calibration mark, a dropper filled past the upper calibration mark, or a household dropper. Furthermore, the droppers that are included with some generic ferrous sulfate products have different scales than the droppers that come with the brand name product. In this case, the order for ferrous sulfate was changed to "elemental iron 15 mg (0.6 mL) 3 times daily" to ensure proper dosing.

Reviewing the dosing instructions for prescription and nonprescription liquid medications with the child's caregiver can help avoid errors. In community pharmacies, all new prescriptions for oral liquid medications (and other new prescriptions that suggest education is warranted) should be placed in a separate area away from other prescriptions. This helps ensure that a pharmacist reviews directions with the caregiver, provides an appropriate measuring device, and demonstrates its use before dispensing the drug. One pharmacy stamps a red "C" for "Counsel" on all such prescription bags to alert the clerk to call a pharmacist when the prescription is being picked up. It is not enough to simply ask if the caregiver has any questions. Reviewing the directions with the caregiver can also alert the pharmacist to inaccurate label directions that may have been overlooked during the checking process.

In inpatient settings, oral liquid medications should be dispensed in unit doses in oral syringes whenever possible. Before pediatric patients are discharged, caregivers should be educated about proper measurement, given an oral syringe when feasible, and reminded to take the syringe to a pharmacy and ask for a measuring demonstration.

If physician offices dispense samples of oral solutions, arrangements should be made with a hospital or community pharmacy for patients to take the samples there to be properly labeled with instructions.

Hypodermic syringes should not be provided to parents for the administration of oral liquids. If the small translucent cap is inadvertently left on one of these syringes during use, the child could choke on it. (It is possible to draw a medication into some syringes and eject it without removing the cap.) Furthermore, oral liquids (e.g., Tylenol, Versed, Augmentin) drawn up in syringes have been inadvertently administered by the IV route.

Only measuring cups or oral syringes should be used to dispense or administer oral liquid medications. Most caps on oral syringes are difficult to dislodge with plunger pressure, but they are easily removed for drug administration. Still, nurses and parents should be cautioned to remove the cap from an oral syringe before drawing fluid into the syringe or forcing fluid into the child's mouth. Syringes should be labeled "Oral Use Only." A liquid medication intended for administration through a small-bore enteral feeding tube with a Luer connection should be dispensed in an oral syringe and transferred into a hypodermic syringe at the time of administration. Alternatively, a Luer-tip adapter can be attached to the oral syringe. Also, Klein-Baker distributes a small-bore feeding tube that is compatible with Baxa and Becton Dickinson oral syringes.

Recommendations for preventing errors in measuring and administering oral liquid medications can be summarized as follows:

1. Always review the dosing instructions for new prescription and nonprescription liquid medications with the child's caregiver. Offer a measuring device, and require a repeat demonstration or spoken acknowledgement of understanding.
2. Remind caregivers to avoid measuring medications with a household spoon.
3. In inpatient settings, dispense liquid medications in oral syringes containing the patient-specific unit dose.
4. Caution nurses and parents to remove syringe caps before drawing fluid into the syringe or placing fluid into the child's mouth.
5. Instruct parents and nurses to use only the dropper that comes with a particular product.

Use of Nonstandard Concentrations and the Rule of 6

It may seem convenient to have medications available in numerous concentrations for patients of different sizes, but this can increase the likelihood that mistakes will be made in calculation and medications will be prepared and dispensed in error. In 2002, the Joint Commission on Accreditation of Healthcare Organizations (JCAHO) established a National Patient Safety Goal (NPSG) that included a requirement to standardize and limit the number of concentrations of high-alert medications. In October 2003, JCAHO confirmed that the requirement applied to continuous infusions of medications for pediatric and neonatal patients.

Simplification and standardization reduce error potential. The use of standardized concentrations of critical care drugs and corresponding charts (which can be made available on preprinted labels) for determining dosages in micrograms per kilogram per minute can help (1) avoid error-prone calculations and use of the wrong diluent or volume, (2) reduce the number of discarded doses and necessary dose preparations, and (3) facilitate the use of premixed IV solutions.

Many pediatric facilities have used the "rule of 6" to prepare continuous infusions of IV medications that are dosed according to the child's weight. According to this formula, from *The Harriet Lane Handbook*, 6 times the child's weight in kilograms equals the amount of drug in milligrams that should be added to 100 mL of solution. The infusion volume in milliliters per hour then equals the dose ordered in micrograms per kilogram per minute. For example, a drug ordered at 10 mcg/kg/minute would equal an infusion rate of 10 mL/hour. (A "rule of 15" also exists, where 15 times the weight in kilograms equals the amount of drug per 250 mL.) Although nurses and house staff physicians may like using this shortcut, it results in wide variation in concentrations.

Furthermore, the rule of 6 may not be consistently followed.[24] Some practitioners may use it while others do not. It may be used in the NICU but not elsewhere. A physician or nurse accustomed to using the rule of 6 might assume that all solutions dosed in micrograms per kilogram per minute are prepared in this fashion. If a solution has not been prepared this way and has a different concentration, these practitioners might adjust the rate inaccurately.

Nurses who routinely use the rule of 6 may recalculate the dose and prepare and hang a new solution at the beginning of their shift if the current solution has not been dosed according to the rule of 6. This practice can unnecessarily introduce errors, including use of the wrong diluent or volume.

The rule of 6 requires mathematical calculation of critical care drug doses, which is always an error-prone process. Errors have been reported when nurses confuse milligrams with milliliters and add the drug to the solution by volume rather than weight (e.g., adding 30 mL instead of 30 mg). Accurate pump settings may also be problematic if milliliters per hour is confused with milliliters per 24 hours.

Hospitals that use the rule of 6 have traditionally had nurses preparing IV solutions on patient care units, an error-prone process that bypasses pharmacy preparation and double-checking. The JCAHO 2004 medication management standards included a new requirement that nurses not prepare nonemergent drug infusions when on-site pharmacy services are available. All sterile medications and IV admixtures are to be prepared by the pharmacy when it is open, with techniques for avoiding contamination and methods that ensure accuracy in preparation and labeling.

In facilities where pharmacy uses the rule of 6 in preparing IV admixtures, errors have occurred because of confusion over whether the patient's weight was in kilograms or pounds. Also, a calculation error in a pharmacy using the rule of 6 may have contributed to an infant's death; a decimal point was misplaced, and a dopamine infusion was prepared at 10 times the concentration that was ordered.

In addition, when admixtures are prepared according to the rule of 6, dosage adjustments can result in fluid overload. For example, if the rate of a dopamine infusion were increased from 5 mcg/kg/minute to 10 mcg/kg/minute, a small infant would receive 10 mL/hour—the infant's total daily fluid requirement—from this medication alone. Therefore, a physician might order an atypical (double or triple) concentration, increasing the likelihood of a dosing error if practitioners are more familiar with rule of 6 dosing concentrations.

Use of the rule of 6 can result in drug waste. Usually, only a portion of the contents of a drug vial is used to prepare solutions in this manner. Either the remaining drug is wasted or single-use containers are inappropriately reused.

The rule of 6 has been controversial for some time.[25] At issue is which is less error-prone: the use of standard concentrations, or the use of a simplified method (the rule of 6) for preparing admixtures and determining flow rate. Despite the best of intentions, the need for calculations increases the risk of error, particularly during times of high stress.

JCAHO has allowed pediatric hospitals and services that use the rule of 6 to apply for exceptions to the NPSG requirement for standard concentrations. A plan to help organizations make the transition from the rule of 6 was developed in collaboration with AAP, Child Health Corporation of America, ISMP, and the National Association of Children's Hospitals and Related Institutes. It is supported by JCAHO's Sentinel Event Advisory Group.[26] Organizations that use the rule of 6 must provide evidence that they are moving toward implementation of standard concentrations, and all organizations must convert to standardized concentrations no later than December 31, 2008.

Exceptions during the transition period can apply only to neonatal or pediatric acute care services. The additional eligibility criteria for exceptions are as follows:

- All (emergent and nonemergent) admixtures are prepared only by pharmacy staff in a sterile environment.
- Calculations of the drug solutions are validated during the preparation.
- The labeling of solution concentration and drug per milliliter is clear to all caregivers, and the solution concentration (amount of drug per unit volume of solution) is clearly indicated on the label.
- If the rule of 6 is used in a pediatric setting but standardized drug concentrations are used in other parts of the hospital, guidance aids are made available to caregivers who may not be familiar with one of these systems.
- If the organization has a NICU, the pharmacy is open 24 hours a day to support the admixture service.
- "Smart" infusion pumps are used. (Smart pumps are designed to recognize prescription errors, dose misinterpretations, and keypad programming errors.)

Many hospitals that have made the transition to standardized concentrations have seen a decrease in medication errors. In 2004, a multidisciplinary team at the University of Maryland Hospital for Children conducted an online national survey of health care providers' practices and opinions on this issue.[27] Of 1,150 pediatric and neonatal critical care providers, 59% were using the rule of 6 and 41% were using standardized concentrations. The University of Maryland team developed a simplified, computerized method for making the transition to standard concentrations.[28] First, ideal standard concentrations were identified through the use of a computer program (Concentration Optimizer) that automatically generated two to four concentrations (based on potential fluid restriction needs) for each drug. Then, a CPOE program for ordering continuous infusions was developed. With only the dose and the patient weight, the CPOE program automatically selects the best concentration from the two to four optimal concentrations. The program generates a printed order containing compounding instructions for the pharmacy, administration instructions for nurses, and a weight-specific dosing chart that displays infusion rates at all dose ranges. The team created a Web site (www.icudrips.org/) for discussion and updates on this subject. A list of the facility's current standard concentrations is at www.icudrips.org/conclist115.pdf.

Recommendations for safe preparation of IV admixtures can be summarized as follows:

1. Standardize the concentrations used for pediatric and neonatal injectable solutions.
2. When preparing IV solutions for pediatric and neonatal patients, use one consistent formula or standard concentration, not the rule of 6.
3. Use commercially available preparations when possible. Allow their availability on patient care units for emergent needs, to avoid preparation of infusions on the patient care unit.
4. Have pharmacy, when on site, prepare all IV admixtures for pediatric and neonatal patients when they are not available commercially.
5. Independently double-check all pediatric and neonatal IV admixtures before dispensing and administering the medications.

Nursing Preparation of IV Admixtures

As a rule, pharmacy should provide all medications in patient-specific unit doses. However, procedures should be established for preparing IV admixtures in emergencies or when pharmacy is unavailable and no commercial preparation exists. Each patient care unit should have a procedure sheet for preparing each admixture, indicating the drug name, number of milligrams or units to be used, type of diluent, and size of the diluent bag. Having a formalized method prevents variation and resultant dosing errors. If certain noncommercial IV admixtures are routinely used and the facility does not have 24-hour pharmacy services, the pharmacy might prepare one or two bags to be available after hours. This is particularly useful when 10% dextrose with various concentrations of sodium chloride is needed. When a rarely used IV admixture is needed, a pharmacist should be called in to prepare it.

IV Administration of Enteral Fluids

IV infusion of nonsterile particulate fluid such as breast milk can cause sepsis, disseminated intravascular coagulation, and emboli to major organs, with sometimes fatal outcomes. This error has been reported several times since 1972.[29-33] Since enteral pumps may not be able to deliver feedings in small enough quantities for neonates, parenteral syringe pumps have been used "off label," which increases the risk for accidental IV administration. In a recent case,[30] an infant received 10 mL of fortified breast milk IV, resulting in respiratory distress and seizures, which were successfully treated. An IV syringe pump for medications had been located on the left side of the baby's incubator, and an identical pump for delivering breast milk via nasogastric tube on the right. Both pumps used identical IV administration tubing. A nurse mistakenly connected a syringe containing breast milk to the IV line.

To prevent such errors, practitioners should

1. Trace the tubing to the point of origin before making any connections or reconnections of tubing,
2. Label tubes, administration sets, and pumps, and
3. Whenever possible, use non-Luer feeding tubes and extension sets, which are available from several manufacturers (e.g., Viasys Healthcare [www.viasys healthcare.com], Neo Devices [www.neodevices.com]), with enteral pumps. The connectors at the distal end of these sets are female and will connect only to the male connector on the systems' feeding tubes. The side ports connect only to an oral syringe. Some manufacturers are adjusting IV syringe pumps to accommodate oral syringes in case very low flow rates are required.

Insulin Dilution

Small doses of short-acting insulin may be ordered as sliding-scale coverage for pediatric patients. For neonates, a commercially available insulin concentration of 100 units/mL may be used for doses of 5 units or greater. When doses less than 5 units are required, the pharmacy must often prepare and label a 10 units/mL concentration, and nurses must use a 1 mL tuberculin syringe with 0.01 mL calibrations to measure the dose and administer the medication.

To avoid errors when insulin must be diluted, hospitals must (1) limit dilution to one concentration, (2) not let vials of diluted insulin leave the pharmacy, and (3) have the pharmacy prepare and deliver individual, patient-specific doses as needed. Stocking multiple concentrations of insulin in the patient care areas is likely to result in errors.

ENSURING STAFF COMPETENCIES

Insufficient knowledge about a drug is one of the leading causes of medication errors.[1] Mechanisms are needed for routinely checking health care providers' competency in this area. Facilities specializing in pediatric and neonatal care are likely to have staff who are well educated about diseases and medication use in that population. Other facilities may have some staff members during daytime hours who are knowledgeable about the dosing of pediatric medications but little support in this area during evenings, nights, and weekends.

Particularly when a new pediatric service is being initiated or an existing service expanded, staff competencies may be inadequate. A pharmacist in a hospital with a recently established pediatric emergency service was asked for ketamine injection to sedate children during procedures. Ketamine is available in vials of 10 mg/mL, 50 mg/mL, and 100 mg/mL. The pharmacist, who had limited knowledge and experience in pediatric dosing, sent 5 mL vials of the 100 mg/mL concentration. The physician, who was accustomed to using 10 mg/mL vials, did not notice the 100 mg/mL concentration and administered the total vial contents of 500 mg instead of 50 mg. The child suffered respiratory arrest but was resuscitated. Before the implementation of any new patient care services, staff must be adequately trained.

Several organizations offer resources to help staff gain or maintain competency in the care of pediatric patients. PPAG, a national organization of pharmacy practitioners who specialize in pediatrics, offers educational programs around the country and has a Web site (www.ppag.org) for posting questions. *Competence Assessment Tools for Health-System Pharmacies,* from the American Society of Health-System Pharmacists, has sections on "Providing Pharmaceutical Care to Neonatal and Infant Patients" and "Providing Pharmaceutical Care to Pediatric and Adolescent Patients." Topics covered are basic terminology, drug disposition in these populations, methods of calculating doses, factors that influence drug administration, the impact of disease processes on dosing, the IV delivery systems used, and precautions for reducing the risk of drug-related problems. The 2004 edition can be purchased at https://shop.ashp.org/timssnet/products/tnt_products.cfm?primary_id=P739&action=long.

To ensure staff competency

1. New services for pediatric and neonatal patients should be designed with careful planning to develop staff competencies for the entire team, including nurses, pharmacists, and support staff, before the service is opened and continually thereafter.
2. Resources should be available for maintaining competency in pediatric and neonatal pharmacology.

3. Assessment of math competencies should be part of the initial interview process for all employees who use math in calculating doses or preparing medications. In particular, all pharmacy technicians, residents, and pharmacists should be required to take a math test as part of the job application process.

4. Pharmacists who cover evenings, nights, and weekends should, as part of their orientation and ongoing training, complete short rotations on neonatal or pediatric units if providing services to this population.

MEDICATION SAFETY IN PEDIATRIC EMERGENCIES

In pediatric emergencies, medication errors can occur during ordering, dosing, preparation, and administration.[34] In the early 1990s, James Broselow, a family physician in rural North Carolina, experienced the stress felt by emergency care providers attempting to resuscitate a child. In searching for a way to provide consistent care in pediatric emergencies, he realized that endotracheal tube size could be keyed to the child's length. He subsequently found that dosages of many emergency medications could also be based on the child's length. He created the Broselow Pediatric Emergency Tape, which uses a specific color for each range of children's body length (height). Within each color area, the tape lists equipment sizes and weight-based doses of commonly used emergency medications. In simulated pediatric resuscitations, use of the Broselow tape has significantly reduced deviation from recommended dosage ranges.[35] The tape is now found in most emergency departments (EDs) around the world.

The Broselow tape has been revised over the years, and it is important to ensure that every ED has the most recent version. ISMP has found that many facilities still use versions from the mid-1990s. The 1998 version listed volumetric doses for quick reference, and clinicians sometimes administered the incorrect dose because concentrations of the drugs in the "crash" cart did not match the concentrations listed on the tape. Concentrations of medications kept in crash carts should be standardized, but the 2002 edition of the tape avoids potential confusion by listing only the weight-based dose (e.g., in milligrams or milliequivalents) for most drugs that are administered by IV push. The exception is epinephrine, for which the concentration (1:10,000 and 1:1,000), the dose in milligrams, and the dose by volume all are listed.

Clinicians have expressed concern about inconsistency in the expression of doses in the 2002 edition of the tape. While weight-based doses are given for IV push medications, doses of drugs to be given by continuous infusion are expressed by volume only, with directions for preparing the infusion preceding the volumetric dose. Furthermore, infusions prepared according to the tape are of various concentrations, despite the NPSG requiring standardization. Future editions of the Broselow tape will not include infusions.

Despite this limitation, health care providers should continue to use the tape during pediatric emergencies. In facilities where standard concentrations are used, staff can be temporarily redirected to a titration dosing table for each emergency drug. This way, if the child is subsequently admitted to the hospital, nurses on the patient care unit will be able to adjust the infusion rate according to the standard concentrations.

Hohenhaus et al.[36] observed safety issues during use of the Broselow tape in mock resuscitations. The most common error was improper positioning of the tape for measuring the patient. Also, errors occurred because clinicians believed the drugs listed for a specific indication (e.g., seizure) represented an algorithm for a sequence of drugs; they therefore administered more than one medication from each list rather than selecting one drug from the list. A tool for assessing nurses' competency in the use of the tape is available,[37] and a Web-based educational packet can be found at http://dukehealth1.org/deps/Study_Packet_v2_0.pdf.

Because the Broselow tape helps staff choose the correct size emergency equipment according to the color within which the child's height falls, some crash carts have been set up with color-coded drawers that contain supplies in sizes corresponding to the colors on the tape (see Figure 7-9). In recent years, new colors representing smaller patients have been introduced. A gray zone has been added for patients in the 3 to 5 kg range of estimated weight. However, this new zone corresponds to the pink/red zone equipment drawer in traditional color-coded carts. Furthermore, the zone is not distinctly labeled "gray," unlike the other zones that are labeled "pink," "red," and so on (Figure 17-3). Confusion occurs when a child is assigned to the gray zone, because there is no corresponding gray drawer. Also, crash carts with color-coded drawers that match the colors on the tape have a putty-colored top and bottom drawer, intended for general use, that could be mistaken as gray zone drawers.

The Broselow tape, while a valuable tool, does not address all emergency situations. It is important to have charts with precalculated dosages, according to the child's weight, of additional medications that are commonly used in pediatric emergencies.[38] These "code charts," commonly prepared as spreadsheets, should include weights in 0.5 kg increments from 1 kg to 10 kg. For children over 10 kg, the code charts should be prepared in 1 kg increments up to 40 kg. For children over 40 kg, algorithms for adult dosing are appropriate. The charts must be clearly legible. Some hospitals print an individualized code chart for each patient admitted. More often, however, the charts are copied from a single source and may have been sitting on crash carts for years. They may no longer be legible, or they may have been misplaced from their original location on the crash cart. Routine reviews of the ED should include ensuring that these code charts with precalculated dosages are accessible and legible.

In addition to these pediatric code charts, separate "code boxes" containing medications for neonatal and pediatric patients should be available. As these code boxes are designed, consideration should be given to the appropriate concentrations of the medications and the par levels of each medication. Unnecessarily large quantities may allow for inadvertent administration of an excessive dose. Often, the code boxes are placed inside a crash cart or in opaque boxes. Thus, unless they open the box, staff members are not familiar with the locations and types of medications. Placing a photograph of the contents of pediatric code boxes on top of the crash cart may help in this regard.

Ideally, in an ED, a pharmacist would be available to review orders and prepare medications for administration. This is one of the few areas in the hospital where, traditionally, only the prescriber and the nurse have been involved in medication use. In most other areas, a pharmacist provides a double check by ensuring that medications are ordered and prepared correctly.

Prescribing errors, omission errors, and improper dosage errors are the most frequent types of medication errors in EDs, according to the United States Pharmacopeia (USP).[39] In EDs, only 23% of errors are detected before reaching the patient. The absence of a pharmacist in the ED decreases the likelihood that errors will be caught before they reach patients. Whenever possible, a pharmacist should review medication orders and participate in the preparation and labeling of medications in EDs.

Recommendations for safe medication use in pediatric emergencies can be summarized as follows:

1. Be sure the most recent revision of the Broselow tape is in use.
2. Provide standard concentrations for resuscitation medications stocked in pediatric crash carts.
3. Stock medications and equipment in crash carts in a fashion that facilitates equipment retrieval according to color-coded weight ranges.

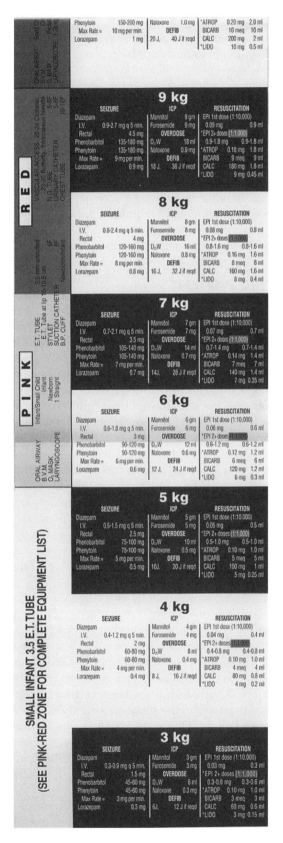

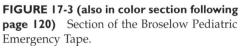

FIGURE 17-3 (also in color section following page 120) Section of the Broselow Pediatric Emergency Tape.

4. In facilities using standard concentrations, redirect staff to titration dosing tables (rather than the Broselow tape) for each emergency drug administered by infusion.

5. Require nurses working with pediatric patients to open crash carts regularly to become familiar with their contents.

6. Hang the Broselow tape with the red arrow, which states "Measure from this End," at the top. Teach staff to remember "red to head" when aligning the tape for measurement.

7. Educate staff in use of the Broselow tape and develop a tool for validating proficiency.

8. For medications used in pediatric codes and drugs that are commonly prescribed in the ED, have charts of precalculated dosages available. Be sure they are updated regularly and reprinted as necessary for legibility.

9. Design code boxes for pediatric and neonatal patients with limited par levels to prevent inadvertent overdoses.

10. Whenever possible, have a pharmacist involved in medication use in the ED.

MEDICATION SAFETY FOR PEDIATRIC PATIENTS IN THE OPERATING ROOM

In general, fewer pharmacy services have been provided in the operating room (OR) than in other inpatient units. Pharmacists do not participate in order review or dispensing in the OR. Spoken orders are common because of the sterile environment, and stat doses may often be ordered because of the preferences of individual surgeons. In many ORs, only a physician, usually the anesthesiologist, participates in the medication-use process; no other health care professionals intervene between prescribing and drug administration.

Pharmacies have used several approaches to improve medication safety in the OR and for pediatric surgical cases in particular.[40] Many spoken and stat orders can be eliminated through the use of physician preference cards. Most surgical cases are scheduled at least 1 day in advance. As cases are scheduled, the OR staff stocks rooms, trays, and kits from a physician's preference card to ensure that instruments and equipment are readily available. Medications (e.g., special preparations of heparin) and solutions for infusion and irrigation can be included on the preference cards and faxed or e-mailed to the pharmacy or entered into a CPOE system. The pharmacist then can review the orders, check for allergies, ensure accurate dosing, provide clear and complete labeling, and prepare and double-check the medication before sending it to the OR. The preparations can be delivered the same day or the next day, eliminating many of the stat and spoken orders.

The anesthesiologist may have access to an ADC, which usually is configured so that the pharmacy can only charge the patient and replace inventory. These systems traditionally have not provided for order review or safety checks. Pharmacies have implemented several strategies for decreasing the risk of error. Pharmacy can prepare and deliver uniform trays for the anesthesia department. These trays contain commonly used medications in a quantity sufficient to meet, but not exceed, the daily requirements, thereby decreasing the risk of inadvertent overdosages. Another strategy has been to prepare weight-based, patient-specific OR packs. For this purpose, the pharmacy receives orders listing the medications needed and the patient's weight. Doses are usually calculated by the anesthesia department and independently double-checked by a pharmacist. A variation of this concept is providing packs for a specific type of procedure (e.g., tonsillectomy and adenoidectomy packs) or according to the intensity of surgery (e.g., level 1, level 2, or level 3 packs).

A frequent source of medication errors in postoperative patients is lack of communication with areas outside the OR. Information about medications administered in the OR often is not readily available to the pharmacy or patient-care units as new medications are ordered, reviewed, and scheduled.

Recommendations for safe medication use in pediatric patients undergoing surgery can be summarized as follows:

1. Avoid the use of spoken orders by using preference cards for surgeons.
2. Prepare uniform trays for the anesthesiologist and deliver them daily from the pharmacy.
3. Prepare weight-based anesthesia packs customized for the individual patient, for a specific surgical procedure, or by intensity of surgery; such packs are more likely to contain the medications and dosages or strengths needed for a pediatric patient.
4. Ensure that information on medications administered in the OR is readily available to the pharmacy and the unit to which the patient is transferred.

ROLE OF AUTOMATION IN PEDIATRIC AND NEONATAL SERVICES

Computerized Prescriber Order Entry

In 1995, Leape, Bates, and colleagues[41] published research showing that 28% of ADEs in adult patients were preventable. The rate of near misses, or potential ADEs, was calculated as 9.1 potential errors for each 1,000 patient days. In 1998, they published an article on the impact of CPOE on serious medication errors,[42] stating that 55% of medication errors could be prevented through CPOE implementation.

Fortescue et al.,[5] rating the effectiveness of 10 strategies for reducing the rate of medication errors in pediatric inpatients, found that the use of ward-based clinical pharmacists and CPOE with decision support had significant potential for reducing errors. In a CPOE system, decision support is provided by rules such as those that ensure checks for drug allergies and interactions. A clinical decision support system (see Chapter 15) should include rules for checking the following:

1. Drug dose based on the patient's weight,
2. Single and cumulative dose limits, including lifetime dosing,
3. Dose limits for combination products (e.g., acetaminophen as an ingredient of multiple products taken by the same patient),
4. Therapeutic duplication, including combination products,
5. Cross-allergies,
6. Contraindications to routes of administration,
7. Food–drug and herbal–drug interactions,
8. Contraindications based on diagnosis, laboratory studies, or radiology studies, and
9. IV incompatibilities.

An important advantage of CPOE in pediatric settings is the decision support system's ability to check the appropriateness of doses on the basis of the patient's weight. The system can be designed to check a dose by using the minimal dose for that medication and a maximum dose determined on the basis of the lowest dosing range for that medication (e.g., for metoclopramide, use 0.1–0.2 mg/kg for gastroesophageal reflux rather than 1 mg/kg for chemotherapy-induced nausea, to avoid using a 10-fold overdose if the patient's diagnosis is not available). Alternatively, decision support can be associated with a diagnosis or an item on the patient's problem list; in this case, minimum and maximum dosages can be associated with a particular diagnosis.

A limitation of decision support for CPOE in pediatric settings is that most commercial drug information updating services provide information about FDA-approved indications only. They do not include information on pediatric dosing outside those indications, and many systems do not allow for customization.

Furthermore, a filtering feature is needed for limiting CPOE systems' ability to accept inappropriate and dangerous medication routes and frequencies. For example, children with orders for IV Solu-Medrol (methlyprednisolone sodium succinate) have been given Depo-Medrol (methylprednisolone acetate) by the IV route. In one case, Depo-Medrol was incorrectly placed in a Solu-Medrol floor stock bin; the nurse administering the drug looked it up under methylprednisolone and found two monographs but thought it was the same drug by two brand names. USP's MEDMARX program has received nearly 50 reports of mix-ups between Solu-Medrol and Depo-Medrol.

Intravascular administration of long-acting penicillin formulations (e.g., penicillin G benzathine or penicillin G procaine) is another example. Some practitioners wrongly believe long-acting injectable penicillins are for IV use. A 1998 survey revealed that 35% of neonatal registered nurses (RNs) and 30% of neonatal nurse practitioners (NNPs) were unable to identify the correct route of administration for penicillin G benzathine, and only 12% of RNs and 20% of NNPs demonstrated correct knowledge about the various types of penicillin G.[43] The labels for penicillin G benzathine and penicillin G procaine now contain a black box warning against IV injection, and bold warnings appear on the carton and syringe of all Bicillin products. Still, practitioners who do not know the correct route of administration for these products could easily overlook the labeling enhancements. It is crucial that CPOE and pharmacy computer systems limit the available routes of administration and prohibit the entry of incorrect routes. It might also be helpful for labels stating "For IM Use Only" to be wrapped around the needle cover of prefilled syringes; a warning that impedes use in this way would have a good chance of being noticed. In addition, if Bicillin products are stocked in ADCs, an alert could be added to the screen when Bicillin is selected.

Labels generated by CPOE or pharmacy systems should be clear and readily understood. The desire to provide a great amount of information on the labels of pediatric medications should be resisted, because a cluttered label can more easily be misinterpreted. If a large amount of information is provided, the font size and the space between fields may have to be reduced, and there may not be room for bold or capitalized characters to highlight critical information. As characters run together, lowercase L can look like the number 1 and the letter O can be interpreted as a zero. Nurses and pharmacists should determine what information is most important and format the system to produce labels that contain only that information.

Recommendations for safe use of CPOE and decision support in pediatric settings can be summarized as follows:

1. Provide dose alerts based on weight (and diagnosis, if possible) in the pharmacy and CPOE systems.
2. Limit the routes of administration and the frequency of dosing available in pharmacy and CPOE systems to only those that are acceptable for each medication.
3. Produce easy-to-read pharmacy-applied labels for unit dose products. (See www.ismp.org/tools/guidelines/default.asp for ISMP guidelines.)

Bar Code Technology

The use of bar code technology in the pediatric setting presents a number of challenges. One of the greatest is the size of the bar code. Traditional linear bar codes are long and need to be relatively flat for scanning. With small patients, flattening the armband to scan the bar code can be difficult. Some bar codes can be switched from a horizontal to a vertical plane for better scanning; in other cases, a change to two-dimensional symbology, such as Data Matrix, may be required.[44]

Affixing a scannable label to syringes may also be an issue. With the small oral and parenteral syringes used to prepare patient-specific unit doses for pediatric patients, placing a bar code label along the barrel may obscure increment markings, but a label wrapped around the syringe is difficult to scan. Since neither of these is a good option, two-dimensional symbology or placing the label as a "flag" on the syringe, with the bar code printed only on the flat section, might be considered.

Nurses in pediatric units traditionally have prepared many medications at the bedside. The use of bar coding to reduce errors requires a robust unit dose dispensing system. Bar-code technology is most beneficial if all medications (e.g., injectable, topical, rectal, oral) can be scanned to be sure the medication reflects the prescriber's order and the "five rights" of drug administration. The initial design and budget for a bar coding system should ensure that adequate resources are available for pharmacy to prepare and affix bar code labels to all medications. Without this commitment, the result can be a mix of bar-coded and non-bar-coded medications, which leads to confusion and to work-arounds to avoid scanning medications that are difficult to scan. Inconsistent use of scanning encourages those administering medications to ignore alerts.

FDA regulations now require bar coding on even the smallest package units. This requirement has discouraged some manufacturers from producing unit dose packages of oral medications, which is particularly problematic for pediatric and neonatal patients. However, commercially available packages with linear bar codes indicating the National Drug Code number are of limited use in the pediatric population because so many medications must be repackaged in doses based on the individual patient's weight. Many participants in an ISMP survey expressed concern about the cost of implementing bar code technology, especially in small, rural hospitals and in pediatric hospitals where so many drugs are not available in unit dose packages.[45]

Patient-specific unit dose dispensing should be fully implemented for pediatric and neonatal patients. Pediatric facilities and services planning for bedside bar code technology should consider the feasibility of scanning identification bands on very small wrists or ankles and bar codes on very small syringes. Plans should include acceptable and safe alternatives.

Automated Dispensing Devices

Many hospitals use ADCs, but this technology has limited utility for pediatric and neonatal areas. The items generally stored in such devices are, for pediatric medications, effectively bulk containers. For example, a 5 mL unit dose cup may contain enough medication for several pediatric doses and require the nurse to calculate the dose, obtain a double check, and draw up the patient-specific dose, a process that is time consuming and error prone. Although standardized doses may be useful for children weighing over 10 kg, doses for smaller patients must be customized.

Availability of medications in ADCs is convenient for nurses and pharmacists, but it is not safer for patients. If these devices are used, the items and quantities should be tailored to the individual pediatric or neonatal unit. Smaller package sizes and limited par levels will reduce the risk of inadvertent overdosage.

Errors have been associated with the use of ADCs in pediatric or neonatal units. In one case, a nurse obtained aminophylline 25 mg/mL from the device and prepared a dose of 11 mL instead of 11 mg for a 2.34 kg neonate. This case also illustrates the dangers of nurses preparing IV solutions without a double check. In another hospital, bulk bottles of midazolam syrup were stocked in the dispensing device. After several calculation errors led to overdosages, the screens on the device were redesigned to provide dose warnings, and dose conversion charts were posted to eliminate the need for calculations. However, an additional overdose occurred when a nurse confused the dose in milligrams with the volume to be administered.

Safety recommendations in regard to the use of ADCs can be summarized as follows:

1. Avoid stocking high-alert medications in ADCs if possible.
2. Stock only pediatric concentrations of oral liquids and injectable medications in pediatric and neonatal ADCs.
3. Limit the variety and quantity of medications in ADCs.
4. Require an independent double check before administration of a high-alert medication removed from an ADC.

ADDITIONAL RESOURCES

Several national organizations have published guidelines for safe medication use in children.

❑ The American Academy of Pediatrics (AAP) has a policy statement titled Prevention of Medication Errors in the Pediatric Inpatient Setting (available at www.pediatrics.org).

❑ The Pediatric Pharmacy Advocacy Group, in collaboration with the Institute for Safe Medication Practices, published Guidelines for Preventing Medication Errors in Pediatrics (www.ppag.org/images/pdf/Guidelines_Peds.pdf).

❑ AAP has guidelines for the administration of medication in schools (http://aappolicy.aap publications.org/cgi/reprint/pediatrics;112/3/697.pdf).

❑ Another resource on medication use in schools (www.fshp.org/Meds_Use_in_School/ MED%20book.qxd.pdf), created by the Florida Society of Health-System Pharmacists, includes sample forms and drug monographs.

❑ The United States Pharmacopeia (USP) has developed Error-Avoidance Recommendations for Medications Used in the Pediatric Population (www.usp.org/patientSafety/resources/ pedRecommnds2003-01-22.html). These recommendations, based on error reports, were reviewed by USP's Pediatric Expert Committee and Safe Medication Use Expert Committee. They can be applied and adapted in various health care settings.

❑ A fact sheet for parents from the Agency for Healthcare Research and Quality, titled 20 Tips to Help Prevent Medical Errors in Children, is available at www.ahrq.gov/consumer/ 20tipkid.pdf.

REFERENCES

1. Levine S. The forgotten patients: establishing pharmacist competency in pediatric therapeutics. *Hosp Pharm.* 2002;37:800–3.
2. Levine S, Cohen MR, Blanchard NR, et al. Guidelines for preventing medication errors in pediatrics. *J Pediatr Pharmacol Ther.* 2001;6:426–42.
3. Gupta A, Waldhauser LK. Adverse drug reactions from birth to early childhood. *Pediatr Clin North Am.* 1997;44:79–92.
4. Kaushal R, Bates DW, Landrigan C, et al. Medication errors and adverse drug events in pediatric inpatients. *JAMA.* 2001;285:2114–20.
5. Fortescue E, Kaushal R, Landrigan CP, et al. Prioritizing strategies for preventing medication errors and adverse drug events in pediatric inpatients. *Pediatrics.* 2003; 111(4 Pt 1):722–9.
6. Institute for Safe Medication Practices. Hospital survey shows much more needs to be done to protect pediatric patients from medication errors. *ISMP Medication Safety Alert!* April 19, 2000;5(8).

7. Nahata MC. Paediatric drug therapy II—drug administration errors. *J Clin Pharm Ther*. 1988;13:399–402.
8. Rosati JR Jr, Nahata MC. Drug administration errors in pediatric patients. *QRB Qual Rev Bull*. 1983;9:212–3.
9. Leff RD, Roberts RJ. Problems in drug therapy in pediatric patients. *Am J Hosp Pharm*. 1987;44:865–70.
10. American Academy of Pediatrics. Guidelines for the ethical conduct of studies to evaluate drugs in pediatric populations. *Pediatrics*. 1995;95:286–94.
11. Hampton T. Pediatric drug studies required by law. *JAMA*. 2004;291:412–3.
12. American Academy of Pediatrics, Committee on Drugs. Guidelines for monitoring and management of pediatric patients during and after sedation for diagnostic and therapeutic procedures. *Pediatrics*. 1992;89:1110–5.
13. American Academy of Pediatrics, Committee on Drugs. Guidelines for monitoring and management of pediatric patients during and after sedation for diagnostic and therapeutic procedures: Addendum. *Pediatrics*. 2002;110:836–8.
14. Institute for Safe Medication Practices. Stop patient harm from chloral hydrate sedation at home. *ISMP Medication Safety Alert!* May 15, 2003;8(10).
15. Potts MS, Phelan KW. Deficiencies in calculations and applied mathematics skills in pediatrics among primary care interns. *Arch Pediatr Adolesc Med*. 1996;150:748–52.
16. Koren G, Barzilay Z, Modan M. Errors in computing drug doses. *Can Med Assoc J*. 1983;129:721–3.
17. Koren G, Barzilay Z, Greenwald M. Tenfold errors in administration of drug doses: a neglected iatrogenic disease in pediatrics. *Pediatrics*. 1986;77:848–9
18. Perlstein PH, Callison C, White M, et al. Errors in drug computations during newborn intensive care. *Am J Dis Child*. 1979;133:376–9.
19. Institute for Safe Medication Practices. Safety briefs. *ISMP Medication Safety Alert!* February 26, 1997;2:1.
20. Clater RW. Pediatric dosing: tips for tots. *Am Pharm*. 1993;NS33(5):55–6.
21. Shirkey HC. Therapeutic orphans [editorial]. *J Pediatr*. 1968;72:119–20.
22. Simon HK. Caregiver knowledge and delivery of a commonly prescribed medication (albuterol) for children. *Arch Pediatr Adolesc Med*. 1999;153(6):615–8.
23. Simon HK, Weinkle DA. Over-the-counter medications. Do parents give what they intend to give? *Arch Pediatr Adolesc Med*. 1997;151(7):654–6.
24. Grissinger M. "Rule of 6" not optimal for patient safety. *P&T*. 2003;28(4):234.
25. Gaffoor M, Vaidya V. Rule of six versus standard drips: the ongoing debate. American Academy of Pediatrics Section on Critical Care newsletter. May 2004:6–7. Available at: http://pedsccm.wustl.edu/ORGMEET/AAP/SOCCMay04.pdf.
26. Joint Commission on Accreditation of Healthcare Organizations. 2006 National Patient Safety Goals FAQs. Available at: www.jointcommission.org/PatientSafety/NationalPatientSafetyGoals/. Accessed June 23, 2006.
27. Gaffoor MI, Hilmas E, Mathews L, et al. National Online Survey of Rule of Six versus Standardized Concentrations. Oral presentation at 2004 Pediatric Critical Care Colloquium. Abstract available at: www.icudrips.org/PCCMsurveyresults.pdf.
28. Vaidya VU, Gaffoor MI, Hilmas E, et al. A Computerized Program for Changing from Rule of Six to Standardized Drips. Poster presentation at 2004 Pediatric Critical Care Colloquium. Available at: www.icudrips.org/PCCMconcopt.pdf.
29. Wallace JR, Payne RW, Mack AJ. Inadvertent IV infusion of milk. *Lancet*. 1972;1(7763):1264–6.
30. Ryan CA, Mohammed I, Murphy B. Normal neurological and developmental outcome after an accidental IV infusion of expressed breast milk in a neonate. *Pediatrics*. 2006;117:236–8.
31. Page L. Diligence, technology prevent IV and feeding tube mix-ups: finding the wrong fit. *Mater Manag Health Care*. 2006;15(4):24–8.
32. Copeland D, Appel J. Implementation of an enteral nutrition and medication administration system utilizing oral syringes in the NICU. *Neonatal Netw*. 2006;25(1):21–4.
33. Institute for Safe Medication Practices. Preventing accidental IV infusion of breast milk in neonates. *ISMP Medication Safety Alert!* June 15, 2006;11:1–2.
34. Kozer E, Seto W, Verjee Z, et al. Prospective observational study on the incidence of medication errors during simulated resuscitation in a paediatric emergency department. *BMJ*. 2004;329:1321.
35. Shah AN, Frush K, Luo X, et al. Effect of an intervention standardization system on pediatric dosing and equipment size determination: a crossover trial involving simulated resuscitation events. *Arch Pediatr Adolesc Med*. 2003;157:229–36.
36. Hohenhaus SM, Frush KS. Pediatric patient safety: common problems in the use of resuscitative aids for simplifying pediatric emergency care. *J Emerg Nurs*. 2004;30(1):49–51.
37. Hohenhaus SM. Assessing competency: the Broselow-Luten resuscitation tape. *J Emerg Nurs*. 2002;28(1):70–2.
38. Levine SR, Holbrook K, O'Connor-Pepe B, et al. Medication safety in the pediatric emergency department. *Hosp Pharm*. 2003;38:426–35, 510.

39. U.S. Pharmacopeia. USP identifies leading medication errors in hospital emergency departments [press release]. March 12, 2003. Available at: www.onlinepressroom.net/uspharm/. Accessed August 29, 2005.

40. Levine SR. Medication safety in the pediatric OR. *Hosp Pharm.* 2002;37:1279–81.

41. Leape L, Bates DW, Cullen J, et al. Systems analysis of adverse drug events. *JAMA.* 1995;274:35–43.

42. Bates DW, Leape LL, Cullen DJ, et al. Effect of computerized physician order entry and a team intervention on prevention of serious medication errors. *JAMA.* 1998;280:1311–6.

43. Horns KM, Gills MB. Neonatal nurse knowledge of penicillin therapy. *The NANN Pages: National Association of Neonatal Nurses.* October 1998.

44. Neuenschwander M, Cohen M, Vaida AJ, et al. Practical guide to bar coding for patient medication safety. *Am J Health Syst Pharm.* 2003;60:768–79.

45. Institute for Safe Medication Practices. ISMP survey shows drug companies providing fewer unit dose packaged medications. *ISMP Medication Safety Alert!* March 6, 2002;7(5).

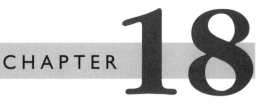

CHAPTER

PREVENTING MEDICATION ERRORS WITH IMMUNOLOGIC DRUGS

John D. Grabenstein and Michael R. Cohen

Vaccines, antibodies, and other immunologic drugs are just as likely as other drugs to be involved in medication errors. In the framework of system-based causes (Chapter 4), this chapter discusses errors with immunologic products and describes some unique consequences of errors with these medications. As shown in the examples provided, a single error can involve the failure of multiple features of the drug delivery system.

DRUG LABELING, PACKAGING, AND NOMENCLATURE

Look-Alike or Confusing Labeling and Packaging

On several occasions, pediatric-strength diphtheria–tetanus toxoids (DT) has been confused with adult-strength tetanus–diphtheria toxoids (Td). Td contains a lower dose of diphtheria toxoid than does DT; this lower dose is given to adults to avoid reactions at the injection site. The lowercase "d" and uppercase "D" are intended to reflect the relative doses, which are inversely proportional to age. Mix-ups have occurred because the product names are similar and the package labels do not clearly distinguish the two, especially when both products are supplied by the same manufacturer (Figure 18-1). Another example was the package of pediatric diphtheria and tetanus toxoids adsorbed purogenated vaccine, formerly manufactured by Lederle (Wyeth-Ayerst); the notation "For Pediatric Use" was not prominently placed (Figure 18-2). The drug name and the term "Purogenated" appeared in large, bold print, but "For Pediatric Use" was in smaller, lighter print, located between the larger drug name and "Purogenated." (In the package insert, however, "For Pediatric Use" appeared in large, bold letters.)

Mix-ups can also be expected with the new adult and adolescent vaccine products that add low-dose acellular pertussis vaccine to Td. The preferred abbreviation for this product name is Tdap, which can easily be misread as DtaP, an abbreviation for the diphtheria–tetanus–acellular pertussis vaccine formulation routinely given to infants and young children. Furthermore, practitioners often pronounce Tdap as "tee-dap," which can be hard to distinguish from the "dee-tap" pronunciation of DTaP.

Health care providers' lack of knowledge about the different vaccine forms can contribute to errors. The consequences may be a painful arm for the adult given a DT or DTaP injection, or inadequate protection for the child given Td or Tdap.[1] Health care workers may also be unaware that two forms of monovalent tetanus toxoid are available: fluid and adsorbed.[2]

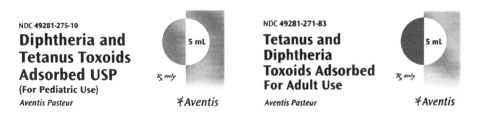

FIGURE 18-1 (also in color section following page 120) The package labels make adult and pediatric vaccines difficult to differentiate.

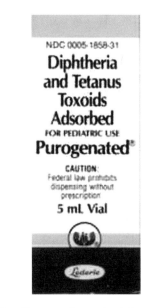

FIGURE 18-2 Is "Purogenated" really more important than "For Pediatric Use"?

Because the official names of combination vaccines are so long, it may be helpful to use proprietary names to reduce confusion. Brand names for DTaP in the United States are Daptacel, Infanrix, and Tripedia. Brand names for Tdap are Adacel and Boostrix. Errors can occur even when brand names are used, however. For example, Infanrix (DTaP) was used when Pediarix (pentavalent DtaP–hepatitis B–poliovirus vaccine) was desired. Contributing to this mix-up was a nurse's inadequate knowledge about a newly licensed vaccine combination. Health care providers need ongoing education about new vaccine products and changes in recommended immunization schedules.

Other errors have occurred because vaccine distributors shipped the wrong product. In one case, a hospital had ordered a supply of influenza virus vaccine USP trivalent types A and B (zonal purified, subvirion) for administration to children under 13 years of age. When the vaccine arrived, the invoice matched the request for the subvirion product. However, the distributor had accidentally shipped both zonal purified, whole virion (intended for patients 13 years and older) and zonal purified, subvirion (intended for patients 6 months and older). The two products' labeling and packaging were quite similar. The pharmacy staff did not notice the shipping error and inadvertently dispensed a combination of whole virion and subvirion products to the flu clinic, which served children under 13 years of age. At least two children received the whole virion product and developed flu-like symptoms, including fever over 101°F. Later, nurses administering the vaccine noticed the error.

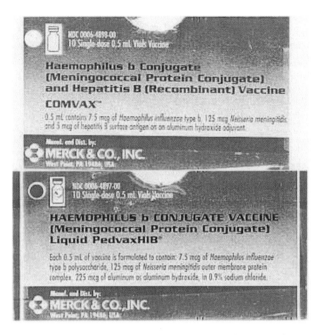

FIGURE 18-3 (also in color section following page 120) PedvaxHIB (Haemophilus b conjugate vaccine) and Comvax (Haemophilus b conjugate and hepatitis B recombinant vaccine) packages.

Mix-ups have also occurred because of the strikingly similar labeling and packaging of Merck's PedvaxHIB (Haemophilus b conjugate vaccine) and Comvax (Haemophilus b conjugate and hepatitis B recombinant vaccine). Both packages are the same size and shape and have a striped and shaded turquoise background with the drug name printed in black and label information in white (Figure 18-3). Both product names have "Haemophilus b conjugate" on the first line and "meningococcal protein conjugate" on the second line. The third line of product information, which distinguishes one product from the other, is not prominent or eye-catching. The vial tops are different colors (blue for PedvaxHIB and clear for Comvax), but this difference is not helpful, especially while the vials remain in the carton. The look-alike packaging of these two products has led to administration of the wrong vaccine to dozens of children. The complexity of Haemophilus b (Hib) vaccine products and schedules also presents opportunities for error. Four inequivalent vaccines are available, with different administration schedules.

It is helpful to place auxiliary warning stickers on vaccine products as they enter the drug inventory. Alerts can be built into hospital and community pharmacy computer systems to warn pharmacists about the potential for mix-ups. Institutions may choose to color code the labels and vial caps to prevent confusion among the products, but errors may still occur.

Errors have occurred in many clinics and hospitals when nurses injected tetanus toxoid or Td intradermally because they mistook the vials for purified protein derivative (PPD, tuberculin for skin testing). The resulting indurations ranged from 30 mm to 60 mm in diameter. For some of the patients, isoniazid was prescribed to treat nonexistent tuberculosis. When the diagnosis was questioned and tuberculin tests were reapplied, the results were negative. Inquiry revealed that Td and PPD had been stored on the same refrigerator shelf and that the packages, both from the same manufacturer, looked quite similar.[3,4] The package design may distract practitioners from careful reading of the labels. The number 5 appears in a circle on the front label panel of all the products in Figure 18-4. On the PPD labels, the 5 indicates 5 TU (tuberculin units); on the vaccine labels, it indicates 5 mL.

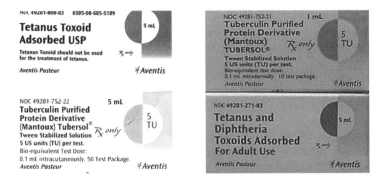

FIGURE 18-4 (also in color section following page 120)   All of these products are stored in the refrigerator and may be located side by side. Limited availability of Td in single-dose syringes forces providers to purchase multidose vials, further contributing to the problem.

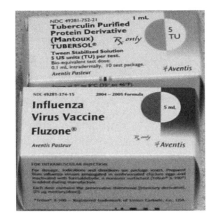

FIGURE 18-5   A manufacturer's similar packages of influenza virus vaccine and tuberculin purified protein derivative.

Similar mix-ups have been reported with PPD and influenza vaccine packages from the same manufacturer (Figure 18-5).[5] In one case, a nurse injected Tubersol (PPD) 0.5 mL into a patient's deltoid muscle instead of Fluzone. The error was discovered when, during documentation of the lot number and expiration date, it became apparent that the numbers were inconsistent with previous documentation for Fluzone injection. The nurse stated that similar packaging of the products contributed to the error. In another case, a hospital employee was given PPD by intramuscular injection instead of the influenza vaccine. Again, look-alike packaging played a role in the error.

The risk of confusing Td and PPD, or PPD and flu vaccine, can be reduced by purchasing these products from different manufacturers. When possible, only one vaccine should be stocked on patient care units, with other vaccines dispensed from pharmacy as needed. Where multiple vaccines are needed (e.g., in the emergency department), stickers can be affixed to the outer carton to help avoid mix-ups. When vaccine names appear on computer screens for prescribing or product selection, the entries should be separated to ensure that they do not appear sequential, and the full vaccine name, not just the abbreviation, should be listed.

TABLE 18-1   Sound-Alike and Look-Alike Names of Vaccines and Other Products

---

Acel-Imune, Acelluvax, Actacel,[a] Actimmune[b]
ActHIB, ActHIB–DTP
Alferon N, Alkeran, Imferon, interferon[b]
Candin, Cantil,[b] Vantin[b]
Combivax,[c,d] Recombivax HB
Engerix-B, Infanrix, Twinrix
Flu-Imune,[d] Pnu-Imune 23[d]
Imogam, Imovax, Imovax Rabies
Ipol, Opol, Optipol, Pediopol, Poliovax[b]
Leukeran, Leukine, Prokine, Proleukin[b]
Neupogen, Pnu-Imune[b]
Pentacel,[e] Pentasure[e]
Tetracel,[e] Tetramune
Tine Test, T.R.U.E. Test[b]
Tri-Immunol, Tripedia
Varicella immune globulin, varicella-zoster immune globulin
Varivax, VZIG

---

[a] Canadian.
[b] Product is vastly different from the others listed.
[c] Belgian.
[d] Formerly marketed.
[e] Trademarked but not yet licensed by the Food and Drug Administration.

Look-Alike and Sound-Alike Names

Many of the common names used to refer to vaccines look or sound alike: varicella and vaccinia, hepatitis A and hepatitis B, *Haemophilus influenzae* and viral influenza,[6] and Hib and hepatitis B. In addition, many vaccine products have look-alike and sound-alike proprietary names; examples are listed in Table 18-1. These names can be confused when spoken, as well as when written.

Confusion about names can result in the administration of a vaccine to someone who is already immune. Usually this is harmless, but adverse effects can occur at the injection site in immune persons given certain vaccines, such as those for tetanus and pneumococcus.[2,7]

Comvax, a combination vaccine against Hib and hepatitis B virus, should never be referred to as "H and H" vaccine, because that nickname could also apply to GlaxoSmith-Kline's Twinrix hepatitis A–hepatitis B vaccine. Similarly, Twinrix should never be called the "A and B" vaccine, because it could then be confused with the influenza vaccine whose label reads "Influenza Virus Vaccine, Trivalent, Types A and B."

Similar names of a series of hyperimmune globulins have presented a risk for error. These were formerly distributed by Bayer Corporation and called BayHep B, BayRab, BayRho-D, and BayTet.[2,8] In 2005 the product line was divested to Talecris Biotherapeutics, which returned to the earlier proprietary names, with an S/D suffix added to reflect solvent-detergent virucidal processing steps during manufacturing: HyperHep B S/D, HyperRab S/D, HyperRho S/D, and HyperTet S/D.

For patients of certain ages, Tripedia diphtheria–tetanus–acellular pertussis vaccine can be used as the diluent for the powdered ActHIB brand of Hib vaccine. The combination of Tripedia and ActHIB, marketed under the trade name TriHIBit, can be confused with ProHIBiT, a different brand of Hib vaccine that does not involve the combination of Tripedia and ActHIB.

Health care workers have confused the vaccine against measles with that against "German measles" (rubella). Adding to the confusion is the use of "rubeola" as a synonym for measles, a practice that should be discouraged.

DON'T CONFUSE VARICELLA VIRUS VACCINE WITH VARICELLA-ZOSTER IMMUNE GLOBULIN

To prevent or attenuate illness from chickenpox, varicella-zoster immune globulin (VZIG) should be given intramuscularly, within 4 days of significant exposure, to susceptible pregnant women or others at elevated risk for severe disease or complications. However, some pregnant women have accidentally received varicella virus vaccine (Varivax). The labeling of this live, attenuated virus product notes that use is contraindicated in pregnancy and that pregnancy should be avoided for 3 months after vaccination. According to the Centers for Disease Control and Prevention (CDC), the risk of congenital abnormality from infection with wild varicella-zoster virus is about 2% during weeks 13 to 20 of pregnancy. Despite warnings from CDC and the Institute for Safe Medication Practices (ISMP), this mix-up continues to occur.

CDC and Merck, the vaccine's manufacturer, established the Varivax Pregnancy Registry to monitor cases of immunization just before or during pregnancy. Of 600 reports in the registry, 22 involved erroneous administration of the vaccine to women who should have received VZIG.[10] Follow-up was possible in 17 of these cases. Two pregnancies ended in a first-trimester spontaneous abortion and one involved a male infant with unilateral renal dysplasia. In at least nine cases (in four emergency departments, two pediatricians' offices, and two obstetricians' offices), VZIG was properly prescribed but Varivax was given. The Food and Drug Administration (FDA) is aware of a case where a patient erroneously received Varivax when varicella antibody testing was ordered.

Regulators, manufacturers, and others concerned with medication safety need to continually educate clinicians about this problem. The primary indication for VZIG in pregnant women is to prevent complications of varicella in the mother, rather than to protect the infant. Administration of VZIG to susceptible pregnant women has not been found to prevent viremia, fetal infection, congenital varicella syndrome, or neonatal varicella.

Practitioners should read the package insert for appropriate indications for use. However, stronger warnings are needed in the product labeling to draw attention to the problem. ISMP is suggesting to FDA that an alert be placed on the package label, with reference to the package insert for details. Pending that change, practitioners should affix their own warning labels to the product. Furthermore, computer screens should warn practitioners about error potential, and varicella products should be stored separately in the pharmacy and patient care units (e.g., the emergency department). Obtaining a careful pregnancy history on all women of childbearing age for whom these products are ordered can also avert problems. Information about the Varivax Pregnancy Registry is available at www.cdc.gov/mmwr/preview/mmwrhtml/00040693.htm.

Similarly, varicella vaccine has been confused with varicella-zoster immune globulin (VZIG). At least 22 pregnant women have received varicella vaccine in error (sidebar, above).[9,10] Infection with wild varicella-zoster virus during the first half of pregnancy can result in congenital varicella syndrome, characterized by limb atrophy, extremity skin scarring, eye involvement, and brain damage. In one reported case, twin infants died after the mother received VZIG intravenously.[11] Such errors are more likely when a product is first introduced.

Mumps skin test antigen (MSTA, formerly available from Aventis Pasteur) and mumps vaccine (Mumpsvax, Merck) have been confused repeatedly. System failures related to nomenclature and distribution contribute to this error.[12] Such errors can also result from rapid staff turnover and lack of training.

Confusing Suffixes

Dispensing errors can occur because of confusing suffixes. In one case, a supply system inadvertently sent Imovax Rabies I.D. Vaccine (a pre-exposure rabies vaccine formulation) instead of Imovax Rabies Vaccine (a pre-exposure and post-exposure vaccine). The error was caught after the patient had received Imovax Rabies I.D. for two of the five doses. The patient suffered no ill effects. In another example, early proprietary names for some monoclonal antibodies varied only in their suffixes, even though the products had drastically different uses.[2]

Traditionally, the brand-name suffixes *-mune* and *-gam* have referred only to vaccines and hyperimmune antibodies, respectively, manufactured by Lederle Laboratories, a division of Wyeth. Two product names may cause confusion, however: Viramune is the Roxane Laboratories brand of nevirapine, a reverse transcriptase inhibitor used for the treatment of human immunodeficiency virus (HIV) infection; and Zagam is the Sanofi Aventis brand of sparfloxacin, a quinolone antimicrobial.

In 2004, the California Department of Health Services began distributing botulinum immune globulin with the proprietary name BabyBIG. The product is approved for treatment of infant botulism caused by type A or B *Clostridium botulinum,* and the trademark identifies the target population. This product has limited distribution because of the rarity of botulism cases and the scarcity of supply. However, because of the BIG in the name, this product could be confused with the much more familiar hepatitis B immune globulin, often referred to as HBIG. BabyBIG should be prescribed by its generic name, and the patient's diagnosis should be provided in communication about the product with nurses and dispensing pharmacists.

Expiration Dates

The Food and Drug Administration (FDA) has issued no requirements or guidance on the presentation or placement of expiration dates on packages. Manufacturers may use small fonts and confusing formats. For example, the poliovirus vaccine inactivated (IPOL) manufactured by Aventis Pasteur lists the expiration date as day/month/year. U.S. citizens, accustomed to a month/day/year format, could be confused by an expiration date of 06 MAR 04 and misinterpret it as March 4, 2006, instead of March 6, 2004. FDA should mandate the use of one uniform sequence for expiration dates.

UNCLEAR COMMUNICATION

Although abbreviations are a well-known source of medication errors,[13–16] many vaccines are commonly identified by abbreviations. For example, "DTP" is commonly understood to refer to diphtheria–tetanus–pertussis vaccine, but in some practice sites it is used as shorthand for a sedative cocktail of Demerol, Thorazine, and Phenergan. Several children for whom the sedative mixture was prescribed have been vaccinated instead. "MR" is another ambiguous abbreviation. To some, it means measles–rubella vaccine (as in Merck's M-R-VAX II); to others, it means mumps–rubella vaccine (as in Merck's Biavax II). Prescribers must make their intentions clear. The sidebar starting on page 500 discusses the Centers for Disease Control and Prevention (CDC) list of standard abbreviations, reports clinicians' experiences with vaccine abbreviations, and offers recommendations.

Orders can be unclear because of poor handwriting. As discussed in other chapters, a handwritten "U" for units can be mistaken for a zero (0) or four (4). Because decimal points may not be written or seen clearly, trailing zeroes should not be used after a decimal point, but a zero should always precede a decimal point for amounts less than 1. Both an abbreviation and unclear handwriting made an order for "TB × 1" ambiguous. The physician intended the patient to receive a tuberculin skin test. A pharmacist had the order rewritten to avoid potential administration of "Td × 1," a single dose of tetanus–diphtheria toxoids.

VACCINE ABBREVIATIONS CAN BE MISUNDERSTOOD

The Institute for Safe Medication Practices (ISMP) strongly discourages the use of abbreviations for drug names. However, to prevent misinterpretation of the ad hoc (coined) vaccine abbreviations that are used in patient records, the Centers for Disease Control and Prevention (CDC) recommends the adoption and use of uniform, standard abbreviations for vaccine names.

CDC believes this will promote accuracy, consistency, and convenience and will prevent errors and ambiguity in vaccine labeling, medical practice, record keeping, written communications, and scientific publications. In addition, the peel-off stickers supplied with vaccines for documenting lot numbers in the patient record are too small to contain the full names of some vaccines and the full names of manufacturers or distributors; standard abbreviations would be helpful for this purpose.

This rationale for abbreviation use may appear sound at first glance, but the CDC list (www.cdc.gov/nip/visi/prototypes/vaxabbrev.htm) contains more than 300 vaccines, each with a main root abbreviation for the type of vaccine, and many with optional specifiers for distinguishing among vaccines used for the same disease. Table 18-2 gives examples. The more complex specifiers are intended for use in scientific publications; simpler specifiers, if any, are proposed for use in medical records. Even without the optional specifiers, about 150 vaccine types appear on the list. Errors due to the similarity of abbreviations, failure to recall the correct abbreviation, or misinterpretation for other reasons are certainly possible.

Many clinicians use just a handful of the more common vaccines on the CDC list, but abbreviations can still cause confusion. The USP–ISMP Medication Errors Reporting program and USP's MEDMARX database contain many instances of this. A few examples are mix-ups between Hib and HBV, Hib and HBV_{ig}, HBV_{ig} and HBV, DTP and DT, and DT and Td. Uses of ad hoc abbreviations, such as "H flu" for *Haemophilus influenzae* type b (misinterpreted as influenza vaccine), have also led to errors.

In France and French-speaking parts of Canada, DTP refers to *vaccin diphtérique-tétanique-poliomyélitique*, or diphtheria–tetanus–poliomyelitis vaccine; and diphtheria–tetanus–pertussis vaccine is abbreviated DCT (*diphtérique-coquelucheux-tétanique*). In German-speaking countries, "typhus vaccine" refers to a vaccine against *Salmonella typhi*, the cause of typhoid fever, not to one against *Rickettsia prowazekii*, the cause of epidemic typhus.

ISMP surveyed health care providers in 2003 about errors related to vaccine abbreviations. Of nearly 100 clinicians participating, 42% said they had experienced errors stemming from vaccine abbreviations in handwritten orders in the past 2 years. One in three had encountered errors associated with abbreviations used on immunization records, and one in four reported that abbreviations on vaccine protocols or schedules had contributed to errors. Only 17% of respondents were aware of errors that resulted from vaccine abbreviations used on pharmacy or manufacturer product labels.

Nearly two-thirds (63%) of the respondents believed standard abbreviations should be used for vaccines, but only 55% of all respondents believed this would reduce the risk of errors. Participants were split on whether CDC's uniform abbreviations should fall into two categories: one for clinical settings and the other for scientific publications. However, most agreed that the vaccine's full generic name (and brand name, if needed) should be listed on immunization schedules (91%), computer screens (85%), preprinted orders and protocols (85%), and immunization forms (81%). Those who opposed this suggestion thought space is too limited, especially on immunization forms. Responses were mixed on whether standard abbreviations should be used on peel-off stickers and for combination vaccine products.

It remains to be seen whether uniform abbreviations will help reduce errors. As noted by several vaccine experts responding to the survey, the CDC list is cumbersome because it includes vaccines in the early phases of research (e.g., Hanta vaccine) and products used more commonly in the past (e.g., oral polio vaccine, which is no longer distributed in the United States; typhus vaccine, for which U.S. distribution stopped in the 1970s). A shorter list with the most commonly used vaccines would be more helpful.

The survey suggests that vaccine abbreviations in handwritten orders pose the greatest risk. Clinicians should consider the use of preprinted order forms for the most common vaccines

TABLE 18-2 Selected Vaccine Abbreviations from CDC

Abbreviation	Full Vaccine Name
TOX	Toxoplasmosis (*Toxoplasma gondii*) vaccine
TET$_{ig}$	Tetanus immune globulin
Td	Tetanus toxoid, and diphtheria toxoid (reduced antigen quantity for adults) vaccine, for adult use
DT	Diphtheria toxoid, and tetanus toxoid, adsorbed, for pediatric use
DTP	Diphtheria toxoid, tetanus toxoid, and pertussis (antigens unspecified) vaccine
DTP$_a$	Diphtheria toxoid, tetanus toxoid, and acellular pertussis vaccine, for pediatric use
D$_r$TP$_{ar}$	Diphtheria toxoid (reduced antigen quantity for adults), tetanus toxoid, and acellular pertussis (reduced antigen quantity for adults) vaccine, for adult use
DTP-HIB	Diphtheria toxoid, tetanus toxoid, pertussis (antigens unspecified), and *Haemophilus influenzae* type b conjugate vaccine
HBV	Hepatitis B vaccine
HBV$_{ig}$	Hepatitis B immune globulin
INF	Influenza vaccine, not otherwise specified
INF$_s$	Influenza virus vaccine, split virion
IPV or POL$_{IPV}$	Poliovirus inactivated (injectable) vaccine
PNU	Pneumococcal (*Streptococcus pneumoniae*) vaccine, not otherwise specified
PNU$_{cn}$	Pneumococcal (*Streptococcus pneumoniae*) conjugate vaccine, not otherwise specified

in their facilities. Each vaccine's full generic name (and brand name, if needed) should be listed on these forms and on computer screens. Immunization forms could be redesigned to leave enough space for full vaccine names. Facilities could also create their own vaccine schedules if published tables and protocols do not include the full names.

Facilities that permit the use of vaccine abbreviations should follow the CDC recommendations. To reinforce the correct use of abbreviations, both the full generic name and the uniform abbreviation should be listed in all electronic and preprinted media. If wallet-sized immunization cards are given to patients, the CDC abbreviations should be used on these so that all health care providers can understand them. Patients can also be given a larger copy of the immunization record with the full vaccine names.

Spoken orders for vaccines should be discouraged because of the many sound-alike vaccine names. An 8-week-old infant was given Recombivax HB (hepatitis B vaccine, recombinant) instead of Comvax (Haemophilus b conjugate vaccine with hepatitis B vaccine) after a nurse misheard the spoken order. If spoken orders must be used, they should always be read back to the prescriber for clarification. Numbers in the teens should be repeated by pronouncing each digit; for example, 16 should be repeated as "one-six" to avoid confusion with the number 60. Another confirmation method is that used by ship captains: One person says, "Set heading 1-2-3," and the other responds, "Heading set 1-2-3, aye."

LACK OF PATIENT INFORMATION

Nearly all children need immunization with the DTP vaccine. A few children who have had a serious adverse reaction to DTP vaccine should not receive the pertussis component but instead should be given pediatric-strength DT. It is possible that some children have received DTP rather than DT vaccine because the person giving the vaccine was uninformed about a prior adverse event. Failure to communicate such information can occur when pediatricians refer patients to local health departments for immunization, when charts are not marked adequately, when patients and parents are not queried about previous adverse events, and when clinicians do not make efforts to identify true adverse events after immunization.

Health care providers usually are meticulous about ensuring that young children are immunized according to the recommended schedule. However, providers may not be so diligent in obtaining information about adults' immunization status. The following sidebar gives recommendations for improving the rate of pneumococcal vaccine administration to elderly patients.

IMPROVE THE PNEUMOCOCCAL VACCINE ADMINISTRATION RATE

A common category of error is the omission of medications. When many people fail to receive a needed medication, such as pneumococcal vaccine, it is a systems problem. The health care system has not taken full advantage of all available opportunities, including hospitalization, to immunize adult patients. The result is that thousands of lives are needlessly lost each year.

The Centers for Medicare & Medicaid Services (CMS) asked hospitals to submit data by August 2004 on 10 quality measures, one of which is the percentage of pneumonia patients age 65 and older who were screened for pneumococcal vaccine status and, if indicated, were given the vaccine prior to discharge. This is a National Quality Forum-endorsed standard for hospital care, as well as one of the core measures used for reporting in the Joint Commission on Accreditation of Healthcare Organizations National Voluntary Hospital Initiative. Although reporting this measure to CMS is voluntary, linkage to a financial incentive has led to widespread participation by hospitals. Since hospitals have begun tracking this measure, practitioners have reported difficulties with the immunization screening process as well as failure to give the vaccine after it has been prescribed.

Inefficient screening process. Most hospitals rely on nurses to screen patients upon admission. Typically, assessment protocols and checklists are used to determine whether the patient should be immunized. Patients who need the immunization can receive it under a standing order, without further physician approval. The most frequent problems with the screening process are confusion about whether to immunize patients who are unsure about prior immunization and whether to reimmunize patients who received the vaccine in the past. One hospital reported that nurses can forget to screen patients if the protocol or checklist is not part of the patient's admission documents or screens.

Omitted vaccine administration. Even when the screening process is satisfactory, practitioners have reported that prescribed immunizations are sometimes not administered. One hospital reported that, almost every day, single-dose vials of pneumococcal vaccine (dispensed for individual patients) are returned to the pharmacy unopened. The labeling of pneumococcal vaccine recommends deferring administration if the patient has any febrile respiratory illness or acute respiratory or other active infection, except when withholding the agent entails an even greater risk. Thus, nurses were giving the vaccine just before discharge. Another hospital reported that the vaccine was given on the day of discharge to avoid the possibility that a febrile reaction to the vaccine would increase the patient's length of stay.

Giving the vaccine on the day of discharge has several disadvantages. First, it is a hectic time for the patient and the nurse. Furthermore, the vaccine administration date and time cannot be scheduled on the medication administration record (MAR) when the patient's discharge date is unknown. Without an administration date, the vaccine can be overlooked, even if there is a notation to give it on the day of discharge. Also, the pharmacist will not know when to dispense the vaccine, so the nurse must call the pharmacy on the day of discharge. This can lead to multiple calls to the pharmacy and even multiple requests for the vaccine. The patient may be discharged before the medication arrives on the unit or may be kept waiting for the vaccine's arrival. Some hospitals provide the vaccine as unit-based stock so it is readily available on the day of discharge. One pharmacist pointed out, however, that omitted doses might not be easily noticed if the vaccine were available in unit-based stock.

Recommendations for preventing underuse or overuse of the pneumococcal vaccine:

❑ **Follow protocols.** Ensure a consistent screening and administration process through physician-approved protocols that do not require individual physician approval for each eligible patient. Be sure the protocol and associated forms are part of the patient's admission documents/screens.

❑ **Define candidates.** Include all patients 65 and older and those under 65 with risk factors (e.g., diabetes, chronic kidney or liver disease), not just patients with pneumonia, in the pneumococcal vaccine screening process. Seek the input of infectious diseases physicians in regard to possible contraindications to immunization. Ensure that the process is clear on whether to include patients who have been previously vaccinated or are poor historians.

❑ **Administer earlier.** To reduce the risk of omitting administration, consider giving the vaccine before the day of discharge. Hospitals have reported success with giving the vaccine on the day it is ordered as long as the patient is not critically ill. One hospital reported an increase in vaccine administration from 43% (vaccine given on day of discharge) to 92% (vaccine given on day 2 of hospitalization or upon transfer from a critical care unit). No adverse effects of giving the vaccine on day 2 were noted. However, one patient had been discharged before day 2 (the screening criteria included all patients over 65), and another patient was discharged directly from a critical care unit.

❑ **Use reminders.** If technology allows, print a daily report listing all vaccines scheduled for administration on that day and their status so that any deferred vaccines can be rescheduled. If the medical staff decides the vaccine must be given on the day of discharge, add a reminder on the discharge order sheets used by nurses and physicians.

❑ **Prevent unnecessary revaccination.** Provide patients with written information about the vaccine and a wallet-size card documenting the vaccination date. If the patient has been vaccinated, inform the patient's primary care provider (PCP). One hospital faxes a completed vaccination form to the PCP's office after the vaccine has been given (not when it is ordered) and keeps the original with the patient's MAR. If possible, ask information technology staff to maintain a running list of patients who have been vaccinated on a shared pharmacy/nursing/physician drive; this can be used if the patient is unsure, although it can eliminate unnecessary duplicate doses only within that health system.

PROBLEMS WITH PREPARATION, DOSING, AND ADMINISTRATION

Many reported errors with immunologic drugs involve product preparation and dose measurement. Although overdoses are most common, underdoses have also occurred.

Hepatitis B vaccine may be the immunologic agent most commonly associated with errors. The recommended dosage depends on the patient's age and health status and the brand of vaccine used. Two brands are available; even though the doses are different, both brands are equally safe and effective when administered according to the product labeling.[2] Over a 2-year period at one hospital, 1,400 newborns were given the wrong vaccine and left vulnerable to hepatitis B. They received an amount that was correct for one of the products but was only half the appropriate amount of the product that was used. One reason for the error was that when the hospital changed from one brand to the other, its preprinted order forms had not been updated. As a corrective measure, the pharmacy decided to dispense prefilled single-dose syringes. It also expanded its educational programs.[17] In another case, a warehouse released the dialysis form of Recombivax-HB (40 mcg/mL) rather than the standard concentration (10 mcg/mL) because the technician did not know the product was available in two concentrations.

The informal terminology used for different concentrations of PPD of tuberculin is another source of error. The terms *first*, *intermediate*, and *second strength* were used years ago to describe concentrations of 1, 5, and 250 tuberculin units (TU) per 0.1 mL, respectively. Errors stemming from these imprecise terms can be significant. Too high a dose can lead to severe cutaneous reactions. Tuberculin products should always be described by numerical concentration. Few pharmacies need to routinely stock 1 TU and 250 TU PPD. These concentrations can be specially procured when individual patients need them.

When health professionals misinterpreted the package inserts for two forms of lyophilized Hib vaccine powder, OmniHIB (no longer available) and ActHIB, patients did not receive the intended immunizations. According to a posting on an electronic bulletin board, the clinicians misconstrued the following statement in the 1998 *Physicians' Desk Reference*:[18]

> Haemophilus b Conjugate Vaccine (Tetanus Toxoid Conjugate)–OmniHIB (distributed by SmithKline Beecham Pharmaceuticals) is identical to Haemophilus b Conjugate Vaccine (Tetanus Toxoid Conjugate)–ActHIB....

The information was misinterpreted to mean that the complete packages were identical. In fact, OmniHIB powder was distributed with a saline diluent, whereas ActHIB powder was distributed with fluid DTP vaccine under the name "ActHIB/DTP." When these professionals administered OmniHIB, they thought they were protecting their patients against four diseases; in reality, they were giving only Hib vaccine. After this error was discovered, many children had to be given additional immunizations.

Including the name of the protein used to conjugate polysaccharide antigens (tetanus toxoid in the preceding example of Hib vaccine products; alternatively, a diphtheria or meningococcal protein[2]) introduces additional opportunity for error. These carrier proteins do not induce immunity to tetanus, diphtheria, or meningococcal disease; the presence of these words must not be considered an indicator of the protection conferred. Furthermore, the sheer length of the official name clutters drug packages and labels, making the key ingredients harder to identify.

Manufacturers of biotechnology products have used different systems for measuring potency at various developmental stages of these medications, leading to confusion and potential for error. For example, the current international standard of potency for interferon beta-1b (Betaseron) supersedes a standard developed by the National Institutes of Health (NIH) for native interferon beta. Doses of 1.6 million international units and 8 million international units in the international system are equivalent to 9 million international units and 45 million international units, respectively, in the NIH system. For aldesleukin (Proleukin), the labeling refers to international units but two other potency systems have been used: One Roche unit is approximately equivalent to 3 international units; one Cetus unit is approximately equivalent to 6 international units. Several potency systems are also in use for botulinum toxin.[19]

Possibly as a result of a pharmacy compounding error, two children with leukemia developed BCG (bacillus Calmette-Guérin)-associated meningitis.[12] Neither child had been given BCG as therapy, and neither had ever been vaccinated with BCG. One explanation is that BCG bacteria contaminated a container of methotrexate in the chemotherapy compounding area. When the methotrexate was administered intrathecally, the BCG may have been introduced across the blood–brain barrier. Extensive review of pharmacy techniques failed to identify any means by which contamination might have occurred, but genomic DNA from the vaccine strain matched BCG bacteria found in the patients' cerebrospinal fluid. In response, the hospital designated one compounding area solely for the preparation of BCG.

Allergen extracts and Hymenoptera venoms are initially administered to allergic patients at extremely low doses. Therapy then continues with progressively higher doses. If a patient is challenged with too high a dose too soon, the results can be fatal. Double-check systems are essential at each step in the compounding process to minimize transcription errors, inaccurate calculations or measurements, and transposition of vials or labels.[2,20,21] A uniform color-coding system, with different vial cap colors for designating dilutional strength, has been recommended (www.aaaai.org/members/allied_health/riskmanagement.stm).

STANDARDIZATION, STORAGE, AND DISTRIBUTION

Unsafe Storage and Handling

If adult-strength Td is prescribed but DTP is delivered, the error is in the drug distribution system. Was there no Td on hand? Were both products stored in the refrigerator but in the wrong locations? Did the person who took the DTP out of the proper bin in the refrigerator not understand the distinction between the products? A related case involved the administration of Hib vaccine that had been inadvertently stored in the location designated for measles–mumps–rubella vaccine. Changing the way in which vaccines are purchased and stored can prevent such errors.

In an error that was repeated dozens of times, health care workers selected the neuromuscular blocker pancuronium instead of influenza vaccine from the refrigerator. No harm was done to the patients, who were given 0.5 mL of pancuronium. Labels similar in color and vials similar in shape contributed to this error, which was an example of confirmation bias. The practitioners relied on familiar evidence (the color or shape of the vial) and ignored contrary evidence (the name on the container). Health care professionals can reduce errors of this type by repeating to themselves the name of the drug as they prepare to select it ("I need 0.5 mL of adult Td") and then reading the container label ("I see 0.5 mL of adult-strength Td in my hand").[7,22,23]

Several instances in which pancuronium or succinylcholine was used to reconstitute vaccine powders have been reported.[24,25] One way to prevent this is to ensure that neuromuscular blocking agents are not easily accessible. They should be stored in a location away from other medications. A clearly visible warning label (e.g., "Warning: Paralyzing Agent") can be affixed to the package.

Inadvertent administration of veterinary vaccines to humans has been reported. A teenager ingested live Newcastle disease vaccine intended for chickens. After induced catharsis, the patient remained asymptomatic and did not seroconvert. In another instance, a woman was exposed to infectious bursal disease vaccine intended for chickens. Her exposure consisted of skin contact and inhalation of aerosolized vaccine. Her symptoms were treated, and she recovered. Other cases have been reported; the common element in all of them was inappropriate handling of the vaccines in an agricultural setting.[26]

In Yemen, insulin was dispensed instead of BCG vaccine during a government-sponsored tuberculosis prevention campaign,[27] and 21 children died. Apparently, a medical worker sent insulin instead of vaccine to the site at which the vaccinations were administered. Quality assurance measures are an essential element of every step of mass vaccination programs, because a single error can affect many people.

Vaccine Shortages

When a vaccine—most notably, the influenza vaccine—is in short supply, health care providers try to use the existing supply sparingly. Criteria should be established for determining which patients have priority for immunization, and unnecessary waste of the product should be avoided. But policies for conserving product can backfire if not communicated clearly. In one case, 25 ROTC cadets were given a twofold overdose of the anthrax vaccine after providers were warned to use the drug sparingly. Those administering the vaccine had been told, "Draw up the exact amount of product to avoid any waste; for example, draw the vaccine up to the 1 mL mark and not any further." The volume of the correct dose was 0.5 mL, but the example was taken literally and 1 mL was given.

Formulary Control

Control over product selection can deter medication errors. For example, if fluid tetanus toxoid or 250 TU PPD is not kept in stock or is segregated from normal storage locations, errors can be averted. Prefilled syringes should be stocked only if the labels are distinctive. During mass immunization programs, syringes should be prefilled from vials only if each syringe is properly labeled.

ENVIRONMENTAL FACTORS

As with other medications, errors with vaccines can be related to environmental stresses. For example, two employees were to receive immunizations at an occupational health clinic. One was to be vaccinated against hepatitis B virus, and the other was to be immunized with Td, but both received hepatitis B vaccine. This error may have occurred because the clinic nurse was distracted by a telephone call or a visitor. Alternatively, it may have resulted from a lapse in attention, from stress, or from miscommunication.[28]

Because of personnel turnover or inadequate staffing, health care workers administering vaccines may lack experience in the proper technique. For example, learning proper technique for intradermal injection requires practice; thus, a medication intended for intradermal use may accidentally be injected subcutaneously.

ADMINISTRATION ROUTES AND TECHNIQUE

Errors with vaccines can occur because of confusion about or inexperience with the correct route of administration. A vaccine intended for intramuscular injection may be inadvertently administered by the subcutaneous route. Since a medication injected subcutaneously is absorbed more slowly than an equivalent volume injected intramuscularly, this may result in reduced antibody titers,[2] but revaccination is usually not warranted. Shallow subcutaneous injection may lead to larger injection-site reactions than would deeper injection into a muscle.

Hepatitis B vaccine can be effective intradermally at a lower dose than when administered IM.[29,30] However, CDC does not recommend the intradermal route because of concerns about improper technique.

BCG vaccine has caused serious injection-site reactions when given IM.[31] BCG vaccines are intended for administration by scarification (percutaneously with a multiple-puncture device) or intradermally; the vaccine for intradermal injection is not available in the United States.

In a case reported to the U.S. Pharmacopeia (USP) Drug Product Quality Review program, oral attenuated poliovirus vaccine was injected IM. No harm came to the patient, but the proper dose was delayed. In other cases, BCG vaccine intended for scarification has been injected intradermally.[32,33] Similar packaging and labeling may have contributed to these errors.

Until the 1980s, most antibody products were administered intramuscularly, but an increasing number are now given intravenously.[2] If a product intended for IM use is injected

IV, intravascular antigen–antibody complexes can result. This may have contributed to the deaths of twin newborn infants given varicella-zoster immune globulin IV rather than IM.

Vaccines have been adulterated when vials were contaminated or needles or syringes reused.[34–36] DTP and measles vaccine vials have been contaminated with streptococci and staphylococci. Hepatitis B virus or HIV could also be transmitted by contaminated vials or equipment; of particular concern is inadequate maintenance of jet injectors.

Meticulous technique must be used during mass immunizations against influenza and other diseases. Health-system vaccine practices should be closely regulated and inspected. In 1997, the medical director of Monroe, Connecticut, resigned after administering contaminated vaccines to 468 people. He used fresh needles when preparing doses of the vaccine from multiple-dose vials, but he did not always change syringes between patients. In the process, blood aspirated into a syringe during one patient's injection may have contaminated another patient's injection. The physician claimed to be unaware that the method he used was improper.

A CDC report described physicians in Washington, D.C., and Bucks County, Pennsylvania, who injected patients and drew up the next patient's dose with the same needle but changed the needle before injecting the next patient.[35] These examples provide evidence of inattention to appropriate infection control procedures and potential medication errors during vaccination programs.

RISK MANAGEMENT AND QUALITY PROCESSES

Reviewing reports of errors at other sites is useful in a health care organization's quality improvement and error prevention efforts. The Institute for Safe Medication Practices (ISMP), FDA, and USP publish accounts of errors in professional journals and newsletters. Research findings should also be evaluated for application in the practice setting. For example, a report on 221 cases of erroneous administration of childhood vaccines described the following deviations from the manufacturers' recommendations:[37] off schedule (27%), error in reconstitution (24%), outside the recommended age range (19%), inappropriate interval between doses (15%), wrong vaccine (13%), use beyond potency or expiration date (2%), and use despite contraindication (<1%). No adverse events related to erroneous administration were recognized. Such information is valuable in prioritizing safety efforts.

The importance of reporting errors cannot be overemphasized. Errors that remain undetected or unreported can affect hundreds of patients. Everyone involved in the medication-use process must acknowledge that even the most experienced health care professionals make errors.[38] Hospitals and other institutions need to create open, guilt-free systems in which preventing errors takes precedence over blaming and punishing employees for errors that have occurred. Employees must have an opportunity to communicate their error prevention ideas. Regular feedback to staff on reported errors is an essential part of risk management.

IMPLICATIONS FOR HEALTH CARE PRACTITIONERS

Inadequate immunization is one of the greatest risks to human health. Many illnesses can be prevented through widespread use of vaccines.[2,38] Vaccines are expected to perform minor miracles by conferring immunity for a year, a decade, or more. By the same token, the consequences of an error, such as vulnerability to a preventable infection, may also be felt for a long time.

Flynn and Barker note in Chapter 2 that the average hospitalized patient experiences at least one medication error per day. To prevent errors with immunologic agents, health professionals should participate in the selection of these products for use in their practice sites. The potential for mix-ups should be considered in the storage of these products. Up-to-date reference materials on each agent should be available, and staff should be educated about proper use. As with other medications, double-checking and independent checking can eliminate many errors.

Maximum use of unit dose packaging helps reduce errors. The added cost of packaging is outweighed by increased patient safety. Preprinted forms or computer order sets can help ensure patient safety, but only if they are routinely revised as conditions warrant. The fact that children are more vulnerable to the effects of medication errors than adults must always be borne in mind. Finally, patient counseling is essential in the prevention of errors with immunologic and other drug products.

REFERENCES

1. Smith G, Norman A, Banks J. Management of school leavers given a diphtheria and tetanus vaccine intended for children instead of the intended low dose preparation. *Commun Dis Rep CDR Rev.* 1997;7:R67–8.
2. Grabenstein JD. *ImmunoFacts: Vaccines & Immunologic Drugs, 30th revision.* St Louis: Wolters Kluwer Health; 2005.
3. Cohen MR. Tetanus toxoid vaccines used for PPD. *Hosp Pharm.* 2005;39:932–9,953.
4. Centers for Disease Control and Prevention. Inadvertent intradermal administration of tetanus toxoid-containing vaccines instead of tuberculosis skin tests. *MMWR Morb Mortal Wkly Rep.* 2004;53:662, 664.
5. Cohen MR. PPD and flu vaccine: Don't get stuck with this mix-up. *Hosp Pharm.* 2005;40:12–3.
6. Cohen MR. Confusing Haemophilus b conjugate vaccine with influenza vaccine. *Hosp Pharm.* 2003;38:110.
7. Davis NM, Cohen MR, Teplitsky B. Look-alike and sound-alike drug names: the problem and the solution. *Hosp Pharm.* 1992;27:95–8, 102–5, 108–10.
8. Cohen MR. "Bay" this and "Bay" that. *Hosp Pharm.* 1997;32:836.
9. Centers for Disease Control and Prevention. Unintentional administration of varicella virus vaccine—United States, 1996. *MMWR Morb Mortal Wkly Rep.* 1996;45:1017–8.
10. Wise RP, Braun MM, Seward JF, et al. Pharmacoepidemiologic implications of erroneous varicella vaccinations in pregnancy through confusion with varicella zoster immune globulin. *Pharmacoepidemiol Drug Saf.* 2002;11:651–4.
11. Bhambhani V, Kumar N, Puliyel JM. Death of twins after intravenous varicella zoster immunoglobulin. *Ann Pharmacother.* 2005;39:198–9.
12. Stone MM, Vannier AM, Storch SK, et al. Meningitis due to iatrogenic BCG infection in two immunocompromised children. *N Engl J Med.* 1995;333:561–3.
13. Cohen MR. Play it safe. Don't use these abbreviations. *Nursing 87.* July 1987;17:46–7.
14. Davis NM. *Medical Abbreviations: 12,000 Conveniences at the Expense of Communications & Safety.* 8th ed. Huntingdon Valley, Pa: Davis Associates; 1997.
15. Grabenstein JD. The importance of up-to-date Vaccine Information Statements. *Hosp Pharm.* 1999;34:1072–3, 1076-8, 1081–2, 1085–7.
16. Grabenstein JD. The Vaccine Identification Standards Initiative (VISI): towards clearer labels and common nomenclature. *Hosp Pharm.* 2002;37:58, 60, 62–4, 67–8, 71–2, 74.
17. Cohen MR. Insufficient dose of hepatitis B vaccine given to 1400 newborns; formalin accidents. *Hosp Pharm.* 1995;30:938–9.
18. *Physicians' Desk Reference.* Montvale, NJ: Medical Economics; 1998:2848.
19. Pearce LB, First ER, Borodic GE. Botulinum toxin potency: a mystery resolved by the median paralysis. *J R Soc Med.* 1994;87:571–2.
20. Grabenstein JD. Immunotherapy for Hymenoptera insects: bees, wasps, hornets, and fire ants. *Hosp Pharm.* 1992;27:883, 887–90, 905.
21. Grabenstein JD. Allergen-extract compounding by pharmacists. *Hosp Pharm.* 1992;27:145, 149–53, 1615.
22. Cohen MR. Drug product characteristics that foster drug-use-system errors. *Am J Health Syst Pharm.* 1995;52: 395–9.
23. Cohen MR. To prevent mix-ups, learn to talk to yourself. *Hosp Pharm.* 1996;31:184, 187–8.
24. World Health Organization. Vaccine supply and quality: surveillance of adverse events following immunization. *Wkly Epidemiol Rec.* 1996;71:237–42.
25. Cohen MR. Prevent mix-ups between vaccines and neuromuscular blockers. *Hosp Pharm.* 2003;38:109–10.
26. Crosby AD, Geller RJ. Human effects of veterinary biological products [published correction appears in *Vet Hum Toxicol.* 1987;29:24]. *Vet Hum Toxicol.* 1986;28:552–3, 569.

27. Institute for Safe Medication Practices. What makes you think it couldn't happen here? *ISMP Medication Safety Alert!* June 4, 1997;2(11).

28. Davis NM, Cohen MR. Sterile cockpit. *Am Pharm*. 1995;35(12):11.

29. King JW, Taylor EM, Crow SD, et al. Comparison of the immunogenicity of hepatitis B vaccine administered intradermally and intramuscularly. *Rev Infect Dis*. 1990;12:1035.

30. Woodruff BA, Moyer LA, Bryan JP, et al. Intradermal vaccination for hepatitis B. *Clin Infect Dis*. 1992;15:1063–6.

31. Shuster JS. ISMP adverse drug reactions: adverse reaction due to wrong route of administration. *Hosp Pharm*. 2001;36:1039.

32. Miles MM, Shaw RJ. Effect of inadvertent intradermal administration of high-dose percutaneous BCG vaccine [letter]. *Br Med J*. 1996;312:1205.

33. Puliyel JM, Hughes A, Chiswick ML, et al. Adverse local reactions from accidental BCG overdose in infants. *Br Med J*. 1996;313:528–9.

34. Stetler HC, Garbe PL, Dwyer DM, et al. Outbreaks of group A streptococcal abscesses following diphtheria-tetanus toxoid-pertussis vaccination. *Pediatrics*. 1985;75:299–303.

35. Centers for Disease Control and Prevention. Improper infection-control practices during employee vaccination programs—District of Columbia and Pennsylvania, 1993. *MMWR Morb Mortal Wkly Rep*. 1993;42:969–71.

36. Centers for Disease Control. Hepatitis B associated with jet gun injection—California. *MMWR Morb Mortal Wkly Rep*. 1986;35:272–6.

37. Derrough TF, Kitchin NRE. Occurrence of adverse events following inadvertent administration of childhood vaccines. *Vaccine*. 2002;21:53–9.

38. Cohen MR. Save lives: improve the pneumococcal vaccine administration rate. *Hosp Pharm*. 2004;39:1142–3.

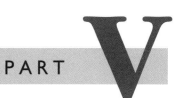

REDUCING RISKS AND CREATING A JUST CULTURE OF SAFETY

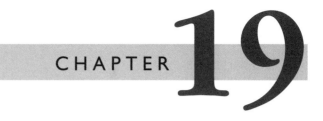

CHAPTER 19

MEDICATION ERROR REPORTING SYSTEMS

Judy L. Smetzer and Michael R. Cohen

Providing the best possible patient care in a safe, compassionate environment is a common goal for all health professionals.[1] Error-reporting systems promote this goal by helping health professionals, organizations, and safety agencies learn about

- *Potential risks:* Risks hidden in the processes used to provide patient care,
- *Actual errors:* Errors that occur during patient care,
- *Causes of errors:* Underlying weaknesses in the systems and processes of care that explain why an error happened, and
- *Prevention:* Ways of preventing recurrent events and, ultimately, patient harm.[2]

Error-reporting programs must be an essential part of any strategy to reduce injuries during patient care, because understanding the types of injuries and their causes is key to the development of effective preventive measures.[3]

Humans can learn from the experiences of others—from mistakes as well as successes.[4] Yet some health professionals have been reluctant to report their mistakes.[3] Not long ago, many felt too embarrassed or ashamed to divulge a medication error. Individuals and facilities were so fearful of legal exposure that there was an unwritten, unspoken, but clearly understood rule: Silence is golden.[4] But times are changing. Health professionals now recognize that admitting and openly discussing errors allows us to better analyze a situation, more appropriately predict behavior, and more safely and reliably design systems and processes that are resistant to errors. Many are beginning to realize that *not* reporting errors incurs greater liability than reporting them.

Developing internal systems for reporting and tracking errors within a health care organization is a first step toward medication safety, but it is not enough. Contributing to external reporting systems facilitates large-scale tracking and trend analysis. Information must be shared with other health care practitioners, drug manufacturers, equipment and technology vendors, the Food and Drug Administration (FDA), and all health care stakeholders who can help design safer systems and processes.[2] External reporting systems can influence the development of best practices, standards of care, error-resistant products, and fail-safe systems. Error reporting can also save unnecessary health care expenditures by helping to prevent repeat errors.[4]

Data from reporting programs highlight areas of vulnerability in the way care is provided. But collecting reports is just the first step in reducing errors. Reporting programs have value only if they lead to changes that reduce errors and improve patient care.[5] Sufficient resources must be devoted to analyzing the data to understand the causes of errors.

DEFINITIONS

Adverse drug event (ADE): Any injury resulting from medical intervention related to a drug.[6]

Preventable ADE: ADE that results from an error or equipment failure.[7]

Error: The failure of a planned action to be completed as intended (i.e., error of execution) or the use of a wrong plan to achieve an aim (i.e., error of planning).[6]

Medication error: Any preventable event that may cause or lead to inappropriate medication use or to patient harm while the medication is in the control of the health care professional, patient, or consumer. Such events may be related to professional practice; health care products, procedures, and systems, including prescribing; order communication; product labeling, packaging, and nomenclature; compounding; dispensing; distribution; administration; education; monitoring; or use.[8] A broader definition is any error that occurs in the medication-use process.[9]

Products included in the definition of medication error: Oral, injectable, intranasal, sublingual, transdermal, and topical medications; anesthetic agents and gases; radiopharmaceuticals and radiopaque contrast media; blood-fraction medications; intravenous fluids; dialysis fluids; respiratory therapy agents; investigational medications; medication samples; medications brought into a health care facility by patients; and other chemical or biological substances.

Close call or near miss: A medication error that was detected and corrected before it reached the patient. (The Agency for Healthcare Research and Quality [AHRQ] describes a near miss as an event or situation that did not produce patient injury, but only because of chance. By this definition, a near miss includes events that may have reached the patient. The AHRQ definition has caused confusion, since most believe a near miss is an error detected before it reached the patient.)

Reducing the frequency of errors requires a shift away from a punitive approach. After an error has been made or reported, the focus should be on identifying error-prone aspects of the medication-use process and improving system safety and reliability.[4]

This chapter examines the roles of internal and external medication error-reporting systems in improving patient safety, and the differences between mandatory and voluntary reporting systems. Examples of voluntary and mandatory systems are used to illustrate their respective strengths and weaknesses. Practitioners' perspectives on error reporting are presented. The chapter ends with a list of qualities of successful error reporting programs.

PURPOSE OF REPORTING SYSTEMS

Error-reporting systems provide organizations and safety agencies with information on adverse drug events (ADEs), medication errors, close calls or near misses (defined above), and other medication safety risks. Although organizations may collect such information in other ways, robust reporting systems are an invaluable resource for learning about hazards related to medication use.

According to the 1999 Institute of Medicine (IOM) report *To Err Is Human*,[6] reporting programs must satisfy two primary purposes: (1) hold providers accountable for performance and patient safety and (2) provide information that leads to new knowledge and improved patient safety. Most health professionals would agree that the main goal of reporting is learning how to improve care. As noted by James Bagian, MD, director of the Veterans Affairs National Center for Patient Safety, error-reporting programs uncover how someone who was trying to do the job correctly ended up with a bad outcome.[10] But IOM's call to hold hospitals accountable for safe practices has met with resistance, since this typically involves public disclosure of ADEs.[3]

Health care organizations' internal error reporting systems are used for improving the management of individual patients, obtaining timely medical advice, providing a record of events, and obtaining immediate legal counsel. External reporting systems (i.e., reports to a safety agency not affiliated with the organization) allow learning from events outside the organization. Ideally, when an error occurs, it is internally reported and investigated to uncover the causes, changes are made to prevent a recurrence within the health system, and the error, its causes, and error-reduction strategies are reported to an external program, which can

- Generate widespread alerts, from even a few reports, about newly recognized hazards (e.g., a new drug with confusing labeling),
- Widely disseminate new methods being used to prevent errors at individual locations, and
- Uncover trends and hazards that require attention and recommend best practices for all health care stakeholders (e.g., health care providers, health professionals, the pharmaceutical industry, medication information and device vendors).[3]

RESPONSIBILITY FOR REPORTING

The best person to report an error or other event is the individual who was involved in it or who discovered or witnessed the problem. Most medication error reports are submitted by pharmacists and nurses, who are often in the best position to identify hazardous situations and detect errors, especially those that originate during prescribing. However, physicians, dentists, podiatrists, physician assistants, pharmacy technicians, nurse practitioners, unit coordinators, medics and paramedics, clinical laboratory technicians, medical and paramedical students, respiratory therapists, pharmaceutical companies, and medical information and device vendors all have roles in the medication-use process and responsibility for reporting ADEs, errors, close calls, or hazards involving medications to internal and external reporting programs.

Health care consumers may report suspected medication errors to the facility in which they occurred; when a medication error or other medication-related concern is identified, the facility should investigate thoroughly. Consumers may also report to external voluntary error-reporting programs; many important issues related to medications and drug-use systems have been revealed in this manner. Consumer concerns can also be directed to the appropriate licensing board.

REPORTABLE EVENTS, CONDITIONS, AND PRIORITIES

Clear, consistent terminology must be used in reporting. Facilities may use terms such as "unusual occurrence," "variance," "medication error," or "incident" to refer to ADEs. Because the word "incident" has acquired the connotation of "crisis," many organizations prefer the word "event."

The American Hospital Association (AHA) defines an event as "any happening which is not consistent with the routine operation of the hospital (or health care organization) or the routine care of a particular patient."[11] This definition is purposely broad in order to accommodate all potentially reportable occurrences. Nevertheless, reporting programs must clearly define the types of events and conditions that should be reported. Focus groups of nurses and physicians in 2002 revealed a lack of consensus on the types of events that should be reported, and participants suggested that not knowing what to report was a barrier to reporting.[12] The types of events and conditions that should be reported to internal and external reporting programs are listed on page 517. Staff members should be provided with examples in each category to clarify what is desired. The American College of Surgeons estimates that 40% to 60% of all adverse occurrences could be identified through a reporting system that lists the specific events to be reported.[13]

Some external reporting systems, especially those that mandate reporting, accept only serious medication errors that have resulted in (or could have resulted in) patient harm. However, near-miss events and newly recognized hazardous conditions that could lead to errors represent critical elements of a reporting program from the standpoint of error prevention. Therefore, programs that request all types of reports are much better equipped to learn about underlying system-based causes of medication errors. These less serious events are often rooted in the same system-based problems that could eventually result in harmful medication errors. Including these events and conditions in a reporting program allows health professionals to take a proactive role in identifying system failures and helps to prevent errors *before* actual patient harm occurs. In addition, it may be more comfortable and productive for staff to report events or conditions that have not yet resulted in patient harm; the emotional toll of harming a patient can be devastating, as discussed in Chapter 3.

To obtain additional information on a particular problem, both internal and external reporting systems may ask participants to report *specific* conditions, hazards, or errors. Reporters may believe that the organization already knows about a problem and thus may not take time to report what they have encountered. To gain perspective on a particular condition or error type, reporting systems may ask participants to report all issues involving this topic. Such stimulated reporting on a particular topic enhances a program's capacity to learn about safety issues and recommend system changes.

REPORTING MECHANISMS

Today's integrated health care systems may include several acute care facilities, as well as physician group practices, ambulatory care clinics, home health services, assisted living centers, nursing homes, and other health care businesses. The staff of each of these entities needs to understand both the system's overall internal event reporting system and alternative, informal ways to report events. For example, an acute care hospital may use a telephone hotline and a reporting form different from those used by a mental health facility. Staff in physician practices and pharmacies may prefer to make oral reports directly to risk managers.

Maintaining informal lines of communication between reporting program staff and reporters helps to personalize the program and enhance reporters' trust and confidence in those who receive the reports. Event-reporting mechanisms should be flexible enough to include both formal and informal ways of accepting information in oral, written, and electronic form. Especially for external reporting systems, reports may be submitted by e-mail. The organization that maintains the reporting program should track the relative use and effectiveness of reporting mechanisms and make adjustments as necessary.

Many liability insurers provide their clients with forms or electronic formats that can be used in internal reporting programs. Some accept facility-specific forms or electronic formats for internal reporting, if they meet specific criteria. External reporting systems may also provide event-reporting forms or electronic formats. Some provide software that must be purchased or for which a licensing fee must be paid. External reporting systems that require a voluntary financial commitment for software can be expected to have fewer participants than systems with no fee for participation.

CONDITIONS AND EVENTS REPORTABLE TO ERROR REPORTING SYSTEMS

Risk: Hazardous conditions that could lead to an error, such as

- ❑ Products with look-alike packaging or names
- ❑ Ambiguous product labels
- ❑ Error-prone medication delivery devices (e.g., pumps)
- ❑ Error-prone functions in computerized prescriber order entry systems
- ❑ Unsafe environmental conditions (e.g., noise, poor lighting, clutter)
- ❑ Staffing shortages that result in excessive workload and fatigue
- ❑ Intimidating behaviors
- ❑ Out-of-date drug references
- ❑ Use of error-prone abbreviations
- ❑ Medication-related device hazards

Near misses/close calls: Errors that were intercepted and corrected before reaching the patient, such as

- ❑ Prescribing errors that were detected and corrected (pharmacy interventions/nurse interventions)
- ❑ Errors detected by independent double checks
- ❑ Dispensing or drug administration errors intercepted by bar coding
- ❑ Drug administration errors intercepted by infusion pumps with "smart" technology
- ❑ Dispensing errors intercepted by nurses
- ❑ Errors detected by patients before administration

Errors, no harm: Errors that reach the patient but do not cause harm

- ❑ Includes errors that do not result in change in patient monitoring or care

Errors, harm: Errors that reach the patient and cause harm

- ❑ Includes errors that result in any change in the level of care or monitoring
- ❑ Includes all levels of harm, from a rash to death

WHEN TO REPORT

Most organizations with internal reporting systems require immediate reporting of ADEs that may cause serious harm or threaten the life of a patient. For less severe events, reporting policies vary. The best approach is to immediately report every incident to a supervisor, no matter how insignificant it seems.

Immediate reporting has two advantages. First, ADEs that initially do not appear to be serious may, in fact, be so. In reporting an event immediately, the individual is not relying on independent judgment about its potential severity. Second, immediate reporting gives the supervisor an opportunity to ask questions while the event is fresh in the reporter's mind.

On the other hand, reports that are hastily prepared because of unrealistic time frames may be incomplete and may not contain information that would identify system failures. A better approach is to require immediate oral reporting of ADEs to a supervisor (and to risk management personnel, if potentially harmful). Final reports can then be forwarded to risk management after all necessary information has been gathered, no later than 1 week after the event. If additional time is needed to gather information, the report should state this.

The benefit of external voluntary reporting systems is enhanced if ADEs and medication errors are reported after all information has been gathered and the event has been investigated to determine the underlying causes of the error. However, external mandatory reporting systems typically have specific time frames for reporting ADEs; thus, all the information may not be available at the time of reporting.

WHAT INFORMATION TO REPORT

The most useful reports include a factual description of the event (what happened and the patient outcome), plus explanatory information, often in separate documentation.

A complete description of what happened, or of the hazard if an actual event did not happen, should be provided. Reports of events involving problematic labeling or packaging should include manufacturers' names to ensure proper product identification. The report should describe any additional patient monitoring or testing performed as a result of the event, additional medications administered as a result of the event (e.g., reversal agents, antihistamines, medications to treat symptoms), other treatment necessary to preclude harm, and actual patient harm, regardless of severity.

The explanatory information should describe

- *How it happened:* The conditions that led to an event or that pose a hazard,
- *What normally happens:* How the processes involved in the event normally happen and how the risks in carrying out those processes were managed before the event,
- *Why it happened:* The system-based causes of the event or hazardous condition,
- *At-risk behaviors:* Any behaviors staff engaged in as a work-around or a means to cut a corner, incentives for the work-around or cut corner (often caused by system problems), and the prevalence of the work-around or cut corner by other like staff, and
- *How to prevent it:* How systems or processes can be changed to prevent similar events or to reduce or eliminate the hazardous condition.

Information about causative factors is crucial. Figure 19-1 shows an event-reporting form containing questions to elicit causes. Without information about the underlying causes of an error, the report holds little value for improving medication safety.

For internal reporting, many organizations prefer that staff document the causative factors and prevention strategies as part of their quality improvement efforts, separating this documentation from the factual description of the event. This may better protect the event analysis from discovery during a lawsuit, depending on the state's statutes on evidentiary protection. The factual description of the event should never contain personal or professional conclusions, opinions, accusations, criticisms, or admissions. Patients' names should not be included in reports submitted to external reporting systems.

CATEGORIZING REPORTS

Error reports should be categorized according to the severity of patient outcome. Figure 19-2 shows an index for this purpose from the National Coordinating Council for Medication Error Reporting and Prevention (NCCMERP). The index considers factors such as whether the error reached the patient and, if the patient was harmed, to what degree. NCCMERP also provides an algorithm for selecting the proper category for each error report.[14]

ISMP ASSESS–ERR™ Medication System Worksheet

Patient MR# _____   Incident # _____
  (if error reached patient)   √ if no callback identified: _____

Date of error: _____   Date information obtained: _____   Patient age: _____

Drug(s) involved in error:_____

Nonformulary drug(s)?	☐ Yes	☐ No
Drug sample(s)?	☐ Yes	☐ No
Drug(s) packaged in unit dose/unit of use?	☐ Yes	☐ No
Drug(s) dispensed from pharmacy?	☐ Yes	☐ No
Error within 24 hours of admission, transfer, or after discharge?	☐ Yes	☐ No
Did the error reach the patient?	☐ Yes	☐ No

Source of IV solution: ☐ Manufacturer premixed solution ☐ Pharmacy IV admixture ☐ Nursing IV admixture

Brief description of the event: (what, when, and why)

_____
_____
_____

Possible causes	Y/N	Comments
Critical patient information missing? (e.g., age, weight, allergies, vital signs, lab values, pregnancy, patient identity, location, renal/liver impairment, diagnoses)		
Critical drug information missing? (e.g., outdated/absent references, inadequate computer screening, inaccessible pharmacist, uncontrolled drug formulary)		
Miscommunication of drug order? (e.g., illegible, ambiguous, incomplete, misheard, or misunderstood orders, intimidation/faulty interaction)		
Drug name, label, packaging problem? (e.g., look/sound-alike names, look-alike packaging, unclear/absent labeling, faulty drug identification)		
Drug storage or delivery problem? (e.g., slow turnaround time, inaccurate delivery, doses missing or expired, multiple concentrations, placed in wrong bin, unnecessary access to quantity/concentration of medications)		
Drug delivery device problem? (e.g., poor device design, misprogramming, free-flow, mixed-up lines, IV administration of oral liquid medication)		
Environmental, staffing, or workflow problems? (e.g., lighting, noise, clutter, interruptions, staffing deficiencies, excessive workload, inefficient workflow, employee safety, fatigue)		
Lack of staff education? (e.g., competency validation, new or unfamiliar drugs/devices, orientation process, feedback about errors/prevention)		
Patient education problem? (e.g., lack of information, noncompliance, not encouraged to ask questions, lack of investigating patient inquiries)		
Lack of quality control or independent check systems? (e.g., equipment quality control checks, independent checks for high-alert drugs/high-risk patient population drugs)		

FIGURE 19-1   ISMP ASSESS–ERR worksheet (continued on page 520). © 2005, Institute for Safe Medication Practices.

What normally happens? (Provide a brief description of how the processes involved in the event normally happen and how the risks in carrying out those processes were managed before the event.)

_____
_____
_____

Explanation of at-risk behaviors: (Provide a brief description of any behaviors staff engaged in as a work-around or a means to cut a corner, incentives for the work-around or the cut corner [often caused by system problems], and the prevalence of the work-around or cut corner by other similar staff.)

_____
_____
_____

Did the patient require any of the following actions after the error that you would not have done if the event had not occurred?

☐ Testing   ☐ Additional observation   ☐ Gave antidote   ☐ Care escalated   ☐ Additional LOS   ☐ Other_____
                                                                          (transferred, etc.)

Patient outcome:

_____

FIGURE 19-1 (continued)   ISMP ASSESS–ERR worksheet. © 2005, Institute for Safe Medication Practices.

Categorizing reports according to patient outcome can help organizations monitor patient harm and prioritize their medication safety activities. However, all event reports—even reports of hazardous conditions or errors that do not reach the patient—hold valuable information about systemic weaknesses that could eventually lead to patient harm. For the purposes of learning and change, an event report that falls into NCCMERP category A (hazard, but no error) is equally important as an event report in category I (error, harm). All reports should be fully investigated and acted upon.

MANDATORY REPORTING PROGRAMS

The 1999 IOM report[6] suggested that the two stated purposes of reporting systems, learning and accountability, are not incompatible. The authors acknowledged, however, that it might be difficult to satisfy both purposes simultaneously. While noting that voluntary reporting systems are more effective for learning about adverse events and improving patient safety, the report stated that mandatory reporting of serious events and disincentives for unsafe care may be needed to hold providers accountable. Thus, both mandatory and voluntary reporting systems were recommended.

The IOM recommendation for mandatory reporting systems sparked controversy.[15] Many national associations, including the Institute for Safe Medication Practices (ISMP), AHA, and the American Medical Association, raised strong objections, stating that mandatory reporting would fail to promote either accountability or learning.[3,16] Instead, they believed reporting would be stifled by heightened fear of damaged reputations and legal liability.[3]

Both mandatory and voluntary reporting systems are currently operating in the United States. Evaluating how well these programs meet the goals of learning and accountability can provide guidance for designing an ideal reporting system.[17]

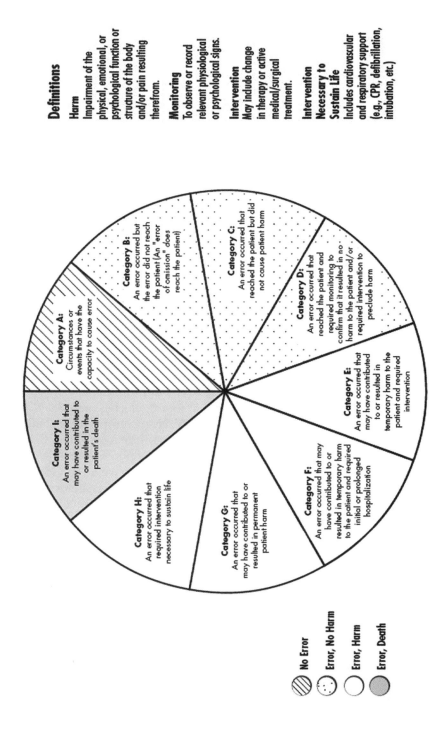

Definitions

Harm

Impairment of the physical, emotional, or psychological function or structure of the body and/or pain resulting therefrom.

Monitoring

To observe or record relevant physiological or psychological signs.

Intervention

May include change in therapy or active medical/surgical treatment.

Intervention Necessary to Sustain Life

Includes cardiovascular and respiratory support (e.g., CPR, defibrillation, intubation, etc.)

Category A:
Circumstances or events that have the capacity to cause error

Category B:
An error occurred but the error did not reach the patient (An "error of omission" does reach the patient)

Category C:
An error occurred that reached the patient but did not cause patient harm

Category D:
An error occurred that reached the patient and required monitoring to confirm that it resulted in no harm to the patient and/or required intervention to preclude harm

Category E:
An error occurred that may have contributed to or resulted in temporary harm to the patient and required intervention

Category F:
An error occurred that may have contributed to or resulted in temporary harm to the patient and required initial or prolonged hospitalization

Category G:
An error occurred that may have contributed to or resulted in permanent patient harm

Category H:
An error occurred that required intervention necessary to sustain life

Category I:
An error occurred that may have contributed to or resulted in the patient's death

No Error

Error, No Harm

Error, Harm

Error, Death

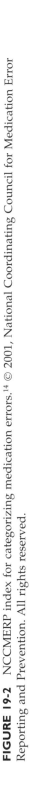

FIGURE 19-2 NCCMERP index for categorizing medication errors.[14] © 2001, National Coordinating Council for Medication Error Reporting and Prevention. All rights reserved.

Limited Success of Mandatory Programs

Mandatory reporting systems typically are run by state departments of health that require reporting the most serious events related to patient safety and by licensing boards that require reporting individual errors. Most mandatory reporting programs have not been entirely successful. Although such systems have the potential to produce useful data, compliance with reporting requirements has been inconsistent, as evidenced by significant variation in the volume of reports and the amount of useful information received. Such underreporting is understandable, given that disclosure has often exposed organizations and individuals to financial penalties, punitive actions concerning professional and organizational licenses, and legal and public scrutiny.

Health care practitioners perceive many of the mandatory systems as less than credible because they tend to assign blame rather than identify and correct the system-based causes of errors. Blame typically underpins accountability systems and may be a disincentive to reckless behavior. However, blame also discourages reporting and is a powerful barrier to collaborative problem solving. The inclination to blame individuals is rooted in *hindsight bias,* a tendency to simplify a problem once all the facts and outcomes are known. Hindsight bias obscures the reality that the situation faced by an individual at the time of an event is very different from what is perceived afterward. The events typically reported to mandatory systems have resulted in serious harm, and outcome-based event analysis is especially prone to hindsight bias.

Any reporting program that has at its core the punishment of health care practitioners and organizations is bound to fail in terms of gaining new knowledge about errors and holding providers accountable for patient safety. Punishment may be warranted in rare instances for illegal or malicious behavior, but mandatory reporting in today's health systems results in punitive measures whether or not punishment is warranted. Thus, mandatory reporting has had the overall effect of suppressing error reporting and inhibiting open discussion about errors and their system-based causes. In truth, all reporting is voluntary; to escape the threat of punishment, mandates to report may be disregarded.[18]

Practitioners may not be afraid to report errors internally. However, health systems can do little to protect individuals from the typical effects of disclosure to external mandatory programs: fear, financial penalties, punitive actions concerning licenses, and legal and public scrutiny. Thus, external mandatory reporting systems can have an inhibitory effect on health systems' internal reporting programs. Health-system leaders cannot make it safe for staff to disclose errors, when the most serious errors must be reported to mandatory programs that punish individuals or the health system.

Reports to existing mandatory systems typically are submitted by a designated person within a health care organization, who is not necessarily one of the frontline practitioners most familiar with the error. Such reports describe what happened but not necessarily why it happened. The person designated to report to a mandatory system is often under considerable pressure to minimize the organization's exposure to liability and public distrust. Therefore, information crucial for effective analysis may be overlooked, unavailable at the time of the report, or excluded. Any program that is not based on the reports of frontline practitioners may be a waste of resources, since information needed to identify system-based causes of error and preventive strategies may be absent.

Most mandatory programs have been less than successful in synthesizing and analyzing reported information and recommending broad system improvements to enhance patient safety.[6] Those running such programs may lack expertise in the system-based causes of errors and the most effective means of improving systems. Important information that could lead to successful error reduction strategies may be overlooked.

Mandatory State Programs

Fewer than half of the U.S. states have mandatory reporting systems.[3] The types of events that must be reported vary from state to state. Some reporting requirements are specific to events, such as brain injury.[6] Others are more general. For instance, California requires reporting "unusual occurrences that threaten the welfare, safety, or health of patients, personnel, or visitors."[6] Unanticipated death is the only event required to be reported in all state programs.[3]

State health departments sometimes investigate serious events, but health professionals and health systems rarely receive feedback about hazards, errors, or error prevention because so little analysis of events occurs. Licensing boards publish information about professionals sanctioned for making errors, often in the midst of a list of sanctions for illegal activities. Health departments typically make some findings public but insulate detailed information from legal discovery.[3,19]

The number of reports received by state programs varies widely. New York received 28,689 reports in 2001[20] and Pennsylvania received more than 200,000 reports during 15 months in 2004 and 2005,[21,22] but few states receive more than 100 reports annually.[3,19] The Colorado and New York state programs publish aggregate health-system-specific data, and other states make this information available upon request. A few state reporting systems (e.g., Colorado, Kansas, Massachusetts, New York, Pennsylvania) send out periodic alerts or newsletters.[3,19]

There is little evidence that existing mandatory reporting programs have improved patient safety. There have been anecdotal reports of changes made after state investigations of serious events, but no controlled studies.[3] Research is needed on how the information provided in state newsletters and advisories is used and whether mandatory reporting programs prompt health care providers to make safety changes that they would not otherwise have made.

It may not be the mandatory nature of these programs that has made them unsuccessful in gaining the public's confidence, learning about the causes of error, and enhancing patient safety. More likely, the lack of success lies in the design of the reporting systems, the punitive culture in which they function, and the ineffective use of data submitted.[17]

Patient Safety Centers

The departments of health in six states have recently acknowledged that to improve patient safety, less punitive and more collaborative efforts must be established and coordinated across all agencies of state government. To this end, the six states have developed patient safety centers that reflect promising changes in the structure, processes, and outcomes of mandatory reporting programs. These centers provide a model for more effective mandatory reporting systems, although demonstrating their impact continues to be difficult.

Florida, Maryland, Pennsylvania, Oregon, Massachusetts, and New York have developed patient safety centers during the past 5 years.[23] Most are still in their infancy; the New York and Pennsylvania centers have existed the longest. Responding in part to broad issues such as affordable health care and malpractice reform, the legislatures in these states authorized or endorsed the centers, distinguishing them from other statewide patient safety programs. The centers' functions vary, but all aim to educate providers about patient safety best practices, develop collaborative relationships among patient safety stakeholders, and educate consumers about patient safety.[23]

Each patient safety center has a governing board and uses consumers in an advisory capacity.[23] Most of the centers work autonomously, with little or no state regulatory control (Table 19-1); however, the New York center operates within the department of health and

TABLE 19-1 State Patient Safety Centers

Center	Autonomy	Reporting System within Center	Relationship to State Mandatory Reporting Program	Unique Uses of Patient Safety Data
Florida Patient Safety Corporation	State assisted in start-up activities, but center is designed to be independent of state regulatory departments.	Confidential, voluntary reporting system for near misses, to augment state mandatory reporting system.	Analyzes reports submitted to state mandatory reporting system.	■ Examines ways of rewarding providers who implement evidence-based medical practices. ■ Will recommend core patient safety competencies for health professional curricula.
Maryland Patient Safety Center	Independent of state regulatory departments.	Confidential, voluntary reporting system for near misses and adverse events that do not cause harm, to augment state mandatory reporting system.	Sharing data from state mandatory reporting system about serious and fatal adverse events with center is being considered; however, data collected by center will not be shared with state.	■ Plans to coordinate educational activities between center and state agency responsible for mandatory reporting system. ■ Publicly discloses which facilities participate in reporting systems.
Betsy Lehman Center for Patient Safety and Medical Error Reduction (Massachusetts)	Housed within executive office of Department of Public Health but not under control of any state agency (however, executive director of center is also assistant commissioner of Department of Public Health).	Pursing possibility of a voluntary, confidential reporting system for near misses and complications.	No sharing of information between center and state mandatory reporting system except to extent that information is otherwise public.	■ Developed ombudsman program to work with patients, families, and consumers on patient-safety-related problems. ■ Collaborates with statewide Coalition for the Prevention of Medical Errors, which serves as advisory committee to center's board. ■ Works with state professional licensing bodies and Coalition for the Prevention of Medical Errors to address health-system and individual practitioner accountability in a less punitive manner.

New York Center for Patient Safety	Operates as state agency within Department of Health, subject to all reporting and administrative requirements.	Has legislative authority to start a confidential, voluntary reporting system but has not done so yet.	Uses aggregate information from state mandatory reporting program to identify areas in need of quality improvement.	■ Administers award program to recognize patient safety leaders of various types of health care facilities. ■ Plans to recommend statewide medical safety goals and publish hospital report card to track progress toward goals.
Oregon Patient Safety Commission	Semi-independent state agency with no regulatory functions, free of most administrative oversight from state.	Confidential, voluntary reporting system for serious adverse events.	No state mandatory reporting system exists. If voluntary reporting system does not succeed, a mandatory reporting system will be considered in 2007. No information from center's voluntary reporting system will be shared with any state regulatory agency.	■ Publicly discloses which facilities participate in reporting systems.
Pennsylvania Patient Safety Authority (PSA)	Independent state agency with no regulatory functions or administrative oversight, but must comply with certain administrative rules regarding personnel and reporting requirements.	Mandatory, confidential reporting system for serious events, near misses, and infrastructure failures. To reduce reporting burden, system uses a single Web-based portal for submission of all reports.	Reporting system automatically directs reports of serious events and near misses to PSA and reports of serious events and infrastructure failures to department of health.	■ PSA and health department collaborate to develop patient safety protocols; for facilities that implement the protocols, medical malpractice insurance premiums may be reduced. ■ Statute provides for a discount in medical malpractice premiums for facilities that demonstrate a reduction in serious events.

Source: Reference 23.

is subject to reporting and administrative requirements.[24] All the centers are required to submit periodic progress reports to legislative or executive bodies. Most of the centers disclose, or plan to disclose, some information to the public.[23] Maryland, New York, and Pennsylvania post consumer information on their Web sites, and Massachusetts plans to do so.[23]

Five of the six states with patient safety centers operate mandatory reporting systems for serious adverse events within their regulatory agencies. Oregon is the exception; it is establishing a confidential, voluntary reporting system for serious adverse events.[23] The centers in Florida, New York, and Pennsylvania help analyze data from the state mandatory reporting systems. The Pennsylvania patient safety center is responsible for developing and administering a mandatory reporting system to replace a previous system administered by a state regulatory agency.[22] To complement mandatory reporting systems, the centers in Florida and Maryland have established voluntary reporting programs for less serious errors.[23] Pennsylvania includes less serious events in its mandatory reporting program.[22] Despite efforts to separate the centers from state regulatory processes and to protect data, health care providers may still be hesitant to report events or hazards.[23]

Pennsylvania's Unique Program

Pennsylvania has a new program that combines attributes of mandatory and voluntary systems. Since June 2004, the mandatory Pennsylvania Patient Safety Reporting System (PA-PSRS) has required the reporting of close calls and near misses as well as serious adverse events.[10,22] All licensed hospitals, birthing centers, and ambulatory surgical facilities must report both "serious events" (actual adverse events) and "incidents" (near misses).

The Pennsylvania program borrows from the successful aviation model of event reporting, in that a separate, independent, nonregulatory state agency analyzes reports for learning purposes.[10] That body, the Patient Safety Authority (PSA), derives all its data from PA-PSRS. PSA is not permitted to collect any identifiable information on practitioners or patients, although the location of the event may be included in the report.[22] All information is confidential, and no information about individual facilities or providers is made public. The program offers whistleblower protection, as well as provisions for health care workers to submit anonymous reports if they believe facilities are not acting appropriately in response to a serious event.[22]

The patient safety officers in each Pennsylvania health care institution can use PA-PSRS to monitor progress in improving safety at their facilities.[22] The system provides tools that individual facilities can use to track and evaluate occurrences and to prepare reports for internal risk management activities.

Among the state programs, Pennsylvania's PA-PSRS is unique in its capacity for expert analysis.[10] PSA developed PA-PSRS to replace a previous mandatory reporting system. The program was developed under the direction of ECRI, a company that is widely known for its investigative work with medical devices but employs clinical support staff to analyze other types of medical error. As a subcontractor to ECRI in this effort, ISMP is primarily responsible for analyzing medication-related errors and adverse drug reactions reported to the system, identifying problems, and suggesting solutions to prevent future serious medication events. The program has provided ISMP and other safety experts with new information about the sources and causes of medication errors and a better understanding of the frequency or potential for harm associated with particular types of errors.

PSA provides facilities with a quarterly publication, *Patient Safety Advisory*, based on the analysis of errors and near misses; supplements are published as needed. Issues have featured, for example, strategies for reducing the risk of overdose from multiple transdermal patches;[25] a trend in insulin overdoses caused by confusion between two types of syringes;[26] guidance on reducing the risk of "wrong drug" errors, focusing on errors related to look-alike or sound-alike drug names (e.g., alprazolam and lorazepam);[27] and confusing drug name suffixes that had been reported to the system.[28]

Most of the trends identified in Pennsylvania in 2004 were consistent with national data.[22] About one-fourth of the reported medication errors involved one or more high-alert medications; two of three harmful events involved one or more high-alert medications.[22] PSA provided strategies for minimizing risk associated with high-alert medications in the September 2004 *Advisory.*[29] About 30% of hospitals responding to a survey in 2004 indicated that they have implemented patient safety protocols as a result of specific articles in the *Advisory* newsletters.[22]

Health systems in Pennsylvania have complained that PA-PSRS requires extra work because the system is not interfaced with their existing information systems.[10] In response, PSA is helping willing facilities to construct interfaces between PA-PSRS and existing internal error and risk management reporting programs so that data need to be entered only once.

VOLUNTARY REPORTING PROGRAMS

Voluntary reporting systems have generally been more successful than mandatory systems. Most reports to voluntary systems come from frontline practitioners who can describe the specific conditions that led to the event, which facilitates analysis of the system-based causes. Because detailed information is provided, conclusions can be drawn without waiting for a large number of reports of similar events. The information can be used promptly to create a road map for improvements by health care organizations and other stakeholders such as medical device manufacturers, pharmaceutical companies, automation technology companies, and health care reimbursement systems.

Another advantage of voluntary systems is the trust that develops between the reporters and recipients. When the information is swiftly and confidentially used to develop recommendations for safe practice, the value of reporting is obvious. Table 19-2 lists elements that encourage reporting by health care personnel.

In addition, voluntary systems are perceived as credible because they operate independent of regulatory and accrediting bodies and other stakeholders. Thus, they can analyze the information without conflict of interest or pressure from political, economic, or marketplace forces.

Perhaps the most important factor in the success of voluntary reporting systems is their nonpunitive approach to error reduction. Underlying this approach is the recognition that human error is inevitable because people cannot consistently outperform unsafe systems that constrain them. In voluntary programs, event analysis is system or process oriented rather than outcome oriented, and error reduction efforts are not targeted at the individual—the least manageable link in the error chain. Rather, efforts are aimed at strengthening the systems in which practitioners work, to make it difficult or impossible to err.

USP-ISMP Medication Errors Reporting Program

The nationwide, voluntary United States Pharmacopoeia (USP)–ISMP Medication Errors Reporting Program (MERP) originated in 1975 from a column on medication safety in the journal *Hospital Pharmacy.* The column encouraged pharmacists to report errors and safety hazards to its author, Michael R. Cohen, and these reports laid the groundwork on which ISMP was founded. USP now operates the reporting program in cooperation with ISMP, which receives all MERP reports, provides expert analysis of reports and aggregate data,

TABLE 19-2   Elements Identified by ISMP That Encourage Error Reporting

Leadership (board, executive, administrative, management, and supervisory leaders)
The organization's mission, vision, values, and strategic goals emphasize patient safety.
Leaders demonstrate a passion for preventing harm to patients and an interest in learning about risk, errors, and patient harm.
Leaders are present in work areas to learn firsthand about barriers to safe care.
Leaders demonstrate positive attitudes about the capabilities of the organization and the quality of individual workers' efforts.
Leaders view errors as a measure of system performance, not staff performance. They acknowledge human fallibility and the high-risk nature of health care, and they focus on the risk of system failure, not individual failure.
When errors occur, leaders share responsibility. They do not discipline individuals who report or commit errors, except in cases of criminal action, mistakes while under the influence of drugs or alcohol, and willful recklessness with an intent to harm patients.

Process
Workers are provided with clear definitions of medication errors, near misses, and hazards, and examples of the types of errors, near misses, and hazards that should be reported.
Workers have easy methods, including informal pathways, for reporting errors, near misses, and hazards.
Guidelines are provided for identifying events for which root cause analysis would be appropriate and useful.
The error-reporting process (with examples) is covered during orientation for all staff; new staff members are assigned a mentor to assist with error reporting and are required to report at least one safety hazard during the orientation period.
Error and hazard reporting are included as core elements in all workers' job descriptions and performance evaluations.

Change
Leaders act on error and hazard reports by fixing system-level vulnerabilities rather than punishing individuals.
Leaders empower staff to correct safety hazards; they support system enhancements suggested by staff for reducing the risk of harmful errors.
Leaders act on reports of errors and hazards outside the organization by making system changes to reduce the risk of similar errors.

Communication
Confidentiality is ensured for the identity of reporters and of patients and staff involved in errors, as well as the location of events.
Information about reporters and individuals involved in errors is redacted after reports are fully investigated.
Information collected during investigation of an error is protected from legal discovery.
Communication channels exist for sharing lessons learned from error analysis and root cause analysis (e.g., storyboards, newsletters, staff meetings, educational presentations, daily safety huddles), as well as for sharing memorable error stories and error-reduction strategies across departments.
Pathways exist for disseminating data to demonstrate safety problems and ensure that actions taken have been successful in reducing risk, error, and patient harm.

Reward
Mechanisms have been established for thanking and rewarding staff who report errors or hazards, and care settings that demonstrate measurable improvements in patient safety.

and disseminates the findings to the health care community and consumers. When appropriate, ISMP interacts with manufacturers, FDA, and regulatory and accrediting agencies to urge changes aimed at reducing the risk of serious harm from medication errors.

Individual health care professionals submit confidential reports of an actual error, near miss, or hazardous condition to MERP. Often, reporters are willing to provide supplemental materials such as photographs and redacted orders. The reporting process is described on page 529. Reporters make themselves available to answer questions during the investigation by USP or ISMP staff. Health professionals who report do so in the hope that the

MAKING A REPORT TO THE USP-ISMP MEDICATION ERRORS REPORTING PROGRAM

Health care practitioners or consumers can report a medication error or a hazardous condition that could lead to errors by

Telephone: Call ISMP at 800-FAIL-SAF(E) (800-324-5723).

Fax: Fax ISMP at 215-914-1492, or USP at 301-816-8532. Reporting forms are available at https://secure.usp.org/patientSafety/mer/merform.html.

E-mail: Send a message to ismpinfo@ismp.org.

Internet: Report to ISMP or USP in confidence via secure online forms at http://www.ismp.org/Pages/communications.asp or https://secure.usp.org/patientSafety/mer/merform.html.

U.S. Mail: Send reports to ISMP, 1800 Byberry Road, Suite 810, Huntingdon Valley, PA 19006; or to USP CAPS, 12601 Twinbrook Parkway, Rockville, MD 20852-1790.

Each report is treated confidentially. The identity of the reporter is not revealed; however, ISMP or USP staff may contact reporters for additional information as necessary to learn about the underlying causes of the error. Anonymous reporting is also an option.

Reporters should describe the hazard or error, including the sequence of events and the work environment in which it occurred or could occur (e.g., during a code, a change of shift, or when the pharmacy was closed). They should answer the following questions:

- ❑ Was the medication administered to or used by the patient?
- ❑ What was the patient outcome (e.g., death, injury or impairment, adverse reaction)?
- ❑ When and how was the error discovered, and by whom (e.g., nurse, physician, pharmacist, technician)?
- ❑ Where did the error occur (e.g., hospital, nursing home, outpatient or community pharmacy, patient's home)?
- ❑ What level of staff (e.g., pharmacist, nurse, technician) made the initial error?
- ❑ Was the error unwittingly perpetuated by another practitioner?
- ❑ Had the patient received counseling on proper use of the medication?
- ❑ What product was involved (if applicable)? Who is the manufacturer? What was the dosage form, strength, concentration, and type and size of the container?

ISMP staff is available to assist reporters between 9 am and 5 pm Eastern Time, Monday through Friday. Call 1-800-FAIL-SAF(E) for help, or e-mail ISMP at ismpinfo@ismp.org.

information they provide will lead to changes by others to prevent future errors and patient harm. Some state boards of pharmacy submit errors reported to them, giving the program insight into problems occurring nationwide.

The 2006 IOM report *Preventing Medication Errors*[9] suggests that it might be more conducive to learning if practice-related medication errors were reported initially to USP or MERP, which automatically passes on all such error reports to the FDA MedWatch program. Although FDA does not usually assert jurisdiction over practice issues or health care system failures, it is concerned with issues relating to product nomenclature, labeling, and packaging; reports on these issues are among those shared with FDA. Product-related reports are also sent to the manufacturer. Reporters' names and locations are never made public by ISMP or USP. Their names may be shared with FDA, ECRI, or the product manufacturer if the reporters specifically grant permission. Staff from USP, ISMP, and FDA may contact reporters for additional information, but reports can also be submitted anonymously.

Since MERP's inception more than 30 years ago, reporters have had no reason to fear retaliation or reprimand for reporting an error. Because MERP is independent of regulatory and accrediting bodies, it can objectively determine the causes of errors and their solutions

TABLE 19-3 Reports Submitted to USP-ISMP Medication Errors Reporting Program (MERP) in 2004

Category	%
A (circumstances that have the capacity to cause an error)	22
B (error occurred but did not reach the patient)	21
C (error reached the patient but did not cause harm)	33
D (error required monitoring to confirm that no harm occurred, or intervention to preclude harm)	8
E (error contributed to or resulted in temporary harm and required intervention)	10
F (error contributed to or resulted in temporary harm and required initial or prolonged hospitalization)	3
G (error may have contributed to or resulted in permanent harm)	1
H (error required intervention to sustain life)	1
I (error may have contributed to or resulted in death)	1

USP = United States Pharmacopeia; ISMP = Institute for Safe Medication Practices.
Data provided by USP and printed with permission.

but has no authority to discipline, regulate, or mandate implementation of the expert recommendations that stem from the error analysis.

Although MERP data cannot be used to determine the prevalence of medication errors, analysis of the reports provides information about the types, causes, and prevention of errors. Because the number of reports is relatively small, USP and ISMP can perform individual investigations and follow-up that would not be possible in programs that collect hundreds of thousands of reports each year. Because MERP is based on shared accountability for errors, without blame for individual practitioners, trust and respect have developed between USP-ISMP and the reporters, and this has enhanced the quality and quantity of reports.

Analysis of Reports to MERP

MERP's focus is on learning from reported events or hazards and preventing future errors through system-based solutions that can be extrapolated to all health care settings. An interdisciplinary team at ISMP analyzes each MERP report to determine the system-based causes of errors and identify trends.

In 2004, 57% of the reports submitted to MERP documented errors that reached the patient (Table 19-3). Thirteen percent of the errors that reached patients resulted in temporary harm; 2% resulted in permanent harm; and 1% resulted in death.

Hazards that could lead to errors accounted for 43% of the reports; these reports are important because hazards may lead to actual errors that harm patients. Recent guidelines from the World Health Organization's World Alliance for Patient Safety[30] cited MERP's success in capturing new and unsuspected hazards (e.g., previously unrecognized complications associated with the use of a medication). The document noted that direct human review of incoming reports can preclude the need for a large number of events to be reported before a problem is recognized.

Most of the errors submitted to MERP in 2004 involved either the wrong drug or the wrong dose, and many originated during prescribing (Table 19-4). Problems related to a product's labeling, packaging, or nomenclature played a role in 39% of the errors.

The contributing factors most frequently cited in the error reports were unsafe staffing and environmental conditions (Table 19-5). The work environment in general was the most frequently cited contributing factor (38%), followed closely by a busy, chaotic work area (32%). Poor communication during handoffs at shift change and inadequate space and lighting were also cited as contributing factors. The most common staffing issue associated with errors was an understaffed work area (16%) (Table 19-5). Reporters also cited the

TABLE 19-4   Types of Errors Reported to MERP in 2004

Description[a]	%
Unauthorized/wrong drug	48
Improper dose/quantity	35
Prescribing error	11
Wrong patient	4
Wrong dosage form	4
Dose omission	4
Wrong route	3
Wrong time	2
Deteriorated/outdated product	2
Wrong drug preparation	2

MERP = U.S. Pharmacopeia (USP)–Institute for Safe Medication Practices Medication Errors Reporting Program.

[a] Some reports contained more than one type of error.

Data provided by USP and printed with permission.

TABLE 19-5   Environmental and Staffing Conditions Contributing to Errors in 2004

Contributing Factor[a]	%
Environmental Conditions	
Work environment (general)	38
Busy work area	32
Handoffs at shift change	3
Not enough space	3
Not enough lighting	3
Staffing Conditions	
Short staffing	16
No 24-hour pharmacy	2
Floating staff	2
Agency/temporary staff	2
Overworked (extra hours/days)	1

[a] Some reports contained more than one contributing factor; not all potential contributing factors are included.

Data provided by U.S. Pharmacopeia and printed with permission.

lack of 24-hour pharmacy services, the use of floating or agency staff, and fatigue from overtime hours as factors that contributed to the errors.

About a dozen pharmaceutical products were repeatedly involved in the harmful errors reported to MERP in 2004 (Table 19-6). Many of these products are on a list of high-alert medications compiled through careful assessment of catastrophic errors nationwide in the past decade. A few drugs currently not considered high-alert medications were among the leading products involved in harmful errors in 2004; their high volume of use may be one reason. They were as follows:

- Lipitor and Zocor: Harm was most often due to drug–drug interactions, contraindications, and adverse effects such as rhabdomyolysis.

TABLE 19-6 Leading Products Involved
in Harmful Errors in 2004[a]

Product	%
Epinephrine[b]	4
Lipitor (atorvastatin)	4
Phenergan (promethazine)	4
Seroquel (quetiapine)	3
Tamoxifen citrate	3
Clonidine[b]	3
Coumadin (warfarin)	3
Diflucan (fluconazole)	3
Lithium[b]	3
Metoprolol[b]	3
Morphine sulfate	3
Paxil (paroxetine)	3
Phenobarbital	3
Potassium chloride	3
Primidone	3
Serzone (nefazodone)	3
Zocor (simvastatin)	3

[a] Based on reports of harmful errors (category E–I) involving one or more products.
[b] Includes all dosage forms and formulations.

Data provided by U.S. Pharmacopeia and printed with permission.

- Phenergan: Harm was most often due to IV or accidental intra-arterial administration.
- Seroquel and Serzone: Harm was most often due to mix-ups between these two drugs, which sometimes resulted in adverse effects such as rhabdomyolysis.
- Clonidine: Harm was most often due to mix-ups with other drugs with similar names (e.g., Klonopin and clonazepam, colchicine).
- Diflucan: Harm was most often due to confusion regarding dosing instructions (e.g., 2.5 tsp instead of 2.5 mL).
- Lithium: Harm was most often due to drug interactions.
- Metoprolol: Harm was most often dose related, particularly when different formulations were confused (e.g., Toprol and Toprol XL).

Impact of MERP

MERP has had a demonstrable nationwide impact on medication safety in the following five areas (see Appendix A for examples):

1. **Early warning system.** When ISMP learns about serious hazards from the MERP database, it immediately disseminates this information through nationwide alerts sent electronically to health care providers and releases sent to the lay and health care media describing the safety issue and recommending error-reduction strategies. The biweekly *ISMP Medication Safety Alert!* newsletter also contains timely hazard reports.

2. **Learning.** In addition to the immediate notification of hazards uncovered through MERP, ISMP uses the MERP data to help individuals and organizations learn about error prevention through memorable stories and detailed analysis of the causes of error. Also,

practitioners who report errors or serve on an ISMP editorial review board or advisory panel share error prevention strategies, and occasional practitioner surveys provide insight on patient safety trends.

Knowledge gained through MERP is presented in educational programs, teleconferences, and the ISMP newsletters and Web site. The *ISMP Medication Safety Alert!* acute care edition, started in 1996, reaches most U.S. hospitals, as well as accrediting and regulatory agencies, academic settings, health care product vendors, and many health care providers both nationally and internationally. ISMP encourages subscribing organizations to distribute copies to their employees and to use the articles, with proper citation, in their internal publications.

The success of this newsletter led to editions for ambulatory care workers, acute care nurses, and consumers. A 2004 survey suggested that through these publications plus regular features in 19 professional journals and newsletters, information from MERP reaches nearly 3.5 million readers worldwide.[31] The lay press uses the newsletters for articles about health care hazards and how to avoid them. Reading about errors stimulates additional reporting and ideas for error reduction.

3. Change. Anecdotal reports and aggregate survey data show that the information provided in ISMP newsletters stimulates practice and system changes by individuals and health care organizations. ISMP has also had considerable success in encouraging the pharmaceutical industry, medication device manufacturers, and health care information vendors to make changes in their products after error potential has been uncovered.

4. Standards. When applicable, what is learned from MERP is shared with regulatory agencies, accrediting bodies, federal agencies, product vendors, and health care purchasing groups to help them establish appropriate safety practices as standards. Staff at JCAHO, the National Quality Forum, FDA, and state health departments routinely read ISMP newsletters and interact with ISMP staff. Many recommendations stemming from MERP findings have been adopted as standards, National Patient Safety Goals (NPSGs), practice guidelines, and best practices. The response by these organizations has further encouraged the health care community at large to adopt recommendations from the newsletters.

MERP has also had an impact on USP's standards and drug information database.[4] For example, labeling changes were required for concentrated electrolytes and vincristine after reports of fatal errors with these drugs. Information on particularly harmful errors reported to MERP has been included under a "Caution" subheading in the "Dosage Forms" section of *USP Drug Information* monographs; examples include warnings about potentially fatal errors with colchicine, cisplatin, carboplatin, chloral hydrate, and esmolol.

5. Public policy. ISMP and USP use information from MERP to promote changes in public policy, such as state and federal legislative efforts to enhance medication safety.

FDA MedWatch

FDA's MedWatch voluntary reporting program receives reports from health professionals and consumers about serious ADEs, potential and actual product use errors, and product quality problems associated with the use of FDA-regulated drugs, biologics (including human cells, tissues, and cellular and tissue-based products), medical devices (including in vitro diagnostics), special nutritional products, and cosmetics.[32] MedWatch does not accept reports involving vaccines; these should be sent instead to the Vaccine Adverse Event Reporting System, a joint program of FDA and the Centers for Disease Control and Prevention.[33]

FDA and the pharmaceutical industry work together to monitor new products for problems, and the first hint of a problem often surfaces through a clinician's report to

MedWatch.[34] A broader drug safety program, the Adverse Event Reporting System, combines the voluntary reports from MedWatch and required reports from manufacturers to identify previously unrecognized events that are potentially serious.[35]

Health care professionals and the public can submit reports to MedWatch (also known as the FDA Safety Information and Adverse Event Reporting Program) by mail, fax (1-800-FDA-0178), telephone (1-800-FDA-1088), or the Internet (www.fda.gov/medwatch/report/hcp.htm). Suspicion, not proof, that a drug may be related to a serious event is reason enough to submit a report. Health professionals who plan to submit an adverse event case report for publication should notify MedWatch concurrently.[34]

In 2004, FDA received 422,889 reports of suspected drug-related adverse events.[35] Of these, only 5% (21,493) were voluntary reports of errors and ADEs to the MedWatch program; the remaining reports came from manufacturers. Many of the medication error reports came to FDA's attention through MERP.

All MERP data are shared with FDA, and the reporters' name are divulged with their permission. FDA reviews product-related errors reported to MERP, but not practice-related medication errors, such as administration of a drug to the wrong patient. ISMP is able to review reports submitted to MedWatch, but federal statutes prohibit FDA from sharing the reporter's identity. Thus, ISMP can follow up with reporters only through a third party within FDA. Furthermore, the narrative reports submitted to MedWatch are not available electronically, although elements of the MedWatch data are periodically available on the FDA Web site. For these reasons, more could be learned about medication safety if errors were reported to MERP and adverse drug reactions to MedWatch.

Reports from both MedWatch and MERP are analyzed by pharmacists and support personnel in FDA's Division of Medication Errors and Technical Support (DMETS) to provide feedback on error prevention.[36] DMETS reviews about 300 medication errors each month; about half are due to error-prone labeling such as look-alike labeling, poor package design, confusing instructions for use, and confusing drug names.[35] Causes and contributing factors are investigated, and recommendations for label or packaging revisions are offered.

In addition to medication-related information, MedWatch disseminates new medical product safety alerts, recalls, withdrawals, and important labeling changes through its Web site and through e-mail notification of health care professionals, institutions, the public, and MedWatch partners such as professional societies, health agencies, and patient and consumer groups. Subscription to e-mail notification is free. In 2004, more than 50,000 individuals and 160 MedWatch partner organizations received 50 safety alerts on drugs and therapeutic biologic products, and 25 to 70 safety-related drug product labeling changes each month, mostly related to newly recognized adverse effects uncovered during postmarketing surveillance.[36]

Joint Commission Sentinel Event Reporting Program

In 1996, JCAHO began asking accredited health care organizations to identify and voluntarily report all sentinel events within the facility. JCAHO defines a sentinel event as "an unexpected occurrence involving death or serious physical or psychological injury, or the risk thereof."[37] The phrase "or the risk thereof" refers to any process variation whose recurrence would carry a significant chance of a serious adverse outcome. The sentinel event policy requires organizations to investigate root causes within 45 days of becoming aware of an event, implement strategies to prevent recurrence of such events, and monitor the effectiveness of these strategies.

Although JCAHO says reporting is not required, the program is not entirely voluntary. If a health system fails to report an event and JCAHO learns about it from another source,

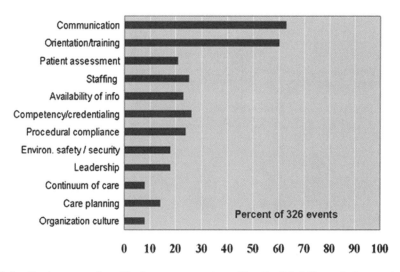

FIGURE 19-3 Root causes of medication errors reviewed by the Joint Commission on Accreditation of Healthcare Organizations (JCAHO), 1995–2004. Reprinted with permission from JCAHO.

the health system must conduct a root cause analysis within the specified time or risk being placed on "accreditation watch" status, with public disclosure of its potential loss of accreditation.[3,38] Whether an organization voluntarily reports an event or JCAHO learns about it from another source, the expected response, time frame, and review procedure are the same.[38] JCAHO provides expertise in analyzing the information about an event and validates, in on-site surveys, that system-based changes have been made to prevent recurrence. However, reporting programs that have the authority to mandate actions after an adverse event inhibit disclosure of errors and lessen the amount of knowledge that can be gained from the reporting system.

In 1995 through 2005, JCAHO reviewed 3,548 sentinel events.[39] During that period, 66% of the events were reported directly to JCAHO; the remainder came to JCAHO's attention through surveys; complaints by patients, families, and employees; reports from state agencies or the Centers for Medicare & Medicaid Services; and the media. JCAHO's sentinel event database contains data on the review of sentinel events, root cause analyses, action plans, and follow-up activities. The most frequently reported events include patient suicides (13.1%), wrong-site surgery (12.8%), operative or postoperative complications (12.5%), and medication errors (10.1%). The most common root causes of medication-related sentinel events in 1995 through 2004 were communication failures, inadequate orientation or training of staff, inaccurate patient assessment, staffing issues, and unavailable information (Figure 19-3).

JCAHO's *Sentinel Event Alert* newsletter contains information learned from the reporting program and recommendations for reducing the risk of similar events.[40] Topics covered in the *Alert* have included removing concentrated potassium chloride vials from patient care units,[41] recognizing and safeguarding high-alert medications,[42] eliminating infusion pumps without free-flow protection,[43] reducing errors with look-alike and sound-alike medication names,[44] prohibiting error-prone abbreviations,[45] avoiding patient-controlled analgesia by proxy,[46] and preventing intrathecal vincristine administration.[47] JCAHO also uses aggregate data on root causes and risk reduction strategies for frequently occurring sentinel events in its development of NPSGs and related standards.[40,48]

Some events of the types publicized in the *Sentinel Event Alert* or addressed in NPSGs have decreased as a percentage of all sentinel events[39]—most notably, events related to

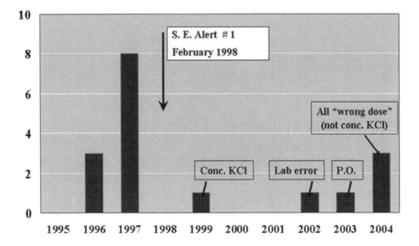

FIGURE 19-4   Sentinel events involving concentrated potassium chloride for injection. Reprinted with permission from the Joint Commission on Accreditation of Healthcare Organizations.

the appropriate storage and handling of concentrated potassium chloride for injection.[49] Eight deaths related to this product were reported in 1997; from 2000 to the present, none have been reported (Figure 19-4). It is important to remember that these numbers reflect reported sentinel events and most likely represent a small fraction of all such events occurring in health care organizations. Still, the data support sharing lessons learned from sentinel events as a way of reducing such events. Compliance rates have also risen steadily for processes related to the NPSGs.[39]

USP MEDMARX

USP's MEDMARX system allows subscribing hospitals and health systems to upload data from their internal reports of medication hazards, errors, and adverse drug reactions; track their own data for quality improvement purposes; and learn about errors reported by other facilities.[50] Reporting to this Internet-based system, launched in 1998, is anonymous and standardized.

Standardized MEDMARX definitions allow data to be aggregated for comparison with demographically similar facilities.[51] Identifying the source of MEDMARX reports is not possible, although USP program administrators can use a coded e-mail notification system to contact the reporting health system for additional information about a hazard or event.[52] Facilities pay an annual licensing fee to use MEDMARX. As of 2005, there were about 800 subscribing facilities.[50] ISMP does not have access to the MEDMARX database but periodically receives reports on the data from USP staff upon request.

USP's Center for the Advancement of Patient Safety (CAPS) analyzes the MEDMARX data for the purpose of developing educational programs and products focused on reporting, understanding, and preventing errors.[50] CAPS uses MEDMARX findings and other sources to propose standards, guidelines, and recommendations for improving medication use and advancing public health.

Since 2001, USP has published annual reports of aggregate MEDMARX data that include the types of errors, causes, contributing factors, products involved, and actions taken.[53] (See Appendix B for topics featured in the annual reports.) Several other USP publications disseminate information from MEDMARX and MERP.[54] The monthly *CAPSLink* electronic newsletter provides brief summaries of safety-related news, with hyperlinks for additional information; each issue contains MEDMARX and MERP findings related to a particular problem. The quarterly *USP Quality Review* newsletter provides analysis and recommendations based on reports to MEDMARX and MERP. *Practitioner's Reporting News* provides periodic summaries of reported data on specific topics.

Veterans Affairs Patient Safety Reporting System

All staff in Department of Veterans Affairs (VA) medical facilities are invited to voluntarily report events or concerns, including those about medication hazards and errors, to the VA's external Patient Safety Reporting System (PSRS), which was established in 2002.[55] Reports are submitted by U.S. Mail; a standardized form collects narrative descriptions of the event or safety problem. PSRS does not replace the VA health system's internal reporting system; it is an independent, complementary system for identifying safety vulnerabilities that VA staff may not feel comfortable reporting to the internal system.[56,57]

PSRS is the most striking example of a health care system's adoption of the aviation industry model of safety reporting.[10] The VA entered an agreement with the National Aeronautics and Space Administration (NASA) in 2000 to jointly develop, and then independently run, the reporting program, thereby applying 30 years of experience with NASA's successful Aviation Safety Reporting System (ASRS).[55]

The guiding principles of PSRS are voluntary participation, confidentiality protection, and nonpunitive reporting. Reports are considered confidential and privileged quality assurance documents under NASA's control and are fully protected under federal statutes (Title 38 United States Code 5705).[55] No disciplinary action is taken related to any reported patient safety issue. Events involving criminal actions, purposefully unsafe acts, and alleged or suspected patient abuse are not considered protected information or immune from disciplinary action; reports of such events are not accepted by PSRS. Reporters are encouraged to include identifying information so that they can be contacted if additional information is needed about the causes of the event. However, once a report is deemed complete, the record is stripped of all identifying information, including the names and locations of the reporter and persons involved in the event.[57]

In the program's first 2½ years of operation, 400 reports were received—a small number compared with the 140,000 reports submitted to the VA's internal reporting system in its first 5 years.[57] The number may be small because not all employees are familiar with the program.[10] However, PSRS may be viewed as a gauge of how well the internal reporting system is working.[57] The internal system, which is also confidential and nonpunitive, appears to have a high level of trust,[56,58] which may lessen the frequency of reporting to PSRS.

When reports are filed with PSRS, a team of trained NASA patient safety experts, including physicians, nurses, and a pharmacist, categorize them and determine their value for identifying safety vulnerabilities in systems and procedures.[57] Reporters are contacted for additional information that may be needed to understand the safety issue. The NASA team does not provide detailed solutions to the safety issues, in contrast to the root cause analysis performed on internally reported events.[55]

If an alarming trend is identified, VA facilities are immediately alerted to the safety problem through systemwide distribution of a patient safety bulletin, which does not identify the source of the problem. In its first 2 years, PSRS issued 10 such bulletins, which were not disseminated outside the VA health system.[57] Other safety trends and excerpts of actual reports are disseminated in a quarterly newsletter, *Feedback*, similar to the ASRS monthly *Callback*. The most frequently discussed problems related to medication safety—dispensing and administration safety hazards and wrong doses—were covered in the spring 2005 issue.[59] In 2002 through 2005, the newsletter covered hazards in prescribing controlled substances, accidental administration of repeat doses, dispensing errors and reporters' suggestions for prevention, allergies to contrast media, look-alike and spelled-alike drug names, and dosing errors with decimal points. The newsletter is publicly available on the PSRS Web site (http://psrs.arc.nasa.gov/).[55]

PSRS reports have been combined with reports from the VA's internal reporting system and root cause analysis program to verify, better understand, and prioritize patient safety issues and determine appropriate actions.[57] PSRS findings might also be used to conduct further research.

DISCLOSURE OF ERROR REPORTS

Public Disclosure

Health care providers have a clear moral and ethical obligation to disclose medical errors promptly to the patients and families who are victims of errors (see Chapter 20). However, public disclosure of medical errors and information uncovered during their investigation is widely debated. Three-fourths of Americans believe health care providers should be required to divulge this information publicly.[3,6,60] Some believe public disclosure is necessary to drive improvements.[3,19] Others think widespread public disclosure of specific adverse events would drive error reporting underground, weakening patient safety efforts.[17]

There is an appropriate place for public disclosure of patient safety issues. The public has a right to expect health care organizations to respond to evidence of safety hazards by taking whatever steps are necessary to make potential errors difficult or impossible to commit.[6] The public also has a right to be informed about unsafe conditions, and a right to expect companies that produce medical devices, pharmaceutical products, health care computer systems, and related products and services to do their part in error-proofing health care. Providers and companies should be held accountable for implementing safety strategies that grow out of expert analysis of reported adverse events and scientific research.

Accountability may not require the release of all patient safety information, but the public wants evidence that health care providers are putting patient safety first.[3] Reporting systems should not have the power to mandate the implementation of recommendations arising from their analysis of adverse events. However, regulatory agencies, accrediting bodies, federal agencies, and health care purchasing groups should evaluate such recommendations and adopt them as standards if efficacy can be established and the cost benefit of adoption is favorable. If health care organizations and companies do not comply with safety standards adopted by accrediting and regulatory bodies or other oversight agencies, public disclosure should be considered so that consumers can make safer and more informed health care decisions.[17] Disclosure of an organization's compliance with safety standards is more useful to consumers making health care decisions than is disclosure of sentinel events. An alternative to disclosing compliance is an annual report summarizing events and actions taken, like the reports issued by some state reporting programs.[3,19] These approaches would provide the public with evidence of accountability for medical errors.

Legal Disclosure

Reporting errors can have adverse consequences for the reporter. Reporting systems that incorporate incentives and safeguards are likely to be perceived as trustworthy and to receive more and better data. One of the greatest incentives for reporting is the offer of confidentiality and evidentiary protection for the information submitted.[17]

Most states have some level of legal protection for information submitted to internal reporting programs operated for quality improvement purposes.[61] However, the absence of federal protection of error reports and other patient safety data has discouraged the submission of information to external reporting programs and to safety experts such as ISMP.[17] Furthermore, protections offered by state statutes may be waived if information is shared outside the quality assurance processes of a health care organization.

Many safety experts, including ISMP, have long held that information developed in connection with external reporting systems should be privileged for purposes of federal and state judicial proceedings in civil matters, and for purposes of federal and state administrative proceedings, including with respect to discovery, subpoenas, testimony, or any other form of disclosure.[62] IOM's *To Err Is Human* report[6] recommended federal legislation to extend this protection to patient safety and quality data collected and analyzed by health care organizations for internal use or shared with others for purposes of improving safety and quality.

Prompted by this IOM recommendation and advocacy efforts by national safety experts, Congress enacted the Patient Safety and Quality Improvement Act of 2005 to encourage greater participation in external medical (and medication) error reporting systems.[63] The act calls for the establishment of certified, independent patient safety organizations (PSOs) that would receive confidential data such as error reports, analyze the data, and disseminate recommendations for reducing risk. Work is under way to define the certification process for PSOs. Information received by PSOs cannot be used as evidence in civil or administrative legal proceedings. The elimination of this legal barrier is expected to create a more favorable environment for reporting safety hazards and errors; the act lessens the threat of litigation without compromising patients' rights to legal remedies in the event of a harmful error.

PRACTITIONERS' PERSPECTIVES ON REPORTING

Responses to a 2002 ISMP survey by more than 300 staff-level clinicians (36% of the respondents), middle managers (48%), and administrators (16%) suggest that more effort is needed to promote voluntary reporting to both internal and external programs.[64] Nearly two-thirds of the respondents (64%) were pharmacists; 32% were nurses, 3% were physicians, and 1% were pharmacy technicians. As expected, respondents reported safety issues more frequently to internal than to external programs (Table 19-7). Just 1 in 10 respondents reported to MERP in 2002.

The types of reports most frequently submitted differed between internal and external programs. The events most frequently reported to internal programs were medication errors that did not reach patients or those that reached patients but caused no harm. Hazardous conditions that could cause errors were reported infrequently to internal programs but were the issue most frequently reported to MERP. Harmful errors were more often reported to internal than to external programs. Half of the respondents had reported at least one harmful error within their organization, but only 1 in 10 had reported a harmful error to MERP or MedWatch. Adverse drug reactions were reported frequently to internal programs and far less frequently to MedWatch (Table 19-7); this suggests that the MedWatch database may lack crucial postmarketing surveillance data.

Nine in 10 survey respondents said they were motivated to report errors to internal and external programs by the belief that the information would be used to enhance patient safety (Table 19-8). Similar percentages of respondents cited avoiding needless tragedies as a reason for reporting to internal programs and to MERP; far fewer cited this reason for reporting to MedWatch. About half of the respondents felt rewarded for reporting to

TABLE 19-7 Percentages of Survey Respondents Who Reported Medication Errors or Patient Safety Issues[64]

| Type of Error or Other Safety Issue | Frequency of Reporting to Each Program (0, 1–5, or >5 Reports) | | | | | | | | |
| | Internal Systemwide | | | ISMP-USP MERP (external) | | | FDA MedWatch (external) | | |
	0	1–5	>5	0	1–5	>5	0	1–5	>5
Adverse drug reaction	25	31	44	82	15	3	57	36	7
Hazardous condition that could lead to error	25	44	31	80	18	2	88	11	1
Error that did not reach patient	20	33	47	88	10	2	95	4	0
Error that reached patient but caused no harm	21	34	44	88	11	2	93	6	0
Error that caused patient harm	50	35	15	88	10	2	86	14	1

ISMP = Institute for Safe Medication Practices; USP = United States Pharmacopeia; MERP = Medication Errors Reporting Program; FDA = Food and Drug Administration.

TABLE 19-8 Motivations for Reporting Medication Errors and Safety Issues[64,a]

| Motivational Factor | Reporting Program | | |
	Internal Systemwide	ISMP-USP MERP (external)	FDA MedWatch (external)
My superior mandates that I report.	71	25	30
I'm granted amnesty if I report an error.	49	38	40
I feel rewarded for reporting.	53	58	49
The information is used to enhance safety.	95	90	89
I want others to know about the problem so needless tragedies can be prevented.	98	91	50
The reporting program is easy to use.	72	67	61
I trust that my name will be kept confidential.	65	77	71

ISMP = Institute for Safe Medication Practices; USP = United States Pharmacopeia; MERP = Medication Errors Reporting Program; FDA = Food and Drug Administration.

[a] Percentages of respondents who said they were motivated by each factor.

MERP, and fewer for reporting to internal programs or MedWatch. More must be done to reward clinicians for voluntary reporting. Compared with internal programs and MedWatch, a greater percentage of respondents (77%) trusted that their names would remain confidential when reporting to MERP.

Although the respondents noted more promotion of internal than of external reporting (Table 19-9), the results indicated insufficient promotion of all reporting programs. Only two-thirds of respondents said accrediting bodies, risk managers, and quality improvement staff frequently promoted internal reporting; fewer said middle managers and staff educators did so. Organizational trustees or senior leaders were among the least likely to encourage staff to report errors internally. Thirty-nine percent of respondents cited frequent promotion of reporting to MERP by professional organizations and professional publications and newsletters. More than half of the respondents said their middle managers, professional licensing bodies, risk managers, and quality improvement staff had never promoted reporting to MERP. Medical and drug product vendors, staff and academic educators, government agencies, and trustees and senior leaders were the least likely to promote reporting to MERP.

TABLE 19-9 Percentages of Survey Respondents Who Observed Promotion of Reporting[64]

Entity Observed Promoting Reporting	Frequency of Promotion of Reporting Program[a]								
	Internal Systemwide			ISMP-USP MERP (external)			FDA MedWatch (external)		
	F	S	N	F	S	N	F	S	N
Trustees/senior leaders	30	39	31	17	20	63	11	26	63
Middle managers	47	42	11	14	28	57	11	29	60
Risk manager	60	22	18	20	22	58	16	25	60
Quality improvement professional	60	21	18	18	27	55	16	24	60
Patient/medication safety officer	57	20	22	20	27	53	16	29	55
Staff educators	39	33	27	11	18	71	8	20	72
Professional licensing bodies	30	33	37	16	28	56	16	28	56
Professional organizations	50	28	22	39	29	32	35	30	35
Professional journals/newsletters	58	26	16	39	27	35	36	36	28
Local/federal government	22	35	43	10	29	61	10	32	58
Accrediting bodies	62	20	18	34	28	38	35	26	39
Academic educators	20	34	46	13	18	69	13	21	67
Drug/medical product vendors	10	35	55	6	21	72	9	22	70

ISMP = Institute for Safe Medication Practices; USP = United States Pharmacopeia; MERP = Medication Errors Reporting Program; FDA = Food and Drug Administration.

[a] F = frequently; S = sometimes; N = never.

MedWatch was promoted less frequently than the other reporting programs. One in three respondents had frequently witnessed ongoing promotion of MedWatch by accrediting bodies, professional publications and newsletters, and professional organizations. Local and federal government agencies were among the least frequent entities to promote this government-run program, closely followed by staff and academic educators, medical and drug product vendors, and middle managers.

The survey results suggest that stakeholders in patient safety must take more time to encourage frontline practitioners to report issues to internal and external programs. Legal impediments are probably one reason clinicians are infrequently encouraged to voluntarily report errors, especially harmful ones, to external programs. The 2005 legislation protecting this information from disclosure may lead to an increase in reporting and thus to greater knowledge about medication errors. The lack of encouragement for reporting noted in the survey may reflect limited knowledge of voluntary external reporting programs, especially among academic and staff educators, trustees and senior leaders, middle managers, and professional licensing boards. This is particularly unsettling, since these individuals are often in the best position to influence public policy, mentor clinicians, and ensure that future generations of practitioners understand the value of internal and external voluntary error reporting programs. The 2006 IOM report[9] recommends that error reporting be promoted more aggressively by all stakeholders and that a national taxonomy be used for data storage and analysis so the information can be aggregated and used to shape health policy at the national level.

CONCLUSION

Voluntary reporting systems have been useful for gaining new information about preventable adverse events, analyzing the data, understanding the causation of errors, and sharing that knowledge. It is up to the health care community to use the knowledge to enhance patient safety, and some organizations are doing so. However, some have lacked the necessary leadership, attention, and resources for the task.

TABLE 19-10 Comparison of Characteristics of External Error-Reporting Systems

Attributes of Successful External Error-Reporting Systems	JCAHO Sentinel Event Reporting System	FDA MedWatch	ISMP-USP Medication Errors Reporting Program	USP MEDMARX	VA Patient Safety Reporting System	Pennsylvania Patient Safety Reporting System
National: The reporting system is national in scope and participation.	X	X	X	X		
Voluntary: Participants are not required to report to the system.		X	X	X	X	
Unrestricted: The system encourages unrestricted reporting within the program specialty (e.g., anesthesia, medical devices, medications) of serious and fatal events caused by error, near misses, and hazardous conditions that could lead to error.		X	X	X	X	X
Confidential: The identities of the patient, reporter, and organization are never revealed to a third party without permission.		X	X	X	X	
Nonpunitive: Reporters do not fear retaliation or punishment from others as a result of reporting.		X	X	X	X	
Practitioner-based: The system receives reports firsthand from practitioners involved in errors or working under hazardous conditions.		X	X		X	
Easy to use: Reporters do not find the reporting process cumbersome.		X	X	X	X	X
Free to use: Reporting to the system requires no fee.	X[a]	X	X		X	
Receives causal information: The program receives adequate information from reporters about the underlying causes of errors and allows program staff to follow up directly with reporters if questions arise during analysis.	X		X	X[b]	X	X[b]
Independent: The reporting system is independent of regulatory, accrediting, or other bodies with the power to enforce change or punish the reporter or organization.			X	X		
Objective: The reporting system is objective regarding findings and recommendations.	X	X	X	X	X	X

Attribute							
Credible: Reports are analyzed by safety experts who understand the clinical setting and who are trained to recognize underlying systems causes.	X	X	X	X	X	X	X
Systems-oriented: Recommendations focus on proven safety practices that target changes in systems, processes, or products, rather than on individual performance.	X	X	X	X	X	X	X
Timely: Reports are analyzed promptly, and recommendations are rapidly disseminated to those who need to know, especially when serious hazards are identified.	X	X		X	X	X	X
Responsive: The agency that receives reports is capable of disseminating recommendations, and	X	X	X	X	X	X	X
Participating organizations attempt to implement recommendations when possible (i.e., the organizational culture supports this).	X	X	X	X	X	X	X
Motivating: The agency that receives reports provides positive incentives for reporting.			X		X	X	
Supported: The program has the (nonfinancial) support of the health care community it targets.	X	X	X	X	X	X	X
Funded: The program is adequately funded to achieve the above attributes.	X	X	X		X	X	X
Offer protection: The program offers evidentiary protection for the error and safety information reported to it.	X	X	X	X	X	X	X
Fosters collaboration: The system fosters confidential collaboration with other health care reporting systems.	X	X	X	X	X		X

JCAHO = Joint Commission on Accreditation of Healthcare Organizations; FDA = Food and Drug Administration; ISMP = Institution for Safe Medication Practices; USP = United States Pharmacopeia; VA = Department of Veterans Affairs.

[a] Accreditation fees apply but are not directly related to reporting.
[b] Partial.

Source: References 1, 3, 17, 62, 65, 66.

The missing link in improving patient safety is widespread adoption of proven error reduction strategies identified through internal analysis of adverse events, external analysis of voluntarily submitted reports, and scientific research.[17] JCAHO's creation of NPSGs holds promise for gaining compliance with safety recommendations, many stemming from voluntary reporting systems. The adoption of a similar approach by state departments of health, professional boards, professional residency program accreditors, and other regulatory agencies could further capitalize on what is learned through voluntary reporting systems.

Table 19-10 presents characteristics identified by patient safety experts as essential for a successful reporting program.[1,3,17,62,65,66] The table indicates which characteristics the reporting programs described in this chapter possess. Programs that strive for these characteristics have the best chance of improving patient safety.

REFERENCES

1. Cohen MR. Why error reporting systems should be voluntary [editorial]. *BMJ*. 2000;320;728–9.
2. Institute for Safe Medication Practices. *Mosby's Nursing PDQ for Medication Safety*. St Louis: Mosby; 2005.
3. Leape LL. Reporting adverse events. *N Engl J Med*. 2002;347:1633–8.
4. Cousins DD, Calnan R. Medication error reporting systems. In: Cohen MR, ed. *Medication Errors*. Sudbury, Mass: Jones and Bartlett; 1999:18.1–18.20.
5. American Hospital Association. Improving care & increasing affordability. Available at: www.aha.org/aha/annual_meeting/content/05_qualitypatientsafety.pdf. Accessed August 31, 2005.
6. Kohn LT, Corrigan JM, Donaldson MS, eds. *To Err Is Human: Building a Safer Health System*. Washington, DC: National Academies Press; 2000.
7. Leape LL, Lawthers AG, Brennan TA, et al. Preventing medical injury. *Qual Rev Bull*. 1993;19:144–9.
8. National Coordinating Council for Medication Error Reporting and Prevention. What is a medication error? Available at: www.nccmerp.org/aboutMedErrors.html. Accessed July 19, 2005.
9. Committee on Identifying and Preventing Medication Errors; Aspden P, Wolcott J, Bootman JL, et al., eds. *Preventing Medication Errors*. Washington, DC: National Academies Press; 2006. Prepublication copy available at http://darwin.nap.edu/books/0309101476/html/R2.html. Accessed July 21, 2006.
10. Sinco P. Air course one. What medicine can learn from aviation safety. *The DO*. April 2004:34–42.
11. ECRI. Event reporting. *Issues in Continuing Care Risk Management*. March 2001:1–10.
12. Jeffe DB, Dunagan WC, Garbutt MB, et al. Using focus groups to understand physicians' and nurses' perspectives on error reporting in hospitals. *Jt Comm J Qual Saf*. 2004;30:471–9.
13. Health care initiatives in hospital risk management. Report to the Honorable Ron Wyden, U.S. House of Representatives. Washington, DC: General Accounting Office; July 1989.
14. National Coordinating Council for Medication Error Reporting and Prevention. Types of medication errors. Available at: www.nccmerp.org/medErrorCatIndex.html. Accessed July 20, 2005.
15. Pear R. Experts cast doubt on medical reporting plan. *New York Times*. February 23, 2000:A-12.
16. Kaufman M. Clinton seeks medical error reports: proposal to reduce mistakes includes mandatory disclosure, lawsuit shield. *Washington Post*. February 22, 2000:A2.
17. Institute for Safe Medication Practices. Discussion paper on adverse event and error reporting in healthcare. January 24, 2000. Available at: www.ismp.org/Tools/whitepapers/concept.asp.
18. Billings C. Presentation to Subcommittee on Creating an External Environment for Quality Healthcare. Jan 29, 1999.
19. Rosenthal J, Booth M, Flowers L, et al. Current state programs addressing medical errors: an analysis of mandatory reporting and other initiatives. Portland, Me: National Academy for State Health Policy; January 2001.
20. New York Patient Occurrence Reporting and Tracking System: annual report 2000/2001. Albany: New York State Department of Health; 2003. Available at: www.health.state.ny.us/nysdoh/hospital/nyports/annual_report/2000-2001/annual_report.htm. Accessed August 31, 2005.
21. Rebinowitz A. Personal communication to ISMP. October 25, 2005.
22. Patient Safety Authority 2004 annual report. April 24, 2005. Available at: www.psa.state.pa.us/psa/lib/psa/annual_reports/psa_annual_report_for_2004_-_final_elec_version.pdf. Accessed August 31, 2005.
23. Rosenthal J, Booth M. The Flood Tide forum. State patient safety centers: a new approach to promote patient safety. October 8, 2004. Portland, Me: National Academy for State Health Policy. Available at: www.nashp.org/Files/final_web_report_11.01.04.pdf. Accessed October 24, 2005.

24. Center for Consumer Health Care Information–Patient Safety Center. DOH initiatives. Available at: www.health.state.ny.us/nysdoh/healthinfo/pscdohi.htm. Accessed October 24, 2005.

25. Patient Safety Authority. Risk of overdose from multiple transdermal patches. *Patient Safety Advisory.* September 2004;1(3):11. Available at: www.psa.state.pa.us/psa/lib/psa/advisories/sept_2004_advisory_v1_n3.pdf. Accessed October 27, 2005.

26. Patient Safety Authority. Overdoses caused by confusion between insulin and tuberculin syringes. *Patient Safety Advisory–Supplementary Advisory.* 2004;1 (Suppl 1). Available at: www.psa.state.pa.us/psa/lib/psa/advisories/pa-psrs_supplementary_advisory_v1_s1.pdf. Accessed October 27, 2005.

27. Patient Safety Authority. Medications linked to drug name confusion. *Patient Safety Advisory.* 2004;1(4):7. Available at: www.psa.state.pa.us/psa/lib/psa/advisories/dec_2004_advisory_v1_n4.pdf. Accessed October 27, 2005.

28. Patient Safety Authority. Drug name suffix confusion is a constant source of errors. *Patient Safety Advisory.* 2004;1(4):17. Available at: www.psa.state.pa.us/psa/lib/psa/advisories/dec_2004_advisory_v1_n4.pdf. Accessed October 27, 2005.

29. Patient Safety Authority. Focus on high-alert medications. *Patient Safety Advisory.* 2004;1(3):6. Available at: www.psa.state.pa.us/psa/lib/psa/advisories/sept_2004_advisory_v1_n3.pdf. Accessed October 27, 2005.

30. World Alliance for Patient Safety. *WHO Draft Guidelines for Adverse Event Reporting and Learning Systems: From Information to Action.* Geneva: World Health Organization; 2005.

31. Institute for Safe Medication Practices. Your "lessons learned" now heard by over 3.5 million! *ISMP Medication Safety Alert!* 2004;9(19):3.

32. Food and Drug Administration. MedWatch online voluntary reporting form (3500). July 6, 2005. Available at: https://www.accessdata.fda.gov/scripts/medwatch/. Accessed September 1, 2005.

33. Zhou W, Pool V, Iskander JK, et al. Surveillance for safety after immunization: Vaccine Adverse Event Reporting System (VAERS)—United States, 1991–2001. *MMWR.* 2003;52(SS-01):1–24.

34. Goldman SA, Kennedy DL. MedWatch: FDA's Medical Products Reporting Program, a joint effort toward improved public health. *Postgrad Med.* 1998;103(3):13–26. Available at: www.postgradmed.com/issues/1998/03_98/edmar98.htm.

35. Food and Drug Administration, Center for Drug Evaluation and Research (CDER). CDER report to the nation: 2004. August 22, 2005. Available at: www.fda.gov/cder/reports/rtn/2004/rtn2004-3.htm#Highlights. Accessed September 1, 2005.

36. Center for Drug Evaluation and Research (CDER). Medication errors. April 26, 2005. Available at: www.fda.gov/cder/drug/MedErrors/default.htm. Accessed September 1, 2005.

37. Joint Commission on Accreditation of Healthcare Organizations. Sentinel event. Available at: www.jointcommission.org/SentinelEvents/. Accessed June 23,2006.

38. Joint Commission on Accreditation of Healthcare Organizations. Sentinel event policy and procedures. Available at: www.jointcommission.org/SentinelEvents/PolicyandProcedures/se_pp.htm. Accessed June 23, 2006.

39. Joint Commission on Accreditation of Healthcare Organizations. Sentinel event statistics—December 31, 2005. Available at: www.jointcommission.org/SentinelEvents/Statistics/. Accessed June 23, 2006.

40. Joint Commission on Accreditation of Healthcare Organizations. Sentinel Event Alert. Available at: www.jointcommission.org/SentinelEvents/SentinelEventAlert/. Accessed June 23, 2006.

41. Joint Commission on Accreditation of Healthcare Organizations. Sentinel Event Alert. Medication error prevention—potassium chloride. February 27, 1998. Available at: www.jointcommission.org/SentinelEvents/SentinelEventAlert/sea_1.htm. Accessed June 23, 2006.

42. Joint Commission on Accreditation of Healthcare Organizations. Sentinel Event Alert. High-alert medications and patient safety. November 19, 1999. Available at: www.jointcommission.org/SentinelEvents/SentinelEventAlert/sea_11.htm. Accessed June 23, 2006.

43. Joint Commission on Accreditation of Healthcare Organizations. Sentinel Event Alert. Infusion pumps: preventing future adverse events. November 30, 2000. Available at: www.jointcommission.org/SentinelEvents/SentinelEventAlert/sea_15.htm. Accessed June 23, 2006.

44. Joint Commission on Accreditation of Healthcare Organizations. Sentinel Event Alert. Look-alike, sound-alike drug names. May 2001. Available at: www.jointcommission.org/SentinelEvents/SentinelEventAlert/sea_19.htm. Accessed June 23, 2006.

45. Joint Commission on Accreditation of Healthcare Organizations. Sentinel Event Alert. Medication errors related to potentially dangerous abbreviations. September 2001. Available at: www.jointcommission.org/SentinelEvents/SentinelEventAlert/sea_23.htm. Accessed June 23, 2006.

46. Joint Commission on Accreditation of Healthcare Organizations. Sentinel Event Alert. Patient controlled analgesia by proxy. December 20, 2004. Available at: www.jointcommission.org/SentinelEvents/SentinelEventAlert/sea_33.htm. Accessed June 23, 2006.

47. Joint Commission on Accreditation of Healthcare Organizations. Sentinel Event Alert. Preventing vincristine administration errors. July 14, 2005. Available at: www.jointcommission.org/SentinelEvents/SentinelEventAlert/sea_34.htm. Accessed June 23, 2006.

48. Joint Commission on Accreditation of Healthcare Organizations. Introduction to National Patient Safety Goals. Available at: www.jointcommission.org/PatientSafety/NationalPatientSafetyGoals/npsg_intro.htm. Accessed June 23, 2006.

49. Joint Commission on Accreditation of Healthcare Organizations. Sentinel Event Alert. Making an impact on healthcare. April 21, 2000. Available at: www.jointcommission.org/SentinelEvents/SentinelEventAlert/sea_13.htm. Accessed June 23, 2006.

50. Cousins D. Personal communication to Judy Smetzer. September 8, 2005.

51. Santell JP, Cousins D. Documenting and reducing medication errors. *US Pharm.* 2003;28:07. Available at: www.uspharmacist.com/index.asp?show=article&page=8_1120.htm.

52. United States Pharmacopeial Convention, Inc. MEDMARX features and benefits. Available at: www.usp.org/patientSafety/MEDMARX/featuresBens.html. Accessed September 21, 2005.

53. United States Pharmacopeial Convention, Inc. MEDMARX data reports product information. Available at: www.usp.org/products/MEDMARX/. Accessed September 21, 2005.

54. United States Pharmacopeial Convention, Inc. Patient safety newsletters. Available at: www.usp.org/patientSafety/newsletters/. Accessed September 21, 2005.

55. Patient Safety Reporting System. Available at: http://psrs.arc.nasa.gov/. Last updated March 9, 2006.

56. Mears D. James P. Bagian on patient safety initiatives. *J Healthc Qual.* 2002;24:15–16, 24.

57. The Commonwealth Fund. Case study: NASA/VA Patient Safety Reporting System. October 2004. Available at: www.cmwf.org/tools/tools_show.htm?doc_id=257033.

58. Bagian JP, Lee C, Gosbee J, et al. Developing and deploying a patient safety program in a large health care delivery system: you can't fix what you don't know about. *Jt Comm J Qual Improv.* 2001;27:522–32.

59. National Aeronautics and Space Administration. Exercising the "rights." *Patient Safety Feedback.* Spring 2005;3(4):1. Available at: http://psrs.arc.nasa.gov/web_docs/Feedback_v3_4.pdf. Accessed October 17, 2005.

60. Kaiser Family Foundation. National survey on Americans as health care consumers. Washington, DC: Agency for Healthcare Research and Quality; December 2000.

61. Flowers L, Riley T. State-based mandatory reporting of medical errors: an analysis of the legal and policy issues. Portland, Me: National Academy for State Health Policy; March 2001.

62. National Coordinating Council on Medication Error Reporting and Prevention (NCCMERP). NCC MERP supports principles for patient safety reporting programs [press release]. November 25, 2003. Available at: www.nccmerp.org/press/press2003-11-25.html. Accessed August 10, 2005.

63. Agency for Healthcare Research and Quality. The Patient Safety and Quality Improvement Act of 2005. Available at: www.ahrq.gov/qual/psoact.htm. Accessed June 20, 2006.

64. Institute for Safe Medication Practices (ISMP). Reports are in, or are they? Awareness of medication error reporting programs needs boost. *ISMP Medication Safety Alert!* February 6, 2003;8(3).

65. Connell L. Statement before the Subcommittee on Oversight and Investigations, Committee on Veterans Affairs. Washington, DC: U.S. House of Representatives; 2000.

66. Gaynes R, Richards C, Edwards J, et al. Feeding back surveillance data to prevent hospital-acquired infections. *Emerg Infect Dis.* 2001;7:295–8.

APPENDIX A

IMPACT OF UNITED STATES PHARMACOPEIA (USP)–INSTITUTE FOR SAFE MEDICATION PRACTICES (ISMP) MEDICATION ERRORS REPORTING PROGRAM (MERP)

1. Early warning system

ISMP issues nationwide hazard alerts and press releases based on reports to MERP.

- Fatal events involving concentrated electrolytes (1996)
- Fatal errors due to mix-ups between lipid-based and conventional products (1998)
- Fatal dosing errors stemming from confusion about labeling of Cerebyx (fosphenytoin) containers (leads to label changes) (1998)
- Methotrexate overdoses due to inadvertent administration daily instead of weekly (2002)
- Call for nationwide replacement of Brethine (terbutaline) ampuls with vials to avoid potentially fatal mix-ups with look-alike ampuls of Methergine (methylergonovine) (2004)

- Risk of acetaminophen overdoses in children if parents or health care providers fail to recognize that different dosage strengths are available (2003)
- Dangerous practice of "PCA by proxy" and other risks associated with patient-controlled analgesia (PCA) (2003)
- Call for definitive action by the Food and Drug Administration (FDA) and manufacturers on long-standing labeling and packaging problems that have led to serious errors (e.g., look-alike vaccine packaging, look-alike low-density polyethylene containers, concentrated liquid morphine without a prominent warning) (2004)
- Fatal misconnections between IV ports and blood pressure device hoses, air supply hoses, oxygen tubing, and other forms of medical tubing (2004)
- Risk of methemoglobinemia associated with benzocaine spray products (2004)
- Fatal overdosages from transdermal fentanyl patches (2005)
- Use of same brand name for different drugs in different countries, causing harm in some cases (2005)

2. Learning

ISMP disseminates information on error-prone trends identified through MERP, with strategies for error reduction.

- Published first list of error-prone drug abbreviations identified from error reports (1987)[1]
- Published first mention in medical literature of dangers of free-flow infusion pumps (1992)[2]
- Published first scholarly article on application of failure mode and effects analysis in health care[3]
- Published nation's first high-alert drug list, based on surveys and error reports (1998)[4]
- Launched biweekly *ISMP Medication Safety Alert!* newsletter to share (blinded) error stories and error-reduction strategies (1996); three additional newsletters launched for nurses, community pharmacy, and consumers (2002–2003)
- Disseminated first ISMP Medication Safety Self Assessment for Hospitals (2001)[5] and follow-up self-assessment (2004), derived in large part from analysis of error reports to MERP
- Launched first certificate program in medication safety, offered as part of Temple University's Doctor of Pharmacy program, using blinded error reports to teach students (2000)

3. Change

ISMP successfully advocates changes in packaging, labeling, and nomenclature based on analysis of error reports.

- Convened a national meeting that resulted in a federal requirement for black caps and closures and warning statements on potassium chloride concentrate for injection to prevent confusion with other injectable drugs (1987)
- Influenced an update of USP standards to require special warning labels on vincristine about fatal intrathecal administration (1991)
- Advocacy led to required maximum dose statement on cisplatin vial caps and seals (1997)
- Filed a petition with the United States Adopted Names Council that led to renaming amrinone as inamrinone to prevent further confusion with amiodarone (2000)
- Influenced Eli Lilly and Company to revise its labels on Zyprexa (olanzapine) containers using tall-man letters to help prevent further mix-ups with Zyrtec (cetirizine) containers (2003)
- Influenced Abbott Laboratories to revise the background colors on labetalol injection vials and cartons to prevent further mix-ups with Dopram vials from ESI Lederle (2003)
- Influenced Abbott Laboratories Hospital Products Division to revise labels of its pre-mixed lidocaine product to give it a unique appearance and to print important information on both sides of the IV overwrap (2003)

- Influenced BD Medical Systems to remove tip caps on its hypodermic syringes to eliminate the risk of accidental choking if used, against the manufacturer's advice, for oral liquid medications (2003)
- Advocacy led to a revised label on Mayne Pharma's hydromorphone vials so it is clear that only 1 mL (2 mg) is available in the 2 mL size vials (2005)
- Influenced McNeil Consumer & Specialty Pharmaceuticals to recall several Tylenol (acetaminophen) products because of confusing labels that could lead to dosing errors (2005)
- Influenced Janssen to change the brand name of Reminyl (galantamine hydrobromide) to Razadyne to prevent further mix-ups with Amaryl (glimepiride) (2005)

4. Standards

ISMP advocates national guidelines, standards, and goals based on analysis of reported errors.

- Convened a national forum on preventing harmful and fatal chemotherapy errors (1995); recommendations were later published (1996)[6]
- Began a formal campaign that spurred the Veterans Health Administration and the Joint Commission on Accreditation of Healthcare Organizations (JCAHO) to urge removal of potassium chloride concentrate for injection from all patient care areas (1997)
- Prepared test cases of medication safety alerts for computerized prescriber order entry, based on reported errors; these are used in efforts by First Consulting Group and Leapfrog Group to improve medical quality, safety, and outcomes (1999)
- Spurred FDA to ask pharmaceutical companies to use tall-man lettering for labeling of 20 generic drug name pairs prone to confusion (2001)
- Issued, in conjunction with the Pediatric Pharmacy Advocacy Group, pediatric pharmacy medication safety guidelines (2002)
- JCAHO adopted recommendations from ISMP's list of error-prone medication abbreviations, symbols, and dose designations for use in its National Patient Safety Goals (NPSGs) (2002)
- JCAHO adopted for use in its NPSGs recommendations from ISMP's list of look-alike and sound-alike drug names, gathered from error reports, and related error-reduction strategies (2004)
- JCAHO adopted for use in its NPSGs ISMP's recommendation to prohibit use of infusion pumps without protection against accidental free-flow (2003); the goal was later retired after widespread compliance by accredited organizations (2006)
- JCAHO responded to repeated descriptions of errors related to unlabeled products on the sterile field by issuing an NPSG to help improve labeling practices (2006)

5. Public policy

ISMP advocates changes in public policy based on findings from MERP.

- Appeared on the first segment of the first Dateline show on ABC television to discuss fatal medication errors, bringing national attention to the issue (1992)
- Held the first Global Conference on Medication Error Reporting Programs with U.S. and international experts (1994)
- Partnered with the American Hospital Association (AHA) in a national initiative to improve medication safety; ISMP staff met with President Clinton and participated in White House press briefing to announce the national initiative (1999)
- Met with Senate and House staff, testified in Senate committee hearings, and presented a Senate staff briefing with AHA and the American Pharmaceutical Association (APhA) (1999); this, along with ongoing USP and ISMP advocacy, contributed to passage in 2005 of legislation offering evidentiary protection of patient safety data and error reports submitted to patient safety organizations (1999)
- Published a discussion paper on adverse event and error reporting in health care, which served as a conceptual model for error reporting position statements by leading health care organizations (2000)[7]

- Testified at an FDA public meeting, and issued a white paper, using findings from MERP to support the need for bar codes on unit dose packages of medications (2002)[8]

More information on MERP's impact, including organizational changes and individual practice changes that resulted from publication of blinded error reports and error-reduction strategies, can be found at www.ismp.org/about/MERPimpact.asp.

1. Cohen MR. Play it safe: don't use these abbreviations. *Nursing.* 1987;17(7):46–7.
2. Cohen MR, Davis NM. Free flow associated with electronic infusion devices: an underestimated danger. *Hosp Pharm.* 1992;27:384–90.
3. Cohen MR, Senders JD, Davis NM. Failure mode and effects analysis: a novel approach to avoiding dangerous medication errors and accidents. *Hosp Pharm.* 1994;29:319–24, 326–8, 330.
4. Cohen MR, Proulx SM, Crawford SY. Survey of hospital systems and common serious medication errors. *J Healthc Risk Manag.* 1998;18(1):16–27.
5. Smetzer JL, Vaida AJ, Cohen MR, et al. Findings from the ISMP Medication Safety Self Assessment for Hospitals. *Jt Com J Qual Saf.* 2003;29:586–97.
6. Cohen MR, Anderson RW, Attilio RM, et al. Preventing medication errors in cancer chemotherapy. *Am J Health Syst Pharm.* 1996;53:737–46.
7. Institute for Safe Medication Practices. Discussion paper on adverse event and error reporting in healthcare. Jan 24, 2000. Available at: www.ismp.org/Tools/whitepapers/concept.asp.
8. Institute for Safe Medication Practices. A call to action: safeguard drug administration within 2 years! Bar coding of unit doses can reduce medication errors. November 2002. Available at: www.ismp.org/MSAarticles/WhitepaperBarCodding.htm.

APPENDIX B

EXAMPLES OF FINDINGS FROM U.S. PHARMACOPEIA MEDMARX REPORTING SYSTEM, 1999–2004

1. Technology Errors[1]

- Nearly 20% of hospital and health-system medication errors involved computerization or automation, particularly computer entry, computerized prescriber order entry (CPOE), and automated dispensing devices (ADDs).
- Errors involving ADDs were the 10th leading type of error; 1.3% of those errors led to patient harm.
- Wrong dose errors were reported twice as often when associated with ADDs.
- Errors in computer entry were the fourth leading proximate cause of errors, representing about 12% of all errors.
- Most computer entry errors occurred in either the transcribing/documenting phase or the dispensing phase of medication use.
- Distractions were the leading contributory factor and were involved in more than half of the errors associated with computer entry.
- Facilities that had implemented CPOE reported fewer harmful errors.
- Dosing errors (extra dose, wrong dose, and omission) accounted for half of the CPOE errors.

2. High-Alert Medications[2]

- Eight of the 10 products most often involved in harmful medication errors are considered high-alert medications; errors with these eight products represented 35% of all harmful medication errors.

- The high-alert medications that have most frequently caused harm to hospitalized patients include insulin, morphine, heparin, potassium chloride, warfarin, and hydromorphone.

3. Errors in Specialty Populations[3,4]

- One-third of medication errors in hospitals involved geriatric patients.
- Nearly 10% of prescribing errors involving geriatric patients were harmful.
- The type of medication errors most harmful to older patients was administration by the wrong route, such as IV administration of tube feeding.
- Errors harm geriatric patients (3.5%) and pediatric patients (6%) more frequently than the general population (1.7%).
- Half of pediatric medication errors occurred during the administration phase.

4. Errors Related to Joint Commission on Accreditation of Healthcare Organizations National Patient Safety Goals[2]

- Misidentification or "wrong patient" errors contributed to 5% of errors and occurred in every phase of the medication-use process.
- Communication issues were the third leading proximate causes of errors.
- About 9% of errors involving infusion pumps resulted in harm.

5. Errors in Specialty Locations[5]

- The emergency department (ED) was the fifth leading location for medication errors.
- More than 5% of medication errors that occurred in the ED led to patient harm.
- Distractions were the leading contributing factor for medication errors that occurred in the ED.
- The most common drugs involved in harmful errors in the ED included heparin (8%), ceftriaxone (3%), insulin (3%), meperidine (2%), and levofloxacin (2%).

1. Computer entry a leading cause of medication errors. Rockville, Md: United States Pharmacopeial Convention, Inc; December 20, 2004. Available at: www.usp.org/aboutUSP/media/.
2. USP's hospital medication error report supports key patient safety goals. Rockville, Md: United States Pharmacopeial Convention, Inc; December 8, 2003. Available at: www.usp.org/aboutUSP/media/.
3. More than one-third of hospital medication errors that reach the patient involve seniors. Rockville, Md: United States Pharmacopeial Convention, Inc; November 18, 2003. Available at: www.usp.org/aboutUSP/media/.
4. Santell JP, Cousins DD, Hicks R, et al. Pediatric population requires vigilance to ensure safety [USP Drug Safety Review]. *Drug Top* (Health System Edition). July 26, 2004. Available at: www.usp.org/pdf/EN/patientSafety/drugSafetyReview2004-07-26.pdf.
5. Hicks R, Camp S. Medication errors in the emergency department [USP Drug Safety Review]. *Drug Top* (Health System Edition). February 23, 2004. Available at: www.usp.org/pdf/EN/patientSafety/drugSafetyReview2004-02-23.pdf.

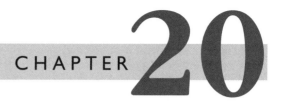

CHAPTER 20

DISCLOSING MEDICATION ERRORS TO PATIENTS AND FAMILIES

Nancy R. Tuohy and Judy L. Smetzer

In the past decade, the American public has grown more aware of the prevalence and consequences of medical error. Professional health care organizations and patient advocacy groups have agreed that disclosing unanticipated outcomes and errors to patients is the ethical thing to do. But the process of disclosure is an emotional experience for both clinician and patient, and health care practitioners and organizations have been hesitant to embrace a process for full disclosure to patients and families.

WHAT CONSTITUTES SUCCESSFUL DISCLOSURE?

According to standards of the Joint Commission on Accreditation of Healthcare Organizations (JCAHO), successful disclosure is evidenced by ensuring that patients and families are informed about the outcomes of medical care, including unanticipated outcomes.[1] Additional elements of successful disclosure of unanticipated events may include the following:[2]

- Absence of litigation,
- Understanding by the patient and family that mistakes are unavoidable,
- Calming of the patient and family's anger in the wake of an adverse outcome, and
- Absence of media coverage or, in the event of media coverage, positive portrayal of the practitioners and the organization.

The overarching goal of the process should be for practitioners and organizations to learn from all adverse events and use them as opportunities for improvements in both the systems of care and patient communication.

PATIENTS' PERSPECTIVE

The National Patient Safety Foundation (NPSF) believes patients and families are entitled to a prompt explanation of how a health care injury occurred and the short-term and long-term effects of that injury. According to NPSF, when an error has contributed to injury, "the patient and the family or representative should receive a truthful and compassionate explanation about the error and the remedies available to the patient."[3] Patients and families would certainly agree with this principle, although they may lack confidence that they will receive a truthful and compassionate explanation.

551

Disclosure is made more difficult when patients do not trust their physicians. In 2001, the Commonwealth Fund found that only 69% of patients had a great deal of confidence in their physician.[4] Patients and families know that errors happen, and they want their health care providers to develop systems for avoiding medical errors. In the event of an error, they want detailed explanations and sincere apologies.[5] Yet, when an error occurs, health care practitioners often distance themselves from patients, choose to speak only about the facts, and refrain from discussing the system elements that contributed to the error and steps that will be taken to avoid the same error in the future.

In a national survey of consumers in 2004,[6]

- 92% of respondents believed the reporting of medical errors should be required,
- 88% believed physicians should be required to tell them if a preventable error resulting in serious harm was made in their own care, and
- 63% believed hospital reports of serious medical errors should be released to the public.

About one-third (34%) of the respondents had experienced medical errors, but only 28% had been told by a physician or other health professional that an error had been made. Only 54% of all respondents believed that the physician would be very or somewhat likely to tell them a preventable error resulting in serious harm had been made in their care.

The survey respondents believed the following would be helpful in reducing medical errors:

- Giving physicians more time to spend with patients (79%),
- Requiring hospitals to develop systems for avoiding errors (72%), and
- Better training of health professionals (72%).

Only 21% believed more malpractice lawsuits would be very effective in reducing medical errors.

These results are consistent with those in prior surveys of patient attitudes about error and disclosure. In a 1999 survey, 98% of patients desired to be informed of all errors, even minor ones; their expressed desire for information increased in proportion to the seriousness of the outcome.[7] Focus group discussions have indicated that patients understand medical errors are inevitable but that they unanimously desire to be told about any error causing harm.[8] Focus group patients expressed differing opinions about the disclosure of near misses (errors that are caught before they reach the patient). Some thought that being told about near misses would provide reassurance that the systems in place to prevent errors were working. Others preferred not to be told about near misses, thinking that it would only add to their fears of medical error.[8]

HEALTH CARE PROVIDERS' PERSPECTIVE

Studies have demonstrated physicians' reluctance to disclose errors to patients.[9-11] In one survey of physicians and patients, 60% of physicians and 92% of patients believed patients should always be told about complications.[11] In focus groups, physicians have expressed the belief that errors causing harm should be disclosed unless the harm is trivial or the patient is unable to understand the error.[8] These physician groups did not think near misses should be disclosed, believing that near misses were "their problem" and not the patient's. These physicians defined errors as deviations from the accepted standard of care, whereas patients had a much broader definition of error that included all unpreventable adverse events. Patients also included poor service quality and low interpersonal skills of practitioners in their definition of medical error.

In a survey of risk managers, more than half reported that they would always disclose death or serious injury due to error.[12] However, when presented with actual clinical scenarios, they were much less likely to disclose preventable harm than unpreventable harm of comparable severity. Risk managers who believed disclosure increased the risk of malpractice litigation were significantly more likely to show a preference for disclosing unpreventable harm over preventable harm.

EXPERIENCE WITH A FULL DISCLOSURE POLICY

The most widely publicized example of a hospital with a full disclosure policy is the Veterans Affairs (VA) Medical Center in Lexington, Kentucky.[13] After losing more than $1.5 million in malpractice judgments, the Lexington center decided in 1987 to adopt a full disclosure policy with equitable compensation for actual losses due to errors. Full disclosure did not cause a flood of lawsuits, and payments for claims were moderate. More than 10 years after implementing its full disclosure policy, the center's economic outcomes were positive.

The center notifies patients and families of accidents, possible negligence, or malpractice as soon as possible after facts are known. The policy has led to numerous settlements, including many that probably would not have resulted in claims if the hospital had not honestly disclosed the errors. The center offers assistance in filing claims and has found that this diminishes patients' anger and desire for retribution.

In addition, because of the voluntary provision of clinical information to attorneys, the center has seen a tendency for plaintiffs' attorneys to negotiate a settlement on the basis of monetary losses rather than on the basis of judgments with a punitive element. Compared with other VA medical centers at the time, the Lexington facility was in the top quartile for number of claims filed but in the bottom quartile for payments.

An article reviewing the Lexington center's experience concluded that "an honest and forthright risk management policy that puts the patient's interests first may be relatively inexpensive because it allows avoidance of lawsuit preparation, litigation, court judgments, and settlements at trial."[13] Intangible benefits, such as maintaining a positive reputation, also accrued.

Full disclosure is now required at all VA facilities. The VA policy calls for a face-to-face meeting with the patient and family, the VA chief of staff, the quality manager, the quality management nurse, and the facility director. The patient and family are given all the details of the event and the names of persons involved. The emphasis is on the regret of the institution and the personnel involved and on what action is being taken to prevent similar events.

However, as noted in the review article, the VA health care system is different from most facilities in the private sector. It is, in effect, a closed system that can offer free universal health coverage, free corrective treatment, and monthly disability payments to its patients. VA practitioners are protected from personal liability and pay no malpractice premiums. Most private sector hospitals and practitioners are dependent upon third-party payers for patient services and on private malpractice insurers.

LEGAL CONCERNS

Fear of legal liability has been cited as the greatest barrier to full disclosure of error.[12] Private sector health care organizations remain uncertain about the implications of full disclosure to patients, since a patient could use the information provided to pursue litigation. However, research has shown that the perceived risk of litigation may be exaggerated. There is anecdotal evidence from several private sector hospitals that pro-active disclosure does not result in more lawsuits.[12]

Most lawsuits are motivated not by negligence but by poor communication between patients and their caregivers, a breakdown in trust between providers and patients, suspicion of a cover-up, or a desire for revenge when an event is not immediately disclosed but is later discovered.[5,14] Nondisclosure has been associated with a more negative emotional response to an event.[15]

A feeling of betrayal is one of the most frequently cited reasons for pursuing legal action.[14-16] The following example illustrates the important role that feelings of betrayal can play in a lawsuit.

The mother of a child who was blind, mute, and suffering from cerebral palsy brought suit against the child's health care providers. She ultimately became a spokesperson on the issue of disclosing medical errors, providing testimony before Congress in 2002. The child's condition was caused by a brain hemorrhage secondary to a lung puncture during fluid aspiration, but the error was not disclosed to the child's parents. Three years later, an obstetrician discovered the error while investigating information provided by the mother in preparation for the birth of her second child. During congressional testimony, the mother stated, "I was able to accept the fact that a human being made a serious mistake, but I felt betrayed, hurt, and angry toward the hospital who had lied to us and continued to lie to us for 3 years."[17]

An editorial commenting on a study of health plan members' views about disclosure of medical error stated, "Patients seeking advice from a lawyer…after a harmful medical error should be no more surprising than patients seeking the services of a physician if they were hurt in a road or workplace accident."[18] Yet, the threat of litigation is strong enough that practitioners are still reticent to speak openly about errors—and even more fearful of offering an apology.[8]

An apology or expression of sympathy is often viewed as an admission of guilt. However, according to a popular book on negotiating,[19] "On many occasions an apology can defuse emotions effectively, even when you do not acknowledge personal responsibility for the action or admit an intention to harm. An apology may be one of the least costly and most rewarding investments you can make." Several states (Pennsylvania, Texas, California, Florida, and Massachusetts) have adopted statutes that specifically protect "benevolent gestures" such as expressions of sympathy from use as evidence of culpability in legal cases.

In contrast, outright admission of fault is admissible in court, so it may be more appropriate to say, "I'm sorry this happened to you" than "I'm sorry we did this to you."[20] Discussion among the disclosure team should include the risks and benefits of the type of apology to be offered in the individual situation.

Disclosure does not protect a facility or practitioner from legal action, but it may satisfy emotional needs that, if left unmet, would trigger a lawsuit. In addition, offering monetary and other fair compensation for injuries could lead toward a settlement rather than a trial. Even if the case goes to trial, juries may adjust awards downward if it is evident that the facility has made efforts to be open and honest with the patient and family throughout the disclosure process.[21]

PERSONAL BARRIERS

Traditionally, when a harmful error occurs, there is a sense of failure, damage to reputation, and loss of trust among colleagues, as well as fear of retribution, punitive action within the organization, and legal action by the patient. Unexpected, harmful outcomes violate the principle *primum non nocere* (first, do no harm). The goal of doing no harm is a laudable one for health professionals, but it places upon them the impossible burden of perfection. Clinicians cannot escape human fallibility, but when they are involved in a harmful error, they feel an enormous sense of failure. (See Chapter 3 for more on health care practitioners' emotional response to error.)

Despite the increasing adoption of a systems-based model of the causes of error, practitioners involved in a harmful error cannot help responding emotionally. Some of their reactions, such as the following, can become barriers to successful disclosure of errors to patients:[2]

- Fear of retribution from the recipient of the news,
- Fear of retribution from colleagues or peers,
- Fear of conducting the conversation poorly,
- Fear of having to handle the recipients' emotions as well as their own emotions,
- Belief that the disclosure is unnecessary,
- Belief that disclosure is primarily a factual conversation and not a complex interpersonal conversation,
- Unfounded belief that the outcome is not related to direct action on the part of the discloser (i.e., no direct involvement in the event and therefore no involvement in the disclosure process), and
- Unfounded belief that the outcome would potentially have occurred even in the absence of the error or intervention (i.e., that the outcome was due to the disease state).

Despite these fears and negative beliefs, practitioners who have emotional support during and after disclosure may be more comfortable with their patients afterward.[20] Effective policies and scenario-based training sessions can help practitioners develop coping mechanisms and communication skills to support them through the disclosure process.

WHAT TO DISCLOSE?

JCAHO standards call for disclosing unanticipated outcomes, but they do not specifically address the disclosure of error.[1] The causes of some unanticipated outcomes are a challenge to discover, and it can be difficult to determine the role, if any, of error. Barron and Kuczewski[22] suggest the following criteria for determining disclosability:

1. The outcome would not be included in a reasonable informed consent process, would not be expected during usual treatment, or both; and
2. It is not possible to exclude error, human or system, from the cause of the outcome.

Using these criteria, the event must be considered unanticipated, and therefore must be disclosed, if error is suspected.

Baron and Kuczewski believe near misses, since they are not related to an outcome, are not required to be disclosed to patients. Health care organizations should have a policy requiring practitioners to report near misses internally, but it can be argued that disclosure of a near miss is not needed for the patient to make treatment choices, and that it may create additional anxieties for the patient.[8,22] An opposing argument favors formal disclosure of a near miss if the patient has become aware of it.[22]

A tougher question is whether to disclose an error that reached the patient but caused no harm. Arguments can be made for both disclosing and not disclosing benign errors. If additional monitoring, observation, or treatment is needed to detect, reduce, or eliminate the risk of harm, health care organizations may feel an obligation to disclose the error to the patient even though it is ultimately found to be benign. However, health care providers may choose not to disclose benign errors if no treatment or precautionary measures are necessary and if harm from the error is not a possibility.

WHO SHOULD DISCLOSE THE ERROR?

Once an organization defines what will be disclosed to patients, a decision must be made about who will be involved in the disclosure process. The team members involved in the disclosure of error to patients can vary according to the circumstances. However, the presence of the attending physician, even if he or she is not the leader of the discussion, is of utmost importance to the patient.[2] The best communicator may or may not be this physician, but the physician's absence can detract from a full explanation of the event, information on short-term and long-term effects, and options for remedy.

Both clinicians and risk managers should be involved in the disclosure process. Some physicians, thinking risk managers are not in favor of disclosing errors to patients, are reluctant to seek them out when faced with disclosure decisions.[23,24] They believe risk managers may be concerned that practitioners will admit fault and accept responsibility unnecessarily, putting the organization at risk; or that practitioners will become defensive and anger the patient and family, leading to litigation.[25]

In the VA system, risk managers are seen as having primary responsibility for disclosure. However, Wu,[26] a noted author on this topic, believes the primary responsibility more naturally falls to the physician. Regardless of the party with primary responsibility, risk managers, physicians, and other practitioners should work together to develop a disclosure policy and a communication model that work best for their facility.

MODELS OF DISCLOSURE

Different models may be followed in disclosing errors to patients. The choice of model depends upon the organization size, the organizational culture, and the needs of the clinicians involved. The American Society for Healthcare Risk Management (ASHRM) suggests the following models:[2]

- For small organizations: One person designated by the organization and trained to have effective disclosure communication skills;
- For small to medium-sized organizations with sufficient staff to participate and coach other staff: A team of individuals who are trained in effective disclosure skills and communication of the policies;
- For medium to large organizations, especially to establish physician buy-in: A train-the-trainer model, in which a large group of practitioners and other individuals undergo disclosure training and in turn become trainers and role models for staff;
- For organizations with a mature culture of patient safety and widespread clinician buy-in: The just-in-time coaching model requires that the clinician at the site of the event, who has a relationship with the patient, disclose the error to the patient, with guidance from an in-house coach who meets with the clinician just before the patient discussion.

For all organizations, certain factors should always be considered in the disclosure process. The organization must comply with all state and federal reporting requirements, as well as JCAHO standards if applicable. The sidebar on page 558 suggests issues for consideration in the development of a plan for responding to various errors, including their disclosure to patients.

AVAILABLE TOOLS

Guidance on the disclosure process is available. The Minnesota Hospital and Healthcare Partnership offers a communication policy framework that individual facilities are encouraged to modify to meet their specific needs.[27] It advises risk managers to review all disclosure policies with individual malpractice insurance carriers. It suggests that discussion with the patient and family include

- An expression of regret and apology,
- The nature of the accident, including time, place, and circumstances,
- The proximate cause, if known,
- Definite and potential consequences to the patient,
- Actions taken to treat any consequences of the accident,
- Who will oversee the ongoing care of the patient,
- Plans for investigation or review of the incident,
- Other parties informed of the event,
- Actions taken to identify systems-related causes and related preventive efforts,
- Who will oversee ongoing communication with the patient or representative,
- Contact information for individuals at the facility who can answer the family's questions,
- Contact information of agencies with which the patient or representative can communicate about the event,
- The process for obtaining support and counseling from the facility and from external resources, and
- The process for discussing compensation for harm.

A sample policy for disclosure of serious events is available on the Institute for Healthcare Improvement Web site.[28] It covers what to disclose, who should disclose the information to patients and families, how disclosure should occur, documenting disclosure, and offering just compensation for injuries.

STAFF EDUCATION AND SUPPORT

Health care organizations must define any terms surrounding medical error and disclosure in proactive, positive language. Some prefer the term "communication policy" to "disclosure policy."[2] Staff education should emphasize use of the appropriate terms and should promote active learning about the barriers to open and honest medical error communication through case studies and role play. The organizational leadership should provide debriefing sessions and private support counseling for staff members involved in an error and in the disclosure.

Leaders must create a culture of safety that supports both the reporting of errors by practitioners and the subsequent disclosure of errors and unanticipated outcomes to patients. After the release of *To Err Is Human* in 2000,[29] the health care community pledged to work toward a culture of patient safety. This has proved to be a challenge, especially in regard to reporting and disclosing errors and unanticipated outcomes. Within health care organizations, individual practitioners remain cautious when disclosing errors to colleagues or superiors or even through anonymous reporting systems. A culture supportive of disclosing errors to patients and families must first eliminate practitioners' fear of reporting errors.

CONCLUSION

Much of the research on disclosure of medical errors is based on hypothetical situations or recall of past experiences, and health care facilities may view this as inadequate evidence for implementing a proactive full disclosure policy. With the advent of JCAHO and state requirements for disclosure, more research on the outcomes of actual cases can be expected. The findings will likely add to the evidence that in both human and financial terms, it pays to be honest with patients.

PREPARING FOR A DAMAGING MEDICATION ERROR

All practice sites should have a plan of action for responding to serious errors, especially errors that result in patient harm or death. The plan should address how, in the event of an incident, the organization should interact with patients, families, and outside organizations, including state and federal regulatory authorities and accrediting bodies. Since it is not uncommon for serious medical errors to receive press coverage, the plan should also address interaction with the media. If this is not handled properly, the result may be long-lasting damage to the health system's reputation and community relations. Managers, attorneys, public relations specialists, and risk managers need to be involved in the development of the overall plan. Key individuals, such as the chief executive officer, manager of the pharmacy, director of nursing, and chief of the medical staff, should be consulted. The following issues need to be addressed:

- ❑ How will the patient and family be informed about the error?
- ❑ How should staff interact with patients and families involved in adverse events?
- ❑ What procedures must be undertaken for safeguarding applicable documents and involved containers and equipment?
- ❑ How should the risk manager's immediate review and investigation be carried out?
- ❑ In the event of inquiry from the news media, how can the health care organization provide useful and accurate information to the public without breaching patient confidentiality?
- ❑ How will internal public relations activities be conducted so that staff knows the incident is being addressed properly?
- ❑ What process will be used to ensure that appropriate immediate and long-term organizational actions are taken to reduce the risk of future errors?
- ❑ If a product or device is defectively labeled, packaged, or designed, what steps should be undertaken to prevent future errors (i.e., should the product be removed, or the brand or package type changed)?
- ❑ What are the internal and external notification processes (e.g., FDA MedWatch, USP-ISMP Medication Errors Reporting Program, manufacturers, state department of health, coroner, professional staff)?
- ❑ How will the practice site accommodate visits from or reviews by regulatory agencies and other investigative bodies?
- ❑ What sort of psychological counseling and other forms of support are available for all involved in the incident?

In the investigation that immediately follows a serious error, it is important to learn as much as possible about the nature of the incident and exactly how it happened. Investigations must focus on system and process deficiencies, not on an individual's knowledge deficit or performance failures.

Source: September 24, 1997, *ISMP Medication Safety Alert!*

REFERENCES

1. Ethics, rights, and responsibilities (RI) standard RI.290. In: *Comprehensive Accreditation Manual for Hospitals: The Official Handbook.* Oakbrook Terrace, Ill: Joint Commission on Accreditation of Healthcare Organizations; 2004.
2. Disclosure of unanticipated events: the next step in better communication with patients. Chicago: American Society for Healthcare Risk Management; 2003. Available at: www.hospitalconnect.com/ashrm/resources/monograph.html. Accessed May 26, 2005.
3. Talking to patients about health care injury: statement of principle. McLean, Va: National Patient Safety Foundation; 2000. Available at: www.npsf.org/html/statement.html. Accessed May 26, 2005.
4. Davis K, Schoenbaum SC, Collins KS, et al. Room for improvement: patients report on the quality of their health care. New York: The Commonwealth Fund; 2002. Available at: www.cmwf.org/surveys/surveys_show.htm?doc_id=228171. Accessed May 26, 2005.
5. Mazor KM, Simon SR, Yood RA, et al. Health plan members' views about disclosure of medical errors. *Ann Intern Med.* 2004;140:409–19.
6. Kaiser Family Foundation. National survey on consumers' experiences with patient safety and quality information, summary and chartpack. Cambridge, Mass: Agency for Healthcare Research and Quality, Harvard School of Public Health; 2004. Available at: www.kff.org/kaiserpolls/7209.cfm. Accessed May 26, 2005.
7. Whitman AB, Park DM, Hardin SB. How do patients want physicians to handle mistakes? A survey of internal medicine patients in an academic setting. *Arch Intern Med.* 1996;156:2565–9.
8. Gallagher TH, Waterman AD, Ebers AG, et al. Patients' and physicians' attitudes regarding the disclosure of medical errors. *JAMA.* 2003;289:1001–7.
9. Wu AW, Folkman S, McPhee SJ, et al. Do house officers learn from their mistakes? *JAMA.* 1991;265:2089–94.
10. Andrews LB, Stocking C, Krizek T, et al. An alternative strategy for studying adverse events in medical care. *Lancet.* 1997;349:309–13.
11. Hingorani M, Wong T, Vafidis G. Patients' and doctors' attitudes to amount of information given after unintended injury during treatment: cross sectional, questionnaire survey. *BMJ.* 1999;318:640–1.
12. Lamb RM, Studdert DM, Bohmer RMJ, et al. Hospital disclosure practices: results of a national survey. *Health Aff.* 2003;22(2):73–83.
13. Kraman SS, Hamm G. Risk management: extreme honesty may be the best policy. *Ann Intern Med.* 1999;131:963–7.
14. Hickson GB, Clayton EW, Githens PB, et al. Factors that prompted families to file medical malpractice claims following prenatal injuries. *JAMA.* 1992;267:1359–63.
15. Green JA. Minimizing malpractice risks by role clarification. The confusing transition from tort to contract. *Ann Intern Med.* 1998;109:234–41.
16. Institute for Safe Medication Practices. Full and timely disclosure of errors to patients: honesty is the best policy. *ISMP Medication Safety Alert!* February 23, 2000;5(4).
17. Ring W. Lawmaker ponders medical errors. *Philadelphia Inquirer.* February 17, 2000.
18. Frenkel DN, Liebman CB. Words that heal. *Ann Intern Med.* 2004;140:482–3.
19. Fisher R, Ury W. *Getting to Yes: Negotiating an Argument without Giving In.* The Harvard Negotiation Project. New York: Penguin Books; 1991:32.
20. Liebman CB, Hyman CS. A mediation skills model to manage disclosure of errors and adverse events to patients. *Health Aff.* 2004;23(4):22–32.
21. Ferguson C. Re: Disclosure to patients and families [electronic message board posting]. Posted March 27, 2003. Available at: www.ihi.org/IHI/forums/ShowPost.aspx?PostID=672. Accessed May 26, 2005.
22. Barron WM, Kuczewski MG. Unanticipated harm to patients: deciding when to disclose outcomes. *Jt Comm J Qual Saf.* 2003;29:551–5.
23. Porto GG. The risk manager's role in disclosure of medical error: seeing ourselves as others see us. *J Healthc Risk Manag.* 2001;21(4):19–24.
24. Woods M. Physician apologies could prevent lawsuits. *Scripps Howard News Service.* November 22, 2000.
25. O'Connell D, Keller VF. Communication: a risk management tool. *J Clin Outcomes Manag.* 1999;6(10):35–8.
26. Wu AW. Handling hospital errors: is disclosure the best defense? *Ann Intern Med.* 1999;131:970–2.
27. Communicating outcomes to patients. St Paul, Minn: Minnesota Hospital and Healthcare Partnership; 2002. Available at: www.mnhospitals.org/inc/data/pdfs/outcomes.pdf. Accessed May 26, 2005.
28. Serious Event Disclosure Policy. Wentworth-Douglass Hospital, Dover, NH. Available at: www.ihi.org/IHI/Topics/PatientSafety/SafetyGeneral/Tools/SeriousEventDisclosurePolicyWentworthDouglass.htm. Accessed May 26, 2005.
29. Kohn LT, Corrigan JM, Donaldson MS, eds. *To Err Is Human: Building a Safer Health System.* Washington, DC: National Academies Press; 2000.

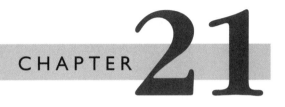

CHAPTER **21**

HEALTH CARE FAILURE MODE AND EFFECTS ANALYSIS

Part I: Introduction to Failure Mode and Effects Analysis

J. W. Senders and S. J. Senders

Part II: An Application of Failure Mode and Effects Analysis

Judy L. Smetzer and Michael R. Cohen

Part III: Veterans Health Administration Approach to Failure Mode and Effects Analysis

Mary Burkhardt, Joseph DeRosier, Erik Stalhandske, and James Bagian

I
INTRODUCTION TO FAILURE MODE AND EFFECTS ANALYSIS

The purpose of failure mode analysis (FMA) is to discover the potential risks in a product or system by identifying all the ways in which it might fail. FMA can be used not only to predict failures but also to analyze why they occur. The term failure mode may refer to specific types of failure (e.g., fractures, burns, or deviations from expected values) or to degrees of failure (e.g., catastrophic, partial, or minimal).

FMA was first used in the engineering field in the early 1960s.[1] By the mid-1970s, it had become a standard term in electronics, structural and mechanical engineering, chemistry, and the aerospace industry.

Failure mode and effects analysis (FMEA), also introduced in the 1960s, is a risk assessment method based on the simultaneous analysis of failure modes, their consequences, and their associated risk factors. Like FMA, it can be used not only in the design stage (to prevent failures or mitigate their consequences) but also in post hoc analysis. Because it is concerned with the effects of failure, FMEA has been used most extensively in areas characterized by high risk, such as nuclear power plant operations, or by high cost, such as the weapons and aerospace industries.

Both FMA and FMEA have been used to reduce the frequency and consequences of failures. The two forms of analysis, however, have different genealogies: FMA is an outgrowth of quality control concerns, whereas FMEA stems from risk assessment.

The human factor has long been recognized as an aspect of system failures. Work on integrating human factors into FMA and FMEA began in the early 1960s[2-4] and, as evidenced by this chapter, has continued into the 21st century. Applications of FMEA to patient safety began in the early 1990s.[5]

FAILURE ANALYSIS

Failure analysis is a central activity of human culture. The search for explanations of all events, especially negative ones, is central to human understanding of order.

Historically, failure analyses were constructed from a linear perspective. In that approach, one needed only to retrace the chain of events until the fault was found. Such analyses were well suited to preindustrial mechanical and engineering failures. Because artisan production was sequential, most failures could be traced to particular events, techniques, or materials.

Industrial and mass production, by contrast, generally involves numerous subsystems in the production of a single product. Its development called for a new, systemic type of failure analysis. No longer could failures necessarily be traced to a single event; combined effects had to be considered. Moreover, the growing market for reliable industrial products, and the increasing complexity of the products themselves, demanded systemic analyses of both production and product failures. The rise of the military as the preeminent consumer of industrial products encouraged the rapid development of systemic analysis.

FMA and FMEA both use what could be called systemic, as opposed to linear-narrative, analysis. Systemic analysis does not demand that events take the form of a single story; instead, it requires a simultaneous imagining of all possible stories. Neither FMA nor FMEA refers to a specific method; instead, they define terms of inquiry. FMA asks, "What has failed, what could fail, and how?" FMEA asks, "Given the various possibilities for failure, what are the potential consequences of each?"

To apply FMA and FMEA, one must first define failure. In general, a failure is said to occur if a component or a collection of components of a system behaves in a way that is not included in its specified performance criteria. Fundamental to FMA and FMEA is an analysis of the system in question, including a detailed specification of all possible sites of failure—components, subsystems, processes, interactions, and functions. Each site must then be analyzed in terms of possible failure modes and, if they are available, the probabilities of those failures. Finally, for each identifiable site of failure, one must identify the consequences and calculate the associated cost.

HUMAN ERROR AND FMEA

Failures in mechanical, material, and production processes are amenable to systemic analysis. It seems clear that careful examination of a system can reveal the various kinds of failure that can occur. Further, there is general acceptance of the idea that if a failure occurs, one can calculate its consequences, provided that one is aware of the interaction between the elements involved.

Human failures, by contrast, are burdened by historical and cultural habit that equates human error with blame, a concept better suited to linear-narrative than to systemic analysis.[6] An estimated 70% to 90% of all accidents result from human error.

It is astonishing that methods commonly applied to the nonhuman components of systems are not applied to humans, the major source of system failure. This lack stems from the view that human errors are unpredictable. Such is not the case. Human errors are not drawn from an infinite set of possibilities. Instead, they are drawn from the limited set of meaningful things that an individual can do in any defined situation. These actions can be termed the affordances of the work environment. Because the spectrum of errors is limited, they are theoretically capable of a priori discovery and analysis. To draw from a time-honored example, Murphy's law asserts: "If something can go wrong, it will." The task in the first instance is to discover what can be done wrong; in the second, to predict what would happen when it is done. These observations could serve, in short, as the basis of an FMEA that factors in human error.

APPLYING FMEA TO MEDICATION ERROR PREVENTION

FMEA acknowledges that errors are inevitable and predictable. It anticipates errors and designs a system that will minimize their impact. Thus, FMEA that factors in human error can be applied to medication error prevention. For each medication, FMEA asks what will happen if a health care provider

- Mistakes one medication for another because of the packaging,
- Administers the wrong amount of drug,
- Gives a drug to the wrong patient,
- Administers a drug by the wrong route or at the wrong rate,
- Omits a dose,
- Gives a drug at the wrong time, or
- Takes any other action that may produce a medication misadventure.

In some cases, FMEA reveals that the patient can tolerate the error or that the error will be intercepted by the checks and balances built into the health system's quality improvement processes. In other cases, FMEA reveals that specific steps must be put in place to address potential errors with significant impact—errors that are intolerable. Figure 21-1 illustrates how FMEA creates "error traps" that will prevent accidents and ensure patient safety.[7]

What would happen if we were to apply FMEA to devices, prescriptions, packages, labels, and instructions? If we follow a medication or a drug administration device from

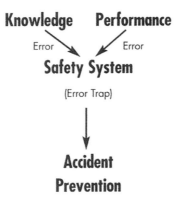

FIGURE 21-1 Failure mode and effects analysis recognizes that human errors related to deficiencies in knowledge or performance are inevitable. Enhancing the safety system (designing error traps) can prevent errors from becoming accidents.

the point of manufacture to the patient, it becomes evident that there are many opportunities to select an incorrect product and substitute it for the correct one. Each opportunity for incorrect selection is an opportunity to examine the consequences (the effects) of that selection and to estimate the associated risk. For example, predicting the outcome of administering an incorrect medication is a matter of pharmacology and physiology. Given the status of the patient, if the correct medication is withheld and a specified incorrect medication administered, it is possible, within limits, to predict the consequences.

Some medications are relatively benign. Their misuse does not lead to illness or death. Some patients are not in a physiological state in which failure to use the correct medication will lead to illness or death. If both are true, the error will be of little consequence. Take, for example, a patient who was supposed to receive ear drops. The physician wrote "OD" (for once a day). The nurse read it as "OD" (right eye) and instilled the ear drops into the patient's right eye. It was only when the patient was about to leave the office and asked the nurse when he would receive his ear drops that the error was discovered.

In this instance, the substance given to the patient was pharmacologically benign, and the delay in administering the ear drops led to no discernible effect. In another context, the same kind of error could have been lethal or permanently injurious. This problem originated with the use of an abbreviation. FMEA suggests that there should be a set of error-prone abbreviations that should never be used, or that all abbreviations should be forbidden in prescription writing (although the latter is impractical).

A second type of error involves packaging. For example, prefilled 5 mL syringes of 20% lidocaine 1,000 mg were substituted for similar syringes containing a 2% concentration, sometimes with fatal outcomes. Although syringe redesign was an obvious remedy, the concentrated product stayed on the market until the early 1990s. No effort was made to redesign the syringe so that the 20% concentration could be used only for IV admixture preparation and not for direct bolus injection. Information about the likelihood of this error was not rapidly disseminated. By the time the product was removed from the market, 12 years had passed and about 100 deaths had occurred since the error was first reported.

Mechanical design errors are also common. Improper assembly of infusion pumps has led to free-flow of medications into patients. This has happened so often that it should be possible to know virtually all the ways in which such devices can be misassembled. FMEA would reveal that if the reservoir is improperly clamped, it can still appear to be properly seated, and free-flow can occur if the pump is operated in that state. The FMEA approach emphasizes that if one person has done something incorrectly, it is probable that another person will do the same thing. Yet manufacturers and regulatory agencies often resist suggestions that redesign is needed. Each reported misuse of a drug or device provides information for identifying potential errors with that medication or device as well as with all medications similarly packaged, labeled, or prescribed and all similar devices.

LEARNING ABOUT POTENTIAL FAILURE MODES FROM REPORTED ERRORS

The range of human error is not infinite; errors are limited to the affordances of the situation. It is difficult, however, for even the most experienced analyst to imagine everything that someone might do incorrectly. Therefore, it is critically important to develop a uniform and rational system of reporting errors, including those that have not resulted in patient injury. A database of error modes will assist in analyzing the kinds of misuses that human ingenuity can devise. The Institute for Safe Medication Practices (ISMP) is collecting this information in the United States, Canada, and Spain.

A standard approach to reducing failures in mechanical and electronic systems is the introduction of redundancy into critical subsystems. Applying the same approach to reducing human errors, multiple sensory channels could be used for error prevention. For example, the packaging of dangerous products could feel different from that of other products; the outside of a vial or preloaded syringe could be bumpy, rough, or square, or have a combination of these tactile characteristics. Before the adoption of such a distinguishing characteristic, however, a complete statistical analysis should be performed of the accidents that the measure is designed to prevent. This would make it possible to assess the benefits and compare them with the costs.

Errors will continue to be made. Accidents, on the other hand, can largely be prevented by intelligent and imaginative use of cues announcing that an error has occurred and enabling correction of the error before damage has been done. Where possible, physical design should be used to prevent error from being translated into injury.

CONCLUSION

Methods such as FMEA, used for the detection and reduction of accidents resulting from machine failures, can also be effective in reducing health care failures if human factors are taken into account. Using FMEA to anticipate and prevent errors can make the medication-use process safer.

REFERENCES

1. Kimball EW. Failure Analysis. Proceedings of National Symposium on Reliability and Quality Control, Washington, DC; 1962:117–28.
2. Meister D. The Prediction and Measurement of Human Reliability. Presented at the IAS Aerospace Systems Reliability Symposium, Salt Lake City, Utah, April 16–18, 1962.
3. Brady JS, Daily A. Evaluation of personnel performance in complex systems. Atlas Crew Procedures Laboratory Technical Memorandum. Space Laboratory Report GM 6300.5-1431; April 1961.
4. Shapero A. Human engineering testing and malfunction data collection in weapon systems test programs. Wright Air Development Division Technical Report 60-36. Dayton, Ohio; Wright Air Development Division; February 1960.
5. Hahn HA. Human factors issues in qualitative and quantitative safety analysis. Submitted to the Russian Institute, Los Alamos National Laboratory, NM; 1993.
6. Denning PJ. Human error and the search for blame. RIACS Technical Report TR-89.46; 1989.
7. Cohen MR, Senders J, Davis NM. Failure mode and effects analysis: a novel approach to avoiding dangerous medication errors and accidents. *Hosp Pharm.* 1994;29:319–30.

II
AN APPLICATION OF FAILURE MODE
AND EFFECTS ANALYSIS

FMEA is a technique used to prevent process or product problems before they occur.[1–4] In health care, the concept of before-the-fact evaluation of the potential for failure is relatively new. More commonly, root cause analysis is performed after an error, especially after a sentinel event that has harmed a patient. Although root cause analysis after such an event is essential, analyzing processes and products before bad things can happen is an equally important component of a comprehensive medication error reduction strategy.

FMEA proactively identifies ways in which products or processes can fail, why they might fail, and how they can be made safer. Its goal is to stimulate the environment to bring potential problems to the surface so they can be minimized or eliminated. FMEA can be thought of as a technique in which pessimists can play an important role in bringing about positive change. When it is used in designing new processes or before using new products, it increases the likelihood of their success. It also fosters the necessary team orientation for interdisciplinary work.

FMEA is performed by an interdisciplinary team to ensure that all steps in processes are identified and their interrelatedness to each other, to other processes, and to each discipline is clearly understood. As a result, participants in FMEA develop a clear understanding of all the work processes involved. This enhances interdisciplinary communication and collaboration, which is especially important during implementation of a process that has been revised through FMEA.

Since 2001, when the Joint Commission on Accreditation of Healthcare Organizations instituted a requirement for proactive risk assessment, many health care organizations have successfully used FMEA.[3,4] The method is logical and straightforward:[2]

- Choose a high-risk process or product vulnerable to error.
- Assemble an interdisciplinary team.
- Describe and document the current process.
- Determine potential areas where errors may occur.
- Decide if the potential errors are unacceptable, on the basis of how likely they are to occur and to cause patient harm.
- Prioritize and take action to eliminate or reduce unacceptable errors.
- Make sure the actions have been successful.

An FMEA for patient-controlled analgesia (PCA) illustrates use of the method (Table 21-1). To conduct this FMEA, an interdisciplinary team of practitioners determined the processes, subprocesses, and tasks associated with PCA prescribing, dispensing, administration, and monitoring. For example, in the prescribing phase, a physician has to assess the patient, choose an analgesic and mode of delivery, and prescribe the analgesic.

After the processes, subprocesses, and tasks were identified, the team determined all that could go wrong (the potential failures) during each step. For the prescriber's tasks in this example, the failure modes were as follows:

- Assess the patient: Inaccurate pain assessment
- Choose an analgesic: Wrong analgesic selected
- Prescribe the analgesic: Wrong dose, route, or frequency prescribed; proper patient monitoring not ordered; analgesic prescribed for the wrong patient; no order received

The next step was to think about the causes of these failures—why they might happen. This step is needed because it would be difficult to predict the probability of a failure, or determine how frequently it might occur, without first considering how it might happen. The following potential causes of failure in the physician's selection of an analgesic were identified:

- The patient's clinical situation (e.g., age, renal function, allergies) may not be considered.
- The patient's tolerance to opioids may not be considered.
- Standard PCA protocols may not be available or followed.
- Concomitant use of other analgesics may not be considered.
- There may be a shortage of the desired analgesic, forcing selection of a less than optimal agent.
- The physician may have a knowledge deficit regarding the safest and most appropriate analgesic to use with PCA.
- The patient may not be an appropriate candidate for PCA.

TABLE 21-1 Failure Mode and Effects Analysis (FMEA) for Patient-Controlled Analgesia (PCA)

Process, Subprocesses, and Tasks	Failure Modes (What Might Happen)	Causes (Why It Happens)	Effects	Severity	Probability	Hazard Score	Strategies to Reduce Failure Modes
Prescribing							
Assess patient	Inaccurate pain assessment	Cultural influences; patient unable to articulate	Poor pain control	2	4	8	Standard scale to help assess pain; training on cultural influences
Choose analgesic and mode of delivery	Wrong analgesic selected	Clinical situation (e.g., age, renal function, allergies) not considered; tolerance to opiates not considered; standard PCA protocols not followed (or not available); concomitant use of other analgesics not considered; drug shortage; knowledge deficit; improper selection of patients appropriate for PCA	Improper dosing; improper drug; allergic response; improper use of substitute drug	4	3	12	Computerized prescriber order entry (CPOE) with decision support; clinical pharmacy program; standard PCA protocol with education on use; point-of-use access to drug information; feedback mechanism on drug shortages, with information on substitute drugs available; selection criteria for PCA patients
Prescribe analgesic	Wrong dose (loading, PCA, constant, lock-out), route, frequency	Knowledge deficit; mental slip; wrong selection from list; information about drug not available	Overdose; underdose; adverse drug reaction (ADR)	4	3	12	CPOE with decision support; clinical pharmacy program; standard PCA protocols
	Proper patient monitoring not ordered	Knowledge deficit; mental slip	Failure to detect problems early to prevent harm	4	3	12	Standard PCA order sets with monitoring guidelines
	Prescribed for wrong patient	Similar patient names; patient identifier not clear; name does not appear on screen during medication ordering	Wrong patient receives inappropriate drug and dose; ADR; allergic response	3	3	9	Match therapy to patient condition; alerts for look-alike patient names; visible demographic information on order form or screen
	No order received	Unable to reach covering physician	Poor pain control	2	2	4	Proper physician coverage and communication channels

TABLE 21-1 Failure Mode and Effects Analysis (FMEA) for Patient-Controlled Analgesia (PCA) (continued)

Process, Subprocesses, and Tasks	Failure Modes (What Might Happen)	Causes (Why It Happens)	Effects	Severity	Probability	Hazard Score	Strategies to Reduce Failure Modes
Dispensing							
Send order to pharmacy	Order not received/ processed in pharmacy	Unaware of order on unit; medication used from floor stock, so order not sent; order entered onto wrong form or screen; spoken orders not documented	Drug therapy omitted; overdose; underdose; ADR; allergic response if wrong drug used	3	3	9	Flagging system for new orders; policy to send all orders to pharmacy; physician review of new orders with unit staff; shift chart checks; standard process for receipt and documentation of spoken orders
	Delay in receiving or processing order	Order not flagged; inefficient process for sending orders to pharmacy; order not seen/misplaced after reaching pharmacy	Delay in dispensing drug; use of floor stock before pharmacy order screening; delay of drug therapy	3	4	12	As above; standard, efficient process for pharmacy order receipt; timely review and triage of orders received in pharmacy
Enter order into computer	Order misunderstood	Illegible order; use of abbreviations, trailing zeroes, naked decimal doses; spoken orders; look-alike drug names; order copy unclear	Overdose, underdose; allergic response; ADR; delay in therapy; poor pain control	3	4	12	CPOE; preprinted orders; prohibit dangerous abbreviations, dose expressions, nonurgent spoken orders; fax original order to pharmacy; seek clarification directly with prescriber
	Order entered incorrectly	Design of software; computer mnemonics; look-alike drugs; failure/absence of double check	Same as above	3	3	9	User-friendly order entry process; look-alike drug alerts; double-check process for order entry
	Order entered into wrong patient profile/wrong encounter	Poor presentation of patient demographics (fax interference, light imprint, order copy unclear); look-alike names	Same as above	3	3	9	CPOE; vivid demographics on order forms/screens; high-quality fax machines; routine maintenance; view-only access to prior patient encounters; alerts for look-alike names

Process step	Failure mode	Cause	Effect	Severity	Probability	Score	Actions
Produce label	Standard directions (concentration, mixing instructions) in computer wrong	Use of substitute drug because of shortage; overlooking default directions in computer when changing processes	Overdose, underdose; poor pain control	3	2	6	Checklist/testing to ensure revisions in electronic/print when changing processes/drugs; quick access to information on substitute drugs
	Label inaccurate	Inaccurate order entry	Overdose, underdose; wrong route; ADR	3	3	9	As above for "Enter order into computer"
	Label unclear	Ambiguous information; poor quality of printer	Same as above; delay in therapy; poor pain control	3	3	9	High-quality laser printer; improve presentation of label information, with nursing input
	Label not printed	Equipment malfunction; improper interface with pharmacy computer	Missed therapy; delay in therapy; poor pain control	2	1	2	Routine equipment maintenance and performance testing
Prepare medication	Wrong drug	Look-alike products stored near each other; drug shortage; knowledge deficit	ADR; overdose; underdose; allergic reaction; poor pain control	4	3	12	Separate look-alike products; PCA protocols; feedback mechanism on drug shortages with information on substitute drugs available; readily available mixing protocols; compounding log of ingredients with lot numbers; independent double check
	Wrong diluent	Same as above	ADR; toxicity from diluent	3	3	9	Same as above
	Wrong dilution or concentration	Knowledge deficit; calculation error	Overdose; underdose; poor pain control	4	3	12	PCA protocols; independent double check for all calculations
Check medication before distribution	Check not completed	Inadequate staffing patterns	Potential error not detected	3	3	9	Adequate staffing patterns
	Check inadequate	Same as above; environmental factors (distractions, space, lighting, noise); inefficient workflow; human factors	Same as above	3	3	9	As above; environmental and workflow improvements; mental warm-ups before checking to increase task focus; use of spoken checks

TABLE 21-1 Failure Mode and Effects Analysis (FMEA) for Patient-Controlled Analgesia (PCA) (continued)

Process, Subprocesses, and Tasks	Failure Modes (What Might Happen)	Causes (Why It Happens)	Effects	Severity	Probability	Hazard Score	Strategies to Reduce Failure Modes
Deliver medication to patient care unit	Delay in distribution	Inadequate staffing or equipment used for delivery of drugs; inefficient drug delivery system; delivery equipment mechanical failure; shared delivery system	Delay in drug therapy; use of floor stock before pharmacy order screening	3	4	12	Establish dedicated delivery system under direct control of pharmacy; use dedicated staff and equipment for medication delivery; routine maintenance and update of equipment
	Delivered to wrong unit	Inadequate, untimely interface with admission/transfer information	Same as above; omitted doses; unneeded doses on wrong unit (possible administration to wrong patient)	3	3	9	Timely and seamless communication of admissions/transfers to pharmacy
Administration							
Receive order and transcribe onto medication administration record (MAR)	Order or MAR misunderstood	Illegible order; use of abbreviations, trailing zeroes, naked decimal doses; spoken orders; look-alike drug names; knowledge deficit	Overdose, underdose; allergic response; ADR; delay in therapy; poor pain control	3	4	12	CPOE; preprinted orders; prohibit dangerous abbreviations and dose expressions, nonurgent spoken orders; seek clarification directly from prescriber/chart; staff training on typical drugs used for PCA
	Order transcribed onto MAR incorrectly	Same as above; too many sections/pages of MAR; lack of support staff training; distractions; failure/absence of double check; knowledge deficit	Same as above	3	3	9	Same as above; pharmacy computer-generated MAR; staff training; environment free of distractions; user-friendly MAR; consistent double-check process

Process	Failure mode	Cause	Effect				Recommended actions
Obtain PCA infusion pump	Order transcribed onto wrong MAR	Look-alike patient names; poor presentation of patient demographics on MAR; order transcribed before patient identifier added	Same as above	2	3	6	Look-alike name alerts; vivid demographics on MAR forms; high-quality imprint machines
	No pump available	Inadequate supply; hoarding; bottlenecks in cleaning process	Delay in therapy; poor pain control; use of improper pump/no pump; overdose, underdose	3	3	9	Purchase adequate supply of pumps; central distribution center; efficient cleaning process
	Wrong pump selected	As above; knowledge deficit	Delay in therapy; poor pain control	2	2	4	As above; staff training
Obtain PCA medication	Cannot find dispensed medication	Pharmacy delivery problem; no communication to nurse that medication was delivered	Delay in therapy; poor pain control	2	2	4	Efficient pharmacy delivery process and communication
	Wrong drug	Look-alike products stored near each other (automated dispensing cabinets, floor stock, refrigerator); drug shortage; knowledge deficit	ADR; overdose; underdose; allergic reaction; poor pain control	4	3	12	Separate look-alike products; PCA protocols; feedback mechanism on drug shortages, with information on substitute drugs available; independent double check
	Wrong concentration	Same as above; unnecessary multiple concentrations available; knowledge deficit; calculation error	Overdose; underdose; poor pain control	4	3	12	Same as above; use one standard concentration (use auxiliary warning labels if using different concentration, and have pharmacy dispense the drug); PCA protocols; independent double check
	Error during compounding (wrong drug, wrong diluent, wrong concentration)	Unfamiliarity with IV admixture; no pharmacy service at night; failure of double check	ADR; overdose; underdose; allergic reaction; poor pain control	4	4	16	Full pharmacy IV admixture service; purchase prefilled syringes/cassettes from manufacturer

TABLE 21-1 Failure Mode and Effects Analysis (FMEA) for Patient-Controlled Analgesia (PCA) (continued)

Process, Subprocesses, and Tasks	Failure Modes (What Might Happen)	Causes (Why It Happens)	Effects	Severity	Probability	Hazard Score	Strategies to Reduce Failure Modes
Program pump	Pump mis-programmed (flow rate, concentration, lock-out, loading dose)	Design flaw in pump (e.g., Abbott LifeCare PCA pump) that makes programming error-prone; lack of standard concentrations; failure to limit variety of products used; knowledge deficit; confusion between units of measure (milligrams versus micrograms); mechanical failure	Overdose; underdose; poor pain control	4	3	12	Purchase pumps that are easy to program: use FMEA process to determine potential failure modes of pumps to guide purchasing decisions; limit variety of pumps; train staff on use of new pumps; minimize variety of products used for PCA; standardize concentrations used; PCA protocols; independent double check at bedside
Check medication and pump settings before administration	Check not completed	Inadequate staffing patterns; lack of priority for the check; previous successful violations; check process not integrated into the way care is delivered	Potential error not detected and likely to reach the patient	4	3	12	Adequate staffing patterns; engage staff in culture of safety; understand causes for prior successful violations and take action to eliminate barriers to consistent checks; build check processes into the care delivery model in use
	Check inadequate	Same as above; environmental factors (distractions, space, lighting, noise); inefficient workflow; human factors; check at bedside (to ensure correct pump settings, patient, line attachments) not completed	Same as above	4	3	12	As above; environmental and workflow improvements; mental warm-ups before checking to increase task focus; use of spoken checks; check performed at bedside

Process	Failure mode	Cause	Effects				Actions
Administer PCA	Wrong patient	Failure of double check at bedside; failure to check/absent name bracelet; ordered for wrong patient or transcribed on wrong MAR	Overdose, underdose; allergic response; ADR; delay in therapy; poor pain control	3	3	9	As above under "Check medication and pump settings before administration"; match patient therapy with condition; patient education
	Wrong route	Catheter attachment confusion; failure of double check at bedside	ADR; poor pain control	4	2	8	As above under "Check medication and pump settings before administration"; label proximal ends of lines near insertion ports
	Wrong dose	Failure of double check; family/nurse activation instead of patient activation; inadequate patient/family education before use; improper use on patients who cannot activate their own PCA; patient/staff/family tampering (drug diversion, criminal intent); patient misuse (e.g., accidental activation due to confusion with call bell)	Overdose; underdose; ADR; poor pain control	4	3	12	As above under "Check medication and pump settings before administration"; patient selection criteria for appropriate use of PCA; staff education; patient education before use (e.g., during surgical preadmission process); inaccessible medication in locked pump with electronic recording of transitions; clear differentiation between call bell and activation button
	Wrong flow rate	Failure of double check; pump not protected from free-flow; mechanical failure; insufficient preventive maintenance of pump; inaccurate pump calibration; insufficient power source for pump	Same as above	4	3	12	As above under "Check medication and pump settings before administration"; proper selection and maintenance of pumps; use of pumps protected from free-flow; backup power source for pump

TABLE 21-1 Failure Mode and Effects Analysis (FMEA) for Patient-Controlled Analgesia (PCA) (continued)

Process, Subprocesses, and Tasks	Failure Modes (What Might Happen)	Causes (Why It Happens)	Effects	Severity	Probability	Hazard Score	Strategies to Reduce Failure Modes
Document PCA	Drug administration not documented	Human factors; environmental distractions; workload; inefficient process; multiple MAR pages/screens	Inability to properly evaluate pain management; duplicate therapy	3	2	6	Establish user-friendly MAR; review documentation before end of each shift to ensure completeness; use flow sheets at bedside to document PCA (and patient monitoring parameters)
Monitoring							
Monitor effects of medication	Insufficient monitoring of effects of PCA	Workload; knowledge deficit; monitoring parameters not ordered; ineffective communication between caregivers; cultural influences	Failure to recognize the consequences of an error before patient harm occurs; inability to evaluate pain management; poor pain control	3	3	9	Standard order sets with monitoring guidelines; standard scale to help assess pain; training on cultural influences; proper staffing patterns and safe workload; use flow sheet at bedside to document PCA and patient monitoring parameters

TABLE 21-2   Hazard Scoring Matrix for Failure Mode and Effects Analysis[a,b]

Probability[c]	Severity of Effect[d]			
	Catastrophic (4)	Major (3)	Moderate (2)	Minor (1)
Frequent (4)	16	12	8	4
Occasional (3)	12	9	6	3
Uncommon (2)	8	6	4	2
Remote (1)	4	3	2	1

[a] Scoring method adapted from the Veterans Health Administration National Center for Patient Safety's Health-care Failure Mode and Effects Analysis.

[b] Hazard score = severity score × probability score; scores of 8 or higher should be given the highest priority.

[c] Probability scores are defined as follows:
Remote: Unlikely to occur (may happen sometime in 5 to 30 years).
Uncommon: Possible to occur (may happen sometime in 2 to 5 years).
Occasional: Probably will occur (may happen several times in 1 to 2 years).
Frequent: Likely to occur immediately or within a short period (may happen several times in 1 year).

[d] Severity scores are defined as follows (see Table 21-5 for additional operational definitions):
Minor patient outcome: No injury, nor increased length of stay, nor increased level of care.
Moderate patient outcome: Increased length of stay or increased level of care for one or two patients.
Major patient outcome: Permanent lessening of bodily functioning (sensory, motor, physiological, or intellectual), disfigurement, surgical intervention required, increased length of stay for three or more patients, increased level of care for three or more patients.
Catastrophic patient outcome: death or major permanent loss of function (sensory, motor, physiological, intellectual), suicide, rape, hemolytic transfusion reaction, surgery or procedure on the wrong patient or wrong part of body, infant abduction or discharge to wrong family.

Next, the potential effects of the failures were considered. This included not only direct effects on the patient but also effects on other parts of the process that, through a domino effect, could allow the error to reach the patient. The team members used both objective data (literature citations, past experiences, accurate measurements) and subjective beliefs to guide their decisions about the possible effects of choosing the wrong analgesic. Using the scoring grid shown in Table 21-2, the team believed the severity of the effect on the patient would be high, so a severity score of 4 (catastrophic effect) was selected. The team members believed the failure would occur several times in 1 to 2 years, so a probability score of 3 (occasional) was selected. The hazard score (sometimes called a risk priority number) was then obtained by multiplying the severity and probability scores ($4 \times 3 = 12$).

Finally, because the hazard score was relatively high, the team identified factors that could reduce the occurrence of the failure (choosing the wrong analgesic):

- Computerized prescriber order entry system with decision support (e.g., capacity to detect dose limits, contraindicated analgesics);
- Clinical pharmacy program that fosters pharmacist participation in the selection of analgesics;
- Standard PCA protocol with education on use;
- Point-of-use access to drug information for prescribers;
- Feedback mechanism on drug shortages, with information on substitute drugs available; and
- Selection criteria for appropriate PCA patients.

This example uses just one of several FMEA methods available to health care providers. Other methods, such as that described in Part III of this chapter, follow a similar pattern, with minor differences in the determination of causative factors and hazard score. Regardless of which method is used, the basic purpose and steps are the same.

REFERENCES

1. Failure mode and effects analysis can help guide error prevention efforts. *ISMP Medication Safety Alert!* October 17, 2001;6(21):1.
2. ECRI failure mode and effects analysis. *Healthcare Risk Control System.* May 2004(suppl).
3. *Failure Mode and Effects Analysis in Health Care: Proactive Risk Reduction.* Oakbrook Terrace, Ill: Joint Commission on Accreditation of Healthcare Organizations; 2002.
4. Institute for Healthcare Improvement. Failure mode and effects analysis tools. Available at: www.ihi.org/IHI/Topics/PatientSafety/MedicationSystems/Tools/Failure+Modes+and+Effects+Analysis+%28FMEA%29+Tool+%28IHI+Tool%29.htm. Accessed May 21, 2005.

III
VETERANS HEALTH ADMINISTRATION APPROACH TO FAILURE MODE AND EFFECTS ANALYSIS

Healthcare Failure Mode and Effects Analysis (HFMEA[SM]), developed by the Department of Veterans Affairs (VA) National Center for Patient Safety (NCPS), is a customized approach to FMEA. It combines FMEA and hazard analysis and critical control point (HACCP) concepts with tools and definitions from the VA's root cause analysis (RCA) process. HFMEA involves a multidisciplinary team, process and subprocess flow diagramming, failure mode and failure mode cause identification, a hazard-scoring matrix, and a decision tree algorithm for identifying and prioritizing system vulnerabilities. As part of the process, actions and outcome measures are developed, and management must concur to ensure follow-through on action items.

The development of HFMEA began with a review of the FMEA system that has been successfully used in industry, but NCPS found that the generic definitions used for severity, occurrence, and detectability needed to be modified for use in evaluating health care processes. It was difficult to stratify the failure modes and causes, since most processes in health care can result in harm to the patient.

In searching for a proactive analysis tool developed specifically for evaluating processes, the NCPS staff reviewed the HACCP system developed by the National Advisory Committee on Microbiological Criteria for Foods,[1] whose participants include the U.S. Department of Agriculture and the Food and Drug Administration (FDA). HACCP was developed by FDA to protect the food supply from biological and chemical contamination and from physical hazards. It involves conducting hazard analysis, determining the critical control points, and establishing critical limits, monitoring procedures, corrective actions, verification procedures, and record-keeping and documentation procedures. HACCP incorporates questions to probe for food system vulnerabilities and a decision tree to help the user identify critical control points. HACCP was not directly applicable to health care because of its focus on food processing and handling and non-health-care questions, but the HACCP concept of a decision tree was adopted for HFMEA.

Prioritization is important in any proactive risk assessment. As part of its RCA process, NCPS had developed a safety assessment code (SAC) to prioritize adverse events and close calls. The SAC definitions for severity and probability (occurrence) are well known by patient safety managers within the VA and were adapted for use in HFMEA.

As shown in Table 21-3, the prospective risk analysis system developed by NCPS includes concepts of the FMEA model from industry and the HACCP model from food safety, as well as tools and concepts that are integral to the VA NCPS program (e.g., SAC, triage cards, parts of the RCA process).[2] Table 21-4 compares RCA and HFMEA.

TABLE 21-3   Sources of Concepts Used in HFMEA

Concept	HFMEA	FMEA	HAACP	VA RCA
Team membership	X	X		X
Diagramming process	X	X		
Failure modes and causes	X	X		
Hazard score matrix	X			X
Severity and probability definitions	X			X
Decision tree	X		X	
Actions and outcomes	X		X	X
Responsible person and management concurrence	X			X

HFMEA = Healthcare Failure Mode and Effects Analysis, the Department of Veterans Affairs (VA) customized approach to FMEA; HAACP = hazard analysis and critical control point concepts; VA RCA = VA root cause analysis process.

TABLE 21-4   Comparison of HFMEA and RCA

Similarities	Differences
Interdisciplinary team	Diagram of processes (HFMEA) versus diagram of chronological steps in the progress of one event (RCA)
Develop flow diagram	
Focus on system issues	Prospective (what if) analysis (HFMEA) versus retrospective (RCA)
Scoring matrix (severity/probability)	
Use of triage/triggering questions, cause-and-effect diagram, and brainstorming	Choose topic for evaluation in HFMEA; sentinel event is topic in RCA
	Include detectability and criticality in evaluation (HFMEA)
	Emphasis on proactive testing and intervention (HFMEA) versus reactive remedies

HFMEA = Healthcare Failure Mode and Effects Analysis developed by the Department of Veterans Affairs National Center for Patient Safety; RCA = root cause analysis.

HFMEA STEPS AND DEFINITIONS

The steps in HFMEA, each described in the following sections, are

1. Select a topic,
2. Assemble the team,
3. Graphically describe the process,
4. Conduct a hazard analysis, and
5. Develop actions and outcome measures.

Working definitions of the terms used are as follows:

Detectability: The likelihood of detecting a failure before it materially affects completion of the task.

Effective control measure: A barrier that eliminates or substantially reduces the likelihood of a hazardous event occurring. For example, an anesthesiology machine may prevent cross-connection of medical gases through the use of pin indexing and connectors that have different threads.

Event diagram: A chronological flow diagram of a series of steps that occurred in the progress of a specific event (used with RCA).

Failure mode: The different ways that a particular process or subprocess step can fail to accomplish its intended purpose. These can be thought of as "what could happen." For example, if the subprocess step is capturing known drug allergies, failure modes could include not recording drug allergies, recording the information incompletely, or recording it incorrectly.

Failure mode cause: The root cause of the failure. This can be thought of as "why a failure could happen." An example of a cause for computer failure might be "infected with virus" or "hard drive failure." A cause is what must be directly remedied.

Failure mode effect: The outcome of the failure for the system or process. Failure mode effects can be local or global; local effects generally are less severe than global ones. The failure mode effect is measured through HFMEA by the severity and probability ratings.

Hazard analysis: A systematic technique for identifying the dangers of specific tasks and processes in order to reduce the risk of injury or failure.

Probability: Also known as occurrence, this is the rating scale representing the number of times (how often) an event occurs.

Process diagram: A diagram of the usual subprocesses or steps followed in a system or process. It is the way things are normally done (used with HFMEA) or ideally done (for comparison). It can be thought of as the directions given to someone new to a particular task or job: "First do this, which involves the following specific activities. Then proceed to...."

Severity: The rating scale that defines the seriousness of the effect should the failure or failure mode occur.

Single-point weakness: Also known as criticality, this is a step in the process so critical that its failure will result in system failure or in an adverse event. For example, momentary interruption of the power supply would result in loss of data.

Selecting a Topic

The selection of a topic for HFMEA is critical. If the topic is too broad, teams will become bogged down in process and subprocess details. If the focus is too narrow, the results can be trivial and have little positive impact. It is best for the patient safety officer (PSO) or medication safety manager (position titles vary), in conjunction with the quality manager or risk manager, to select the topic. Selection should be based on the corporate knowledge of the organization's PSO and leadership, reports of adverse events, and high-risk areas identified by the Joint Commission on Accreditation of Healthcare Organizations (JCAHO) through sentinel event alerts.

JCAHO advises that hospitals, in choosing a topic for proactive risk assessment (sidebar, page 579), use available information about sentinel events known to occur in health care institutions that provide similar care and services.[3] The topic selected for HFMEA should be worth the investment of resources by the institution, and the reason for the choice should be justifiable to an auditor or board member. Some potential topics related to the medication-use process are allergy information processing, proper execution of stat orders, chemotherapy processes, administration of patient-controlled analgesia, hypoglycemia or hyperglycemia management protocols, anticoagulant bridging processes, and addition of new drugs to the drug file.

Once a topic is selected, the PSO should complete a rough flow diagram outlining the primary steps in the process as used in that hospital. The PSO should then select five or six steps or a discrete portion of the process that will be the focus of the HFMEA. For example, in Figure 21-2, step 6 of the narcotic use process was selected. NCPS has found

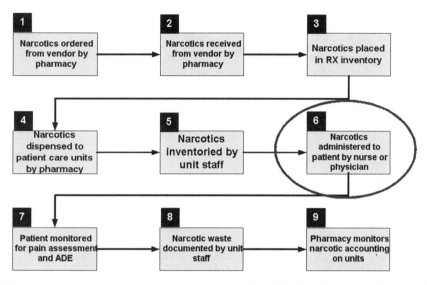

FIGURE 21-2 Identifying steps in the process selected for HFMEA (Healthcare Failure Mode and Effects Analysis, developed by the Department of Veterans Affairs National Center for Patient Safety), which in this example is a hospital's process for narcotic use.

PROACTIVE RISK ASSESSMENT AS AN ACCREDITATION STANDARD

The Joint Commission on Accreditation of Healthcare Organizations (JCAHO) influences the provision of care through its standards for accreditation. Although JCAHO accreditation is voluntary, almost all hospitals seek it. JCAHO's leadership standard LD 4.40 requires proactive risk assessment. The intent statement for this standard requires leaders of each accredited program to select at least one high-risk process for assessment each year. The medication system is high volume, high risk, and problem prone, making it an excellent choice for proactive risk assessment.

Health care professionals work in environments with complex human–machine interactions and exchanges of information and materials; therefore, they understand the need for proactively evaluating processes of care. Since the health care mission includes not harming patients, proactive risk assessment makes sense.

The LD 4.40 patient safety standard reads as follows: "Leaders ensure that an ongoing, proactive program for identifying risks to patient safety and reducing medical/health care errors is defined and implemented."[3] In the required risk assessment, failure modes and their possible effects must be identified. The most critical effects must be analyzed to determine what systems issues allow these effects to occur, and serious issues must be mitigated. HFMEA accomplishes this.

---

that narrowing the scope of the review provides a higher quality analysis that yields specific and effective actions. The team can analyze other parts of the process later, if relevant.

Forming a Team

The HFMEA team should be multidisciplinary. In the VA, a team has six to eight members. Having at least two subject matter experts on the team improves the likelihood that the analysis has technical merit. If a subject matter expert cannot attend a scheduled team

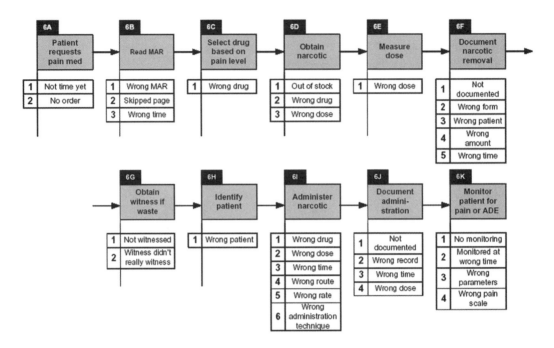

FIGURE 21-3 Subprocess steps (6A through 6K) in the narcotic use process. Failure modes are listed below each step.

meeting, a person with similar expertise in the subject can substitute. If additional subject matter expertise is required, individuals who are not on the team but possess the needed expertise can be consulted.

One team member serves as a team leader and one as the team recorder. It is helpful to designate a team leader who has skills in group process and can make sure the team functions effectively. The team recorder should be computer literate and expert in word processing, spreadsheet, and flow diagramming software. Usually, the PSO serves as an adviser to keep the team on track and a consultant to answer questions about the process, as well as helping the leader accomplish necessary tasks.

The multidisciplinary nature of the team ensures that various viewpoints are considered. Having a subject matter expert helps the team gain insight into how the process is actually performed. Conversely, having people who do not know the process ensures critical review of accepted standards and practices and identification of potential vulnerabilities that others might miss.

Graphically Describing the Process

Next, the process flow diagram is developed and verified. It is helpful to number the process and subprocess steps on the flow diagram (Figure 21-3).

Conducting a Hazard Analysis

The next step is to conduct a hazard analysis for the selected part of the process, listing and numbering all potential failure modes for each subprocess, as shown in Figure 21-3. The team should use various methods for identifying potential failure modes, including the NCPS triage cards for RCA, brainstorming, and cause-and-effect diagramming.

TABLE 21-5 HFMEA Operational Definitions of Severity

Type of Outcome	Description
Catastrophic Event *(Traditional FMEA rating of 10—Failure could cause death or injury)*	
Patient	Death or major permanent loss of function (sensory, motor, physiological, or intellectual), suicide, rape, hemolytic transfusion reaction, surgery or procedure on the wrong patient or wrong body part, infant abduction or infant discharge to the wrong family
Visitor	Death, or hospitalization of three or more
Staff	Death, or hospitalization of three or more
Equipment or facility	Damage equal to or more than $250,000
Fire	Any fire that grows larger than an incipient stage
Major Event *(Traditional FMEA rating of 7—Failure causes a high degree of customer dissatisfaction)*	
Patient	Permanent lessening of bodily functioning (sensory, motor, physiological, or intellectual), disfigurement, surgical intervention required, increased length of stay for three or more patients, increased level of care for three or more patients
Visitor	Hospitalization of one or two visitors
Staff	Hospitalization of one or two staff, or three or more staff experiencing lost time or restricted-duty injuries or illnesses
Equipment or facility	Damage equal to or more than $100,000
Fire	Not applicable—See Moderate and Catastrophic
Moderate Event *(Traditional FMEA rating of 4—Failure can be overcome with modifications to the process or product, but there is minor performance loss)*	
Patient	Increased length of stay, or increased level of care for one or two patients
Visitor	Evaluation and treatment for one or two visitors (less than hospitalization)
Staff	Medical expenses, lost time, or restricted-duty injuries or illness for one or two staff
Equipment or facility	Damage more than $10,000 but less than $100,000
Fire	Incipient stage or smaller
Minor Event *(Traditional FMEA rating of 1—Failure would not be noticeable to the customer and would not affect delivery of the service or product)*	
Patient	No injury nor increased length of stay nor increased level of care
Visitor	Evaluated and no treatment required, or refused treatment
Staff	First aid treatment only, with no lost time nor restricted-duty injuries nor illnesses
Equipment or facility	Damage less than $10,000 or loss of any utility without adverse patient outcome (e.g., power, natural gas, electricity, water, communications, transport, heat/air conditioning)
Fire	Not applicable—See Moderate and Catastrophic

Next, the team determines the severity and probability of the potential failure mode and the resulting hazard score, as shown in the matrix in Table 21-2. Severity is a measure of the potential effect of the failure mode—in other words, what would the impact be on patients or patient care if this should happen? Table 21-5 lists specific operational definitions for the categories of severity.

After the hazard score is determined, a decision tree (Figure 21-4) is used to determine the course of action. A separate worksheet (Table 21-6) is completed for each failure mode

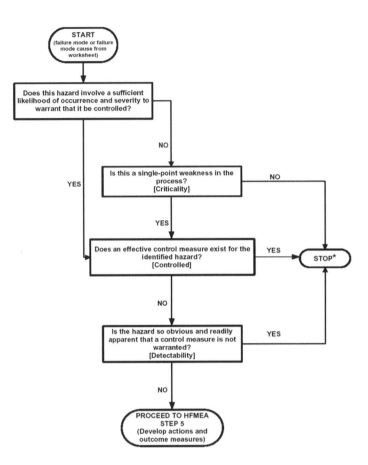

FIGURE 21-4 Hazard analysis decision tree. The rationale for all "stop" decisions is to be documented on the worksheet.

identified. The team completes the scoring for each failure mode before moving on to failure mode causes. If the hazard score is 8 or higher, the failure mode needs to be assessed.

The team does not need to determine causes for low-hazard failure modes. However, failure modes with low hazard scores are prioritized for action if the hazard is a single-point weakness. Similarly, high hazard scores are de-emphasized if the failure mode has an existing control measure or if it is detectable before the event would occur (i.e., if there is sufficient time to prevent harm to the patient or prevent that failure). One example of a detectable hazard is a missing patient wristband. If sufficient resources exist, a team can choose to remediate all failure modes, even those with low hazard scores.

Developing Actions and Outcome Measures

After proceeding through the decision tree (Figure 21-4), the team is ready to develop a description of actions for each failure mode selected for remediation, identify outcome measures, and identify a single person responsible for completing each action, as done in Table 21-6 for the failure mode "wrong narcotic selected" and its potential causes. In another example, actions for the failure mode cause "poor support from automated systems in confirming known drug allergies" might be "activate drug allergy module/screen in the computerized medical record, and prevent transmittal of prescription order unless allergy questions have been completed." Outcome measures for these actions could include setting a date for checking to ensure that the module has be activated and setting

TABLE 21-6 Failure Mode Worksheet for Selection of Wrong Narcotic

		HFMEA Step 4: Hazard Analysis				Decision Tree Analysis					HFMEA Step 5: Identify Actions and Outcomes			
Failure Mode: First evaluate failure mode before determining potential causes	Potential Causes	Severity	Probability	Hazard Score	Single-Point Weakness?[a]	Existing Control Measure?	Detectability	Proceed?	Action Type (Control, Accept, Eliminate)	Actions or Rationale for Stopping	Outcome Measure	Person Responsible	Management Concurrence
6 C(1) Wrong narcotic selected		Catastrophic	Occasional	12	>	N	N	Y					
	6C(1)a No profile interface on automated dispensing cabinet	Major	Occasional	9	>	N	N	Y	C	Implement bidirectional profile interface to automated dispensing cabinets by 6/1/04	100% of inpatient units will have profile interface by 7/1/04	IRM director	Y
	6C(1)b Drug is available on override in ADM after profile software installation	Major	Occasional	9	>	N	N	Y	C	Restrict the number and types of drugs available on override to emergency drugs and morphine injection	Less than 2% of drugs administered through the ADM will be removed via override studied monthly x 3	P&T chair	Y
	6c(1)c Multiple choices in ADM (i.e., matrix drawers)	Major	Occasional	9	>	N	N	Y	E	Weed out multiple choices of drugs and segregate the high-alert medications into unit dose compartments	Less than 2% of high-alert drugs will be in matrix drawers by 8/1/04 measured monthly x 3	Rx director	Y

HFMEA = Healthcare Failure Mode and Effects Analysis, developed by the Department of Veterans Affairs National Center for Patient Safety; IRM = information resource manager; ADM = automated dispensing machine; P&T = pharmacy and therapeutics committee; Rx = pharmacy.

[a] If the hazard score (see Table 21-2) is 8 or higher, HFMEA continues. HFMEA also continues, regardless of the hazard score, if a single-point weakness is present. Here, the arrow (>) in the single-point weakness column means HFMEA should continue on the basis of the hazard score, whether or not a single-point weakness exists.

a date for testing the system to verify that the allergy questions must be completed prior to order transmittal. A critical step in any proactive analysis model is testing to ensure that the system functions effectively and new vulnerabilities have not been introduced elsewhere in the system.

The commitment of the organization's leadership to each recommended action is needed. If management does not concur with an action, the team should revise it.

THE VA EXPERIENCE

The VA launched the use of HFMEA with a nationwide topic: assessment of hospitals' contingency processes for failure of the electronic bar code medication administration (BCMA) system. All facilities are required to have an up-to-date and well-tested contingency plan for medication administration in the event of a failure of BCMA. This was a complex topic for the facilities' first attempt at HFMEA. Supporting documents and guidelines were prepared by NCPS staff. National calls were made, documents were reviewed, team briefings occurred, and all VA facilities submitted their HFMEA reports to NCPS in the fall of 2002. The organization learned much from the process, and in 2003 the Office of Information (also involved with the HFMEA project) reviewed the best ideas from around the country. The information office released (and currently supports) software to help facilities nationwide to be in constant readiness for management of the medication process during BCMA downtime. Several far-reaching disasters in the past few years (the August 2004 power failure in the Northeast, hurricanes in Virginia, Florida, and the Gulf states) have affected VA facilities, but no facility reported any major problems in safely continuing the pharmaceutical care of veterans.

When the VA developed its proposed HFMEA method and plan for assessing the BCMA contingency process, JCAHO reviewed the process in advance. One caution given was that although this was a large national project, the risk assessment should be facility specific and represent risk to the patients served by that particular facility. It would be unacceptable to take a cookie-cutter approach that did not involve thorough and credible analysis by the facility where the actions were to be applied. This same caution should be applied to failure mode projects shared between health systems.

Although the VA does not require that HFMEA projects be submitted to NCPS, PSOs maintain an informal list of HFMEA projects. The VA has found that once facilities gain experience and recognize the utility of the approach, staff begins to analyze work processes and use HFMEA, often on more than one project per year.

TIPS FOR PERFORMING HFMEA

- ❑ Think of failure modes as "what could go wrong" that would prevent the process or subprocess step from being successfully completed.
- ❑ Think of the failure mode cause as "why" the failure mode would occur.
- ❑ Present failure modes as a problem statement that needs to be corrected (e.g., inadequate printer power supply).
- ❑ In making the process flow diagram, ensure that the team is diagramming steps that actually occur, not the ideal process (unless the ideal is being diagrammed for comparison).
- ❑ Once the team has diagrammed a process, post the flow charts in the work area. Staff on other shifts who do not serve on the team may have ideas for additional steps that have been forgotten or failure modes that no one has suggested.
- ❑ After the team develops the process diagram, have team members visit the work area to observe staff performing the process and verify that their assumptions are correct.

❑ Follow the numbering and lettering format for the process and subprocess diagrams. This is essential for keeping the team organized when it moves on to identifying failure modes.

❑ Chronological event flow diagrams used in RCAs are different from process flow diagrams used in HFMEA. Event diagrams show what actually happened on the day of the event. Process diagrams depict the usual activities needed to complete the task.

❑ For a failure mode or failure mode cause to be classified as "detectable" on the HFMEA decision tree, it must be so visible and obvious that it will be discovered before it interferes with completion of the task or activity.

❑ A single individual should be identified as responsible for follow-up on the corrective actions identified on the HFMEA worksheet.

❑ Use the most recent HFMEA worksheet; check the Internet site (www.patientsafety.gov) for the current version. Remember to conduct the hazard analysis on the failure mode before identifying failure mode causes, so that time is not spent identifying causes when it is not necessary.

❑ Pick projects of manageable size. More improvement can be made in safety through manageable continuous change that is actually implemented than through large, unmanageable projects.

❑ Failure modes can be tough to brainstorm. Teams can use the literature, the facility's own events, ISMP medication safety reports, similar failures from other industries, and the experience of team members. If teams get stuck, they should take a break or use creativity-building exercises to improve the flow of information. Cause-and-effect diagrams can also help by constantly raising the question "why?"

REFERENCES

1. National Advisory Committee on Microbiological Criteria for Foods. Hazard Analysis and Critical Control Point Principles and Application Guidelines, August 1997. Available at: http:/vm.cfsan.fda.gov/~comm./nacmcfp.html. Accessed August 18, 2005.

2. DeRosier J, Stalhandske E, Bagian JP, et al. Using Healthcare Failure Mode and Effect Analysis: the VA National Center for Patient Safety's prospective risk analysis system. *Jt Comm J Qual Improv.* 2002;28(5):248–67, 209.

3. *2005 Comprehensive Accreditation Manual for Hospitals.* Oakbrook Terrace, Ill: Joint Commission on Accreditation of Healthcare Organizations; 2004.

ADDITIONAL READINGS

Apkon M, Leonard J, Probst L, et al. Design of a safer approach to intravenous drug infusions: failure mode effects analysis. *Qual Saf Health Care.* 2004;13(4):265–71.

Benjamin DM. Reducing medication errors and increasing patient safety: case studies in clinical pharmacology. *J Clin Pharmacol.* 2003;43(7):768–83.

Blanchard J, Clinton P, De Lorimier K, et al. FMEA utilization as part of the implementation process of computerized physician order entry in a procedure area. Medinfo. 2004(CD):1529.

Capunzo M, Cavallo P, Boccia G, et al. A FMEA clinical laboratory case study: how to make problems and improvements measurable. *Clin Leadersh Manag Rev.* 2004;18(1):37–41.

Cohen MR, Senders J, Davis NM. Failure mode and effects analysis: a novel approach to avoiding dangerous medication errors and accidents. *Hosp Pharm.* 1994;29(4):319–24, 326–8, 330.

Dailey K. *The FMEA Pocket Handbook.* St Petersburg, Fla: DW Publishing; 2004.

Feldman SE, Roblin DW. Medical accidents in hospital care: applications of failure analysis to hospital quality appraisal. *Jt Comm J Qual Improv.* 1997;23(11):567–80.

Fletcher CE. Failure mode and effects analysis. *J Nurs Adm.* 1997;27(12):19–25.

FMEA (failure mode analysis): a new QI tool to help improve case management processes. *Hosp Case Manag.* 2003;11(3):33–6.

Gano D. *A New Way of Thinking: Apollo Root Cause Analysis. Effective Solutions to Everyday Problems Every Time.* 2nd ed. Yakima, Wash: Apollonian Publications; 2003.

Good J, Blandford A. Incorporating a user-focused failure modes and effects analysis-like technique into the design of safety critical systems. PUMA (Programmable User Modeling Applications). December 18,1997. Available at: www.cs.mdx.ac.uk/puma/.

Grissinger M, Rich D. JCAHO: meeting the standards for patient safety. *J Am Pharm Assoc*. 2002;42(5 Suppl 1):S54–5.

Joint Commission on Accreditation of Healthcare Organizations. *Failure Mode and Effects Analysis in Health Care: Proactive Risk Reduction*. Oakbrook Terrace, Ill: Joint Commission Resources; 2002.

Krouwer JS. An improved failure mode effects analysis for hospitals. *Arch Pathol Lab Med*. 2004;128(6):663–7.

Lerner EJ. An alternative to "launch on hunch." *Aerospace America*. May 1987:40–3.

Marx D. *Patient Safety and the "Just Culture": A Primer for Health Care Executives*. New York: Columbia University; 2001. National Heart, Lung, and Blood Institute Grant RO1 HR53772.

Marx DA, Slonim AD. Assessing patient safety risk before the injury occurs: an introduction to socio-technical probabilistic risk modelling in health care. *Qual Saf Health Care*. 2003;12 Suppl 2:ii33–8.

McDermott RE, Mikulak RJ, Beauregard MR. *The Basics of FMEA*. Portland, Ore: Productivity, Inc; 1996.

McNally KM, Page MA, Sunderland BV. Failure-mode and effects analysis in improving a drug distribution system. *Am J Health Syst Pharm*. 1997;54:171-7.

Palady P. *FMEA Failure Modes & Effects Analysis: Predicting & Preventing Problems Before They Occur*. West Palm Beach, Fla: PT Publications, Inc; 1995.

Passey RD. Foresight begins with FMEA. Delivering accurate risk assessments. *Med Device Technol*. 1999;10(2):88–92.

Ridgway M. Analyzing planned maintenance (PM) inspection data by failure mode and effect analysis methodology. *Biomed Instrum Technol*. 2003;37(3):167–79.

Senders JW. FMEA and RCA: the mantras of modern risk management. *Qual Saf Health Care*. 2004;13(4):249–50.

Spath P. Worst practices used in conducting FMEA projects (part 1). *Hosp Peer Rev*. 2004;29(8):114–6.

Spath PL. Using failure mode and effects analysis to improve patient safety. *AORN J*. 2003;78(1):16–37, 41–4.

Stalhandske E, DeRosier J, Patail B, et al. How to make the most of failure mode and effect analysis. *Biomed Instrum Technol*. 2003;37(2):96–102.

Stamatis DH. *Failure Mode and Effect Analysis: FMEA from Theory to Execution*. 2nd ed. Milwaukee, Wis: ASQC Quality Press; 2003.

Stevens T. Method to the madness. *Industry Week*. November 18, 1996:34.

Weeks WB, Bagian JP. Developing a culture of safety in the Veterans Health Administration. *Eff Clin Pract*. 2000;3(6):270–7.

Williams E, Talley R. The use of failure mode and criticality analysis in a medication error subcommittee. *Hosp Pharm*. 1994;29:331–7.

Woodhouse S, Burney B, Coste K. To err is human: improving patient safety through failure mode and effect analysis. *Clin Leadersh Manag Rev*. 2004;18(1):32–6.

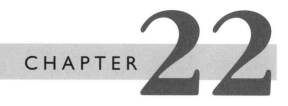

CHAPTER 22

THE CLINICAL BIOETHICS OF SAFE MEDICATION PRACTICES

J. Russell Teagarden

> The status quo is not acceptable and cannot be tolerated any longer. Despite the cost pressures, liability constraints, resistance to change, and other seemingly insurmountable barriers, it is simply not acceptable for patients to be harmed by the same health care system that is supposed to offer healing and comfort.
>
> *Committee on Quality of Health Care in America, Institute of Medicine*[1]

The National Academy of Sciences Institute of Medicine (IOM) challenged the status quo in American health care with the publication of its 2000 report *To Err Is Human: Building a Safer Health System.*[1] IOM's Committee on Quality of Health Care in America was reacting to the accumulating evidence that the number of errors—the number of preventable errors, in particular—was alarmingly high and needed immediate, systematic attention on a large-scale, societal level. The IOM report called for "a national commitment to achieve a threshold improvement in patient safety." Expert committees were formed to begin assessing safety problems in health care in the United States and to issue recommendations for improvement.[1-4]

This work of IOM ushered in a new level of public awareness and concern about safety. IOM called for bringing together "the intrinsic motivation of health care providers, shaped by professional ethics, norms and expectations, [with] factors in the external environment and factors inside health care organizations [that] can...prompt the changes needed to improve patient safety." The assumption was that health care workers would be motivated by their fundamental values to take the actions necessary to improve patient safety.

However, the sole responsibility for improving safe medication practices does not lie with health care professionals, as noted in the widely accepted definition of medication error from the National Coordinating Council for Medication Error Reporting and Prevention:[5]

> A medication error is any preventable event that may cause or lead to inappropriate medication use or patient harm while the medication is in the control of the health care professional, patient, or consumer. Such events may be related to professional practice; health care products, procedures, and systems, including prescribing; order communication; product labeling, packaging, and nomenclature; compounding; dispensing; distribution; administration; education; monitoring; and use.

By this definition, obligations are shared with patients, pharmaceutical and medical device manufacturers, drug distributors, medical system designers, drug safety regulators such as the U.S. Food and Drug Administration (FDA), educators, and the news media. Furthermore, taking responsibility for patient safety is an expectation; it should not be considered voluntary or above and beyond what is expected.

This chapter makes the case that safe medication practices are rooted in clinical bioethics. It discusses links among clinical bioethics concepts, safe medication practices, and current views of health care. The chapter also describes how clinical bioethics concepts can be used to work through issues related to safe medication practices, and how they can help explain and justify the positions taken by individuals and groups at different times.

CLINICAL BIOETHICS

The term "clinical bioethics" is used here to apply to the obligations conferred upon all participants in health care in their professional roles of taking care of individual patients and in their effects on the well-being of populations. "Ethics" refers to all aspects of what human beings owe one another. "Bioethics" refers to ethical issues in any of the fields within the life sciences. This chapter uses the term clinical bioethics to distinguish the obligations owed individual patients or groups by participants in their health care from ethical obligations in basic research functions or ordinary business transactions.

The clinical bioethics concepts discussed here derive from secular perspectives based on the moral reasoning of Western intellectual tradition, as distinguished from nonsecular perspectives drawn from religious doctrine, political systems, cultural norms, and established mores of associations and communities. Secular approaches to bioethics take the form of procedural concepts and justifications in order to be accepted across a broad range of moral viewpoints. Nonsecular perspectives more often include concrete guidance (e.g., directives) and moral sanctions (e.g., eternal damnation).[6]

The elements of secular clinical bioethics include moral theory, principles, rules, and judgments. Codes of ethics are also a common feature. Ethicists and philosophers debate the legitimacy and roles of these elements,[6–9] but these debates are not of concern for the purposes of this chapter. Instead, the chapter uses these elements as a framework for discussion of the obligations of individuals and organizations involved in the health care of patients and patient populations.

MORAL THEORIES

Moral theories provide a general view of a set of moral beliefs, norms, and practices. A moral theory can provide explanations and justifications for its constituent parts (e.g., principles, rules, and judgments) and how and why they relate to one another.[7] Familiarity with different moral theories is helpful in understanding the basis for the positions of others. The moral theories that can be applied to safe medication practices include consequentialist theory, deontological theory, liberal individualism, communitarian theory, ethics of care theory, and pragmatism (Table 22-1).

Consequentialist Theory

Consequentialist theory emphasizes the consequences of specific rules and acts, with judgments determined by the effects on particular groups. Best known among consequentialist approaches is utilitarianism, whose basic thrust is that rules and acts are morally correct when they produce the best state of affairs overall (e.g., the greatest good for the greatest number). Interpreted in the strictest sense, utilitarian theory does not easily

TABLE 22-1   Moral Theories Applicable to Safe Medication Practices

Theory	Description	Example
Consequentialist	Focus is on the net benefit, i.e., the greatest good for the greatest number, without respect for the impact on individuals	Drugs known to be harmful to some people can be approved for sale because of benefits they provide to many
Deontological	Focus is on what is right and what is wrong on the basis of obligations that can be generalized, and consequences can be disregarded	The truth about medication errors cannot be concealed from patients to protect providers and other patients from higher costs that result from process changes to improve safety and from litigation
Liberal individualism	Focus is on the rights of individuals and the obligations that accrue to others to effect those rights or at least not interfere with those rights	Patient claims of rights to be safe from harm caused by preventable errors in a hospital convey requirements for the hospital to implement specific safety measures
Communitarian	Focus is on the traditions, goals, values, social interactions, and practices of particular communities	Health care staff of an institution can possess a common goal of eliminating preventable errors and work toward implementing necessary improvement processes
Ethics of care	Focus is on relationships, emotions, empathy, and other forms of concern rather than on just objective and impartial concepts	Health care staff spend time listening to patients' stories and concerns and integrate them into their care plans
Pragmatism	Focus is on processes involving inquiry, discussion, negotiation, and reflection; judgments and reference to previous cases and experience are encouraged	Decision about the drugs to stock on a nursing unit is based on experience with previous actions and judgments about likely consequences

accommodate fairness and distribution of burdens as they apply to individuals.[7] As put by Rawls,[10] with utilitarianism "there is no reason in principle why the greater gains of some should not compensate for the lesser losses of others.... Utilitarianism does not take seriously the distinction between persons."

Policy-making bodies, legislatures, regulatory agencies, and pharmaceutical and medical device manufacturers often make decisions affecting safe medication practices that are consistent with utilitarian theory. They consider the effects of their decisions on populations and try to achieve the best possible result for the largest number of people, with the knowledge that these decisions could have adverse effects on certain individuals.

Utilitarian theory is at work, for example, when pharmaceutical manufacturers market FDA-approved products with the knowledge that they will be harmful to some individuals but with the hope that they will help many others.[11] A federal government evaluation of drugs approved for marketing between 1976 and 1985 showed that 50% of them were associated with serious risks for adverse drug reactions that manifested only after market availability.[12] Yet, because of favorable benefit-to-risk assessments, few of the drugs were withdrawn from the market. This application of utilitarian theory is well accepted, although arguments are common over what degree of harm to individuals is acceptable when juxtaposed with a certain net benefit to a population.[13]

A more controversial example of the application of this theory is debate about the hazards posed by the brand name of a particular pharmaceutical product. The brand names chosen for pharmaceutical products are known to affect medication safety, and, in general, manufacturers take safety into account when they consider brand names that will advance their marketing objectives. When challenged by practitioners and patient advocacy groups about potential and known hazards of a particular product name, manufacturers applying utilitarian theories consider the effects of a name change on larger groups. For example, manufacturers would give priority to consideration of the effects of the name change on populations of patients, health care professionals, and shareholders (potentially higher costs and confusion related to the change) over the effects on specific individuals.[14] The result might be different actions for different populations. Losec, the original brand name for omeprazole, was changed to Prilosec in the United States because of confusion with Lasix (furosemide), but it was not changed in other countries.[15]

Health care professionals may wonder why regulatory agencies do not require certain safety elements when approving pharmaceutical products. For example, specific requirements for labeling, packaging, or shipping might reduce the potential for certain medication errors. In applying utilitarian theory, however, regulatory agencies could decide that the higher costs associated with the benefits to a few individuals who might be harmed (or who might benefit more) could potentially put the products involved out of the reach of far more people, meaning that fewer would benefit overall. The approach may change for particular medications, because the theory permits revisions. For example, it seemed that the teratogenicity risk of oral isotretinoin for individuals was not acceptable when measured against the benefits to patient populations, but rather than removal of the product from the market, procedures for prescribing and dispensing were put into place.[16] The idea was to lower the risk to individual patients while preserving the benefits to patient populations.

Utilitarian theory can easily be accepted prima facie when presented as greatest good for the greatest number. When the effects on individuals are better understood, it can easily be rejected. Nevertheless, the application of utilitarian theory by pharmaceutical manufacturers and drug safety officials is understandable. If they were to prevent the use of any drug that could harm a few people, many people would be deprived of beneficial drug therapies. The key to applying utilitarian theory to safe medication practices is knowing when population benefits hold primacy over potential adverse effects on individuals, and when they do not. Such assessments are often referred to as "utilitarian calculations."[17]

Deontological Theories

Deontological theories rely less upon the consequences of rules and acts than on the rightness or wrongness of those rules or acts. What is considered morally right or wrong derives from obligations such as not lying, not deceiving, not betraying confidences, and not using people only as a means. If not lying is a generalized obligation, then health care professionals and institutions cannot lie to patients about medication errors, even when telling the truth leaves them open to punitive repercussions. Deontological theories also take into account intentions and motivations. For example, a health care institution that implements certain safe medication practices for the sole purpose of reducing financial liabilities cannot claim the moral high ground for protecting patients. Its actions may produce better patient protections, but that was not the primary motivation; the protections did not result from an attempt to comply with a general obligation for patient protection.[7]

In some respects, deontological theories can be seen as a counterbalance to consequentialist theories. According to deontological theory, some acts and rules cannot be permitted under any circumstances. People who oppose reimportation of prescription drugs because of patient safety concerns can be working under deontological theory. In taking this position, based on pre-existing standards and regulations, they are generalizing an existing obligation to ensure the safety of individual patients.[18] Despite the many benefits of lower-cost prescription drugs to patient populations, payer populations, and society in general, permitting reimportation of products that cannot be guaranteed to meet established safety standards and regulations is not consistent with the general obligation. A consequentialist view would permit prescription drug reimportation, but deontological views would not unless underlying general obligations are met.

As presented above, deontological and consequentialist theories appear to be polar opposites. However, certain aspects of deontological views have been used to modify strict utilitarian approaches. Called "deontological constraints" and "side constraints," these approaches alter utilitarian views by requiring consideration of effects on individuals. They allow limits on what can be done for the greater good when it comes at a cost to individuals.[19] The isotretinoin example can be seen as a deontological constraint. The drug's benefit to the population of users overall is sufficient to justify accepting the harm that can be done to individuals. However, consideration of the potential harm to individuals resulted in requirements to reduce the risk.[16]

Liberal Individualism

People staking out their "rights" are generally working under liberal individualism. Moral theories based on rights arose from motivations to protect individuals from exploitation, oppression, inequity, and various forms of harm that can interfere with a person's pursuit of life plans.[7] The rights most commonly considered in clinical bioethics are patient rights. People frequently insist on their right to health care and on their right to die. Legislators draft patient bills of rights.

A distinguishing feature of rights is that when they are accorded to some person, this implies the obligation of other persons to take action to benefit the rights holder or to at least avoid interfering with the rights holder insofar as it involves the rights accorded.[20] However, since moral theories based on rights usually are not comprehensive and often depend on the strength of their appeal, they can be vulnerable to other theories and opposing rights. For example, the obligations of health care professionals entailed by certain patient rights might be considered a violation of the rights of health care professionals.

Patients in the health care system are often in vulnerable positions and at risk for harm.[1] On the basis of this position, they can claim rights to be free from harm (minimally). But they also have a claim based on the privilege they, as members of the public, extend to health care professionals and institutions through licensing. Therefore, health care professionals and institutions have patient safety obligations on the basis of their licensure. That health care professionals and institutions accrue these obligations is not debatable, although the degree to which they do so (i.e., whether the obligations are too demanding) can be legitimately debated.

Rights-based theories, like deontological theories, can counter purely utilitarian approaches. Consider a requirement to remove concentrated potassium chloride solution for injection from hospital units and permit only the pharmacy to dispense it in diluted form. This requirement could be rejected on utilitarian grounds in situations where very few people are harmed and the inefficiencies and higher costs threaten the best result for the organization overall. However, patients' rights to safe medication practices could trump the utilitarian argument in this case.

Communitarian Theory

Communitarian theories counter liberal individualism (and other theories focused on individuals). These theories, sometimes known collectively as "communitarianism," are derived from the traditions, goals, values, social interactions, and practices of particular communities. The attendant moral views are based on the effects of actions and rules on a community rather than on particular individuals. The degree to which individual rights (i.e., liberalism) are subjugated for a community varies among the communitarian theories. Not all forms reject any amount of autonomy and pluralism. Communitarians can adopt democratic processes that depend on the input of individual members and processes that take into account individual rights.[21]

Communities are probably most often thought of in the form of political units (e.g., towns, counties, states); however, they can be thought of as groups of people brought together by shared goals and purposes. In regard to safe medication practices, then, patients within a health care system could be seen as a community based on their shared interests, goals, and expectations of medication safety. Health care providers and institutions, pharmaceutical and medical device manufacturers, and patient safety and regulatory officials can be thought of as separate communities because, for the most part, they do not share similar goals, values, and expectations in a uniform manner. For example, they may assign different weights to medication safety among all their goals, protestations to the contrary notwithstanding.

The IOM effort to improve safe medication practices draws on communitarian theory by attempting to bring together patients, providers, manufacturers, regulators, and others into one community with a shared goal of improving medication safety. The report also attempted to establish a common set of goals and purposes that set expectations for safe medication practices much higher than they currently are, given the separate communities' competing goals and purposes.[2,4] A community formed around improving medication safety can establish expectations that all the community members align their objectives accordingly and create a culture of safety. Although the concept may seem abstract, it has been realized in the aviation industry. The flying public—a community of travelers—demands a high degree of safety, and the aviation industry has joined this community and continued to advance the safety of air travel.

Ethics of Care Theory

The moral theories described thus far are generally considered impartial and based on universal principles and concepts. Not much room is left for injecting emotion, empathy, compassion, concern, relationships, and other such input. Supporters of ethics of care theory find that the content of other moral theories is inadequate to address all the possible needs of individuals in given situations. This theory has feminist origins and captures the female orientation that places importance on relationships and special needs of particular situations. Advocates of ethics of care theory are quick to reject any notion that only women can apply it; they also reject the notion that there is no place for moral theories that are based on more impartial universal principles and concepts.[22]

Ethics of care theory can be at work, for example, when health care professionals talk to patients about their medications and how to take them in the safest and most effective way. The relationship between the patient and the clinician, and the empathy and concern conveyed, can be important factors in improving medication safety. Other moral theories (best left to bioethicists and philosophers) can be used to justify patient medication counseling, but only ethics of care theory can justify it on the grounds that are most accessible to health care professionals because they are consistent with motivations for entering their chosen fields.

Pragmatism

Moral theories, particularly consequentialist and deontological theories, are considered foundational. Each is associated with a set of principles, rules, and virtues derived mostly from reason. As such, the theories cannot withstand too much alteration in interpretation or application without losing their identity. That is, at some point enough change has occurred that the theory is no longer what it started out to be. For example, attaching several deontological constraints in the application of consequentialist theory would impugn its integrity as a distinct and intact theory.[7] Furthermore, these theories do not easily accommodate experience. Therefore, an approach is needed that lies somewhere between consequentialist and deontological theories and that allows experiences to be considered in moral decision-making. Pragmatism, which has early 20th century American origins, offers a way to involve experience in clinical bioethics issues.[23]

"Clinical pragmatism" is the term used for the application of pragmatism to clinical bioethics. Fins et al.[24] describe pragmatism as "thorough processes of inquiry, discussion, negotiation, and reflective evaluation." Their description does not reject foundational moral theories; they position moral rules and principles as "hypothetical guides that identify a range of reasonable moral choices for the deliberations of patients, families, and clinicians." The requirement for incorporating moral theories and principles with experiences gives pragmatism structure and discipline, but reliance upon moral theories and principles is de-emphasized. The decision-making processes associated with pragmatism and clinical medicine are similar. Thus, wittingly or unwittingly, clinicians making moral judgments are more likely to apply clinical pragmatism than foundational moral theories and principles.[23]

The problem of concentrated potassium chloride solution is illustrative. The consequences have been deadly when potassium chloride solution stored on hospital units has been given by direct IV injection, rather than being diluted and slowly infused. The concentrated solution has been stored on some hospital units to enable rapid and efficient retrieval and eliminate the need to send unit staff to the pharmacy for a diluted solution ready for infusion.[25] Thus the problem: Should the convenience and efficiency of storing concentrated potassium chloride solution on the hospital unit outweigh the relatively rare but deadly error of injecting the concentrated solution? Utilitarianism would put emphasis on the overall good that can come from the decision; thus, the occasional catastrophic outcome is not material. Deontological theories would put emphasis on what is right or wrong on the basis of some generalization such as never countenancing any environmental element that could produce harm to an individual or institution. In liberal individualism, the right of patients to be safe would square off against the rights of clinicians and institutions. Clinical pragmatism, like ethics of care theory in this case, would permit other factors to enter the deliberation. For example, experience from previous situations, considered judgments based on similar cases, and input from all stakeholders (e.g., patients, clinicians, and administrators) could be used. When made in this way, the decision on what to do about concentrated potassium chloride solution would be tested against established moral theories and principles but would also take into account aspects that are highly relevant to the situation. This would ensure that the decision withstands moral scrutiny and is accepted as legitimate by those who are affected by it.

PRINCIPLES

Moral theories cover particular concepts in general terms. Principles have been established that bring guidance from moral theory into clinical bioethics (Table 22-2).[7] Still, critics charge that "principlism" is not sufficiently directive and in fact can cloud the moral clarity provided by theory. They also question whether principles provide useful guidance on moral theories, since principles can be linked to more than one theory.[8] Nonetheless, principles of clinical bioethics can be useful in justifying the ethical imperative for safe medication practices and can help clinicians arrive at good decisions. Four principles

TABLE 22-2   Principles Applicable to Safe Medication Practices

Principle	Description	Example
Nonmalfeasance	Refers to obligations to take actions to prevent harm to some person or persons	Using bar code technology for medication administration to reduce chances for error
Beneficence	Refers to obligation to take actions to benefit some person or persons	Helping patients get access to coverage for medications so that they receive adequate treatment and do not compromise use of the products in a harmful way
Respect for autonomy	Refers to patients' being able to make decisions about their health care and the obligation of health care professionals to ensure that patients have enough information	Patients are informed about safe medication practices they can effect in their own drug therapy
Justice	Refers to the equitable allocation of resources and treatment of one another	Medication error reporting that is nonpunitive and takes into account all possible causes and remedies

commonly used in clinical bioethics are nonmalfeasance, beneficence, respect for autonomy, and justice.

Nonmalfeasance

To health care professionals, "first, do no harm" *(primum non nocere)* has become a mantra. As such, practitioners may not recognize that this is a principle of clinical bioethics that entails obligations to take the actions necessary to prevent harm. Nonmalfeasance is one of the first principles of clinical bioethics and has been a part of Hippocratic tradition for centuries.

Despite this long-established principle, many people continue to be harmed by the health care system. An estimated 98,000 Americans die in hospitals annually because of medical errors, and preventable adverse events occurring in hospitals are among the top 10 causes of death.[1] The principle of nonmalfeasance demands significant attention to making health care safer. It connects "first, do no harm" to deontological, rights-based, and ethics of care theories—to a moral imperative and a corresponding set of obligations.

As it pertains to safe medication practices, the principle of nonmalfeasance implies, at minimum, that health care practitioners must follow professional standards and all policies and procedures directed at patient safety, such as matching patient identification with medication orders through bar coding systems. Beyond this, it requires that health care practitioners be aware of situations that could lead to harm and see that those situations are addressed. This awareness comes from being vigilant at the practice site and keeping up with the clinical literature on safety (e.g., Institute for Safe Medication Practices newsletters). The principle of nonmalfeasance also covers the role of health care practitioners in the safety of groups of people. For example, it compels health care professionals to report medication errors to individual health care system operations and to national reporting systems so safety can be improved for all people.

If nonmalfeasance is perceived to involve only the prevention of any possible harm to any individual or group, many opportunities to do better for an individual or group are precluded. No risk for harm would be tolerated or accepted; the use of the benefit-to-risk analysis would be invalidated. Innovation would be stifled; pharmaceutical and medical device manufacturers, for example, would produce only risk-free products. The aggressiveness of treatment regimens instituted by health care providers would be curtailed; only the most conservative measures, such as bed rest and oral hydration, would be used. Many cancer chemotherapies would never be used. Such a view of the principle of nonmalfeasance would be a misinterpretation, and it would do many patients a disservice. Nonmalfeasance leaves room for, and indeed anticipates, benefit-to-risk assessments. Pharmaceutical manufacturers and patient safety officials are not violating this principle per se if they accept some amount of risk for harm to individuals when it is balanced against the benefits afforded to others. Nor are health care providers violating the principle if they use treatment strategies with known risk for harm when there is a mitigating potential for benefit and the patient has given consent. Anything less than a careful and rigorous assessment of the risks and benefits, however, would be subject to blame, condemnation, and sanction.

In addition to effects on individual patients, nonmalfeasance also applies to effects on others. Certain actions to protect patients against harm could cause harm to health care providers or other populations. It may be too demanding to ask health care professionals and institutions to take on personal risk of harm or to ask organizations or populations to give up benefits to prevent the potential harm to certain individuals. For patient safety, blood may need to be drawn or X-rays taken, but it is probably asking too much of health care providers to carry out these procedures without proper protections and training (because of the risk of harm to themselves). However, if effective protective equipment and training are available, then the risk of harm to health care providers is lowered to a level that makes it difficult to justify refusal to provide patient care. Merck & Co., Inc. cited concerns about patient safety when it withdrew Vioxx (rofecoxib) from the market. The decision also took into account the effects on people who benefit from the drug, as evidenced by references made to the availability of alternatives. The company also had to consider the impact of the decision on its investors. In the end, the benefit-to-risk assessment was most consistent with product withdrawal.[26] In contrast, Roche did not withdraw Accutane (isotretinoin) from the market despite strong evidence for its teratogenetic effects, because the drug is important to many people who have no available alternative. In this case, the potential harm to many from withdrawal of the drug was more important than the potential harm to a few.

Nonmalfeasance, then, is a core principle of clinical bioethics that must be a part of every analysis and decision of every person to whom and every institution in which safe medication practices are relevant. The principle is complex, in that it is not aimed solely at individual patients nor meant to preclude any risk of harm. It calls for benefit-to-risk assessments, and it calls for assessments of risk to all stakeholders.

Beneficence

Many health care providers cite beneficence—perhaps using different words—as the reason they pursued careers in patient care. As used in clinical bioethics, beneficence refers to the moral obligation to take the actions necessary to benefit a person or group. Thus, as nonmalfeasance is a principle requiring actions to prevent negative consequences, beneficence is a principle requiring actions to cause positive consequences.

The notion of beneficence might conjure visions of only great and magnificent acts with huge societal implications, leaving the impression that beneficent acts are the sole province of the mighty and heroic. But this principle is meant to provide guidance on benefiting others, whether in a small matter involving one person or a substantial matter on a societal level. Beneficence applies to all health care professionals in their everyday roles with individual patients and in their leadership roles within their organized professions.

Some ethicists prefer to combine nonmalfeasance and beneficence because they are both meant to enhance the likelihood of a net benefit. Others prefer to consider these two principles separately because they may want to put more weight on the moral importance

TABLE 22-3 Conditions for Obligations Deriving from the Principle of Beneficence

Condition	Description
1	Y is at risk of significant loss of or damage to life or health or some other major interest
2	X's action is needed (singly or in concert with others) to prevent this loss or damage
3	X's action (singly or in concert with others) has a high probability of preventing it
4	X's action would not present significant risks, costs, or burdens to X
5	The benefit that Y can be expected to gain outweighs any harms, costs, or burdens that X is likely to incur

Sources: Adapted from reference 7 and, with permission, from D'Arcy E. *Human Acts: An Essay in their Moral Evaluation.* New York: Oxford University Press; 1963:56–7.

of nonmalfeasance, and because there are situations when these two principles are at odds with one another and need to be reconciled. As it pertains to safe medication practices, the distinction between nonmalfeasance and beneficence can be difficult at times to discern, but it can be important. Arranging the inventory of potentially dangerous products in ways that reduce the chance for mix-ups (e.g., separating sodium chloride from potassium chloride concentrated solutions for injection) could be considered an action taken to reduce harm and thus consistent with nonmalfeasance. Helping a patient get access to a prescription drug through a patient assistance program so that the patient's use of the medication is not modified in some harmful way could be considered an action to provide a benefit to the patient and thus consistent with beneficence.[27] The drug reimportation debate is as an example of how these two principles can be at work on the same issue. People in support of prescription drug reimportation point to the principle of beneficence as a motivating factor because many more people would have access to drugs that are more affordable. Opponents point to nonmalfeasance as a motivating factor because of concerns about safety.[28] Although the distinction between these two principles can be obscure at times, at other times the distinction is necessary in order to prioritize actions on issues of contention in ways that are ethically justifiable.

The principle of beneficence can be very demanding. Without limits, it could result in physical harm, social disruption, and financial ruin, among other adverse consequences to those striving to meet its requirements. This principle can have a powerful effect on people; government officials in some states have felt compelled to circumvent the law to facilitate prescription drug reimportation for citizens in their states.[29,30] This principle clearly is not meant to motivate people to break laws or harm themselves in other ways. A health care professional who is the only known person to be histocompatible with a patient needing a heart transplant would not be expected to be a live donor on the basis of obligations stemming from the principle of beneficence. Beauchamp and Childress[7] have established a set of conditions to help people determine reasonable limits to obligations stemming from the principle of beneficence (Table 22-3). These conditions take into account the severity of the consequences of inaction, the importance of the needed action to the desired outcome and the probability of its success, the benefit-to-risk assessment, and the intensity of demands placed on the person or group bearing the obligation to act.

Respect for Autonomy

People should be free to make decisions or at least to have significant involvement in decisions that affect them. As obvious and inviolable as this idea may seem today, it is contrary to the Hippocratic tradition that dominated for 2,500 years. Physicians decided what was best without the patient's input; other health care professionals (e.g., pharmacists, nurses) behaved accordingly. In the 1960s, the unfettered authority of health care professionals over their patients was rejected—along with many other forms of authority. In health care, the rejection of authority came in the form of the principle of respect for autonomy.[7]

This principle requires that patients have all the information they need to make good decisions. Although it may be tempting to think this principle applies only to informed consent for experiments involving human subjects, the principle is meant to cover all aspects of health care for individual patients, including safe medication practices. As articulated by the IOM Committee on Quality of Health Care in America,[2]

> Ensuring patient safety also requires that patients be informed and participate as fully as they wish and are able. Patients and their families should not be excluded from learning about uncertainty, risks, and treatment choices. The committee believes an informed patient is a safer patient. (p. 45)

Thus entailed are obligations of health care professionals and institutions to proactively provide patients and family members the information they need to participate in benefit-to-risk assessments and to use medications safely and effectively. These obligations extend to educators to prepare health care professionals to perform in these roles; to pharmaceutical manufacturers to provide labeling, packaging, and support materials to enhance patient knowledge; and to health care institutions that provide the staffing and environments to teach patients about safe medication practices.

A reciprocal obligation resides with patients: to seek and use information to ensure medication safety (for themselves and other patients). This obligation includes reporting errors to health care professionals and through available reporting systems. The Committee on Data Standards for Patient Safety has recommended that the Agency for Healthcare Research and Quality encourage and support research to "study the role of patients in the prevention, early detection, and mitigation of harm due to errors."[4] (p. 170) Patients should not rely solely on health care professionals and institutions. They can get good information from a variety of credible consumer-oriented sources: the Institute for Safe Medication Practices (www.ismp.org), Agency for Healthcare Research and Quality (www.ahrq.gov/consumer/), National Patient Safety Foundation (www.npsf.org), and Joint Commission on Accreditation of Healthcare Organizations (www.jointcommission.org/GeneralPublic/).

The principle of respect for autonomy works also to mitigate potentially extreme applications of the principles of nonmalfeasance and beneficence. Nonmalfeasance taken to its literal extreme, as discussed above, could mean no action is taken if there is any risk for adverse consequences. If patients are brought into a benefit-to-risk assessment, they may be willing to tolerate the risk for harm involved (e.g., with cancer chemotherapy). Beneficence taken to its literal extreme becomes paternalism, in which decisions are made on the assumption that "the doctor knows what is best for the patient." The result can be actions that harm the patient or fail to meet the patient's objectives. Patients can be protected against this possibility by being brought into the decision making-process.

Justice

As used in clinical bioethics, the principle of justice is most often focused on health care resource allocation. A real or relative scarcity of resources is apparent in every health care system. This means there will be competition among those who want or need those resources, and thus there will be winners and losers. The principle of justice is used to guide the distribution of limited resources among certain groups.[7,31] The principle of justice has been applied to certain aspects of safe medication practices as well.[32]

Different conceptions of justice have been established. Everyone is familiar with justice as applied in the context of the law of the land and as administered by the courts. More relevant to safe medication practices is Rawls's conception of justice as fairness: "fair terms of social cooperation…given by an agreement entered into by those engaged in it."[33] (p. 15) Rawls's work was aimed broadly at societies, but the concept can be applied to smaller groups. To do so, patients, health care providers and institutions, pharmaceutical and medical device manufacturers, health care safety officials, and payers and administrators must be viewed as participants in a cooperative arrangement (or the communities envisioned by communitarians). Participants join cooperative arrangements because there are benefits, but there are rules that specify fair terms of cooperation. The terms must be reasonable to and accepted by all participants and must include reciprocity or mutuality concepts so that "all who do their part as the recognized rules require are to benefit as specified by a public and agreed-upon standard." (p. 6) The result of this cooperative arrangement is a just culture, and it has been said that a just culture is a safe culture.[32]

An example of how a just culture can improve medication safety involves error reporting. Few will disagree that reporting medication errors is an ethical imperative and an obligation conferred on all participants in health care, including patients, although debate exists about the seriousness and the nature of errors that should be reported.[34] But health care professionals traditionally have been reluctant to report medication (and other) errors because of concerns about being singled out and sanctioned. As stated by Hebert,[35] "Fears of punishment and retribution typically drive adverse event reporting and disclosure underground and prevent learning and improvements in patient safety." Reason and Hobbs[32] refer to this approach as the "person model of human error" and characterize it as "the idea that errors and violations arise solely out of the perversity and unreliability of human nature." A just culture will incorporate a view that there are many aspects to errors, and will establish an environment of trust where blame-free and attributable actions can be distinguished and handled accordingly. Only in a just culture (see Chapter 23) will all participants in health care report errors through local and national reporting systems.

The principle of justice as it applies to resource allocation is also relevant to safe medication practices. Medication safety is advanced by staffing levels, education and training of all participants in health care, availability of reporting systems, and technology, among other factors, all of which come at a cost of time and money. Thus, on both local and societal levels, justice requires that the allocation of resources for health care include needs for medication safety. In 2001, the IOM Committee on the Quality of Health Care in America suggested that about $1 billion should be allocated over 3 to 5 years to address needed improvements in safety issues in health care.[2]

CODES OF ETHICS

For centuries, health care professions have developed and maintained codes of ethics to articulate the moral dimensions of the roles and responsibilities of their members. These codes are meant to provide direction and guidance to the profession's members and to establish expectations for its constituents (e.g., patients, communities).[17]

Interpreting and using codes of ethics in the health professions is not always straightforward. Codes can vary in their degree of specificity. Some provide very clear direction on actions to take in specific situations, whereas others provide only general guidance. Likewise, the consequences of noncompliance with codes of ethics vary. Some sponsors sanction members for not meeting the ethical obligations specified by their code; others use their code as justification for holding someone blameworthy and as a basis for remedial education and training. The interpretation and use of codes of ethics for health care professionals is further complicated by the multiple codes of ethics that can be relevant to any of them at any given time. For example, a health care professional can be subject to codes of ethics from professional organizations, employers, and affiliated communities and religions. Different organizations' codes can be at odds with one another, making it necessary for the health care professional to ascertain which one has primacy in a given situation.

Today's codes of ethics in the health care professions address imperatives related to safe medication practices, but their guidance tends to be general rather than specific. The codes function more as a framework than as an inventory of answers to specific problems. Thus, obligations for safe medication practices must be inferred from the elements of the codes that focus on the needs of patients. For example, pharmacists incur this obligation from the statement in the Code of Ethics for Pharmacists that says the "pharmacist promises to help individuals achieve optimum benefit from their medications."[36] Nurses can locate this obligation in a statement found in the Code of Ethics for Nurses that says, "The nurse promotes, advocates for, and strives to protect the health, safety, and rights of the patients."[37] From what the American Medical Association calls the "principles of medical ethics," physicians can discern a moral obligation for safe medication practices in the statement, "A physician shall, while caring for a patient, regard responsibility to the patient as paramount."[38] In contrast, codes of ethics from earlier times were much more specific on this issue. The Hippocratic Oath requires that the physician swear to keep patients "from harm and wrong." Pharmacists were given explicit direction on how to keep patients from harm, for example, in the stipulation that they not provide powerful substances or poisons to people.[39]

Codes of ethics established by the health care professions often consider the members' obligations to larger communities as well as to individual patients. They give no guidance, however, on how to prioritize one set of obligations over another when the two conflict. As a result, health care professionals are likely to confront particular situations in which an individual patient or a community will win or lose when the relevant code of ethics specifies that obligations are owed to both. It is then left to the health care professional to make a judgment about priorities, using input from moral theories and principles, as well as from considered judgments and experience.

SAFE MEDICATION PRACTICES AND CURRENT VIEWS OF HEALTH CARE

The moral dimensions of safe medication practices are substantiated by the connections between clinical bioethics concepts and current, credible views of health care. The view of health care as proposed by the IOM Committee on Quality of Health Care in America and pharmaceutical care doctrine can be used to make this case.

Medication Safety and the Six Aims of Health Care

In *To Err Is Human*, the Committee on Quality of Health Care in America documented important gaps in health care in the United States. In turn, the committee was charged with proposing strategies for redesigning the health care system to address patient safety. The committee presented six aims for health care: that it should be safe, effective, patient-centered, timely, efficient, and equitable.[2] Each of the six aims entails safe medication practices, and each can be linked to core clinical bioethics concepts.

The aim of *safety* obviously implies safe medication practices. This aim should be interpreted broadly, however, to encompass safety aspects of treatment failures (e.g., poor effectiveness) as well as the occurrence of errors leading to harm. The *effectiveness* aim refers mostly to how clinical decisions are made. It requires that evidence be used in making decisions and specifies that patient values be taken into account. Ensuring effectiveness is important because as the chances for effectiveness diminish, the relative chances for harm increase. *Patient-centeredness*, as described in the committee report, "encompasses qualities of compassion, empathy, and responsiveness to the needs, values, and expressed preferences of the individual patient." This aim requires actions to ensure that patients are relieved of physical and emotional discomfort, which includes being kept safe from harm. *Timeliness* was made a specific aim because delays in health care delivery can have an important impact on safety and effectiveness. *Efficiency* was seen by the committee as an important aim because successfully attacking inefficiencies resulting from overuse will lower the risk of harm from unnecessary interventions. One aspect of the *equity* aim focused on the requirement of treating patients equally without regard to any personal attributes or characteristics such as age, ethnicity, religion, and sexual orientation. Delivering on this aim with respect to safe medication practices means that actions taken to improve medication safety must be applied to all patients. This aim also implies a just system that encourages medication error reporting by not singling out health care professionals for punitive consequences when criminal behavior or ill intent is not involved.

The six aims were not directed only at health care professionals. Health care organizations and institutions, managers, administrators, pharmaceutical and medical device manufacturers, safety officials, professional societies and accrediting organizations, academia, news and broadcast media, and patients all have responsibilities for furthering these aims. Health care organizations and institutions can create the environments and support systems needed for educating patients in safe medication practices and can work to improve the efficiency and timeliness aspects of medication safety. Professional societies and accrediting organizations can set safety-related standards and hold stakeholders accountable. Legislative and regulatory bodies can establish the safe harbors and just processes that would facilitate the reporting of errors. Pharmaceutical and medical device manufacturers can develop and retool products according to safety needs. News and broadcast media can communicate important medication safety messages to consumers. Attempts to produce a health care system reflecting the six aims will not succeed if the effort is shouldered only by professionals working in direct patient care settings.

The committee did not cite particular bioethics concepts to justify any of the six aims of a health care system. But aspects of bioethics theory, principles, and codes underlie the aims, furthering the integration of clinical bioethics into the basic structure of health care. Nonmalfeasance and beneficence are prominent principles in the aims involving safety, effectiveness, patient-centeredness, and timeliness. Respect for autonomy is also at work within these aims because of the importance placed on the patient's role in safe medication practices; patients need to be informed to be effective. Justice is at work in both the efficiency and equity aims, as evidenced in the emphasis placed on securing the resources necessary for a safe and effective health care system and on providing a just process for people who report and react to medication errors. Ethics of care theory can be appreciated in the aim of patient-centeredness, with its emphasis on compassion and empathy. Some aspects of liberal individualism are hinted at in this aim as well, through its reference to expectations patients can have that health care professionals must make efforts to relieve their discomfort. The aims of safety and effectiveness could be justified on the basis of deontological theory, in that they place an emphasis on what is right to do for patients and what obligations are thereby conveyed to all the stakeholders that have been identified. In contrast, the aims of efficiency and equity are more consistent with utilitarian theory because they address patient populations, which could mean that benefits to a certain population can be gained at the expense of particular individuals.

TABLE 22-4 Eight Categories of Drug-Related Problems

Category	Description
Untreated indications	The patient has a medical problem that requires drug therapy (an indication for drug use) but is not receiving a drug for that indication
Improper drug selection	The patient has a drug indication but is taking the wrong drug
Subtherapeutic dosage	The patient has a medical problem that is being treated with too little of the correct drug
Failure to receive drugs	The patient has a medical problem that is the result of his or her not receiving a drug (e.g., for pharmaceutical, psychological, sociological, or economic reasons)
Overdosage	The patient has a medical problem that is being treated with too much of the correct drug (toxicity)
Adverse drug reactions (ADRs)	The patient has a medical problem that is the result of an ADR or adverse effect
Drug interactions	The patient has a medical problem that is the result of a drug–drug, drug–food, or drug–laboratory interaction
Drug use without indication	The patient is taking a drug for no medically valid indication

Source: Adapted with permission from reference 40.

Medication Safety and Pharmaceutical Care

In the practice of pharmaceutical care, the focus is on achieving desired outcomes of drug therapy for patients. Thus, although pharmaceutical care has been referred to as a theory of practice within the pharmacy profession, its concepts apply not only to pharmacists but to all participants in health care.[40]

Pharmaceutical care is organized conceptually around drug-related problems. The outcomes of drug therapy are defined as follows: cure of a disease, reduction or elimination of symptoms, arresting or slowing of a disease process, and preventing a disease or symptoms. Table 22-4 relates these outcomes to eight categories of drug-related problems. It is easy to see the strong link between safe medication practices and these elements of pharmaceutical care. Thus, if pharmaceutical care is accepted as the prevailing mode of drug therapy within health care, safe medication practices have to be accepted as an integral element of health care rather than as tangential.

As with the six aims of a health care system identified by the IOM committee, the definition of pharmaceutical care was not conceived as an ethics tract but clinical bioethics concepts are apparent in its foundation. Pharmaceutical care "is based on a covenant between the patient...and the provider."[40] Such a basis could be derived from ethics of care theory. With its emphasis on the rightness of focusing on drug-related problems, pharmaceutical care has strong links to deontological theory as well, but it does not go so far as to suggest that patients have certain rights that convey absolute duties upon pharmacists or other participants in health care. Pharmaceutical care's emphasis on patient-centeredness, when strictly interpreted, is strong enough to disqualify ethical justifications based on utilitarian or consequentialist theories. A strict interpretation would suggest that the obligations owed to individual patients are without regard to effects on populations; a more liberal interpretation would accommodate the effects of these obligations on populations, at least to the extent that they affect individual patients. For the most part, then, the links between pharmaceutical care and clinical bioethics theories are to theories that place priority on individual patients rather than those (e.g., consequentialist theory) that place priority on the net effects on populations. This emphasis may be more a result of when the doctrine was introduced than of any conscious effort to exclude the possibility that a group could hold primacy over an individual within the scope of pharmaceutical care. Since the doctrine was first published in 1990, codes of ethics have evolved to recognize responsibilities to groups and communities, as well as to recognize that resources available for pharmaceutical care are limited.

The four outcomes and eight drug-related problems around which pharmaceutical care is organized suggest strong links to the bioethics principles of nonmalfeasance and beneficence. Responsibilities for taking action to prevent harm to patients are conveyed by the drug-related problems labeled as overdosage, adverse drug reactions, drug interactions, and drug use without indication. Responsibilities for taking action to ensure that desired outcomes are achieved are conveyed by the drug-related problems labeled as untreated indications, improper drug selection, subtherapeutic dosage, and failure to receive drugs. Despite the emphasis on individual patients in pharmaceutical care, a link to respect for autonomy is not highlighted, but it is implied in the reference to the covenant between the pharmacist and patient.

CONCLUSION

Core clinical bioethics concepts applicable to current views of health care obligate all participants in care to be involved in safe medication practices. Different views of health care could change this imperative. A view could emerge that only diseases or conditions that harm society as a whole (e.g., massive epidemics) be addressed, which would mean the mortality rates associated with diseases like cancer and heart failure would not be a concern as long as birth rates kept pace.[41] Another view could be that health care is like all other consumer products, which would mean leaving consumers to fend for themselves for the most part. Both of these alternatives would diminish obligations to effect safe medication practices. In the current view, however, health care holds a special status over that of ordinary consumer goods, and the needs of individuals are more important than how health care contributes only to the perpetuation of society as a single entity.[42]

The current view of health care involves giving priority to the health needs of individual people while balancing the needs of populations. Further, the current view distinguishes health care from ordinary consumer products and services, and this distinction carries with it a warranty of truth, which means consumers expect that representations of health care products and services are true and not subject to the exaggerations associated with other consumer products.[43] Thus, clinical bioethics applies to current views of health care because these views require consideration of what individuals and populations are owed and how to balance competing priorities.

Because pharmaceuticals can produce great benefit or great harm, safe medication practices are integral to health care. No single overarching moral theory can be referenced to support the ethical justification for safe medication practices. However, several moral theories, principles, rules, and codes provide inspiration and guidance. Further, they require the involvement of all participants in health care in safe medication practices. And they are consistent with, if not a basis for, credible views of health care. Given the obligations to provide health care and the ethical basis for safe medication practices, IOM was correct in saying that "it is simply not acceptable for patients to be harmed by the same health care system that is supposed to offer healing and comfort" and in challenging all participants in health care to overcome "cost pressures, liability constraints, resistance to change, and other seemingly insurmountable barriers" to safe medication practices. This will happen only when all participants in health care understand that safe medication practices are an ethical enterprise.

REFERENCES

1. Kohn LT, Corrigan JM, Donaldson MS, eds. *To Err Is Human: Building a Safer Health System*. Washington, DC: National Academies Press; 2000.
2. Committee on Quality of Health Care in America, Institute of Medicine. *Crossing the Quality Chasm: A New Health System for the 21st Century*. Washington, DC: National Academies Press; 2001.
3. Committee on the Work Environment for Nurses and Patient Safety. Page A, ed. *Keeping Patients Safe: Transforming the Work Environment for Nurses*. Washington, DC: National Academies Press; 2004.
4. Committee on Data Standards for Patient Safety. Aspden P, Corrigan JM, Wolcott J, et al., eds. *Patient Safety: Achieving a New Standard for Care*. Washington, DC: National Academies Press; 2004.
5. National Coordinating Council for Medication Error Reporting and Prevention. What is a medication error? Available at: www.nccmerp.org/aboutMedErrors.html. Accessed December 1, 2004.
6. Engelhardt HT. *The Foundations of Bioethics*. 2nd ed. New York: Oxford University Press; 1996.
7. Beauchamp TL, Childress JF. *Principles of Biomedical Ethics*. 5th ed. New York: Oxford University Press; 2001.
8. Clouser KD, Gert B. A critique of principlism. *J Med Phil*. 1990;15:219–36.
9. Daniels N. *Justice and Justification: Reflective Equilibrium in Theory and Practice*. Cambridge, UK: Cambridge University Press; 1996.
10. Rawls J. Classical utilitarianism. In: Scheffler S, ed. *Consequentialism and Its Critics*. Oxford, UK: Oxford University Press; 1994:14–9.
11. Strom B. Potential for conflict of interest in the evaluation of suspected adverse drug reactions. *JAMA*. 2004;292:2643–6.
12. *FDA Drug Review: Postapproval Risks 1976–1985*. Washington, DC: General Accounting Office; April 26, 1990.
13. FDA's Dr. Graham says other drugs besides Vioxx also pose safety risks. *Scrip*. November 22, 2004.
14. Davis N. Trademarks, the bottom line, and safety. *Hosp Pharm*. 1999;34:1141.
15. Cohen M. Lessons lost by the global pharmaceutical industry. *ISMP Medication Safety Alert!* April 18, 2001.
16. Roche Laboratories. New prescribing procedures for Accutane as of April 10, 2002. Available at: www.rocheusa.com/products/accutane/accutane_prescriber.pdf. Accessed September 12, 2004.
17. Veatch RM, Haddad AM. *Case Studies in Pharmacy Ethics*. New York: Oxford University Press; 1999.
18. Cohen M. The high cost of medications: a bitter pill to swallow. *ISMP Medication Safety Alert!* May 20, 2004.
19. Nozick R. Side constraints. In: Scheffler S, ed. *Consequentialism and Its Critics*. Oxford, UK: Oxford University Press; 1994:134–41.
20. Hart H. Are there any natural rights? *Phil Rev*. 1955;64:175–91.
21. Emanuel EJ. *The Ends of Human Life: Medical Ethics in a Liberal Polity*. Cambridge, Mass: Harvard University Press; 1991.
22. Carse A. Facing up to moral perils: the virtues of care in bioethics. In: Gordan S, Benner P, Noddings N, eds. *Caregiving: Readings in Knowledge, Practice, Ethics, and Politics*. Philadelphia: University of Pennsylvania Press; 1996.
23. Moreno JD. Bioethics is a naturalism. In: McGee G, ed. *Pragmatic Bioethics*. 2nd ed. Cambridge, Mass: MIT Press; 2003:3–16.
24. Fins JJ, Bacchetta MD, Miller FG. Clinical pragmatism: a method of moral problem solving. In: McGee G, ed. *Pragmatic Bioethics*. 2nd ed. Cambridge, Mass: MIT Press; 2003:29–44.
25. Cohen M. Despite knowledge of accidents, opportunities for potassium ADEs persist in some US hospitals. *ISMP Medication Safety Alert!* August 28, 1996.
26. Neilan T. Merck pulls Vioxx painkiller from market, and stock plunges. Available at: www.nytimes.com/2004/09/30/business/30CND-MERCK.html. Accessed October 2, 2004.
27. Cohen M. ISMP Quarterly Action Agenda—March–June 2004. *ISMP Medication Safety Alert!* July 1, 2004.
28. Kaiser Family Foundation. Prescription drug costs. Available at: www.kff.org/rxdrugs/7175.cfm. Accessed October 7, 2004.
29. Haskell M. State to start importation of Rx drugs; Gov. Baldacci defies feds in move to lower drug costs. *Bangor Daily News*. October 1, 2004: 1.
30. Press A. States launch prescription drug program. *New York Times*. Available at: www.nytimes.com/aponline/health/AP-Prescription-Drugs.html. Accessed October 5, 2004.
31. Daniels N, Sabin JE. *Setting Limits Fairly: Can We Learn to Share Medical Resources?* New York: Oxford University Press; 2002.
32. Reason J, Hobbs A. *Managing Maintenance Error: A Practical Guide*. Burlington, Vt: Ashgate; 2003.
33. Rawls J. *Justice as Fairness: A Restatement*. Cambridge, Mass: Belknap Press; 2001.
34. Regents of the University of Michigan. Disclosure. 2002. Available at: www.med.umich.edu/patientsafety/toolkit/disclosure/chapter.pdf#controversy. Accessed October 17, 2004.
35. Hebert P. Disclosure of adverse events and errors in healthcare: an ethical perspective. *Drug Saf*. 2001;24:1095–102.

36. American Pharmacists Association. Code of ethics for pharmacists. Available at: www.aphanet.org. Accessed October 23, 2004.

37. American Nurses Publishing. Code of ethics for nurses with interpretive statements. Available at: http://nursingworld.org/ethics/code/ethicscode150.htm. Accessed October 23, 2004.

38. American Medical Association. Principles of medical ethics. Available at: www.ama-assn.org/apps/pf_new/pf_online?f_n=browse&doc=policyfiles/HnE/E-0.01.HTM&&s_t=&st_p=&nth=1&prev_pol=policyfiles/CEJA-TOC.HTM&nxt_pol=policyfiles/HnE/E-0.01.HTM&. Accessed October 23, 2004.

39. Lawall CH. Pharmaceutical ethics: a historical review of the subject with examples of codes adopted or suggested at different periods, together with a suggested code for adoption by present-day associations. *J Am Pharm Assoc.* 1921;10:895–910, 961–4.

40. Hepler CD, Strand LM. Opportunities and responsibilities in pharmaceutical care. *Am J Hosp Pharm.* 1990;47:533–43.

41. Jonas H. Philosophical reflections on experimenting with human subjects. *Daedalus: J Am Acad Arts Sci.* 1969;98:219–47.

42. Daniels N. Justice, health, and healthcare. *Am J Bioethics.* 2001;1(2):8–16.

43. Illingworth P. Bluffing, puffing and spinning in managed care organizations. *J Med Phil.* 2000;25(1):62–75.

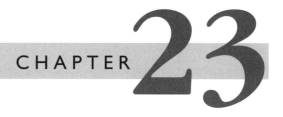

CHAPTER 23

MANAGING MEDICATION RISKS THROUGH A CULTURE OF SAFETY

Judy L. Smetzer

Health care is a highly complex, error-prone industry. From emergency departments to high-volume pharmacies, providing patient care involves nonstop activity and intricate, interdisciplinary processes in which the slightest mistake could spell catastrophe. Other industries, such as chemical manufacturing, nuclear power production, and aviation, are equally prone to errors with potentially dire consequences, yet many of them have better safety records than health care. Leaders in such industries, known as high-reliability organizations (HROs), manage with the goal of safe, reliable performance while acknowledging the complexity of their systems, creating an environment in which workers can openly talk about safety concerns, and successfully handling the unexpected.[1]

The laudable safety record of HROs stems from their culture, in which all levels of the organization share the same safety goals and values.[2] The difference between health care and HROs lies not so much in the tools used to achieve safety, but in a willingness to fully abandon cultural precedents linked to perfect performance, individual autonomy and accountability, ambition, and discipline.[3]

During the past decade, those most involved in the patient safety movement have come to realize that preventing catastrophic events—or, for that matter, any preventable event that causes patient harm—requires more than changing systems and implementing best practices. It also requires a change in our mindset about patient safety, and a change in the underlying culture in which health care is provided, assessed, and improved.

Today, health care leaders can no longer ask staff to work in systems that rely on perfect performance every time. They can no longer believe that autonomous individuals can work as safely as well-trained teams. They can no longer leave patients out of the loop when it comes to their safety. They can no longer turn a blind eye to what all know are common causes of failure, such as fatigue. They can no longer afford to simply pay lip service to patient safety while tacitly supporting productivity goals that encourage shortcuts. They can no longer find merit in disciplining staff for unintentional mistakes that were caused, in large part, by systems outside their direct control. They can no longer assume that "no news is good news" in regard to the prevalence of errors. Most health care providers are now ready to embrace culture changes that will vastly improve patient safety.

DEFINING A CULTURE OF SAFETY

An organization's culture is defined as a pattern of shared basic assumptions about its values (what is important), beliefs (how things work), and behaviors (the way things are done there) that are taught to its workforce in both explicit and implicit ways.[4] Cultural assumptions in an organization typically embody the philosophies of senior leaders. The attitudes and beliefs of individual workers may vary, but knowing the organizational culture helps guide their day-to-day activities. The culture also makes life predictable, because workers know how the leaders will likely react to certain situations.

The definition of a culture of safety in health care is still being refined. The United Kingdom's Health and Safety Commission describes it as follows:

> The safety culture of an organization is the product of individual and group values, attitudes, competencies, and patterns of behavior that determine the commitment to, and the style and proficiency of, an organization's health and safety [efforts]. Organizations with a positive safety culture are characterized by communications founded on mutual trust, by shared perceptions of the importance of safety, and by confidence in the efficacy of preventive measures.[5]

This definition does not identify specific elements of a culture of safety in health care or means of achieving it. However, recurrent themes or characteristics have been identified in HROs:

- Strategic emphasis on safety,
- Mindfulness and resilience,
- Just culture,
- Teamwork and localized decision-making,
- Error-defying systems and redundancy,
- Proactive focus and community involvement,
- Learning culture, and
- Safety measurement.

The safety performance of HROs is based on the combination of all these characteristics. Together, these characteristics form the underpinning of a safety culture with five subcultures:[6,7]

- *Informed culture.* Safety information systems that collect, analyze, and communicate information about risk and errors provide all workers with knowledge of the current factors that determine the safety of the organization as a whole.
- *Reporting culture.* Workers are prepared to report hazards, risks, near misses, and errors, thus arming the organization with an accessible memory of safety information.
- *Just culture.* Workers trust each other, are rewarded for providing safety information, and are clear about their responsibilities regarding safe behavioral choices.
- *Flexible culture.* Workers respect each other's abilities and are adaptable in crisis, often reorganizing themselves to manage impending danger by deferring important decisions to task experts until the crisis is resolved.
- *Learning culture.* Workers possess the willingness and competence to draw responsible conclusions from the organization's safety information systems and make substantial system changes when necessary.

This chapter addresses each identified characteristic of safety in HROs and encourages readers to consider its application in health care and medication safety.

STRATEGIC EMPHASIS ON SAFETY

HROs have a palpable passion for safety, which is grounded in a healthy acknowledgment of the high-risk nature of the business and a preoccupation with the potential for failure. The leaders know that although safety does not guarantee quality, it is an absolute prerequisite for the delivery of high-quality service. It is the way they do business—articulated in specific terms, not safety jargon or buzzwords, and incorporated into strategic plans with generous budgets. Leaders are visible in work areas and hold discussions with the workforce to learn firsthand about the barriers to safe work, and to share strategic goals, build trust, and demonstrate safety priorities. The leaders realize that errors are costly in financial terms, but the strategic emphasis on safety is driven largely by consideration of important societal values, such as freedom from accidental injury, that are part of the organization's culture.

Strategic Plans in Health Care

An organization's strategic goals reflect its mission, values, and priorities and define its intent and vision for the future. Therefore, much can be learned about the organization's culture by examining its strategic plan and assessing the change projects intended to achieve its long-term goals.

Since medication errors represent one of the greatest risks to patients,[2] a health care organization's strategic plan might be expected to include specific medication safety objectives. However, the 2000 Institute for Safe Medication Practices (ISMP) Medication Safety Self Assessment indicated that just 12% of hospital chief executive officers had included such objectives in their overall strategic plans.[8] The 2004 ISMP Medication Safety Self Assessment showed improvement; about half (53%) of the participating hospitals had included medication safety objectives in their strategic plans. The other half, however, apparently have yet to give this crucial patient safety issue the leadership attention it merits. Most likely, the situation is similar in other types of health care facilities.

Medications have an important role in achieving most health care organizations' core mission, so preventing patient harm during the delivery of services should be considered good business.[9] A sizable body of evidence suggests that medication errors are bad business because they are costly in both human and financial terms.[10–14] One study identified an additional cost of $5,857 per adverse drug event,[10] which can be extrapolated to $2.8 million for a 700-bed hospital. Patients also bear financial costs of medication errors, such as loss of income for themselves and for family members providing care.[13,14] A successful business model for health care must focus on medication safety not just because it makes sense financially, but because it is the right thing to do.[9]

Medication Safety Strategic Goals

Strategic goals related to medication safety should be based on an assessment of internal medication-use processes and capabilities, external influences on medication safety, patient needs, and the health care marketplace as it relates to medication use. One tool for identifying organizational strengths, weaknesses, and opportunities for improvement is the ISMP Medication Safety Self Assessment.[15] External influences that might be considered in setting strategic goals include the Joint Commission on Accreditation of Healthcare Organizations (JCAHO) National Patient Safety Goals[16] and medication management standards,[17] the National Quality Forum Safe Practices for Better Healthcare,[18] the Institute for Healthcare Improvement (IHI) 100,000 Lives Campaign,[19] and ISMP's quarterly action agendas.[20]

In selecting strategic goals, the long-term benefits to staff and patients should be carefully considered; the goal should have real value to the organization and its patients.

Goals related to medication safety should be brief, clearly describe where the organization wants to be in the future, integrate well with the organization's other strategic goals, and match the organization's capabilities and culture.[21] Realistic boundaries for each goal should be established; although it may be difficult to reject great ideas for reducing medication errors, the goals should reflect agreed-upon capabilities. The sidebar below gives an example of a goal and change projects necessary to achieve it.

SAMPLE STRATEGIC GOAL[21]

Goal: Involve patients and the local community in medication safety initiatives and medication self-management programs

Boundaries

❏ Specific evidentiary materials that could be used against the hospital in the event of a lawsuit should not be shared with patients.
❏ Proper medical supervision is required for patient self-management programs.

Enduring Advantages

❏ Patients are reassured that the organization is taking effective steps to reduce the risk of medication errors.
❏ Allows patients to play an important role in their own safety.
❏ Allows consumers to make more informed decisions about their health care.
❏ Enhances public perception of the organization's commitment to patient safety.
❏ Increases potential to become the provider of choice for patients, employers, and other purchasers of health care.

Potential Barriers or Threats

❏ Lack of media and community interest in proactive, nonsensational, medication safety information.
❏ Lack of sufficient reimbursement for medical supervision of medication self-management programs for patients.

Change Projects

❏ Quarterly (or more often), submit proactive medication safety information (editorials, feature articles, appearances on radio talk shows) to the local media to educate patients about medication safety, actions taken to reduce the risk of medication errors, and ways patients can help prevent medication errors.
❏ Communicate the hospital's mission, vision, and medication safety initiatives to patients and visitors through internal resources such as videos, televisions in patient rooms, and storyboards in the lobby.
❏ Provide patients and the community with a periodic newsletter covering safe medication practices.
❏ Establish patient responsibilities regarding medication use in the hospital, and review the policy with all patients and families upon admission or during the preadmission process. (Examples include prohibition of taking medications from home, and the expectations patients should have about medications provided in the inpatient setting.)
❏ Invite community representatives to quarterly meetings with nurses, pharmacists, and physicians to regularly solicit their input on medication safety issues.

❑ Hold an annual community health fair to raise awareness of medication safety issues (e.g., poison prevention, safe use of herbal products, safety tips for self administration of nonprescription medications) and to describe error prevention efforts at the hospital.

❑ Establish self-management programs in the community using hand-held monitoring devices for patients who have diabetes or take warfarin.

❑ Define and communicate the means for patients and their families to report concerns about safety, and encourage them to do so (a JCAHO National Patient Safety Goal).

	Timeline										
Milestone	**Mar**	**Apr**	**May**	**Jun**	**Jul**	**Aug**	**Sep**	**Oct**	**Nov**	**Dec**
Patient bill of responsibilities	X									
Community meetings		X		X			X		X	
Editorial to media	X			X			X			X
Consumer newsletter					X					
Consumer reporting system						X				
Self management program—warfarin									X	

Leadership Roles

Leaders play a crucial role not only in setting strategic goals for medication safety but also in executing those goals and maintaining a culture of safety. Table 23-1[22] lists some characteristics identified in senior leaders who manage highly productive, safe, and reliable organizations.

While senior leaders in HROs garner workforce enthusiasm for safety, they know that middle managers convey the culture to frontline workers. If middle managers' behavior supports the message that safety is a top priority, then frontline employees will prioritize their work accordingly.

TABLE 23-1 Characteristics of Senior Leaders in High-Reliability Organizations[22]

Sets well-defined, nonnegotiable, evidence-based goals

Does not postpone action for weeks or months while refining data; instead, looks for action that can be taken on the basis of available information

Garners rapid agreement among managers and staff on goals and timelines for achieving them

Exerts energy in building structures to ensure flawless execution of plans, rather than devising financial incentives, kick-off retreats, motivating campaigns, or other fanfare

Possesses sophisticated knowledge of the cost of poor quality and safety as it relates to complex workflow and variable processes

Insists on execution of plans by managers

Actively engages in improvement efforts firsthand, providing directional leadership regarding measurement, infrastructure management, results reporting, overcoming barriers to execution, and setting the next wave of action plan execution

Supports a culture in which execution of plans is the norm and part of every leader's and manager's day-to-day work but does not consume an excessive amount of effort (execution of plans seems to be hard-wired into the culture)

Succeeds without incentives alone playing a key role

Metes out no observed consequences for failure (but minimizes the potential for failure)

Requires a disciplined format for recording action plans and reporting results (sometimes sophisticated spreadsheets, but more often just a text document or graphic presentation template)

Oversees an intense, frequent, focused review process, requiring all managers to provide detailed reports on the execution of plans, and reserving adequate time for these team activities (may seem tedious to some, but results in flawless execution, a worthy outcome for any extended meeting)

TABLE 23-2   Questions to Ask Staff during WalkRounds[1,23]

1. Were you able to care for your patients this week as safely as possible? If not, why not?
2. Can you describe the unit's ability to work as a team?
3. Have there been incidents that almost caused patient harm but didn't?
4. What do you think the unit could do on a regular basis to improve safety? Would it help to talk about safety concerns, such as near misses and patients with the same name, during report?
5. If you prevent or intercept an error, do you always report it?
6. If you make or report an error, are you concerned about personal consequences?
7. Do you know what happens to the information once you report it?
8. Have you developed any personal practices to avoid making errors (e.g., memory aids, checking)?
9. What specific intervention from leadership would make the work you do safer for patients?
10. What would make these WalkRounds more effective?

The ability to achieve strategic goals and sustain a culture of safety is linked to visible support from high administrative positions and open, two-way communication between senior leaders and workers. Frankel and colleagues[23] demonstrated the success of a tool, called WalkRounds, for connecting senior leadership to patient safety and embedding safety in the culture. A core group of senior executives and vice presidents, patient safety/quality/risk managers, and others (e.g., pharmacist, research assistant, physicians) makes weekly rounds in different areas of the organization to talk with staff about safety. Over time, the team repeatedly visits all clinical units. When the team arrives on a unit, the nurse manager finds one or two nurses who can spare 15 minutes. The unit's physician leaders are also asked to join the group. For high visibility, the leadership group holds the safety discussion with staff in an open area on the unit. The leaders ask questions (such as those in Table 23-2) about patient safety and adverse events and record the comments on a worksheet. At the end of the discussion, a senior leader summarizes the most important issues. Staff members who participated are thanked in an e-mail message and are asked to tell two other staff members about the rounds.

Information shared during the rounds is then analyzed, classified according to contributing factors, and prioritized. A summary report is created monthly for the senior leaders, high-priority issues are addressed, and feedback on how to improve safety is given to the frontline staff during future rounds. This cycle of information, analysis, action, and feedback sustains itself as it continues to engage leadership, educate clinicians and managers, and lead to improvements. Each participant in WalkRounds receives the message that the organization encourages a healthy preoccupation with patient safety, supports and values the skills needed to assess the environment for potential harm, and appreciates and rewards those who report risk and adverse events and make appropriate changes to enhance safety.

Some health care facilities have used the basic concept of WalkRounds to facilitate leadership support for patient safety in other ways. Pronovost et al.[24] described a process in which senior hospital leaders each "adopt" an intensive care unit (ICU) and work with the staff to identify and address safety issues. This process includes asking staff to describe the last patient who could have been harmed if someone had not intervened, and to describe how the next patient on the unit will likely be harmed and actions that could prevent this. Leaders then use this information to plan and fund system changes designed to avoid harmful errors.

MINDFULNESS AND RESILIENCE

Workers in HROs use a vital set of cognitive processes to continuously discover and correct errors, especially under adverse conditions. Collectively termed mindfulness, this characteristic of HROs is driven by a deep, chronic sense of unease that arises from admitting the possibility of failure even with familiar, well-designed, stable processes.[25,26] Workers in HROs pay attention to their work in a more mindful way than workers in less reliable organizations. They expect surprises and consider them a valuable resource because they encourage learning and discovery and discourage complacency or inertia.[25] Workers in HROs are empowered to act on surprises to achieve reliable outcomes. Their ability to deal with the unexpected, even in crises, is largely dependent on the structures and cognitive processes that have been nurtured in their organizations before the unexpected happens, such as

- Preoccupation with system failures that counteracts the usual sense of comfort and complacency that stems from success,
- Reluctance to simplify interpretations of ongoing information about safety,
- Sensitivity to operations on the part of all workers, regardless of their level, particularly those at the frontline of work,
- Cultivation of resilience to improvise and work with existing tools in different ways to solve problems, and
- Deference to expertise; adherence to hierarchies is loosened to allow the person with the most expertise to make decisions.[1,25,27]

Preoccupation with System Failures

Chronic worry about system failure is a characteristic of HROs.[1,25–27] People in HROs are naturally suspicious of quiet periods and reluctant to engage in any activities that are not sensitive to the possibility of error.[25] They ask, "What happens when the system fails?" not "What happens if the system fails?"[1] This preoccupation with failure is interesting, since actual failures in HROs are rare. With few data on actual failures, learning in HROs is accomplished in three ways: by treating any and all failures or near misses as a symptom of systemwide problems, by thoroughly analyzing actual and potential failures, and by counteracting the complacency of success.[25,27]

To increase the flow of information available for learning about safety, HROs encourage and reward error and near-miss reporting. They recognize that the value of remaining fully informed about safety is far greater than any perceived benefit from disciplinary actions. Landau and Chisholm[25,28] emphasized this point more than a decade ago by describing a seaman on a nuclear aircraft carrier who broke a vital rule: He did not keep track of all his tools while working on the landing deck. He subsequently found one of his tools missing and immediately reported it. All aircraft en route to the carrier were redirected to other bases until the tool was found. The next day, the seaman was commended for his disclosure during a formal ceremony—a very different response than would be expected in health care (e.g., if reporting a lost sponge after an operative procedure delayed or postponed other scheduled procedures).

HROs perform in-depth analyses of the information they get. They pay attention to near misses and can clearly see how close they came to a full-blown disaster; less safe organizations consider close calls to be evidence of their successful ability to avoid a disaster.[25] Less safe organizations also tend to localize failures (e.g., the problem is in the ICU, so changes are needed in the ICU). HROs generalize even small failures and consider them a lens for uncovering weaknesses in other vulnerable parts of the system.[25,27] HROs acknowledge that the accumulation of small failures increases the risk of large failures.

Because HROs focus on failures, they avoid potential pitfalls of success, such as complacency, overconfidence, and inertia.[27] They do not expect success to breed success, and managers do not attribute success to their own abilities or the organization as a whole. Instead, they are alert to the danger of drifting into overconfidence and rote work habits during periods of success.[1,25–27]

Reluctance to Simplify Interpretations

Organizations typically handle complex issues by simplifying them, thus ignoring certain aspects. Top management can wind up making decisions based on an oversimplified view of the issue.[27] Seemingly inconsequential details that are ignored can accumulate and come rushing to the forefront as complex problems. HROs resist simplification because it limits the ability to envision all possible undesirable effects and the precautions necessary to avoid them.[1,25,27] They take nothing for granted.

In resisting simplification of safety issues, HROs seek out different points of view and encourage healthy skepticism.[1,25–27] The downside of this is the potential for miscommunication and conflict among workers with differing views. HROs counteract this by placing high value on interpersonal skills, mutual respect, norms that curb arrogance and self importance, and teamwork.[1,25,27] HROs promote trust among people with diverse opinions by fostering the belief that skepticism and diversity are necessary to improve reliability.[25]

Sensitivity to Operations

People in HROs are more likely than those in less reliable organizations to monitor the big picture. Workers are familiar with operations beyond their own jobs. They provide and receive real-time information about current operations and ongoing organizational monitoring.[25,27] Sensitivity to operations means not only that workers have a big picture of current or future operations but that they participate in ongoing assessment to identify problems early. Thus, small problems get undivided attention, and unexpected events are attended to more quickly, seldom growing into large-scale issues.

Commitment to Resilience

While HROs spend an enormous amount of time anticipating system failures and taking steps to prevent them, they devote equal resources to cultivating workers' ability to improvise and cope with unexpected hazards.[25,27] Reliable organizations expect to have problems that cannot be solved by following the usual rules.[1,26] They accept that they cannot foresee everything or fully eliminate human error, technical failures, or system weaknesses. Therefore, they continually build workers' competence to quickly recognize and assess approaching hazards, detect and respond to failures, contain them, and recover from them when necessary.[25–27]

Unlike anticipation, which encourages workers to think before acting to avoid problems, resilience requires workers to act while thinking about a problem that has already occurred. When lives are at stake, informal networks of people quickly organize themselves and pool their knowledge to respond to the crisis.[25] Once the danger is past, the failure is thoroughly analyzed and steps are taken to prevent recurrence.

Deference to Expertise

To manage the unexpected, HROs allow decisions to be made by those with the appropriate expertise, who are not necessarily those with the most seniority or authority.[25,26] In less reliable organizations, important decisions are made by those at the top of the hierarchy. HROs have hierarchies too, but position does not necessarily dictate who is an important decision maker.[25]

When problems arise, workers in HROs follow a more flexible decision-making structure. They rely on a combination of decision makers from all levels of the organization, selected on the basis of worker or team specialization and expertise.[25] When decisions have to be made quickly, those closest to the problem and its resolution are empowered to make important decisions.[25–27] If workers get into situations they do not understand or can no longer manage, they are not afraid to admit they need help. In fact, it is considered a sign of strength and confidence for staff to know when they have reached their limit and enlist help from others, including senior leaders.[27]

JUST CULTURE

HROs have embraced a just set of values and characteristics that support the reporting and investigation of hazards and errors, and the fair handling of workers involved in errors. A just culture does not have a "name, blame, shame, and train" philosophy, nor does it take the position that only "bad apples" are involved in errors; rather, the leaders and workforce support a fierce intolerance of intentional risk taking, and fair treatment of individuals who make errors, regardless of the outcome. Thus, workers trust each other and their leaders, and they report hazards and errors without fear of retribution or embarrassment. The language used in discussing errors is positive; near misses are great catches, errors are opportunities to learn. Leaders demonstrate that all reports, contributions, and concerns about safety are valued, respected, appreciated, and rewarded.

Health Care: Where We Were

Punitive Culture

Before 1990, health care providers often attempted to manage risk, errors, and catastrophic mistakes by exhorting their staffs to work carefully and by retraining, "counseling," or disciplining workers involved in errors. The prevailing thought was that individual workers were fully, and sometimes solely, accountable for the outcomes of patients under their care, even if the processes for achieving those outcomes were not under the workers' direct control.

Perfect performance was expected and was believed to be achievable through education, professionalism, vigilance, and care. The threat of disciplinary action for errors was thought to be a necessary part of maintaining safety. Counseling sessions after an error often focused on perceived weaknesses in the individual worker, with little thought to the system's contribution. Improvement strategies offered to the worker were often goal oriented—"follow the five rights," for example, when a medication error occurred—with little direction about how to achieve the goals or how to make safer behavioral choices.

In many cases, the severity of disciplinary actions was determined by the severity of the undesirable outcome. Some believed that the potential consequences of even a single mistake were enough to justify punitive action; workers who made an error that caused patient harm were thought to be "justly" disciplined. Procedural violations were regarded as simply unacceptable; this provided little insight into their system-based causes. Many believed that bad apples, or bad practitioners, were the cause of frequent or harmful errors, and that weeding them out would result in a safer health care environment.

The effect of such a punitive environment was the exact opposite of the intended result. Fear of retribution, ranging from undue embarrassment to termination of employment or licensure, drove errors underground. Frontline workers were afraid to report their own errors or those of a colleague. Most workers did not even consider reporting hazards that could lead to errors, believing little would be done to remedy them. Instead, they created work-arounds to avoid those minefields. Middle managers and organizational leaders grew content with believing that "no news was good news," thus missing opportunities to learn about existing risks and implement robust system changes to reduce the chance of error.

Blame-Free Culture

In response to the shortcomings of a punitive culture, a shift toward a blame-free, or no-blame, response to errors was occurring by the mid 1990s. It was clearly a step in the right direction,[7] acknowledging human fallibility and the impossibility of perfect performance. It recognized that most unsafe acts were the result of mental slips or lapses, or honest mistakes that were rooted in system, process, technical, or environmental weaknesses that lay dormant in the organization until errors or proactive assessment efforts brought them to light.

In this new culture, there was general agreement that even the most experienced, knowledgeable, vigilant, and caring workers could make mistakes that could lead to patient harm. There was recognition that workers who made honest errors were not truly blameworthy, and that there was little benefit in punishing them for these unintentional acts. A survey of 1,200 health care professionals in 2001 clearly indicated that individual attitudes about errors, disciplinary action, and overall accountability for safety were becoming less punitive; however, practitioners did not fully support an industrywide desire to become wholly nonpunitive.[29-32]

The weakness of a blame-free approach is that it fails to confront individuals who willfully (and often repeatedly) make unsafe behavioral choices, knowingly disregarding a substantial and unjustifiable risk that most peers would recognize as likely leading to a bad outcome.[7,33,34] Although disciplining workers for honest mistakes is counterproductive, a wholly blame-free culture is problematic because of failure to discipline for truly reckless behavioral choices that endanger patients.[6,7,33,34] In such cases, sanctions of an appropriate severity may be warranted. Furthermore, a policy of amnesty for all unsafe acts lacks credibility and opposes many workers' sense of justice. A wholly blame-free culture is not feasible or desirable.

Health Care: Where We Are Going

Just Culture

A new culture is emerging. Drawing from the culture in HROs, it runs counter to an overly punitive culture, yet it addresses the weakness of a wholly blame-free approach. This just culture has been described as follows:[35]

> People often ask, so what is a just culture? There is no short recipe for developing a just culture within an organization. Just culture is part science, part philosophy, and a whole bunch of hard work and commitment. It's a way of doing business—a set of standards by which regulators, employers, and employees can work together to create the best possible outcomes.
>
> On one side of the coin, it is about creating a reporting environment where staff can raise their hand when they have seen a risk, or made a mistake. It is a culture that rewards reporting and puts a high value on open communication—where risks are openly discussed between managers and staff. It is a culture hungry for knowledge.
>
> On the other side of the coin, it is about having a well-established system of accountability. A just culture must recognize that while we as humans are fallible, we do generally have control of our behavioral choices—whether we are an executive, a manager, or a staff member. Just culture flourishes in an organization that understands the concept of shared accountability—that good system design and good behavioral choices of staff together produce good results. It has to be both.

In a just culture, the emphasis is on learning and shared accountability for outcomes. All workers know what is valued in the organization, including safety, and they continually look for risks that pose a threat to those values. They are thoughtful about their behavioral choices and always thinking about the most reliable ways to get the job done right. Managers are always looking for system design features that would give the workforce the very best opportunity to perform well. It is recognized that every endeavor carries the risk of unpredictable human error, but workers are held accountable for the things that are under their control: system design, particularly for the management and administrative team, and behavioral choices for the entire workforce.[36]

This accountability model is not dependent on outcomes. How a worker is judged or treated after an error does not depend on whether patient harm has occurred. Rather, behavioral choices leading to risk or error, which were under the worker's control, form the basis for accountability in a just culture.[33]

Three Behaviors

Three types of behavior can be involved in error: human error (worker did something other than intended), at-risk behavior (unintentional risk taking), and reckless behavior (conscious disregard for a substantial and unjustifiable risk).[33,34] Each type of behavior has a different cause and thus requires a different response.

Human Error

Human error involves unintentional behavior that causes or could have caused an undesirable outcome.[36] An error of execution occurs when a planned action is not completed as intended; an error of planning occurs when the wrong plan is used to achieve an aim.[2,6] Since human error is not predictable and can strike at any moment, it is the weakest link in performance.

Often, human error is a product of system design.[34] Since it arises from weaknesses in the system, it must be managed through process improvements and system or environmental changes. Discipline is not warranted or productive, because the worker did not intend the action or the risk or harm that resulted. The just option is to console the worker and shore up the systems to prevent further errors.[33] As Reason[6] noted, we cannot change the human condition, but we can change the conditions under which humans work.

At-Risk Behavior

Everyone knows that "to err is human," but we tend to forget that "to drift is human," too.[34] Behavioral research shows that we are programmed to drift into unsafe habits, to lose perception of the risk attached to everyday behaviors, or mistakenly believe the risk to be justified.[37] In general, workers are most concerned with the immediate and certain consequences of their behavior—saved time, for example—and undervalue delayed or uncertain consequences, such as patient harm. Their decisions about what is important on a daily list of tasks are based on the immediate desired outcomes.[37] Over time, as perceptions of risk fade away and workers try to do more with less, they take shortcuts and drift away from behaviors they know are safer.[34] Table 23-3 gives examples of at-risk behaviors in the medication-use process.

The reasons workers drift into unsafe behaviors are often rooted in the system. Safe behavioral choices may invoke criticism, and at-risk behaviors may invoke rewards. For example, a nurse who takes longer to administer medications to her patients may be criticized, even if the additional time is attributable to safe practice habits and patient education. But a nurse who is able to handle a half-dozen new admissions in the course of a shift may be admired, and others may follow her example, even if dangerous shortcuts have been taken.

Therein lies the problem. At-risk behaviors can become a normal part of everyday work; they can become so common and seem so inconsequential that perception of their risk fades.[6,25] This is known as normalization of deviance.[6,38] Procedures that are obviously risky become accepted because they have not caused a problem—yet. Workers no longer perceive the risk, or they mistakenly believe the risk is justified.[33] And cutting corners has

TABLE 23-3   Practitioners' At-Risk Behaviors in the Medication Process[34]

Patient Information

Preparing more than one patient's medications or more than one medication at one time

Not using two identifiers (e.g., name, medical record number, birth date) to check patient identity

Using estimated, rather than actual, patient weight

Prescribing, dispensing, or administering medications without checking patients' laboratory values and vital signs

Not checking a patient's allergies before prescribing, dispensing, or administering medications

Not waking the patient for assessments or medications

Not viewing or checking the patient's complete medication profile (or medication administration record [MAR]) before prescribing, dispensing, or administering medications

Drug Information

Prescribing, dispensing, or administering medications without complete knowledge of the medication

Unnecessary use of manual calculations

Not taking the MAR to the patient's bedside when administering medications

Administering medication before pharmacy review of the order

Excessive prescribing of nonformulary medications, or refusal of therapeutic interchange

Not questioning unusually large doses of medications

Writing incomplete discharge instructions

Failing to validate or reconcile the medications and doses the patient states he or she uses at home

Communication

Rushed communication with the next shift or a covering colleague

Intimidation or failure to speak up when there is a question or concern about a medication

Use of error-prone abbreviations, apothecary designations, or dangerous dose designations

Unnecessary use of spoken orders

Not reading back spoken orders

Overuse of stat orders or stat process as a work-around for slow pharmacy service

Providing incomplete orders (e.g., lack of full drug name, route, strength, frequency)

Not questioning incomplete orders

Not communicating important patient information (e.g., allergies, height, weight, chronic and acute diagnoses) to the pharmacy

Documenting medication administration and monitoring parameters at the end of the shift

Not sending all orders to pharmacy (e.g., if they contain no medication orders, or if the prescribed medication is available as unit-based floor stock)

Illegible handwriting

Writing multiple prescriptions on one prescription blank

Labeling, Packaging, Nomenclature

Removing medications from packages before they reach the patient's bedside

Not labeling or poorly labeling syringes, solutions, or other medication packages

Not fully reading the label of a medication ("grab and go") before dispensing, administering, or restocking medications

Storing medications with look-alike labels and packaging beside one another

Placing hospital-prepared or auxiliary labels over important information on the manufacturer's label

Drug Stock, Storage, Distribution

Leaving medications at bedside

Leaving medications in an unlocked storage area

Preparing intravenous admixtures outside the pharmacy

Not notifying physicians, nurses, and other personnel who order and administer drugs of impending and actual drug shortages

Keeping unused medications from discharged patients in patient care areas for potential administration to other patients

Borrowing medications from one patient to administer to another patient

Carrying medications in a uniform or coat pocket

Placing more importance on financial criteria than on safety when procuring medications (e.g., multiple-dose vials versus single-use vials or prefilled syringes)

Failure to dispense medications in unit doses or patient-specific doses

Nonpharmacist access to the pharmacy when closed

TABLE 23-3 Practitioners' At-Risk Behaviors in the Medication Process[34] (continued)

Environment/Staffing Patterns
Managing multiple priorities while carrying out complex processes (e.g., order entry, transcription, drug administration, IV admixture)
Holding (or admitting) overflow patients in inappropriate units or areas
Not notifying management if staffing is inadequate
Failure to adequately supervise or orient staff
Inadequate staffing for patient acuity

Patient Education
Prescribing, administering, or dispensing medications without educating the patient
Disregarding the patient's or caregiver's concerns about a medication's appearance, reactions, or effects, or other expressed worry
Discharging patients without proper education about the medications to take at home

Staff Education
Inadequate orientation of new or agency staff
No organizational incentives to achieve certification or attend continuing education
Lack of a structured and ongoing staff competency program related to medication use

Culture
Sacrificing safety for timeliness
Failure to report and share error information
Organizational culture of secrecy rather than openness about medication errors
Organizational culture of finger pointing rather than system change

Double Checks
Overconfidence in colleague's work (failure to independently double-check thoroughly)
Filling or checking medications by using the label, not the order or prescription
Failure to ask a colleague to double-check manual calculations before proceeding
Failure to ask a colleague to double-check high-alert medications before dispensing/administration
Failure to ask a colleague to double-check high-risk processes (e.g., patient controlled analgesia) before proceeding

Teamwork
Reluctance to consult others or ask for help when indicated
Lack of responsiveness to colleague or patient requests

Technology
Technology work-arounds
Overriding computer alerts without due consideration
Overreliance on technology as a safety tool
Using outdated or poorly maintained technology
Failure to fully engage available technology
Failure to provide education and training on new or updated technology
Inadequate ongoing participation of frontline clinical staff in technology user or planning meetings

---

a cumulative effect.[38] The effect of a single shortcut may seem insignificant, but over time a worker can drift into at-risk behaviors and this, combined with other workers' at-risk behaviors, can spell disaster.

Discouraging at-risk behaviors is one of the most important steps an organization can take to reduce patient harm. The incentives for unsafe behaviors should be uncovered and removed, and stronger incentives for safe behaviors should be created.[34,39] The solution is not to punish those who engage in at-risk behaviors, but to uncover the system-based reasons for their behavior and decrease staff tolerance for risk taking.

Once the incentives for their at-risk behaviors have been addressed, workers should be coached on making better behavioral choices. Marx[40] suggests the following: Never coach workers to not make mistakes; instead, give them a different, realistic behavioral choice that will reduce the risk of errors. The following sidebar offers additional tips for reducing at-risk behaviors.[34,36,39]

MANAGING AT-RISK BEHAVIORS

It is often easier to take risks than to work safely. Risk taking rarely results in patient harm, and it consistently provides rewards—convenience, comfort, and saved time—that encourage additional risk taking.[39] The Institute for Safe Medication Practices has long urged health care practitioners to stop thinking "It (a harmful medication error) won't happen to me." But it has been difficult for practitioners to embrace that attitude when it seems that most such errors really do happen to "the other guy." Motivating people to always choose the safest way to work is an ongoing struggle. Human behavior runs counter to patient safety efforts because the rewards for risk taking are immediate and positive, and the punishment for risk taking is remote and unlikely.[36,39] Even the most highly educated, diligent, and careful practitioners learn to master dangerous shortcuts and engage in at-risk behavior.

We learn at-risk behaviors through experience. Remember when you first learned to prescribe, dispense, or administer medications? Most likely, you were a bit nervous and carefully followed all the safety procedures you had been taught. You gave your undivided attention to the task, sought out information on unfamiliar medications, prepared just one patient's medications at a time or just one IV admixture at a time, always checked the patient's weight and allergies, educated patients about their drug therapy, asked others to double-check your work, provided covering practitioners with detailed reports, and so on. But as the years went by, your complete concentration was no longer needed. Many precautions fell by the wayside, and you probably developed some bad habits and at-risk behaviors.

If you are an experienced physician, for example, you may now assume that you know enough about a medication to prescribe it without looking it up. You may write multiple outpatient prescriptions on the same prescription pad and rush through reports to covering colleagues. You may no longer review inpatients' medication administration records (MARs) each day or write legible orders and discharge instructions. Upon patient admission and transfer, you may supply incomplete orders such as "take home meds" or "resume all meds." You may also have learned to use intimidating behaviors to discourage others from interrupting your busy workday.

If you are an experienced pharmacist, you may not think twice about answering the telephone and managing walk-in requests at the same time you are entering complex medication orders. When patients picking up their prescriptions sign away the option to be counseled, you may feel relieved because your workflow is not disrupted. You may no longer check the patient's full drug profile, allergies, and weight before entering medication orders. You may now fill written medication orders using the label, not the order or prescription, and rush past drug interaction messages you barely notice. You may no longer dispense injectable medications in patient-specific unit doses, or ask another pharmacist to check chemotherapy solutions you prepare.

If you are an experienced nurse, you may think it is acceptable to maintain an unauthorized stash of medications on your unit, prepare IV admixtures instead of waiting for pharmacy to dispense them, and administer medications to patients before pharmacy has reviewed the order. You may borrow another patient's medications for quick administration to your patient and leave medications at the bedside. You may no longer take the patient's MAR to the bedside if you are administering just a prn medication. You may no longer take the time to label all self-prepared syringes or have mathematical dose calculations independently checked by another nurse.

It is frightening how quickly we learn to take these and other important medication-use tasks for granted. In no time at all, we have gone from the safe and controlled processes we learned to unsafe, automatic behaviors. Although we know on some level that patient safety may be at risk, the rewards for our shortcuts encourage their continuation. We may think of our shortcuts as efficiency measures, but these at-risk behaviors often emerge from system-based problems.[34,36,39]

System-based causes. Unnecessarily complex processes provide many opportunities for shortcuts. For example, nurses who must obtain medications from four different storage units—an automated dispensing cabinet, a refrigerator, a patient-specific bin containing pharmacy-dispensed drugs, and a locked storage unit in the patient's room—are more inclined to gather all their patients' medications each day and place them in a more readily accessible area (e.g., a pocket).

Problems with technology are another source of at-risk behaviors. For example, physicians who often must wait for access to a computer terminal for prescribing are more apt to give spoken orders. Pharmacists who must back out of the order entry system to reference a drug or a corresponding laboratory value in an electronic database are more inclined to skip this step when they are busy.

When patient harm results, we tend to focus on the individuals who engaged in at-risk behaviors. We are getting better at identifying the system-based causes of error, but too often we overlook what lies at the root of many system problems: an organizational culture with a high tolerance for at-risk behaviors.

Culture tolerant of risk. Ask yourself whether your culture is tolerant of at-risk behaviors. Does the organization tend to punish safe behavior or reward at-risk behavior?[34,39] Consider the following:

❑ What is your reaction to a pharmacist who takes time to fully investigate a "missing" medication request during the busy morning hours, compared with your reaction to a colleague who unquestioningly sends the drug to the requesting unit? What if you are the nurse waiting for the drug, or the pharmacy supervisor who now has to help enter the huge backlog of orders that resulted? Does efficiently sending the missing medication gain more positive reinforcement than investigating the reason for the request?

❑ How would you react to a physician who asks for help in locating a patient's MAR so she can be sure no medications have been accidentally discontinued upon transfer? What if you are the nurse manager or unit secretary who must help find the MAR while managing other tasks? What if you are the nurse who is using the MAR? Would the physician be appreciated more if she did not try to find the MAR?

❑ What is your reaction to a nurse who takes longer than most to administer medications because he asks colleagues to independently check high-alert drugs before administration? What if you are the person who is asked to help when you have other pressing demands? Is the nurse who does not bother others praised and respected for his ability to work independently?

❑ Are your best (and safest) performers rewarded with extra work? Is the most vocal person on a particular safety issue rewarded with primary responsibility for fixing it? Is the lone pharmacist who always dons a gown and gloves before entering the IV preparation area ridiculed behind her back?

Look closely, and you will find many more examples in which health care workers gain positive regard from co-workers for engaging in at-risk behaviors.

Discipline is unproductive. The use of disciplinary measures when policy is breached will not result in a commitment to safety. It only reminds the worker of the organization's top-down control, and any change in behavior will be temporary.

Increase awareness. It is more important to reduce staff tolerance of at-risk behaviors than to increase compliance with specific safety rules,[39] and reducing tolerance begins with enhancing awareness of at-risk behaviors.[34] It should be possible to identify some at-risk behaviors by analyzing the organization's error reports, especially reports of sentinel events, which give more information about causative factors. For each at-risk behavior, a corresponding safe behavior should be readily apparent. Remember this as you analyze error reports: Although staff reporting errors may not divulge at-risk behaviors without prompting, not all errors involve conscious risk taking.

Learn what supports the behaviors. What consequences may be encouraging the belief that an at-risk behavior produces more positive than negative outcomes—and possibly that there are fewer rewards for the corresponding safe behavior?[34] Identify undesirable consequences that can be reduced or eliminated.

Motivate through feedback and rewards. This is the most difficult step: to align individual and group motivation with avoidance of at-risk behaviors. An organizational priority of efficiency and productivity may misdirect staff motivation. An incentive program based solely on outcomes may inadvertently reward underreporting of errors and injuries; if making and reporting an error or injury causes someone (especially a group) to lose a reward, underreporting results.[39] Emphasize the specific behaviors that lead to patient safety; staff will feel better about the process if the focus is on achievement rather than failure.

To start, consider asking all staff to document one at-risk behavior and one safe behavior each day, and the conditions under which they occurred. Identify antecedents of the at-risk and the safe behaviors. When staff members have learned safe behaviors and factors that facilitate them, they need to practice the safe behaviors until they become ingrained in the system. Safe behaviors should receive ongoing support, encouragement, recognition, and rewards. Everyone who meets behavioral criteria should be rewarded; it is better for many to receive a small reward than for one person to receive a large reward.[39]

Reckless Behavior

In reckless behavior, the worker

- Always perceives the risk he or she is taking,
- Understands that the risk is substantial,
- Behaves intentionally but is unable to justify the behavior through objective risk–benefit analysis (i.e., does not mistakenly believe the risk is justified),
- Knows that others are not engaging in the same behaviors (i.e., the at-risk behavior is not the norm), and
- Makes a conscious choice to disregard the substantial and unjustifiable risk, for subjective reasons that do not meet the usual grounds of social utility.[33]

The difference between at-risk behavior and reckless behavior can be likened to speeding on the highway. Most people drive 5 to 10 miles over the speed limit on a limited-access highway; this is an at-risk behavior that has become the norm. Most drivers feel safe at this speed and can justify the behavior on the basis of the social utility of getting to a destination more quickly. Most drivers would agree, however, that driving 95 miles per hour where the speed limit is 65 is reckless behavior. The risk is substantial and known—most do not feel safe at that speed—and the social utility of arriving more quickly at a destination is no longer justified when weighed against the risk of an accident.

Behaviors are categorized as reckless when the worker realizes the possibility of harm, whether or not harm results.[33] The worker is intentionally taking a risk but not necessarily intending harm. Workers under the influence of alcohol or illegal drugs may know that harm is possible but not intend it. In cases of homicide of a patient or sabotage of the organization, harm is intended.

Health care providers very rarely engage in reckless behavior. A nurse who is too vain to wear reading glasses while administering medications may be exhibiting reckless behavior if she knows the risk she is taking, knows that the risk is substantial, and then consciously disregards the risk, which is unjustifiable. Most workers would not think vanity is a justifiable reason for not wearing reading glasses while administering medications.

Reckless behavior is blameworthy behavior. As such, it should be managed through remedial or disciplinary actions according to the organization's human resources policies.[33]

Proactive Risk Management

Although the 1999 report *To Err Is Human*[2] framed patient safety as freedom from accidental injury, its meaning is broader. Safety also means freedom from substantial and unjustifiable risk, regardless of the actual outcome. A just culture includes not only a robust accountability model, fair to all stakeholders, but a proactive model for addressing system and behavioral risks before events occur.[35]

In a just culture, managers coach workers on the risks posed by behaviors they observe daily. They seek to eliminate the incentives for at-risk behaviors before patients are harmed. They engage the workforce in uncovering and repairing system design flaws before human errors occur. Organizational leaders in a just culture have a duty to address system weaknesses and to fairly manage workers involved in an error. When an error occurs, the most important question is not how to handle the involved workers but what can be done to avoid the next error.[41]

Collaboration of Licensing Bodies, Regulatory Bodies, and Health Care Providers

External influences can make it difficult for health care systems to maintain a just culture. When a patient is harmed, licensing bodies, the legal system, the patient's family, and the media tend to deal with the involved workers in a punitive manner.[1,42]

However, some licensing and regulatory bodies have joined statewide initiatives supporting a just culture. In Minnesota, for example, the Minnesota Hospital Association, Minnesota Alliance for Patient Safety, state department of health, and state licensing boards for medicine, pharmacy, and nursing have joined with hospitals to create and uphold a just culture.[43] North Carolina has begun a similar collaborative effort, and the idea is spreading to other states.

These collaboratives have grown into a just culture community (www.justculture.org) where regulators and organizations from various industries, including health care, come together to learn, share experiences, and use a common set of tools for a common set of issues.[35] Such efforts hold promise for broader adoption of a just culture in health care. Establishing a just culture will not be easy, but it is vital to improving patient safety.[7]

TEAMWORK AND LOCALIZED DECISION-MAKING

In HROs, teams comprising multiple disciplines and levels of workers meet regularly to plan, deliberate, communicate, and evaluate their work. The rigid hierarchical structures that make it difficult for people, regardless of rank or education, to raise concerns and voice opinions have been erased, and there is real collaboration to solve problems. The teams are highly functional; they are not just proficient in technical skills but also adept at avoiding errors caused by failures in communication and decision-making in a dynamic environment.

Because HROs have effective teams, they are able to shift the burden of decisions from top leaders to a more localized decision-making model. Every team member feels empowered to make quick decisions about impending safety issues. On the other hand, workers understand that collaboration with other team members, when time permits, results in higher-quality decisions. Decisions made by teams lead to innovation that cannot be realized without such collaborative interaction.[4,44]

HROs have also established cross-departmental, meaningful feedback systems that keep the teams and entire workforce informed about safety, errors, and causal trends—not just through sophisticated charts and graphs but also through rich stories about safety that can be recalled as a constant reminder and a sound rationale for keeping safety a priority.

Aviation Example of Teams in an HRO

A team can be defined as a distinguishable set of two or more committed individuals with specific roles and complementary skills who interact dynamically to achieve shared and valued goals for which they are mutually accountable.[45,46] Effective teamwork does not come naturally. In HROs, those expected to work in teams are trained in teams via simulation; the education is directly linked to the desired outcome. For example, in aviation, effective team communication is taught through simulations known as crew resource management (CRM).[47] Aviation crew members spend many days together practicing communication and inquiry skills: how to ask questions, ways to seek relevant information, how to advocate for safety and counteract intimidation, how to resolve conflicts, and how to make team decisions. During these and many other training simulations, crew members practice many of the skills, attitudes, and behavioral choices associated with teamwork.

The concept of CRM originated in 1979 in response to the analysis of several airline accidents in which a minor problem, such as a burned out 59 cent bulb on an instrument panel, occupied crew to the extent that they lost sight of the bigger picture of flying the plane and crashed.[27,47,48] If the crew had functioned well as a team, minor technical problems would not have precluded a safe landing. Communication failures ultimately led to the accidents. In 70% of the accidents reviewed, someone in the cockpit knew there was a problem but could not communicate it properly.

Measuring the frequency of airline accidents or near misses might seem to be a logical way to assess the effectiveness of CRM. However, aviation accident rates are extremely low, and near misses are reported voluntarily.[49] Therefore, proxy tools have been used to establish effectiveness.[47,49–51] Assessments by trained observers on more than 2,000 flights showed that after CRM training, the percentage of crew attitudes rated as "above average" (the highest possible score) was significantly higher and the percentage "below average" (the lowest possible score) was lower. Superior pilots demonstrated a shared set of attitudes linked to safety:[49]

- They were aware of their personal limitations.
- They were aware of their diminished decision-making capacity during emergencies.
- They encouraged crew members to question their decisions and actions.
- They were sensitive to the personal problems of other crew members.
- They recognized the need to verbalize plans.
- They understood the need to train other crew members.

Team-related attitudes such as these, along with other core skills, knowledge, and behaviors associated with effective teams in aviation, are also relevant in health care and need to be taught, learned, and practiced in order to improve patient safety.[46,52–55]

Teams in Health Care

The importance of interdisciplinary teams in the delivery of safe, high-quality health care has become increasingly evident in the past 20 years.[56] As in the airline industry before CRM, failed communications and incongruent teamwork account for a large portion of poor clinical outcomes. JCAHO statistics confirm this; communication failures were the most common causes of sentinel events between 1995 and 2005, accounting for nearly 70% of the reported events.[57] In 2005 alone, communication failures played a role in more than 80% of harmful medication errors reported to JCAHO.[58] In a 2004 survey of health care providers by ECRI, 72% of respondents attributed more than half of all errors in health care to a lack of teamwork and communication.[59]

Studies have confirmed that highly functional teams make fewer errors than individuals because variability is reduced, decisions are of higher quality, complex care is better coordinated, and heightened situational awareness allows early detection and mitigation of errors.[1,27] Creative solutions to complex problems can be found as team members integrate their observations and expertise to coordinate, collaborate, and communicate with one another in order to optimize care. The use of redundant or duplicative services can be reduced, and the length of hospital stays can be lessened. Effective teams can increase efficiency, lower costs, and improve safety and clinical outcomes.[46,52–56,60–64] Effective teamwork also results in a more satisfying and rewarding work environment for staff, which helps to attract and retain health care professionals.[1,27]

Given the interdisciplinary nature of most aspects of health care, it could be argued that most care is delivered by teams. However, simply initiating a team structure on individual units or in medical practices does not guarantee that the team will function well, or that it will function well as part of a larger team providing care to the patient throughout the continuum of settings.[65,66] Health care's challenge, therefore, is not whether we will deliver care in teams—the benefits are too numerous to cast aside—but how well we will deliver care in teams.[66]

Barriers to Teamwork in Health Care

Training

Just as individuals need experience and practice to recognize and respond to unexpected situations, teams need to be similarly nurtured.[66] However, members of health care teams are typically trained in separate disciplines and educational programs—often having no team training even within their respective discipline—leaving them unprepared to enter complex collaborative settings and function well as team members.[56,67] They may not appreciate each other's strengths and weaknesses and may not have learned how to cooperate, communicate, and integrate care to ensure that it is continuous and reliable. They may not have acquired the skills necessary to anticipate the needs of other health care providers, evaluate and adjust to their actions, and give and receive feedback. They may lack full understanding of the role each plays in delivering care.

Since 2000, the Institute of Medicine (IOM) has called for educational reform to ensure that health care professionals attain a set of core competencies for working in interdisciplinary teams.[56,67] It has recommended that academic accreditation bodies and professional licensing boards hold accredited training programs and licensed health care professionals accountable for teaching and acquiring team competencies.

In addition, IOM has recommended that health care providers establish interdisciplinary team training programs within their organizations and incorporate proven team management methods.[67] JCAHO standards also address team training within health care organizations. The elements of performance for human resource standard HR.2.30 note that team training methods should be incorporated in ongoing staff education, when appropriate.[17,46]

Nevertheless, a 2004 survey of health care providers by ECRI revealed that less than one-third were providing team training, and of those, just a quarter included physicians and other independent contractors in the training.[59] When it was provided, training did not target high-risk areas such as the emergency department, according to 86% of the respondents. The educational content of the training programs varied considerably. Most respondents who had received team training believed it had improved communication among staff and departments.

Researchers have begun to identify the core competencies necessary for effective inter-disciplinary teamwork in health care. Baker et al.[46] analyzed this research and identified skills, knowledge, and attitudes that are needed to function well as a team member and coordinate day-to-day tasks in health care (Table 23-4). They suggested using these core competencies as a basis for teaching interdisciplinary team skills and evaluating health care workers' team competencies. They believed these competencies are measurable and can be used to predict effective team performance in health care.

Complexity and Autonomy

Another barrier to teamwork in health care is the complexity, variety, and specialization of services provided to a patient from the start of symptoms to the end of an episode of care. A person with a chronic illness interacts with many inpatient and outpatient health care providers. What is conceptualized as teamwork and collaboration in care delivery may actually be uncoordinated, sequential, and autonomous care by individual practition-ers.[67] In *From Chaos to Care: The Promise of Team-Based Medicine,*[65] Lawrence refers to each of these encounters with a single health care provider as a vertical moment. Although individual practitioners may believe their own vertical moments are efficient, the care may seem chaotic and disjointed to patients.

Vertical moments with each caregiver are difficult to integrate into the entire horizontal continuum of care.[65] Even if small health care teams—for example, in a physician's office, in a community pharmacy, in a radiology department, among physicians and nurses on an inpatient unit—are quite functional, connecting these teams to each other is a challenge.

Health care professionals may fail to recognize the lack of care coordination as a problem, in part because medical education emphasizes professional autonomy and indi-vidual accountability—attributes that have been viewed as ideal in assessments of pro-fessionals' character and work ethics.[66,67] Some health care professionals may have diffi-culty abandoning their status and self-image as "craftsmen" rather than "equivalent actors" among team members.[3] Amalberti et al.[3] illustrated this point by comparing sur-geons with airline pilots and anesthesiologists:

> A commercial airline customer neither knows nor cares who the pilot or copilot flying the plane is; a last minute change of captain is not a concern to passengers, as people have grown accustomed to the notion that all pilots are, to an excellent approximation, equivalent to one another in their skills. Patients have a similar attitude toward anesthesiologists when they face surgery. In both cases, the practice is highly standardized, and the professionals involved have, in essence, renounced their individuality in the service of a reliable standard of excellent care. They sell a service instead of individual identity. As a consequence, the risk for catastrophic death in healthy patients undergoing anesthesia is very low, close to 10^{-6} per anesthetic episode (3.4 deaths per million). Conversely, most patients specifically request and can recall the name of their surgeon. Often the patient has chosen the surgeon and believes that the result of surgery could vary according to that choice. (p. 759)

Experience in anesthesiology, the airline industry, and other HROs such as the nuclear power industry shows that a reduction in autonomy and a shared concept of team mem-bers as equivalent actors can improve safety. To improve patient safety, we must move from single solutions crafted by individual practitioners to integrated care teams.[56]

TABLE 23-4 Team Skills, Knowledge, and Attitudes and the Coordinating Mechanisms of Teamwork

Definition	Behavioral Examples	Citations
Team Leadership		
Ability to direct and coordinate the activities of other team members; assess team performance; assign tasks; develop team knowledge, skills, and attitudes; motivate team members; plan and organize; and establish a positive atmosphere	■ Facilitate team problem solving ■ Provide performance expectations and acceptable interaction patterns ■ Synchronize and combine individual team member contributions ■ Seek and evaluate information that impacts team functioning ■ Clarify team member roles ■ Engage in preparatory meetings and feedback sessions with the team	Cannon-Bowers et al.[68] Salas et al.[69] Healey et al.[70] Thomas et al.[55] Flin and Maran[71]
Mutual Performance Monitoring		
Ability to develop common understandings of the team environment and apply appropriate task strategies in order to accurately monitor teammate performance	■ Identify mistakes and lapses in other team members' actions ■ Provide feedback regarding team members' actions in order to facilitate self-correction	McIntyre and Salas[72] Healey et al.[70] Thomas et al.[55]
Backup Behavior		
Ability to anticipate other team members' needs through accurate knowledge about their responsibilities. Ability to shift workload among members to achieve balance during periods of high workload	■ Recognition by potential backup providers that there is a workload distribution problem in their team ■ Shifting of work responsibilities to underutilized team members ■ Completion of the whole task or parts of tasks by other team members	McIntyre and Salas[72] Porter et al.[73]
Adaptability		
Ability to adjust strategies on the basis of information gathered from the environment through the use of compensatory behavior and reallocation of intrateam resources. Altering a course of action or team repertoire in response to changing conditions (internal or external)	■ Identify cues that a change has occurred, assign meaning to that change, and develop a new plan for dealing with the change ■ Identify opportunities for improvement and innovation for habitual or routine practices ■ Remain vigilant to changes in the internal and external environment of the team	Cannon-Bowers et al.[68] Kozlowski et al.[74] Klein and Pierce[75]
Team/Collective Orientation		
Propensity to take others' behavior into account during group interaction, and belief in the importance of team goals over individual members' goals	■ Taking into account alternative solutions provided by teammates and appraising that input to determine what is most appropriate ■ Increased task involvement, information sharing, strategizing, and participatory goal setting	Driskell and Salas[76] Shamir[77] Wagner[78]
Shared Mental Model		
An organizing knowledge structure of the relationships between the task the team is engaged in and how the team members will interact	■ Anticipate and predict each other's needs ■ Identify changes in the team, task, or teammates and implicitly adjust strategies as needed	Cannon-Bowers et al.[68] Klimoski and Mohammed[79] Mathieu et al.[80] Stout et al.[81] Wright et al.[82]

TABLE 23-4   Team Skills, Knowledge, and Attitudes and the Coordinating Mechanisms
of Teamwork (continued)

Definition	Behavioral Examples	Citations
Mutual Trust		
Shared belief that team members will perform their roles and protect the interests of their teammates	▪ Information sharing ▪ Willingness to admit mistakes and accept feedback	Bandow[83] Webber[84]
Closed-Loop Communication		
Exchange of information between a sender and a receiver irrespective of the medium	▪ Following up with team members to ensure the message was received ▪ Acknowledging that a message was received ▪ Clarifying with the sender of the message that the message received is the same as the intended message sent	McIntyre and Salas[72] Healey et al.[70] Thomas et al.[55] Flin and Maran[71] Leonard et al.[85]

Source: Reprinted with permission from reference 46.

Hierarchical Structure

All too often, seasoned health care practitioners feel compelled to warn new staff members about a particularly difficult physician or other practitioner, or even to shield them from that person for as long as possible. This is a telling sign of a culture that tolerates, even fosters, intimidation.

Intimidating behaviors stem from a long-standing hierarchical culture in medicine.[86] This acculturation makes it difficult for health care practitioners to point out safety problems to those in authority. Challenging authority is discouraged, at the expense of losing the valuable input of practitioners, whatever their formal credentials.[67,87]

Being at the top of the hierarchy, physicians may not recognize the need for teamwork; they may not see the hierarchy itself as a problem or a threat to patient safety, even though it clearly impedes communication.[1,25] A survey of operating room (OR) staff illustrated this point.[53] Almost three-fourths (73%) of surgical residents and two-thirds of attending surgeons (64%) reported high levels of teamwork in the OR, compared with 39% of attending anesthesiologists, 28% of surgical nurses, 25% of nurse anesthetists, and 10% of anesthesia residents.

The same study[53] compared the attitudes of surgeons and airline flight crews. About half (59%) of attending surgeons were opposed to steep hierarchies, which was determined by asking whether they thought junior team members should question the decisions of senior team members. In contrast, most airline crew members (94%) preferred flat hierarchies and questioning by subordinates.

Intimidating behaviors are not the exclusive province of physicians, nor are they used only on impressionable new recruits to health care. An ISMP survey of more than 2,000 health care providers suggested that this damaging style of personal interaction is used by various health care professionals, targeting co-workers at all stages of their careers.[88,89] (Chapter 9 includes key findings.)

The ISMP survey provided a glimpse of an apparent culture of disrespect among health care providers. Those who endure ongoing intimidation may subconsciously use intimidating tactics on others, perpetuating this damaging culture. The survey respondents indicated dissatisfaction with their organizations' efforts to handle intimidation. A solution will reveal itself only when health care practitioners and organizations acknowledge the problem, discuss it openly, analyze the causes, and lay the groundwork for change. Recommendations for reducing workplace intimidation are presented on page 627,[86,89–93] followed by tools for assertive communication.[1,27,92]

RECOMMENDATIONS FOR REDUCING WORKPLACE INTIMIDATION[86,89–93]

Establish a steering committee of trustees and senior leaders, middle managers, physicians, pharmacists, nurses, and other staff from diverse areas of the workplace.[90] Define workplace intimidation and list examples of the many forms it can take. This is no easy task, since people's tolerance for certain behaviors varies, but consider this simple definition: not being treated with respect, or, any behavior, no matter how small, that causes another to doubt his or her self-worth. Develop a mission statement that defines the organization's effort to reduce intimidation. The committee should establish an action plan and share it with the workforce, gain full administrative support, and educate providers about the damaging effects of intimidation on patient safety and staff morale.

Create a code of conduct that flows logically from your organization's mission statement.[91] No code can list every possible violation, but be sure to specify both blatantly unacceptable behaviors and those that can subtly undermine team cohesion, staff morale, self-worth, and safety. Convene a diverse group to identify and list positive and negative behaviors in staff interaction. Use this list as the basis for the code of conduct and to develop values statements about staff interaction. Have all existing and new staff sign the code of conduct and values statements upon hire/appointment and annually. Include the code of conduct and values statements in all job descriptions, medical staff bylaws, and performance appraisals.

Survey staff attitudes about intimidation, the kinds of behaviors that seem intimidating, and the levels of intimidation by all health care providers.[91] The survey can also be used to garner information about whether staff feel valued in the organization, how they handle stress and intimidation, how they treat others at work, and secret rules they share with new co-workers about how to interact with (or avoid) certain staff members.

Open the dialogue about workplace intimidation. Hold frank discussions, using objective moderators to keep the conversation productive. The survey results will likely trigger a process of questioning the way health care providers interact with each other. However uncomfortable, opening the dialogue on this issue is crucial to the development of more effective and respectful ways of interacting.

Establish a standard, assertive communication process for use by health care providers conveying important information. For example, consider asking staff to use the first names of colleagues, including physicians, to get their attention when important information must be communicated.[86] Using a colleague's first name can help break down barriers to effective communication. To enhance awareness of intimidating behaviors, consider establishing a code phrase, such as "red light," that can be used to halt the behavior immediately. Stating the problem along with its rationale and a potential solution can also improve assertive communication. Tools for structured communication are presented on pages 628 and 629. If the response from a colleague is not mutually acceptable, follow a conflict resolution process.

Establish a conflict resolution process to communicate effectively and protect patients, not to punish, embarrass, or coerce involved staff. Be sure the process provides an avenue for resolution outside the typical chain of command if the conflict involves a subordinate and supervisor. Following a "two-challenge" rule is one option. Used in highly reliable industries with excellent safety records, this rule calls for communication of critical information twice to the same person; if there is no resolution, the matter is then automatically referred to at least one other person before a final decision is made.

Another tool, used in aviation, is the "most conservative response" rule: In the event of a clinical or operational impasse, the involved parties accept the most conservative (and safest) of the options being considered.[92] If, for example, an emergency department nurse believes an elderly patient with a possible pelvic fracture should be admitted but the physician is planning to discharge the patient, the most conservative response would be admission. Acknowledging that as a starting point, both practitioners should be able to objectively reach the best and safest solution.

Encourage confidential reporting of behavior that intimidates. Provide periodic updates to complainants on how the issue is being addressed.

Enforce zero tolerance for intimidating behaviors, regardless of the offender's standing in the organization. Expect intimidating behaviors to re-emerge, and establish a process for dealing with each reported event.[93] Confront offenders with data, authority, and compassion; punitive responses will not foster interpersonal skills or the desired culture changes.[91] Solicit the offender's side of the story while stressing that regardless of why it happened, the behavior is unacceptable. Offer concrete advice for positive change.

Provide ongoing education that reinforces the organization's commitment to a caring and respectful culture. Use role-playing and vignettes to strengthen skills associated with assertive communication, conflict resolution, and interpersonal interactions. Provide managers with customer service and conflict resolution training, as well as other nonclinical skills necessary to facilitate the desired culture.

Lead by example and surround staff with positive workplace experiences and ever-growing circles of positive relationships.

Reward outstanding examples of collaborative teamwork, respectful communication, and positive interpersonal skills. For example, several times a year, allow staff to select and recognize colleagues, including physicians, who demonstrate superior interpersonal skills, thus establishing role models for the organization.

TOOLS FOR STRUCTURED COMMUNICATION

Using these tools will help health care practitioners communicate clearly and effectively in a timely manner. Their purpose is to standardize the type of information to be communicated and ensure critical thinking about the problem and solution before and while communicating. These techniques will enable practitioners to share a mental model of the clinical plan of care for the patient and what is to be expected. They will promote assertiveness and reduce intimidation with minimal risk of conflict.

SBAR[1]

Useful for communicating a patient's condition that requires immediate attention and action

S̲ituation: Briefly state what the problem is, when it happened or started, and its severity.

B̲ackground: Provide information such as current medications, allergies, lab values (current and previous for comparison), and vital signs.

A̲ssessment: Give your assessment of the situation.

R̲ecommendation: Give your recommendations and state the specific response you are seeking (e.g., patient needs to be seen now, order needs to be changed).

DESCript[92]

Useful for communicating a patient's condition that requires immediate attention and action

D̲escribe: Using objective terms, describe what you observed, heard, or perceived.

E̲xpress: State your concerns, using "I" statements and nonjudgmental terminology.

S̲uggest: Recommend or inquire about a course of action.

C̲onsensus: Gain consensus about the course of action.

STICC[27]

Useful for describing a safety problem and potential solutions to a colleague

S̲ituation: State the problem as you see it.

T̲ask: Describe what you think should be done.

I̲ntent: State why you recommended the specific tasks.

C̲oncern: State what you think needs to be watched or monitored, and how that can be accomplished.

C̲alibrate: Ask the recipient of the information to respond.

Briefings[1]

Useful before the start of procedures (during time-outs), at the beginning of a new workday or shift, and during handoffs in care

- ❑ *Be concise.* Communicate meaningful information as quickly and efficiently as possible.
- ❑ *Ensure two-way communication.* Ask for input from others to clarify information, responsibilities, and understanding and their comfort with any anticipated tasks.
- ❑ *Flatten hierarchies.* Address colleagues by their first names to promote familiarity and comfort with speaking up about perceived problems.
- ❑ *Communicate interest.* Make eye contact with colleagues to show interest and confirm value in their contributions.
- ❑ *Talk about next steps.* Suggest ongoing monitoring when appropriate and plans for next steps.

Debriefings[1]

Useful for assessing team activities after their completion, for the purposes of reward and improvement

- ❑ *Stress positive points.* Keep the tone positive and discuss what the team did well (both individual and team tasks).
- ❑ *Understand learning points.* Consider in detail what was learned while carrying out the activities.
- ❑ *Generate new ideas.* Describe what could be done differently next time.
- ❑ *Identify opportunities for improvement.* Uncover system issues that made the job more difficult or error-prone than necessary.
- ❑ *Assign responsibility.* Identify individuals or teams who will be responsible for agreed-upon system improvements.

ERROR-DEFYING SYSTEMS AND REDUNDANCY

HROs design systems that defy errors, avoiding reliance on human memory and vigilance. They carefully consider human factors, attending to unsafe conditions such as long working hours, excessive workloads, unsafe staffing ratios, sources of distraction, and other environmental conditions known to contribute to errors. HROs do not rely solely on worker education to ensure that systems function properly; instead, they use technology and proven principles of error reduction—forcing functions, fail-safes, standardization, simplification, constraints, and so on—that have demonstrated sustained safety improvement over time. They also have built-in systems of redundancy for critical processes and workers, and recovery plans to minimize loss after an error.

Unresolved Problems

Selecting the best strategy for preventing medication errors is not easy. Even when system-based causes have been identified, the most effective action may not be obvious. A problem that seems to have been solved can reappear months later. Steps taken to remedy the problem may have reduced the risk of an error but not completely prevented it, as in the following case.

Midazolam syrup was used frequently on the hospital's pediatric unit, so bulk bottles of the syrup (2 mg/mL) were stocked in the automated dispensing cabinet (ADC). After several calculation errors led to overdoses, the ADC screen was redesigned to provide dose warnings. Also, dose conversion charts were posted nearby to eliminate the need for calculations. These measures seemed to work for a while, but then another overdose occurred. A child was to receive 6 mg of midazolam. The nurse had used the conversion chart to determine the correct volume of syrup to administer (3 mL). However, a mental slip caused her to confuse the dose in mg (6) as the volume to be administered. She incorrectly drew up 6 mL of syrup and administered 12 mg of midazolam to the child, who was unharmed.

More could have been done to prevent overdoses of midazolam syrup; the pharmacy could have dispensed unit doses, for example. But this error report is typical; it shows that health care providers are on the right road to error prevention but their efforts are not fully reliable. If health care is to become a highly reliable industry, the goal must be to design systems that defy errors, not just reduce the risk of error. The bar must be set higher; the aim must be "six sigma," or near perfection (less than 3.4 defects per million opportunities).

Designing for Reliability

Reliability in health care means providing failure-free care of all patients in a system over time, and of individual patients obtaining care from multiple providers. Reliability is measured by the system's failure rate. For example, a health system that has 1 failure in 10 opportunities (10% failure rate) performs at a 10^{-1} level; a health system that has 1 failure in 100 opportunities (1% failure rate) performs at a 10^{-2} level, and so on.

Studies of adverse events in the United States and abroad suggest that 10^{-1} is the current level of performance in most health care organizations.[67,94–98] In contrast, aviation passenger safety is measured at 10^{-6} and nuclear power plants must demonstrate a design capable of 10^{-6} before they can be built.[94,96]

IHI[96,97] has linked these measures of reliability (10^{-1} to 10^{-6}) to specific design characteristics of systems, particularly the types of safety principles used (see Table 23-5).

10^{-1}. Overall performance at the 10^{-1} level reflects the application of rules (policies), training, and low-level standardization, simplification, and reminders. When faced with problems, many people revert back to these old, familiar ways of handling them. Rules and policies are useful and necessary in organizations, but they alone cannot prevent errors, because human memory and vigilance must be relied upon to remember the rule or policy, apply it to appropriate situations, and carry it out properly. Similarly, staff education is a weak error prevention strategy because it is difficult to ensure training of all existing and new staff, and, again, the application is dependent on correct human performance. Basic simplification and standardization, such as using one type of infusion pump, offers some protection from errors, but more sophisticated strategies are needed for higher levels of reliability.

10^{-2}. Overall performance at the 10^{-2} level reflects systems that have been designed with tools and concepts to compensate for human weaknesses, for the purposes of error-proofing the system, reducing the need for work-arounds, identifying failures, and mitigating harm. Key safety principles include high-level reminders, standardization, and simplification; differentiation; limits and constraints; affordances; redundancies; patient monitoring; and improved access to information.

10^{-3} or better. Overall performance at the 10^{-3} level or better reflects well-designed systems with attention to the structures in which processes work, linkages between care episodes, transfer of information, and identification and elimination of potential critical failures. Using the findings of root cause analysis (RCA) and, particularly, failure mode and effects analysis (FMEA), system weaknesses are identified that exist despite application of 10^{-1} and 10^{-2} strategies. In addition to the safety tools applied at the 10^{-2} level, forcing functions and fail-safes are abundant. (Forcing functions, fail-safes, RCA, and FMEA are important tools at each level of performance, but they are crucial for achieving a level of 10^{-3} or better.)

TABLE 23-5 Key Safety Principles for Designing and Redesigning Systems

Principle	Description	Examples
Simplify	Reduce the number of steps, handoffs, and options without eliminating crucial redundancies	■ Use commercially available premixed solutions instead of preparing IV admixtures ■ Limit drug choice to a single concentration ■ Dispense oral and injectable medications in ready-to-use form (unit dose packages) ■ Transmit orders to nurses and pharmacies electronically (via computerized prescribing) to avoid manual transcription
Externalize or centralize error-prone processes	Transfer error-prone tasks to an external site or centralized area to ensure that they are completed in a distraction-free environment by those who have expertise, and that appropriate quality control steps (e.g., sterility measures, double checks) are carried out	■ Have pharmacy prepare all IV solutions under sterile conditions ■ Use a specialized external service to prepare complicated solutions such as total parenteral nutrition, dialysate, cardioplegic solutions
Differentiate items	Modify the packages and labels of medications to help distinguish them from other medications with look-alike packages or look-alike and sound-alike names	■ Use colored backgrounds to highlight warnings on labels ■ Purchase look-alike medications from different manufacturers to maximize differences in label appearance ■ Use tactile cues such as placing a rubber band on a vial of long-acting insulin to help a vision-impaired patient differentiate it from short-acting insulin
Standardize	Create clinically sound, uniform models of care that should be adhered to when carrying out various functions related to medication use in order to reduce variation and complexity in the processes	■ Use carefully designed preprinted order sets, protocols, and clinical pathways to standardize high-risk processes and the administration of high-alert medications ■ Gain consensus among physicians who treat similar diseases and establish one standard order set for each standardized care process. Standardize the sliding scale used to prescribe insulin coverage and design/use a preprinted order form ■ Standardize to a single concentration and container size whenever possible for all high-alert medications given by IV infusion
Reminders	Provide additional alerts or warnings to make important information highly visible so practitioners remember it while carrying out medication-use processes	■ Set visual and audible alarms on equipment ■ Build reminders into screens on automated dispensing cabinets (ADCs), for example, "measure dose using dropper provided" ■ Affix auxiliary labels to medications or add highlighted notes to medication administration records to remind staff about important functions (e.g., check for pregnancy or cross allergies) ■ Use checklists for complex processes ■ Build reminders for special monitoring into order sets or protocols
Improve access to information	Use active, not passive, means of providing staff and patients with necessary information at the exact time they need it for performing critical tasks related to medication use	■ Provide easy access to quick drug reference tables at the point of drug administration ■ Increase visibility of pharmacists in patient care units for immediate consultation when needed ■ Include a medical librarian on patient rounds to identify important items and follow through with dissemination of education materials and evidence-based practices ■ Use computer order entry systems that merge patient and drug information to provide immediate warnings if unsafe orders are entered

TABLE 23-5 Key Safety Principles for Designing and Redesigning Systems (continued)

Principle	Description	Examples
Limit access or use (constraints)	Use constraints to restrict access to certain medications or error-prone conditions; require special education or conditions for prescribing, dispensing, or administering a particular drug; require special authorization for participation in certain critical tasks related to medication use	▪ Prohibit access of nurses and other nonpharmacy staff to the pharmacy when it is closed ▪ Remove concentrated electrolytes from patient care areas ▪ Store neuromuscular blocking agents in a separate container to limit access ▪ Require special credentialing for use of certain high-alert medications (e.g., chemotherapy, conscious sedation, patient-controlled analgesia [PCA]) ▪ Establish parameters for changing IV therapy to oral therapy as soon as possible ▪ Minimize the variety of medication choices and dose ranges on preprinted order forms
Forcing functions and fail-safes	Use procedures or equipment design features that will (1) prevent something from happening until certain conditions are met (often referred to as lock-and-key design); this is a forcing function or (2) prevent malfunctioning or unintentional operation by reverting back to a predetermined safe state if a failure occurs; this is a fail-safe	▪ Use oral syringes that cannot be connected to IV tubing ports ▪ Use medication ordering programs that cannot process an order unless key information, such as allergies and weight, has been entered ▪ Use ADCs that require pharmacy review of medication orders before access to the drug is provided ▪ Use epidural tubing without access ports ▪ Use PCA pumps with default settings of zero, or the highest possible concentration for the opiates used
Redundancies	Implement duplicate steps in a process to force additional checks in the system. Use more than one qualified and trained staff member to carry out specialized processes to ensure ability to perform critical functions	▪ Perform an independent double check for critical steps in the medication-use process ▪ Use automated check systems, such as bar coding or infusion pumps that sound an alarm when the rate exceeds safe limits (smart pumps) ▪ Ask patients about medication allergies each time medication is administered ▪ Cross-train selected staff to perform critical medication-use functions, and maintain proficiency through ongoing experiences
Patient monitoring	Assess the effects of medication through a constant feedback loop of predetermined patient parameters evaluated at set intervals	▪ Prospectively establish parameters (e.g., vital signs, quality of respirations, capnography, lab tests, observation, neurological signs) for monitoring patients who are receiving high-alert medications ▪ Concurrently monitor patients who are receiving high-alert drugs for medication effects ▪ Retrospectively monitor the effects of medications on groups of patients through chart audits aimed at detecting untoward drug effects (e.g., insulin-induced hypoglycemia, heparin- or warfarin-induced bleeding, chemotherapy-induced leukopenia, use of an antidote to reverse oversedation)
Failure mode and effects analysis (FMEA)	Convene a team to proactively identify ways a process or medication-related equipment can fail, why it might fail, how it might affect patients, and how it can be made safer	▪ Perform FMEA on a new high-alert medication before allowing its use ▪ Perform FMEA on a new infusion pump being considered for purchase ▪ Perform FMEA on a high-risk process or subprocess related to medication use (e.g., order transcription, selection of medications from ADCs, PCA, chemotherapy administration)

TABLE 23-5 Key Safety Principles for Designing and Redesigning Systems (continued)

Principle	Description	Examples
Root cause analysis (RCA)	Convene a team to retrospectively identify the system-based causes of errors	■ Perform RCA on a specific event to learn why it occurred ■ Perform RCA on the use of a particular drug or class of drugs involved most often in potentially harmful errors in the organization to learn why they are happening

Using a Bundle Strategy

When care processes are grouped into bundles of several interventions, health care practitioners are more likely to change work processes and implement them.[99,100] This has been the experience of hospitals working to prevent ventilator-associated pneumonia as part of IHI's 100,000 Lives Campaign. Teams have reported a synergistic effect from adopting the "ventilator bundle"; joining key steps into bundles served as a forcing function on an interdisciplinary level, improving teamwork and dramatically reducing ventilator-associated pneumonia. Additional benefits include decreased costs and improved staff morale.

A bundle strategy can also be applied to medication error prevention, particularly for certain high-risk processes, high-alert medications, and high-risk patient populations. Bundles of critical error-prevention strategies can be created to promote the best safety outcomes possible. Chapter 14 can be used as a resource in identifying potential bundles for high-alert medications. The JCAHO National Patient Safety Goals also provide examples of interventions grouped by desired outcome, such as medication safety and communication.

Bundles should be relatively small; the strategies should be based on error-prevention principles that have been proven or have face validity (page 634).[101–103] They should be treated as a cohesive unit; for success, all the strategies in a bundle must be implemented. According to IHI, the power of bundles lies in their "all or none" nature; if the individual steps are not implemented together, reliability may not improve. IHI also suggests that bundles may change over time as new elements are identified through research or health care providers' experience.

Redundancy

One hallmark of HROs is their high level of redundancy in both safety measures and personnel for the most critical processes.[2] Redundancy allows a system to fail benignly; extra trained staff and equipment are on site to duplicate critical functions and thereby detect and intercept errors before harm occurs.

A system that is only a single failure deep lacks redundancy. For example, many facets of the drug administration process allow no opportunity for a downstream check. An estimated 2% of errors that originate during drug administration are captured and corrected, whereas 48% of prescribing orders are corrected before reaching the patient.[104] Prescribing errors are more amenable to correction because of system checks for a drug's appropriateness and safety before it is administered. To become more reliable, health care organizations need to redesign critical processes that are a single failure deep in order to build in redundancy.

Assuming that errors will happen, HROs plan for recovery after an error. This means making errors visible and easy to reverse, or making irreversible errors difficult to commit.[2] An example of design for recovery is familiar to all computer users: When the user tries to delete a file, the computer ask for confirmation that it should be deleted; if confirmation is given, the deleted file moves to a recycle or trash bin and can still be retrieved until the user actively empties the bin.

CHOOSING ERROR PREVENTION STRATEGIES[101–103]

If you wanted to go skydiving, you would not ask first for scientific evidence that parachutes prevent injury during free-fall.[102] Some people have, without parachutes, survived free-fall uninjured, and some people who did use parachutes have been injured. Still, you would use a parachute when skydiving, even without a single randomized trial showing its effectiveness. In health care, however, clinicians may be reluctant to try any intervention without scientific proof of its efficacy.

This desire for evidence may have grown out of past experience with practices that were abandoned because scientific scrutiny showed they were ineffective or harmful.[103] Like most practitioners, we see the importance of evidence-based medicine. But, when it comes to patient safety, there are significant obstacles to this approach. There is a notable lack of research supporting many obvious error-reduction strategies. A safety program based solely on evidence-based interventions could be ineffective because it does not focus on the most important problems.

Obvious ethical and recruitment difficulties preclude randomized trials of parachute effectiveness, and the same is true for some patient safety interventions. Among other concerns, the size of a trial needed to prove efficacy of a safety practice would be prohibitive. Take, for example, the practice of requiring a leading zero for doses less than one.[103] Perhaps only 1 in 100 clinicians would misread the dose as a whole number if the leading zero were omitted. If this error did occur, it might have a 1 in 5 chance of reaching the patient and a 1 in 10 chance of causing significant harm. If experience tells us that leading zeros reduce the risk of errors, then is such a study needed?

Scientific evidence cannot be the only source of strategies for advancing patient safety. For example, mortality during elective anesthesia has declined 10-fold in the past few decades. This achievement required a broad array of changes in processes, equipment, organizational leadership, education, and teamwork—not one of which had been proven to have a clear-cut impact on mortality.[103] The changes were based on an understanding of human-factors principles and on clear linkage between certain processes and observed adverse events. They were learned from the safety practices of other industries. And they made sense.

In choosing safety strategies, we must make decisions based on common sense and the best available information about human-factors principles, linkage between processes and adverse events, and safety practices in other industries. We must not wait for irrefutable proof of effectiveness—or abandon initiatives such as pharmacy IV admixture systems and computer-generated medication administration records simply because they are not backed by rigorous scientific evidence.

PROACTIVE FOCUS AND COMMUNITY INVOLVEMENT

Learning in HROs occurs not only from within, but also through a search for outside knowledge to improve safety. HROs do not need an accident as a call to action. They consistently engage in proactive risk assessment activities, capitalizing on effective hazard reporting programs and using teams with sophisticated knowledge of systems to test and anticipate the ways things could go wrong. Furthermore, HROs share their knowledge through mentoring, networking, collaborative work, and external reporting systems.

HROs engage the community in their safety efforts. They build positive relationships with the media and respond openly to the public, who may have anxieties about safety within the industry. They are transparent with the public, disclosing information about accidents, errors, and safety hazards and other performance data. They often ask community members to serve on safety panels, where their input is greatly valued and respected.

Sharing Lessons Learned

External error reporting systems (for reporting to a safety agency not affiliated with the organization) allow practitioners and health care organizations to share lessons they have learned in order to help others avoid similar mishaps. Ideally, external reporting programs analyze submitted reports, disseminate alerts on newly recognized hazards, and suggest error-reduction strategies, and organizations receiving the alerts adopt the suggested strategies.

The U.S. Pharmacopoeia (USP)-ISMP Medication Errors Reporting Program (MERP) is the primary external voluntary reporting program for medication safety in the United States. MERP receives some 800 reports annually. Although MERP data cannot be used to determine the prevalence of medication errors, analysis of the reports provides insight into the types, causes, and prevention of errors. In a variety of ways, ISMP broadly disseminates MERP findings to health care providers and consumers; ISMP's newsletters alone have nearly 3.5 million readers worldwide.[105]

Knowledge from Outside

Experience has shown that a medication error reported in one institution will likely occur in other facilities as well. Institutions can use the experiences of others as a road map for improvement.[106] However, many do not seek and use outside information and recommendations for improvement. In 2000 and 2004, ISMP offered a medication safety self-assessment tool for use by U.S. hospitals.[8,107] When asked if an interdisciplinary team routinely analyzes and uses published error experiences to improve medication safety, only 50% of more than 1,600 participating hospitals in 2004 (and 29% in 2000) said they consistently perform this important function.

Practitioners may read published error reports but not truly believe the same errors could happen in their institutions. At some institutions, committees to address errors have a solely internal focus and do not effectively learn about errors occurring elsewhere and their causes. As stated by quality improvement expert W. Edwards Deming, organizations with an internal focus "can learn a lot about ice and know nothing about water."[106]

Process for Proactive Change

Some health care providers have successfully used external sources in identifying risks and implementing proactive changes, thereby averting patient harm. These successful organizations have used the following processes.

Make assignments. Assign one or more practitioners to routinely search the literature for new technologies, evidence-based practices, and published experiences with errors at other organizations. This should be part of the staff member's job description and performance evaluation.

List on agendas. Make proactive change a standing agenda item for discussion by the interdisciplinary team that reviews internal medication safety. Ensure that the team routinely analyzes external information about errors and other patient safety issues to determine the need for change. Set a routine time for the team to meet, at least monthly.

Be prepared for each meeting. Some health care providers have found it helpful to create a worksheet succinctly describing published errors, prevention recommendations, related safeguards in place in the hospital, and new error-reduction strategies that need to be implemented.

Review outside information. Establish a systematic way to review new information, assess the organization's current status in relation to each item, and prioritize the items according to their potential to cause or prevent patient harm.

Plan changes. Determine a workable action plan that includes process and outcome measures for evaluating success and timelines for completion. Some hospitals have found Gantt charts useful for graphically representing the timing, duration, and people responsible for specific tasks in the completion of a project. Assign staff, manager, or leader teams most suitable for the specific actions to ensure that proactive change occurs.

Test and spread the change. First, implement the change on a small scale. Make any necessary revisions uncovered during the test before introducing the change throughout the organization.

ISMP Action Agenda

ISMP offers a quarterly action agenda[20] for hospitals; it describes the most important topics covered during the previous quarter in the *ISMP Medication Safety Alert!* newsletters. Each agenda item describes the problem and gives recommendations for reducing risk, with reference to the newsletter article for additional information. ISMP recommends sharing the action agenda with administrative staff and an interdisciplinary committee at practice sites to stimulate discussion and actions to reduce the risk of errors. The concept of an action agenda can be used in any practice site, including hospital and community pharmacies, long-term care facilities, and home care companies.

Eliminating "Never" Events

Despite the widespread increase in patient safety activities in the past decade, too little attention has been given to reducing the risk of the most serious errors. This may be because such events occur infrequently or because strategies for preventing them have not been tested scientifically.

For example, fatalities from intrathecal administration of IV vincristine continue to be reported, despite recognized strategies for preventing them. Inadvertent administration of oral liquids by the IV route is another example; the use of an inexpensive oral syringe could significantly reduce or eliminate this.

Perhaps a desire to get the most out of allotted patient safety resources has increased health care providers' tolerance for rare but harmful events. Practices that most would consider unsafe have been tolerated simply because there are no data to confirm their danger or prove the effectiveness of safer practices.

Consumers are unlikely to understand health care providers' tolerance of rare but harmful events that should *never* happen. The public would not understand if the risk of an airplane crash were given low priority just because crashes happen infrequently, particularly if pilots were poorly trained or intimidating or used ambiguous abbreviations or unclear spoken orders.

Complacency about the risk of rare but harmful events is indefensible. Prevalence should be considered in prioritizing patient safety efforts, but it certainly should not be the only determinant of whether proactive steps must be taken. When health care providers fail to take relatively simple actions that could prevent harmful errors, consumers have every right to doubt our commitment to safety.

Patient and Community Involvement

Public Opinion about Health Care and Medical Errors

Information in the mass media feeds public opinion about medical error. Press coverage of the issue since 2000 has been unprecedented. One-third of U.S. patients responding to a 2005 survey believed they had been victims of a treatment error, medication error, or lab error.[108] Patients from five other countries included in the survey were less likely to give this response. The rate of reported errors rose sharply as the number of physicians involved in the patient's care increased. Most patients (61% to 83%) in each country said their health care providers did not tell them about the mistakes. Nevertheless, Americans hold their individual physicians and hospitals in high regard; 84% to 93% expressed overall satisfaction with their medical care in a recent survey.[109]

Reaching Out to the Community

Health care providers should take advantage of the increased media scrutiny of medical errors and the public's enduring faith in their health care providers as an opportunity to begin talking with patients and consumers about errors and building stronger relationships with the media. While they work to enhance patient safety in their organizations, practitioners should go outside the walls of their facilities to educate the public about errors, their causes, and how providers and patients together can prevent them.

Practitioners can start by finding a news report of a medical error and responding to the report with a press release, commentary, or editorial on the likely system-based causes of the error and the steps their own facility is taking to prevent similar errors. Local, regional, or state organizations can collaborate in such an effort. Practitioners can speak at local gatherings or host events in their facilities. They can listen to the public's concerns, honestly acknowledge them, and demonstrate their commitment to safety by giving examples of how the facility has made it difficult for staff to err.

Patient Safety Advisories

Educated patients are the safest patients. As discussed in Chapter 13, patients who know what to expect are more alert to potential risks and errors. Although most adult patients believe they have a positive role in their own safety,[110] organizations vary widely in their efforts to educate patients about their role in safety and encourage their contributions.

Most health care providers do give patients printed information (e.g., a brochure or pamphlet, or a handout in patient admission materials) containing general safety tips and encouraging patients to speak up about hazards. The emphasis usually is on direct actions patients can take to help ensure their safety. Although such safety advisories may help reduce errors, their impact has not been well studied. A recent analysis of five national safety advisories suggests that they may have unintended consequences that compromise patient safety efforts.[111] The materials were analyzed by patient safety researchers with academic, clinical, administrative, and consumer backgrounds. Table 23-6, based on this analysis, lists questions for assessing patient safety materials.

Collaborative Efforts

Creating opportunities for patients, community members, and health care providers to work together for safety is key to delivering reliable health care every time to every patient. Yet many organizations keep patients and the community at arm's length when identifying safety problems, analyzing the problems, implementing changes to reduce risk, and measuring the outcome.

Directly involving patients has helped organizations move toward highly reliable health care. Some organizations have included patients and consumers in internal quality improvement and safety initiatives. Chapter 13 describes an early experience with the patient and family advisory council established at the Dana-Farber Cancer Institute.[112] Dana-Farber has continued to expand patient and consumer involvement in safety. In

TABLE 23-6   Self-Assessment Questions for Patient Safety Advisories

Content

Are the safety tips well defined?
People who are ill may be less likely to act on vague safety tips, such as "Ask questions."

Is the basis for the safety tips provided?
Knowing the basis for a safety tip helps patients remember it and use it.

Are the safety tips prioritized?
Receiving a large number of tips can make people feel overburdened or guilty because they cannot act on all
   of them. Telling patients which tips are most important in their case could help improve compliance.

Does the advisory specify what the organization is doing to enhance safety?
A list of safety tips alone may imply that patients are the only ones looking out for their safety.

Is the difference between harm from errors and unpreventable harm covered?
If patients do not understand that some adverse outcomes in health care are not preventable, they may equate
   all bad outcomes with negligence.

Are patients advised how to report hazards and errors?
Patients need a means of reporting perceived risks and errors to their health care providers.

Tone

Is the advisory written from the patient's perspective?
Attempts should be made to learn about patients' beliefs, concerns, and self-perceived information needs, or to
   test the advisory before dissemination.

Do the safety tips require patients to check or challenge health care providers?
Patients may fear being labeled as difficult if they speak up, and staff may be less inclined to interact with
   patients who challenge them, potentially worsening safety risks.

Does the advisory shift responsibility for safe care from the provider to the patient?
This perceived shift of responsibilities is particularly prevalent when there is little evidence that the health care
   provider is also taking steps to improve safety.

Is it implied that patients need to "work around" system deficiencies?
The tone of the advisory could leave patients uncertain about the extent of support they will receive from staff,
   if the message is not collaborative.

Message Reinforcement

Do staff reinforce the safety tips in the advisory and offer patients practical support in carrying them out?
Health care providers may not regularly discuss the safety tips in the advisory with patients and give them
   personal encouragement to follow the tips.

Source: Reference 111.

2004, the organization studied the impact of clinician and patient (consumer) champions
on its patient safety rounds, used to elicit safety concerns.[113] In one phase of the study,
volunteer patients from the adult patient and family advisory council interviewed other
patients currently in treatment about their perceptions of safe care at Dana-Farber. The
council helped develop the interview tool. Many of the safety concerns mentioned by
patients had never been identified by staff. The patient-to-patient interaction increased
patients' willingness to speak up about safety issues and provided new information about
risks and hazards from the patient's perspective.

LEARNING CULTURE

HROs have a strong desire to learn. Learning is not the same as training, which typically
is episodic and passive with little or no link to the desired results. Learning means

enhancing capacity through real-life experiences gained over time. HROs see learning as inseparable from everyday work, and a necessary precursor to change. For the workforce, it is learning reflection and inquiry skills, not training in operational skills, that enables workers to talk about tough issues, including risks and errors, without defensiveness. For leaders, training means trying to make the workforce perform flawlessly, whereas learning means understanding the constraints that keep the staff from flawless work.[44]

HROs use their learning experiences as the basis for change. The leaders know that little change can come from the top alone. They do not see themselves as special people blessed with the ability to command, influence, and bring about change. They know that real change comes from commitment, not management-driven compliance that directs the workforce to "just do it" or be at odds with the boss. They know the workforce is skeptical about "flavor of the month" strategies, and that without a commitment to change, people cling to old habits. They recognize that the workforce holds the power to either change or maintain the status quo. Thus, HROs typically employ leadership communities comprising local line leaders, internal networkers, and managing leaders to drive change.[44]

The local line leaders (frontline workers and managers) are the only ones who can undertake a test of change, evaluate its practicality, see how it fits into the workflow, and ultimately change the way service is delivered. Internal networkers (staff such as physicians who are not limited to a specific department or unit) are used as natural seed carriers of new ideas to generate a sense of urgency to spread the change. Managing leaders support, guide, and fund the changes, and help create urgency to change.

Learning Culture in Health Care

When viewed from the aggregate perspective of all health care provided to all patients, bad outcomes may seem to occur frequently. In individual organizations, however, they occur infrequently. Therefore, the only way to remain consistently mindful of patient safety, learn from failures, and make significant safety improvements is to gather the right kind of data and use that information to drive change. This means creating a robust patient safety information system that collects, analyzes, and disseminates information about errors and near misses within an organization, as well as risks identified proactively both in the organization and externally.[6] This safety information system forms the nucleus of a learning culture in which people convert the lessons they learn into actions to improve safety.[6,114]

A learning culture has been described by human-factors researcher James Reason as an environment in which "those who manage and operate the system have current knowledge about the human, technological, organizational, and environmental factors that determine the safety of the system as a whole" (p. 294).[115] It is a culture that depends on the existence of other key characteristics of a safety culture, most notably

- How organizational leaders apportion blame (just culture),
- How readily workers can adapt to changes (resilience),
- How well teams function (teamwork), and
- To what degree the bearers of bad news are embraced (questioning).[6,115–117]

Just Culture

A learning culture is highly dependent on the willingness of workers to report mistakes and risks that are often interpersonally and interdepartmentally troubling.[116] How an organization handles blame and punishment affects what is reported. An organization cannot learn if its reporting system is flawed, or if workers are uncomfortable discussing and analyzing mistakes.[6]

TABLE 23-7 Behaviors of Adaptive Conformers versus Observant Questioners

What the Worker Faces	Adaptive Conformer	Observant Questioner
Obstacles	Adjusts and improvises without bothering managers or others	Noisy complainer: Remedies immediate situation but also lets managers and others know when the system has failed
Others' errors	Seamlessly corrects errors of others, without confronting them about their error	Nosy interrupter: Asks what others are doing and lets others know they have made a mistake, with the intent of creating learning, not blame
Own errors	Creates an impression of never making mistakes	Self-aware error maker: Lets manager and others know they have made a mistake so everyone can learn; communicates openness to hearing about his or her own errors discovered by others
Subtle opportunities for change	Is committed to the organization and understands the "way things work around here"	Disruptive questioner: Asks, Why do we do things this way? Is there a better way of providing the care?

Adapted, with permission, from reference 117.

Resilience

A learning culture is dependent on workers' ability to understand and react to complex, demanding processes both at typical capacity and during periods of high capacity and stress. Learning fosters the flexibility needed to handle fluctuations in activity levels, intensity, and tempo.[6,114]

Teamwork

Organizational learning occurs best in small groups or teams that are organized and inspired.[116] Whereas individual learning is important to individual performance, collective learning in groups is needed to foster organizational change.

Questioning

Although no one likes to hear bad news, learning organizations value its content and encourage workers to communicate questions and concerns about their work.[116,117] To illustrate the degree of questioning desired from workers in learning organizations, Tucker and Edmondson[116,117] compared "adaptive conformers" with "observant questioners" (Table 23-7). Capable and dedicated workers typically are adaptive conformers, and many managers truthfully would prefer such workers. Without the observant and disruptive questioner, however, collective learning is not possible. It is this type of worker who stimulates debates that identify new sources of hazard and new ways to cope.[6]

Barriers to Learning in Health Care

Reason[6] has stated that of all the elements of a culture of safety, a learning culture is probably the easiest to engineer and the hardest to make work. Edmondson[116] agrees and notes that it is rare for a health care organization to systematically and effectively learn from failures that occur, especially small ones. One barrier is learned helplessness—abandonment of efforts to change because attempts have continually been fruitless. Over time, people simply grow less willing to speak up. The power of observation is suppressed and problems may go unnoticed. When problems are noticed, they may be reasoned away rather than pursued. Because people want to be safe, they look for evidence of safety, not hazards, and they see a smaller number of error reports as a positive factor.[6,116]

Another barrier to learning is a culture in which work-arounds are the dominant response to problems.[6] This is symptomatic of first-order problem solving (short-term fixes) rather than second-order problem solving (systemic fixes).[117]

First-Order and Second-Order Problem Solving

Whereas short-term remedies patch problems temporarily so work can be accomplished, long-term remedies seek to change the underlying systems and processes, thus preventing recurrence. Short-term remedies are reactive to the immediate environment, and long-term remedies are preventive, leading to more reliable care.[118,119]

In first-order problem solving, a worker compensates for a problem by using any means possible to complete a task but does not discover or address underlying causes. The problem therefore reappears and the work-arounds continue, often placing patients at risk.

One study showed that nurses used first-order problem solving to implement short-term fixes for 93% of the failures they encountered.[117] For example, when faced with dwindling or absent floor stock of IV solutions or medications, nurses often borrowed the necessary products from another patient's supply or another unit. When faced with congestion at an ADC, they removed all of their patients' medications for the shift and kept them in various unsecured areas, all mixed together, until needed. Because their primary goal was to continue caring for patients, many nurses interviewed during the study felt gratified that they were able to handle a problem quickly with minimal cost. They did whatever it took to continue patient care. When they needed help in solving a problem, they asked a colleague with whom they were socially close, not necessarily the person best able to correct the problem. This approach helped preserve the nurses' reputations as capable of handling daily challenges, and it helped the nurses avoid unpleasant encounters.

With first-order problem solving, problems are not communicated to those who could investigate their causes and remedy them, so the same problems continue to appear. Nurses in the study spent an average of 33 minutes per 8 hour shift dealing with frequently repeated failures that could have been prevented if they had been brought to the attention of others. First-order problem solving also creates new problems elsewhere—shortages on the units from which medications were borrowed, for example.

Like the previously described quality of resilience, second-order problem solving involves both handling the unexpected problem and taking steps to address its underlying cause. For frontline staff, bringing an issue to the manager's attention may be all that is needed to start an investigation into the causes. In the study of nurses' approach to problems, the nurses communicated problems to their managers or others in a position to help just 7% of the time.[117] It is likely that other health care professionals, such as physicians and pharmacists, behave similarly.

Leadership and Change

A learning culture must be capable of observing, reflecting, creating, and acting. It is the last element, acting, that is most difficult.[6] Leaders and workers must be willing and able to implement the changes found to be necessary by the safety information system. Without action that brings about change and improvement, learning is meaningless. Thus, the challenge of patient safety is linked to the challenge of organizational change.[120]

It is the leaders in an organization, at both the administrative and patient care levels, who inspire organizational learning and change. Table 23-8[6,120–122] lists actions commonly attributed to leaders who do this well.

Theories on change management—or the best way to link learning, change, and improvement—are too numerous to describe here in detail. The following section notes key change management concepts that have been used to improve patient safety.

TABLE 23-8   Leadership Actions that Promote Organizational Learning

---

Create an environment of psychological safety that fosters reporting
Inspire and encourage workers to notice everything and deny nothing
Reward workers who question their work
Provide a compelling vision of patient safety
Challenge the status quo
Create a sense of urgency to learn and change
Build a team-based learning infrastructure
Track down bad news
Shatter assumptions of safe care
Encourage workers to assume the system is dangerous until proven safe, not safe until proven dangerous
Promote the perspective that a near miss is a sign of system vulnerability, not system safety
Elicit commitment, rather than exerting control
Look for multiple explanations for failures
Do not underestimate the importance of social influence on the culture
Believe feedback is important and understand its role in taking action
Act, not just talk, their way into new values
Recognize that expectations energized by strong feelings shape the culture

---

Adapted from references 6 and 120–122.

Challenge the Status Quo

To create a sense of urgency for change, effective leaders routinely challenge the status quo.[120,121] They offer compelling reasons why the status quo is not acceptable and clearly explain change concepts that reflect well-conceived alternatives to "business as usual." They convey the message that maintaining the status quo is far more dangerous than launching into new ways of providing care, and they shatter the erroneous assumption that change is not warranted if the prevalence of harm is low.

Form Guiding Coalition, Communicate Vision

Effective leaders assemble, early in the process, a group with enough power, in terms of titles, information, expertise, reputations, and relationships, to lead the change.[122] A sense of urgency to change within the managerial ranks and a history of teamwork at the top of the organization are key to forming this coalition. Groups without strong line leadership rarely achieve the power necessary to lead change efforts. One of the first tasks of the guiding coalition is to develop a vision of the future that is easy to communicate. Without a vision, the effort can easily dissolve into incompatible projects. According to Kotter,[122] a leading theorist on organizational change, if leaders cannot communicate a vision in 5 minutes or less and get a positive reaction, then the vision is not fully developed.

Use PDSA Cycles

Effective leaders resist the temptation to fall back on familiar but less powerful ways of effecting change, such as education and policy enforcement to gain compliance with existing systems. Instead, they challenge the status quo by planning changes, testing them on a small scale, and using a plan–do–study–act (PDSA) process to spread the change. The leaders understand the need to specifically reserve time to reflect on what was learned from the test, how to build upon it, and how to spread the change throughout the organization.[121] Aggressive time frames for testing changes, learning from the tests, and spreading the change are not altered unnecessarily, but workers are given sufficient time to acclimate to the change. To avoid premature withdrawal of the support needed to sustain change, leaders ensure that resources for the change are in place.

Use Multiple Tactics

Leaders improve the likelihood of successful change by using multiple tactics to solve even simple problems,[121] since problems tend to have multiple causes. For real transformation, multiple components of the system must be targeted at multiple levels, from frontline workers to the top leaders of the organization.[120] With this approach, the organization can attain short-term wins to help convince doubters that the effort is worthwhile.[122] Victory should not be declared, however, until the change has been spread and sustained throughout the organization.

Disable the Trump

Berwick[121] describes a problem commonly faced by teams working for change in an organization: trumping. Those resisting the change suggest that no progress can be made until after other large-scale problems (e.g., the malpractice crisis, inequitable reimbursement systems, unrealistic patient demands, health professional shortages, punitive licensing boards) are solved. The person trumping the effort, especially if he or she is highly regarded in the organization, can divert energy from the change effort. Skillful leaders can regain the energy by disabling the trump, through acknowledging the problem and suggesting ways the organization can make the desired change at the same time it is tackling the large-scale problem.

SAFETY MEASUREMENT

HROs know their safety climate and their level of system performance. They can tell if a change has resulted in improvement, not just through workforce notification of problems, errors, and accidents, but through devoting resources to more accurate ways of detecting risk, errors, and harm. HROs do not simply count the number of accidents (e.g., airline crashes, nuclear meltdowns, chemical spills). Instead, they use standard surveillance plans for systematically uncovering risk, errors, and less-than-optimal outcomes. Tracking their performance over time gives HROs reliable outcome data.

Because they are often less visible, errors in health care may be more difficult to quantify than accidents in HROs. Practitioner reporting uncovers only a fraction of the errors that occur. But measurement is fundamental to improvement. It is needed to answer these essential questions: Do we have a problem? What is the extent of the problem? How will we know if a change results in improvement? How do we compare with others? Four types of measures should be used to answer these questions and improve medication safety: process measures, structural measures, outcome measures, and balancing measures.

Process Measures

These measures help assess performance of core processes in medication use. Measurement identifies variations in carrying out core processes that could lead to undesirable outcomes and patient harm.

Reducing the potential for adverse drug events (ADEs) is key to improving medication safety. Errors that result in serious patient harm are infrequent, but the potential for these catastrophic events lurks within the processes in many organizations. Measuring processes provides data upon which organizations can act to prevent errors.

Process measures can be identified for all facets of medication use, from compliance with safety standards in prescribing to compliance with protocols for monitoring patients' response. To maximize the benefit, high-volume and high-risk processes, or processes associated with high-alert medications, should be targeted for measurement, such as

- Number of pharmacy profiles without allergy information per number of new admission orders,
- Percentage of medication orders with prohibited error-prone abbreviations,
- Percentage of encounters in which two identifiers are not used to verify patient identity before drug administration,
- Time interval between prescribing and administering "stat" medications,
- Number of pharmacy interventions per 100 admissions, and
- Percentage of chemotherapy orders that do not comply with standardized prescribing guidelines (e.g., inclusion of the dose in milligrams per square meter as well as the calculated dose; order for single daily dose, not course dose).

One innovative process measure is the total risk priority number (RPN) of a process that has undergone FMEA.[123] As an organization works to improve the process and reduce the risk or severity of error, the RPN should decrease over time.

Structural Measures

These measures assess the organizational structure in which processes are carried out: the culture, values, leadership, and knowledge. In contrast to process measures, they are not task oriented, but foundational. Examples include

- Percentage of days on which established nurse–patient staffing ratios are maintained,
- Percentage of staffing met with agency staff,
- Percentage of new staff members who achieve 100% on particular competency tests,
- Number of error reports received (the reporting rate helps measure the culture), and
- Percentage of staff reporting a positive safety culture.

The Agency for Healthcare Research and Quality (AHRQ) funded the development of a survey of hospitals' safety culture.[124] The tool collects information about perceptions of safety and frequency of events reported, and yields an overall patient safety grade. It is designed to measure 10 dimensions of a safety culture:

1. Supervisor/manager expectations and actions promoting safety,
2. Organizational learning and continuous improvement,
3. Teamwork within units,
4. Communication and openness,
5. Feedback and communication about errors,
6. Nonpunitive responses to error,
7. Staffing,
8. Hospital management support for patient safety,
9. Teamwork across hospital units, and
10. Hospital handoffs and transitions.

The tool is accompanied by a guidance document that covers sampling, data collection, and analysis of findings. Tools like this can be used to survey a large cross-section of an organization, collecting information from frontline workers that would not otherwise be available to managers, and information from managers that would not otherwise be available to organizational leaders.[1]

Outcome Measures

These measures assess the results of processes—whether efforts to improve medication safety have been successful. Many believe errors are the most useful outcome measure of medication safety, but data on errors typically come from self-reporting, which is highly inaccurate.[125] Errors, including those that cause patient harm, often go undetected, and those that are detected may not be reported. Practitioners may not report errors that are intercepted before reaching the patient unless the organization clearly defines and communicates all situations that should be reported. Once an error has been reported, practitioners may not report similar errors, believing the leadership is aware of the particular problem. Furthermore, reporting is inhibited by failures to remedy reported problems, insufficient feedback about actions taken to prevent recurrence, complex and time-consuming reporting systems, and fear of personal and professional consequences. A focus on error rates derived from spontaneous reporting systems can cause practitioners to report fewer errors.

Errors in medication dispensing and administration can be measured more accurately through observational methods (see Chapter 2).[126] Trained observers watch practitioners prepare and dispense medications (typically in community pharmacies) or administer medications (typically in hospitals). The observer documents exactly what has been dispensed or administered, how and when it was dispensed or administered, and to whom. Comparing this information with the original prescription or order yields the rate of error.

Since this observational method cannot be used to detect prescribing errors, dispensing or administering an excessive dose that conforms to the prescriber's order would not be considered an error, even if the patient was harmed. Another shortcoming of the method is the commitment of staff needed to carry out enough observations for accurate comparisons over time. Despite these limitations, organizations that have used this method have been stunned by the number of errors uncovered and have used the findings to drive change and measure its success.

Harm may be a more reliable outcome measure than errors. ADEs are usually categorized as preventable or nonpreventable. Deeming some ADEs nonpreventable promotes tacit acceptance of harm as a property of the medication system for which practitioners bear no responsibility. Harm is a better measure of medication safety because it is clear and direct, encompasses *all* unintended results, and keeps practitioners focused on improvement.

For example, most hospitals collect data on readmissions. Readmissions due to bleeding from warfarin may not be fully assessed if the focus is on errors alone. If no errors in the patients' care are apparent, these events would likely be tagged as nonpreventable ADEs. But if the focus is on preventing harm in patients who take warfarin, practitioners are more likely to explore ways of reducing the occurrence of bleeding. Thus, the best outcome measure for medication safety is all ADEs (which cause harm), regardless of causation.

One of the most effective ways of collecting data on ADEs is examining patient records for triggers—clues that an ADE may have occurred. When one or more triggers appear, follow-up is needed to confirm whether harm actually occurred. ISMP has developed a list of such triggers,[127] for example

- *Drugs:* Diphenhydramine, vitamin K, flumazenil, glucagon, digoxin immune fab (Digibind), sodium polystyrene sulfonate (Kayexalate);

- *Lab results:* Elevation of a serum drug level, activated partial thromboplastin time, international normalized ratio (INR), or serum creatinine level; low and high blood glucose levels;
- *Other:* Rash, lethargy, falls, abrupt medication stop, transfer to a higher level of care.

Computerized methods using triggers to detect ADEs have proven effective,[128] but they require a high level of automation with customized software linkage to clinical databases, so the initial outlay may be costly. Recently, a relatively low-cost method for using triggers to uncover ADEs has been devised and tested in more than 80 hospitals.[129] The technique, which requires minimal training, appears to increase the rate of ADE detection 50-fold from traditional reporting methods.

Balancing Measures

These measures are used to ensure that a change in one part of the system is not causing problems in another part of the system—as happened, for example, with a change in the process for antiemetic therapy that reduced patients' time in the oncology clinic but also decreased their satisfaction.[112] The patients felt rushed and unable to talk with staff about their diagnosis and treatment. An example of a balancing measure is the percentage of patients or customers reporting satisfaction with a specific change intended to improve safety. Information obtained with this measure might lead to a different way of explaining a change to patients or customers and promoting it to practitioners.

Selecting Measures and Collecting Data

The primary reason for measuring medication safety should be learning how to improve, not issuing rewards or punishment.[121] Measurement systems need not be perfect to gain valuable information. Randomized, double-blind studies, large sample sizes, and complex statistical calculations are not necessary; all that is needed is enough information to take the next step toward improvement.

A systematic measurement process should be followed to ensure that the measures are clear, the purpose and goal of the measurement are as intended, the data collection methods are adequate and feasible, and the data collected are valid, consistent, and reliable.[121,130] The process should include the following steps.

1. Determine the medication safety issue to be measured and improved. External sources of information (e.g., regulators, accrediting bodies, and patient safety organizations such as ISMP) should be used to identify issues that can lead to serious patient harm. Internal sources such as event reports and staff surveys on the extent to which the problem exists should be used to narrow the choices.[130]

2. Search the literature. A literature review will reveal what is known about the area targeted for measurement and improvement and how specific processes are linked to the desired outcomes.[130] These links can be used to determine process and structural measures.

3. Establish aims. Aims must be clearly articulated to answer the question, "What are we trying to accomplish?"[121] Some examples: reduce the volume of "missing" medications by 50%; improve compliance with established turnaround times for stat medications by 30%; reduce the frequency of hypoglycemia in diabetic patients by 40%; reduce the frequency of errors with heparin by 75%; reduce the frequency of errors in pediatric patients by 40%. The more specific the aim, the more likely is the improvement.

To build momentum for change, the aims should be ambitious, making it obvious that the current system is inadequate. (Lesser goals can result in temporary improvements rather than sustainable system changes.) It is important for leaders to regularly communicate and reinforce the aims, in order to keep change and its measurement focused.

4. Construct the measures. Construct process, structural, and outcome measures to assess progress toward the aims. Measures should have clinical relevance and provide useful information about the topic of interest. The measures should be clearly stated to avoid errors in data collection. Most measures will include both a numerator (the number of times a finding, such as an elevated INR, occurred) and a denominator (the total number of opportunities to observe the finding, such as the total number of patients receiving warfarin).

5. Establish a data collection plan. For the plan to be workable, the time commitment must be acceptable to those responsible for collecting the information, analyzing it, communicating the findings, and using the findings to guide changes. The plan should clearly describe the following:[130]

- When the data should be collected,
- How often the data should be collected,
- The setting for data collection, or the target patient/customer population (e.g., diabetic patients, pediatric patients) or unit (e.g., oncology services, ICU),
- The target sample size,
- The source of data
  - Self-reporting (e.g., surveys)
  - Observations
  - Clinical values (e.g., lab values)
  - Medical records
  - Computer databases,
- The method of data collection (e.g., chart review, written instrument, interviews, computer-assisted),
- Responsibilities for data collection, analysis, and dissemination of information,
- The audience for findings of the analysis,
- How the information will be communicated, and
- The person to contact with questions.

6. Test and use the measures. Measures should be tested on a small scale for clarity, adequacy, utility, feasibility, and appropriateness for the intended purpose.[130] If the measure is found acceptable, data collection, analysis, and communication of the findings should proceed.

7. Communicate the findings. After analysis, the data should be disseminated to all who can apply what is learned, change the system or process associated with the measure, or be affected by a change in the system or process.[121,130] The findings can be distributed through memos, posters, storyboards, oral presentations, and other means. Findings should be supported with graphic displays such as the following:[131]

- *Histograms (bar graphs of the distribution of data, showing the degree of variability and skewness).* A histogram might be used to show variability in the past month of turnaround time for stat doses prepared by pharmacy. The histogram could show the number of times delivery falls within specific time spans, such as less than 5 minutes, 6–10 minutes, 11–15 minutes, and so on.
- *Pie charts (displays of data as slices of a circle representing percentages).* A pie chart might be used to show the proportions of medications involved in errors that are removed from ADCs via override, removed from ADCs after pharmacy review of the order, and dispensed from the pharmacy.

- *Pareto charts (displays of data in vertical bar graphs showing the frequency of distribution among variables).* A Pareto chart might be used to determine which problems to solve and in what order; the vertical bars would show the frequency of various causes of medication errors (e.g., lack of patient information, lack of drug information, problems with labeling and packaging, drug storage, the environment, staff training, patient education).
- *Run charts or line graphs (displays of observable data points along connected lines over a specified time period).* These could be used to evaluate a new calling system intended to reduce the number of customers who fail to pick up their prescriptions within 1 week. The weekly numbers could be plotted over 3 months to show changes.
- *Control charts (run charts with statistically determined upper and lower control limits on either side of the average, used most commonly to determine whether a process is under control).* These could be used to track the rate of prescriptions presented for which medications were not immediately available in the pharmacy. The number of times new prescriptions (or refills) were involved each day, week, or month could be plotted to determine whether the drug procurement process is under control.

Benchmarking

Benchmarking refers to the process of identifying practices that yield optimal results and implementing those best practices to improve organizational performance. Effective benchmarking entails both benchmarks and enablers.[132–134] Benchmarks are measures of comparative performance that answer the question, "What is the organization's level of performance?" To improve performance, benchmarking must provide a systematic method for understanding the processes that determine performance. To that end, enablers must be identified. Enablers are the specific practices that lead to exemplary performance; they answer the question, "How do you do it?"

Caution must be used in applying benchmarking to medication safety. The quality and safety of the medication-use process cannot be gauged simply by comparing error rates within an organization or externally. The number of reported errors is more likely to reflect the rigor of the error identification and reporting process than the true error rate. Because many medication errors cause no harm to patients, they remain undetected or unreported. A seemingly high error rate may suggest either unsafe medication practices or an organizational culture that promotes error reporting. Conversely, a low error rate may suggest either successful error prevention strategies or a punitive culture that inhibits reporting. Thus, error rate is usually not a valid benchmark.

Benchmarking should not be seen simply as a process for comparing numbers.[132,134,135] Too often, health care organizations compare medication error rates, despite their lack of meaning, but direct little effort toward identifying enablers of safe medication use. Focused on maintaining a low error rate, organizations give the errors themselves, rather than their correction, disproportionate importance. This promotes an unproductive cycle of underreporting and failure to detect weaknesses in the medication-use system. Low error rates can result in a false sense of security and tacit acceptance of preventable errors.

Benchmarking can be effectively applied to the medication-use process only if objective measurement (such as observational methods or systematic evaluation of errors), rather than spontaneous error reporting alone, is used to identify best practices.[132,134,136,137] Benchmarking must include a method for accurately determining the specific processes that enable the organization to achieve an environment in which medications are safely used. Success is more likely if benchmarking is focused on specific areas of drug therapy (such as insulin therapy or anticoagulant therapy) so that accurate benchmarks (performance measurements) and enablers (practices that lead to exemplary performance) can be more easily identified and implemented.

CONCLUSION

Laying a foundation for a culture of safety in health care takes time, commitment, and practice of the elements described in this chapter. But simply checking off the elements is not a good indication of an organization's progress toward a culture of safety.[6] The organization may have an event reporting program, a reasonably just culture, and a fair amount of measurement and teamwork. It may have succeeded in implementing some important safety measures. However, as Reason notes, "assembling the parts of a machine is not the same thing as making it work" (page 219).[6] It is not enough to possess some of the elements of a culture of safety. A total transformation in the way we perceive and react to risks that threaten patients is needed.

The experiences of HROs provide a useful road map for health care, although some have noted that the work environment, complexity, unpredictability, error-proneness, and consequences of failure are not really similar between health care and other industries. Consider, however, a Navy veteran's description of life on an aircraft carrier:[27]

> Imagine that it's a busy day, and you shrink the San Francisco airport to only one short runway and one ramp and one gate. Make the planes take off and land at the same time, at half the present time interval, rock the runway from side to side, and require that everyone who leaves in the morning returns the same day. Make sure the equipment is so close to the envelope that it's fragile. Then turn off the radar to avoid detection, impose strict controls on the radios, fuel the aircraft in place with their engines running, put an enemy in the air, and scatter live bombs and rockets around. Now wet the whole thing down with sea water and oil, and man it with 20-year-olds, half of whom have never seen an airplane up close. Oh, and by the way, try not to kill anyone (p. 26).

Is the environment in health care any more complex or unpredictable than on an aircraft carrier? Are the working conditions so different? Are the consequences of failure on a carrier any less dire than the consequences of failure in health care? Carriers may seem quite different, but their workers, like those in all HROs, confront and solve the same types of problems that health care practitioners face. The differences are only in the details, not in the character, scope, or urgency of the problems. HROs are a worthy source from which to learn as we begin to maximize our commitment to our patients, our cognizance of the dangers that threaten them, and our competence to handle the unexpected and achieve reliable health care at all times, despite adversity.

REFERENCES

1. Leonard M, Frankel A, Simmonds T, et al. for Foundation of American College of Healthcare Executives. *Achieving Safe and Reliable Healthcare: Strategies and Solutions.* Chicago: Health Administration Press; 2004.
2. Kohn LT, Corrigan JM, Donaldson MS, eds. *To Err Is Human: Building a Safer Health System.* Washington, DC: National Academies Press; 2000.
3. Amalberti R, Auroy Y, Berwick D, et al. Five system barriers to achieving ultrasafe health care. *Ann Intern Med.* 2005;142:756–64.
4. Senge P, Kleiner A, Roberts C, et al. *The Dance of Change.* New York: Doubleday/Currency; 1999.
5. Booth R. Safety culture: concept, measurement and training implications. Proceedings of British Health and Safety Society Spring Conference: Safety Culture and the Management of Risk. April 19–20, 1993, p. 5.
6. Reason J. *Managing the Risks of Organizational Accidents.* Hants, England: Ashgate Publishing Ltd; 1997.
7. GAIN Working Group E, Flight Ops/ATC Ops Safety Information Sharing. A roadmap to a just culture: enhancing the safety of the environment. September 2004. Available at: http://204.108.6.79/products/documents/roadmap%20to%20a%20just%20culture.pdf. Accessed April 7, 2006.
8. Smetzer JL, Vaida AJ, Cohen MR, et al. Findings from the ISMP Medication Safety Self-Assessment for Hospitals. *Jt Comm J Qual Saf.* 2003;29:586–97.

9. Turnbull JE, Mortimer J. The business case for safety. In: Zipperer L, Cushman S, eds. *Lessons in Patient Safety*. Chicago: National Patient Safety Foundation; 2000:21–6.

10. Bates D, Spell N, Cullen D, et al. The cost of adverse events in hospitalized patients. *JAMA*. 1997;277:307–11.

11. Weeks WB, Waldron J, Foster T, et al. The organizational costs of preventable medical errors. *Jt Comm J Qual Saf*. 2001;27:533–9.

12. Schneider P, Gift M, Lee Y, et al. Cost of medication-related problems at a university hospital. *Am J Health Syst Pharm*. 1995;52:2415–8.

13. Thomas E, Studdert DM, Newhouse JP. Costs of medical injuries in Utah and Colorado. *Inquiry*. 1999;36(fall):255–64.

14. Brahams D. Medical errors: a cost burden on society. *Medico-Legal J*. 2000;68(pt 1):1–2.

15. Institute for Safe Medication Practices. 2004 ISMP Medication Safety Self Assessment for Hospitals. Available at: www.ismp.org/selfassessments/Hospital/Intro.asp. Accessed May 11, 2006.

16. Joint Commission on Accreditation of Healthcare Organizations. National Patient Safety Goals for 2006. Available at: www.jointcommission.org/PatientSafety/NationalPatientSafetyGoals/06_npsg_cah.htm. Accessed May 5, 2006.

17. Joint Commission on Accreditation of Healthcare Organizations. *2006 Comprehensive Accreditation Manual for Hospitals*. Oakbrook Terrace, Ill: Joint Commission Resources; 2006.

18. National Quality Forum. The National Quality Forum Safe Practices for Better Healthcare. 2003. Available at: www.qualityforum.org/txsafeexecsumm+order6-8-03PUBLIC.pdf. Accessed February 22, 2006.

19. Institute for Healthcare Improvement. 100k Lives Campaign. Available at: www.ihi.org/IHI/Programs/Campaign/. Accessed February 22, 2006.

20. Institute for Safe Medication Practices. ISMP Quarterly Action Agenda. *ISMP Medication Safety Alert!* Available at: www.ismp.org/Newsletters/acutecare/actionagendas.asp.

21. American Hospital Association, Health Research and Education Trust, Institute for Safe Medication Practices. *Pathways for Medication Safety: Leading a Strategic Planning Effort*. Chicago: American Hospital Association; 2002. Available at: www.ismp.org/Tools/PathwaySection1.pdf.

22. Caldwell C. Six-sigma high performance characteristics: the senior leaders' role—part 3. HealthLeaders News. January 3, 2002. Available at: www.healthleadersmedia.com/view_feature.cfm?content_id=40950. Accessed February 20, 2006.

23. Frankel A, Graydon-Baker E, Neppl C, et al. Patient safety leadership WalkRounds. *Jt Comm J Qual Saf*. 2003;29:16–28.

24. Pronovost PJ, Weast B, Bishop K, et al. Senior executive adopt-a-work unit: a model for safety improvement. *Jt Comm J Qual Saf*. 2004,30:59–68.

25. Weick KE, Sutcliffe KM, Obstfeld D. Organizing for high reliability: processes of collective mindfulness. *Res Organ Behav*. 1999;21:81–123.

26. Reason J. *Managing the Risks of Organizational Accidents*. Burlington, Vt: Ashgate Publishing; 2000.

27. Weick KE, Sutcliffe KM. *Managing the Unexpected: Assuring High Performance in an Age of Complexity*. San Francisco: Jossey-Bass; 2001.

28. Landau M, Chisholm D. The arrogance of optimism: notes on failure avoidance management. *J Contingencies Crisis Manag*. 1995;3:67–80.

29. Institute for Safe Medication Practices. Survey on perceptions regarding a non-punitive culture in healthcare. *ISMP Medication Safety Alert!* June 27, 2001;6(13):1–2.

30. Institute for Safe Medication Practices. ISMP survey on perceptions of a nonpunitive culture produces some surprising results. *ISMP Medication Safety Alert!* August 22, 2001;6(17):1–2.

31. Institute for Safe Medication Practices. ISMP survey on perceptions of a nonpunitive culture—Part II. *ISMP Medication Safety Alert!* September 5, 2001;6(18):1-2.

32. Institute for Safe Medication Practices. ISMP survey on perceptions of a nonpunitive culture—Part III. *ISMP Medication Safety Alert!* September 19, 2001;6(19)1–2.

33. Outcome Engineering. The just culture algorithm-version 1.0. Dallas, Tex: Outcome Engineering, Inc; March 2005. Available at: www.justculture.org/downloads/jc_algorithm05.pdf. Accessed May 5, 2006.

34. Outcome Engineering. An introduction to just culture. Dallas, Tex: Outcome Engineering, Inc; 2005. Available at: www.justculture.org/downloads/jc_overview.pdf. Accessed May 5, 2006.

35. Marx D, Comden SC, Sexhus Z. Our inaugural issue—in recognition of a growing community. *Just Culture Community News and Views*. 2005;1(Nov/Dec):1.

36. Marx D. Patient safety and the "just culture": a primer for health care executives. April 17, 2001. Prepared for Columbia University under a grant provided by the National Heart, Lung, and Blood Institute. Available at: www.mers-tm.net/support/marx_primer.pdf. Accessed May 5, 2006.

37. Marx D, Comden SC, Sexhus Z, eds. Repetitive at-risk behavior—what to do when everyone is doing it. *Just Culture Community News and Views*. 2005;1(Nov/Dec):5–6.

38. Kotulak R. Similarities found to '86 catastrophe. *Chicago Tribune*. August 27, 2003:26.

39. Geller ES. *The Psychology of Safety Handbook*. New York: Lewis Publishers; 2001:33–49.

40. Marx D, Comden SC, Sexhus Z, eds. Coaching for dummies? *Just Culture Community News and Views.* 2005;1(Nov/Dec):6.

41. Marx D, Comden SC, Sexhus Z, eds. Using the JC algorithm: a practice session. *Just Culture Community News and Views.* 2006;2(Jan/Feb):4-6.

42. Institute for Safe Medication Practices. Practitioners anticipate punitive action from licensing boards. *ISMP Medication Safety Alert!* May 19, 2005;10(10):1–2.

43. Marx D, Comden SC, Sexhus Z, eds. The Minnesota journey—an interview with Alison Page, MS, MHA, VP of patient safety, Fairview Health Services. *Just Culture Community News and Views.* 2005;1(Nov/Dec):2–4.

44. Senge P, Kleiner A, Roberts C, et al. *The Fifth Discipline Fieldbook.* New York: Doubleday/Currency;1994.

45. Katzenbach JR, Smith DK. *The Wisdom of Teams: Creating the High-Performance Organization.* New York: Harper Collins; 1993.

46. Baker DP, Salas E, King H, et al. The role of teamwork in professional education of physicians: current status and assessment recommendations. *Jt Comm J Qual Saf.* 2005;31:185–202.

47. Shojania KG, Duncan WB, McDonald KM, et al. Making healthcare safer: a critical analysis of patient safety practices. Evidence report/technology assessment #43 (Prepared by University of California at San Francisco–Stanford University under contract #290-97-0013). AHRQ publication #01-E058. Rockville, Md: Agency for Healthcare Research and Quality; July 2001.

48. Helmreich RL. Managing human error in aviation. *Sci Am.* 1997;277(5):40.

49. Helmreich RL, Wilhelm JA, Gregorich SE, et al. Preliminary results from the evaluation of cockpit resource management training: performance ratings of flight crews. *Aviation Space Environ Med.* 1990;61:576–9.

50. Barker JM, Clothier CC, Woody JR, et al. Crew resource management: a simulator study comparing fixed versus formed crews. *Aviation Space Environ Med.* 1996; 67:3–7.

51. Weigmann DA, Shappell SA. Human error and crew resource management failures in Naval aviation mishaps: a review of US Naval Safety Center data, 1990–96. *Aviation Space Environ Med.* 1999;70:1147–51.

52. Helmreich RL, Foushee HC. Why crew resource management? Empirical and theoretical bases of human factors training in aviation. In: Weiner EL, Kanki BG, Helmreich RL, eds. *Cockpit Resource.* San Diego; Academic Press; 1993:3–45.

53. Sexton JB, Thomas EJ, Helmreich RL. Error, stress, and teamwork in medicine and aviation: cross sectional surveys. *BMJ.* 2000;320:745–9.

54. Gaba DM, Howard SK, Fish KJ, et al. Simulation-based training in anesthesia crisis resource management (ACRM): a decade of experience. *Simulation Gaming.* 2001;32(2):175–93.

55. Thomas EJ, Sexton JB, Helmreich RL. Translating teamwork behaviors from aviation to healthcare: development of behavioral markers for neonatal resuscitation. *Qual Saf Health Care.* 2004;12(Oct suppl):i57-i64.

56. Institute of Medicine. Committee on Health Care Services, Board of Health Care Services. *Health Professions Education: A Bridge to Quality.* Washington, DC: National Academies Press; 2003.

57. Joint Commission on Accreditation of Healthcare Organizations. Root causes of sentinel events. Available at: www.jointcommission.org/SentinelEvents/Statistics/. Accessed April 14, 2006.

58. Joint Commission on Accreditation of Healthcare Organizations. Root causes of medication errors. Available at: www.jointcommission.org/NR/rdonlyres/969F94E2-6908-4A30-A1B4-EFE9BDB23D24/0/se_rc_medication_errors.jpg. Accessed April 14, 2006.

59. Solomon RP, Bruley M, Wallace C, et al., eds. Teamwork training catching on slowly. *Risk Management Reporter* (ECRI); February 2005:3.

60. Bagg JG, Ryan SA, Phelps CE, et al. The association between interdisciplinary collaboration and patient outcomes in medical intensive care units. *Heart Lung.* 1992;21(1):18–24.

61. Risser DT, Rice MM, Salisbury ML, et al. The potential for improved teamwork to reduce medical errors in the emergency department. The MedTeams Research Consortium. *Ann Emerg Med.* 1999;34:373–83.

62. Halamek LP, Kaegi DM, Gaba DM, et al. Time for a new paradigm in pediatric medical education: teaching neonatal resuscitation in a simulated delivery room environment. *Pediatrics.* 2000;106:E45.

63. Silver MP, Antonow JA. Reducing medication errors in hospitals: a peer review organization collaboration. *Jt Comm J Qual Improv.* 2000;26:332–40.

64. Weeks WB, Mills PD, Dittus RS, et al. Using an improvement model to reduce adverse drug events in VA facilities. *Jt Comm J Qual Improv.* 2001;27:243–54.

65. Lawrence D. *From Chaos to Care: The Promise of Team-Based Medicine.* Cambridge, Mass: Perseus; 2002.

66. Schyve PM. Teamwork—the changing nature of professional competence [editorial]. *Jt Comm J Qual Patient Saf.* 2005;31:183–4.

67. Institute of Medicine. Committee on Quality of Health Care in America. *Crossing the Quality Chasm: A New Health System for the 21st Century.* Washington, DC: National Academies Press, 2001.

68. Cannon-Bowers JA, Tannenbaum SI, Salas E, et al. Defining competencies and establishing team training requirements. In: Guzzo RA, Salas E, et al., eds. *Team Effectiveness and Decision-Making in Organizations.* San Francisco: Jossey-Bass; 1995:333–80.

69. Salas E, Burke CS, Stagl KC. Developing teams and team leaders: strategies and principles. In: Demaree RG, Zaccaro SJ, Halpin SM, eds. *Leader Development for Transforming Organizations.* Mahwah, NJ: Erlbaum; 2004.

70. Healey AN, Undre S, Vincent CA. Developing observational measures of performance in surgical teams. *Qual Saf Health Care.* 2004;13(Suppl):i33–i40.

71. Flin R, Maran N. Identifying and training non-technical skills for teams in acute medicine. *Qual Saf Health Care.* 2004;13(Suppl):i80–i84.

72. McIntyre RM, Salas E. Measuring and managing for team performance: emerging principles from complex environments. In: Guzzo RA, Salas E, et al., eds. *Team Effectiveness and Decision Making in Organizations.* Mahwah, NJ: Erlbaum; 1995:9–45.

73. Porter CO, Hollenbeck JR, Ilgen DR, et al. Backing up behaviors in teams: the role of personality and legitimacy of need. *J Appl Psychol.* 2003;88:391–403.

74. Kozlowski SWJ, Gully SM, Nason ER, et al. Developing adaptive teams: a theory of compilation and performance across levels and time. In: Ilgen DR, Pulakos ED, eds. *The Changing Nature of Performance: Implications for Staffing, Motivation, and Development.* San Francisco: Jossey-Bass; 1999:240–92.

75. Klein G, Pierce LG. Adaptive Teams. *Proceedings of the 6th ICCRTS Collaboration in the Information Age, Track 4: C2 Decision Making and Cognitive Analysis;* 2001.

76. Driskell JE, Salas E. Collective behavior and team performance. *Hum Factors.* 1992;34:277–88.

77. Shamir B. Calculations, values, and entities: the sources of collective motivation. *Hum Relations.* 1990;43:313–32.

78. Wagner JA. Studies of individualism–collectivism: effects on cooperation in groups. *Acad Manage J.* 1995;38:152–72.

79. Klimoski R, Mohammed S. Team mental model: construct or metaphor? *J Manage.* 1994;20:403–37.

80. Mathieu JE, Heffner TS, Goodwin GF, et al. The influence of shared mental models on team process and performance. *J Appl Psychol.* 2000;85:273–83.

81. Stout RJ, Cannon-Bowers JA, Salas E. The role of shared mental models in developing team situational awareness: implications for team training. *Training Res J.* 1996;2:85–116.

82. Wright MC, Taekman JM, Endsley MR. Objective measures of situation awareness in a simulated medical environment. *Qual Saf Health Care.* 2004;13(Suppl):i65–i71.

83. Bandow D. Time to create sound teamwork. *J Qual Participation.* 2001;24:41–7.

84. Webber SS. Leadership and trust facilitating cross-functional team success. *J Manage Dev.* 2002;21:201–14.

85. Leonard M, Graham S, Bonacum D. The human factor: the critical importance of effective teamwork and communication in providing safe care. *Qual Saf Health Care.* 2004;13(Suppl):i85–i90.

86. Adubato S. Talk is not cheap when it saves lives. *The Star-Ledger* (Newark, NJ). Feb 15, 2004; Business section:7.

87. Helmreich RL, Schaefer HG. Team performance in the operating room. In: Bogner MS, ed. *Human Error in Medicine.* Hillside, NJ: Erlbaum; 1998.

88. Institute for Safe Medication Practices. Intimidation: practitioners speak up about this unresolved problem (part I). *ISMP Medication Safety Alert!* March 11, 2004;9(5):1–2. Available at: www.ismp.org/Newsletters/acutecare/articles/20040311_2.asp.

89. Institute for Safe Medication Practices. Intimidation: mapping a plan for cultural change in healthcare (part II). *ISMP Medication Safety Alert!* March 25, 2004;9(6):1–2. Available at: www.ismp.org/Newsletters/acute care/articles/20040325.asp.

90. Kaeter M. Medicine confronts workplace abuse. *Minn Med.* 1999;82. Available at: www.mmaonline.net/publications/MnMed1999/February/kaeter.cfm. Accessed May 5, 2006.

91. Sotile WM, Sotile MO. How to shape positive relationships in medical practice and hospitals. *Physician Exec.* Sep/Oct 1999;51–5.

92. Institute for Safe Medication Practices. Message in our mailbox. *ISMP Medication Safety Alert!* September 9, 2004;9(1):3.

93. Aiyegbuis A. Anne's angle [editorial]. *Ment Health Pract.* 2003;7(2):35.

94. Wilson RM, Runciman WB, Gibberd RQ, et al. The quality in Australian health care study. *Med J Aust.* 1995;163;458–71.

95. Vincent C, Neale G, Woloshynowych M. Adverse events in British hospitals; preliminary retrospective record review. *BMJ.* 2001;322:517–9.

96. Nolan T, Resar R, Haraden C, et al. Improving the reliability of health care. Cambridge, Mass: Institute for Healthcare Improvement; 2004. Available at: www.ihi.org/NR/rdonlyres/0BDFE6FD-3491-4226-9C69-ECDF1EB4FA2D/0/ReliabilityWhitePaper2004.pdf. Accessed May 5, 2006.

97. Institute for Healthcare Improvement. Design for healthcare reliability: 10^{-1} and 10^{-2} concepts [PowerPoint presentation]. April 20, 2005. Available at: www.ihi.org/IHI/Topics/Reliability/ReliabilityGeneral/Emerging Content/DesignforHealthCareReliabilityReviewofReliabilityModelandChangeConcepts.htm. Accessed April 26, 2006.

98. Baker GR, Norton PG, Flintoft V, et al. The Canadian Adverse Events Study: the incidence of adverse events among hospital patients in Canada. *Can Med Assoc J.* 2004;170:1678-86.
99. Institute for Healthcare Improvement. Bundle up for safety. Available at: www.ihi.org/IHI/Topics/CriticalCare/IntensiveCare/ImprovementStories/BundleUpforSafety.htm. Accessed April 28, 2006.
100. Resar R, Pronovost P, Haraden C, et al. Using a bundle approach to improve ventilator care processes and reduce ventilator-associated pneumonia. *Jt Comm J Qual Patient Saf.* 2005;31:243–8.
101. Institute for Safe Medication Practices. Evidence-based medicine doesn't preclude common sense. *ISMP Medication Safety Alert!* January 29, 2004;9(2):1–2.
102. Smith CS, Pell JP. Parachute use to prevent death and major trauma related to gravitational challenge: a systematic review of randomized control trials. *BMJ.* 2003;327:1459–61.
103. Leape LL, Berwick MB, Bates DW. What practices will most improve safety? Evidence-based medicine meets patient safety. *JAMA.* 2002;288:501–7.
104. Leape LL, Bates DW, Cullen DJ, et al. Systems analysis of adverse drug events. *JAMA.* 1995,274:35–43.
105. Institute for Safe Medication Practices. Your "lessons learned" now heard by over 3.5 million! *ISMP Medication Safety Alert!* September 23, 2004;9(19):3.
106. Deming WE. *The New Economics.* Cambridge, Mass: Massachusetts Institute of Technology Center for Advanced Engineering Study; 1993.
107. Institute for Safe Medication Practices. 2004 ISMP Medication Safety Self Assessment. Available at: www.ismp.org/selfassessments/Hospital/Intro.asp. Accessed February 23, 2006.
108. Schoen C, Osborn R, Huynh PT, et al. Taking the pulse of health care systems: experiences of patients with health problems in six countries. *Health Aff* Web Exclusive. 2005(November 3):W5-509–W5-525. Available at: www.cmwf.org/publications/publications_show.htm?doc_id=313012. Accessed April 26, 2006.
109. Pentecost MJ. Health care and public opinion. *Permanente J.* 2006;10(2). Available at: http://xnet.kp.org/permanentejournal/summer06/opinion.html. Accessed May 5, 2006.
110. Louis Harris & Associates. Public Opinion of Patient Safety Issues: Research Findings. Prepared for National Patient Safety Foundation at AMA. September 1997. Available at: www.npsf.org/download/1997survey.pdf. Accessed June 16, 2006.
111. Entwistle VA, Mello MM, Brennan TA. Advising patients about patient safety: current initiatives risk shifting responsibility. *Jt Comm J Qual Patient Saf.* 2005;31:483–94.
112. Institute for Safe Medication Practices. Want a savvy participant in your error-prevention program? Put a consumer on your team! *ISMP Medication Safety Alert!* May 17, 2000;5(10):2.
113. Ponte PR, Connor M, DeMarco R, et al. Linking patient and family-centered care and patient safety: the next leap. *Nurs Econ.* 2004;22(4):221–13, 215.
114. Westgard S. Patient safety: can we get there from here? Madison, Wis: Westgard QC. Available at: www.westgard.com/lesson82.htm. Accessed May 5, 2006.
115. Reason JT. Achieving a safe culture: theory and practice. *Work Stress.* 1998;12:293–306.
116. Edmondson AC. Learning from failure in health care: frequent opportunities, pervasive barriers. *Qual Saf Health Care.* 2004;13:ii3–ii9. Available at: http://qhc.bmjjournals.com/cgi/content/full/13/suppl_2/ii3. Accessed April 28, 2006.
117. Tucker AL, Edmondson AC. Why hospitals don't learn from failures: organizational and psychological dynamics that inhibit system change. *Calif Manage Rev.* 2003;45(2):55–72.
118. Hayes RH, Wheelwright SC, Clark KB. *Dynamic Manufacturing: Creating the Learning Organization.* New York: Free Press; 1988.
119. Repenning N, Sterman JD. Capability traps and self-confirming attribution errors in the dynamics of process improvement. *Adm Sci Q.* 2002;47:265–95.
120. Ramanujam R, Keyser DJ, Sirio CA. Making a case for organizational change in patient safety initiatives. *Advances in Patient Safety: From Research to Implementation.* Volume 2. Concepts and Methodology. AHRQ Publication No. 05-0021-2 . Rockville, Md: Agency for Healthcare Research and Quality; 2005.
121. Berwick DM, A primer on leading the improvement of systems. *BMJ.* 1996;312:619–22.
122. Kotter JP. Leading change: why transformation efforts fail. *Harvard Bus Rev.* Mar/Apr 1995:59–67.
123. Institute for Healthcare Improvement. Risk priority number (from failure mode and effects analysis). Available at: www.ihi.org/IHI/Topics/PatientSafety/MedicationSystems/Measures/Risk+Priority+Number+%28from+Failure+Modes+and+Effects+Analysis%29.htm. Accessed April 10, 2006.
124. Agency for Healthcare Research and Quality. Hospital survey on patient safety culture. Pub. No. 04-0041. September 2004. Prepared by Westat under contract No. 290-96-0004. Available at: www.ahrq.gov/qual/hospculture/hospcult.pdf. Accessed May 5, 2006.
125. National Coordinating Council for Medication Error Reporting and Prevention. Using medication error rates to compare health care organizations is of no value. June 11, 2002. Available at: www.nccmerp.org/council/council2002-06-11.html. Accessed May 5, 2006.
126. Barker KN, Flynn EA, Pepper GA. Observation method of detecting medication errors. *Am J Health Syst Pharm.* 2002;59:2314–16.

127. Institute for Safe Medication Practices. ISMP trigger alert list. September 6, 2000. Available at: www.ismp.org/Newsletters/acutecare/articles/20050310_2.asp.

128. Classen DC, Metzger J. Improving medication safety: the measurement conundrum and where to start. *Int J Qual Health Care.* 2003;15:i41–i47.

129. Rozich JD, Haraden CR, Resar RK. Adverse drug event trigger tool: a practical methodology for measuring medication related harm. *Qual Saf Health Care.* 2003;12:194–200.

130. Newhouse RP. The metrics of measuring patient safety. In: Newhouse RP, Poe SS, eds. *Measuring Patient Safety.* Sudbury, Mass: Jones and Bartlett; 2005.

131. Oddo F, ed. *The Memory Jogger II.* Salem, NH: GOAL/QPC; 1994.

132. Joint Commission Resources. Benchmarking exercises: not fit for medication error reduction programs. *Jt Comm Benchmark.* March/April 2005;7(2):1–3.

133. Institute for Safe Medication Practices. Benchmarking—when is it dangerous? *ISMP Medication Safety Alert!* September 9, 1998;3(18):2.

134. Franklin DM. Benchmarking: laying a foundation. *Infusion.* February 2000:32–4.

135. American Society for Healthcare Risk Management. *Health Care Risk Management Benchmarking Primer.* Chicago: American Hospital Association; 1996.

136. Allen EL, Barker KN. Fundamentals of medication error research. *Am J Hosp Pharm.* 1990;47:555–71.

137. Lesar TS. Factors related to errors in medication prescribing. *JAMA.* 1997;277:312–7.

Index

Note: Page numbers followed by *f* or *t* indicate figures and tables, respectively.

C